Atlas of Limb Deformity

Sihe Qin • Wen Tian • Qianyu Zhuang
Baofeng Guo
Editors

Atlas of Limb Deformity

Etiological Classification

Springer

Editors
Sihe Qin
National Research Center for Rehabilitation
Beijing, China

Wen Tian
Beijing Jishuitan Hospital
Beijing, China

Qianyu Zhuang
Peking Union Medical College Hospital
Beijing, China

Baofeng Guo
Department of Orthopedics
Chuiyangliu Hospital affiliated to Tsinghua University
Beijing, China

ISBN 978-981-97-0998-4   ISBN 978-981-97-0999-1 (eBook)
https://doi.org/10.1007/978-981-97-0999-1

This Springer imprint is published by the registered company Springer Nature Singapore Pte Ltd.
The registered company address is: 152 Beach Road, #21-01/04 Gateway East, Singapore 189721, Singapore

Preface

The limbs refer to upper limbs, lower limbs and body, which are the parts below head and outside internal organs of the human body. Just in terms of morphology, the human limbs are also a huge system. Limb deformity is an abnormal structure, shape and function that is different from the normal human standard. Limb deformity can be caused by a variety of factors, including congenital, hereditary, acquired trauma, disease, development abnormalities, aging etc. The obvious motor dysfunction resulting from limb deformity is limb disability. If the limb deformity disability cannot be completely cured, there will be varying degrees of abnormal appearance and dysfunction, which will affect mental health. With the advent of population aging, the number of limb deformities and disabilities caused by bone and joint degeneration has naturally increased.

What are the main causes of limb deformities in the Chinese population? What percentage of the elderly population suffer from limb deformities and disabilities? How to classify the disease types and how to classify the disease conditions? What are the differences in the types of limb deformities between China and Western countries? How to establish the category of limb deformity in the form of real case pictures? There is no monograph or systematic literature to answer these original questions.

This book is based on a database of more than 200 cases of limb deformity surgery in Qin Sihe Orthopaedic Surgery. This book includes contributions from the following authors: Tian Wen, Department of Hand Surgery, Beijing Jishuitan Hospital; Zhuang Ganyu, Department of Spine Surgery, Peking Union Medical College Hospital; and Liang Yijian, Chengdu Third Hospital and Professor Hua Qikai from the First Affiliated Hospital of Guangxi Medical University. This book is divided into 14 chapters and covers 283 diseases. The content embodies the following features:

1. Classification according to anatomical location and etiology of limbs

   It includes four parts: spine, pelvis, limbs, and hands and feet. The etiology involves congenital, genetic, immune, traumatic, and acquired teratogenic diseases. Diseases run through more than a dozen disciplines besides orthopedics, such as genetics, immunity, blood vessels, nerves, endocrinology, skin, and tumors, in order to show the disease spectrum and characteristics of diseases leading to limb deformities in China to the greatest extent and to open a new interdisciplinary research field for future scholars.
2. It reflects the etiology of limb deformities and the characteristics of deformity categories in China.

   Statistical analysis of 36,664 cases of limb deformities, 2,094 cases of different types of congenital limb deformities and the 3,547 cases of severe deformity and disability of lower limbs are all cases of surgical treatment by the author, providing a reflection of the real types of limb deformities, geographical distribution, etiology, disease types, disease classification, and the relationship between limb deformities and gender and age.
3. Real body photos or image pictures show diseases and conditions

   Almost every disease introduced in this book is accompanied by photographs of limb deformities or images of image examination, as well as videos related to the diseases. These disease types are all limb deformity disease types suffered by the Chinese population, which can enable readers to truly understand the clinical manifestations and characteristics of a specific deformity. It can achieve the effect of recognizing diseases by analyzing pictures. The text of the book is concise, which saves clinicians time when searching the literature.

4. The case pictures have a long historical value.

   These case pictures span more than 40 years, which are selected, screened, and systematically sorted out by the author from tens of thousands of cases diagnosed and treated by himself. The cases come from all over the country, including Kashin-Beck disease suffered by Tibetan colleagues living in the Qinghai-Tibet Plateau. More than 280 case pictures of various causes, types, genders, ages, and nationalities to a certain extent represent the "characteristics of diseases and categories of limb deformities in China," which are extremely precious and hold a long historical value.

5. Including and naming new diseases that have not been published or are uncertain in the previous literature.

   Such as congenital genu recurvatum, parasitic fetus and limb deformity, heroin encephalopathy, limb rigidity deformity etc. There are also some diseases named after the conditions treated by Qin Sihe's orthopedic surgery, such as congenital cervical hyperextension deformity, stress genu recurvatum deformity, foot and ankle deformity after organophosphorus pesticide poisoning, developmental subluxation of hip joint caused by hip adductor spasm, congenital talipes equinovarus in adulthood, congenital dislocation of patella in adulthood, developmental dislocation of hip joint in adulthood with delayed treatment, etc. The reason why Qin Sihe named one deformity as two disease types is that if a congenital limb deformity fails to receive effective treatment in infancy, childhood and adolescence, and surgical reconstruction is carried out in adulthood and middle age, in terms of pathological changes, deformity nature and category, patient constitution, degree of dysfunction and surgical reconstruction principles, it has completely become two diseases. This book is specially set up to introduce iatrogenic limb deformities, aiming to remind medical staff to pay attention to the prevention and avoidance of serious complications in clinical work. Whether the author's classification method of etiology and disease is reasonable, and whether the naming and analysis of new diseases are appropriate, we hope to receive corrections from colleagues.

   English scientist Thomas Henry Huxley once said: "Classification helps the brain to operate, the purpose is to conceive and retain the characteristics of classified objects in memory." "Etiological classification of limb deformities" is a huge systematic research project, through the efforts of several clinicians in this book, it can only complete the initial work. Despite the foundational work of "Atlas and Etiological Classification of Limb Deformities," the publication of this book fills a significant gap by providing the global medical community with a understanding of the real spectrum and classification methods of limb deformities in China. It is our hope that this book will medical professionals to cultivate this medical and social discipline, ultimately contributing to the betterment of public health.

   We would like to extend our gratitude to Liu Yuxin and Yang Meng from the Department of Orthopaedics. Zhang Junming is responsible for the arrangement, translation, and proofreading of this book. We are grateful to the patients with limb deformities who have kindly allowed doctors to take photos to record their conditions, which served as the basis for the achievement of this book.

Beijing, China Sihe Qin
Beijing, China Wen Tian
Beijing, China Qianyu Zhuang
Beijing, China Baofeng Guo

Synopsis

This book is the first monograph on the classification and category of etiology, clinical manifestations, diagnosis, and orthopedic principles of different types of limb deformities in China. A total of 284 diseases were recorded based on the statistical analysis of 36664 cases of limb deformities in the orthopaedic surgery department of Qin Sihe, combining cases from other relevant experts. It is divided into congenital deformity of lower limb; genetic and genetic defects; dysplasia, rheumatic immunity, and degenerative deformities; tumor-related deformities; vascular, blood, and lymphoid diseases related deformities; neurogenic diseases; infectious diseases; traumatic sequelae; spinal cord deformity; congenital upper limb and hand deformities associated with genetic abnormality; and acquired upper limb and hand deformities caused by comprehensive causes. The relativity of the definition of limb deformity, the cognitive history of human beings on limb deformity and disability spanning thousands of years, and the characteristics and classification methods of the diseases category of limb deformity in the Chinese population are expounded in this book. Furthermore, the dynamic nature of the occurrence and development of limb deformity is analyzed from the perspectives of biological evolution and auxology. Finally, the author puts forward an ecological law, stating that the reconstruction of limb appearance and function should be based on imitating nature.

Contents

Contributors

Zhuosong Bai Department of Orthopaedics, Peking Union Medical College Hospital, Beijing, China

Zhiwei Fang Department of Bone and Soft Tissue Tumor, Peking University Cancer Hospital, Key laboratory of Carcinogenesis and Translational Research (Ministry of Education/Beijing), Beijing, China

Baofeng Guo Department of Orthopedics, Chuiyangliu Hospital affiliated to Tsinghua University, Beijing, China

Qikai Hua Department of Bone and Joint Surgery, the First Affiliated Hospital of Guangxi Medical University, Nanning, Guangxi, China

Shaofeng Jiao Department of Orthopaedics, Rehabilitation Hospital of the National Research Center for Rehabilitation Technical Aids, Beijing, China

Shu Li Department of Bone and Soft Tissue Tumor, Peking University Cancer Hospital, Key laboratory of Carcinogenesis and Translational Research (Ministry of Education/Beijing), Beijing, China

Yijian Liang Department of Orthopaedics, The Third People's Hospital of Chengdu, Southwest Jiao Tong University, Chengdu, Sichuan, China

Yueju Liu Department of Orthopaedic Trauma, The Third Hospital of Hebei Medical University, Shijiazhuang, Hebei, China

Yue Peng Department of Orthopedic Surgery, Peking Union Medical College Hospital, Chinese Academy of Medical Sciences and Peking Union Medical College, Beijing, China

Sihe Qin Department of Orthopaedics, Rehabilitation Hospital of the National Research Center for Rehabilitation Technical Aids, Beijing, China

Lei Shi Department of Orthopaedics, Rehabilitation Hospital of the National Research Center for Rehabilitation Technical Aids, Beijing, China

Wen Tian Beijing Jishuitan Hospital, Beijing, China

Yilan Wang Qinsihe Orthopedics Institute, Beijing, China

Jiancheng Zang Department of Hand and Foot Surgery, Beijing University of Chinese Medicine Third Affiliated Hospital, Beijing, China

Dingwei Zhang Department of Orthopedic Surgery, Central Hospital of Mianyang, Mianyang, Sichuan, China

Jianguo Zhang Department of Orthopaedics, Peking Union Medical College Hospital, Beijing, China

Junming Zhang Department of Orthopaedics, Rehabilitation Hospital, National Research Center for Rehabilitation, Beijing, China

Wenyao Zhong Department of Hand Surgery, Beijing Jishuitan Hospital, Beijing, China

Qianyu Zhuang Peking Union Medical College Hospital, Beijing, China

Translators

Junming Zhang Department of Orthopaedics, Rehabilitation Hospital, National Research Center for Rehabilitation, Beijing, China

General Introduction

1

Sihe Qin, Yueju Liu, Junming Zhang, Yilan Wang, and Baofeng Guo

1.1 Brief History of Human Limb Deformity Cognition

1.1.1 Relativity of the Definition of Limb Deformity

Deformity refers to any defect state that deviates from the normal anatomical structure and morphology, which is a problem that every living body may face, and is also one of the common problems that plague human health. However, people in different times, different countries, different nationalities, and different cultural backgrounds have great differences in their understanding of limb deformities. For example, Mongolians have a high incidence of mild genu varum deformity in horse riding since childhood, which is not considered abnormal by their own people. In order to meet the local custom of "women's beauty standards," Chinese women's foot binding custom has led to the lifelong disability of countless women's feet for thousands of years, but it is euphemistically called "three-inch golden lotus" (Fig. 1.1). There is a long-necked ethnic group in northern Myanmar that also shows a long neck through the deformity of the collarbone and scapula caused by pressure, which is considered to be a sign of beauty (Fig. 1.2). In the eighteenth century, the upper class in Europe liked beautiful women with slender waists, which led some women to remove the 11th and 12th ribs for the sake of "slender waists and protruding breasts" (Fig. 1.3).

1.1.2 Ancient Egyptians' Understanding of Limb Deformity and Disability

The ancient Egyptians held a positive attitude toward the physically disabled, and physical deformities may be regarded as a positive sign of divinity. They believed that some physically deformed people were messengers sent by the gods, and they arranged sacrifices to communicate with the gods. In addition, dwarfism (achondroplasia) has gained a respected status (Fig. 1.4). They follow strict ethical behavior and also recommend respect and tolerance for the disabled: no ridicule of the blind, no teasing of the midgets, no interference with the lame. Don't laugh at a man in God's hands, and if he makes a mistake, don't glare at him. The ancients left many real stone carvings, bones with incomplete osteogenesis, sculptures, and even mummies of disabled people with limb deformities. Researchers found bones with incomplete osteogenesis in

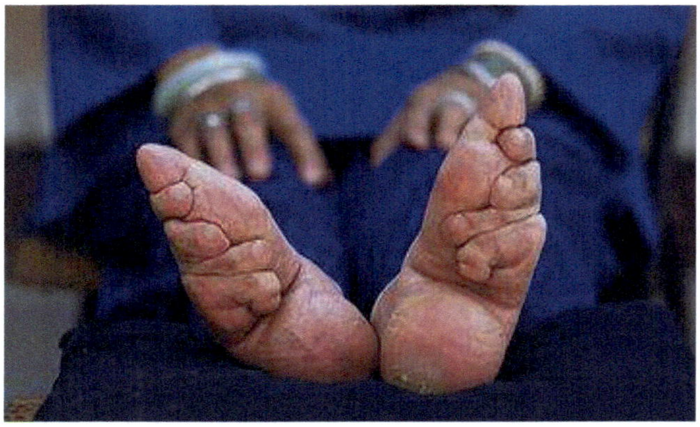

Fig. 1.1 Foot deformity of Chinese women after foot binding, who can only walk with heel load

S. Qin (✉)
Department of Orthopaedics, Rehabilitation Hospital of the National Research Center for Rehabilitation Technical Aids, Beijing, China

Y. Liu
Department of Orthopaedic Trauma, The Third Hospital of Hebei Medical University, Shijiazhuang, Hebei, China

J. Zhang
Department of Orthopaedics, Rehabilitation Hospital, National Research Center for Rehabilitation, Beijing, China

Y. Wang
Qinsihe Orthopedics Institute, Beijing, China

B. Guo
Department of Orthopedics, Chuiyangliu Hospital affiliated to Tsinghua University, Beijing, China

S. Qin et al. (eds.), *Atlas of Limb Deformity*, https://doi.org/10.1007/978-981-97-0999-1_1

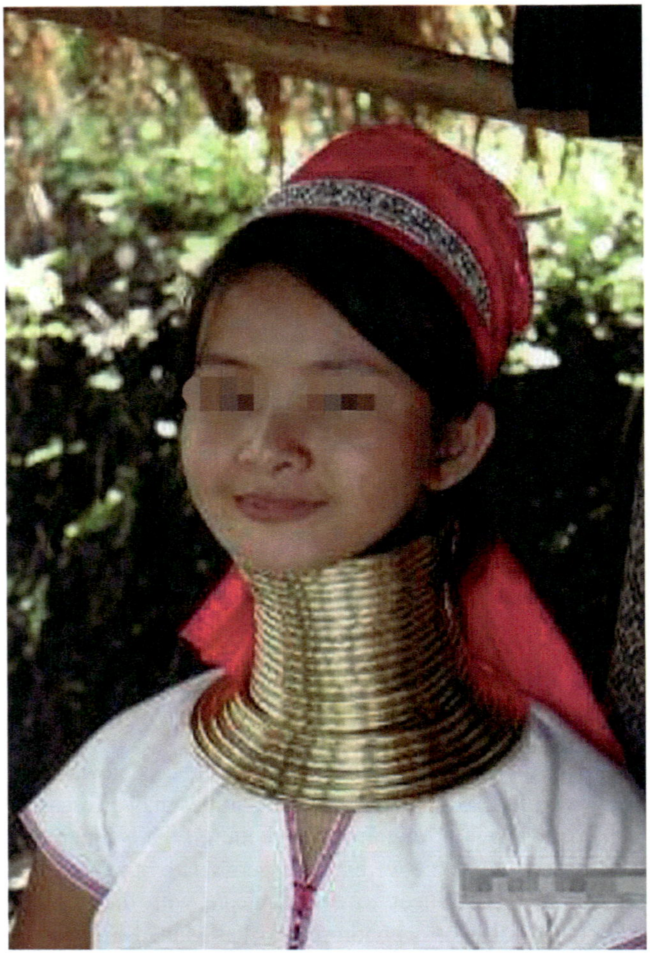

Fig. 1.2 Since childhood, the neck is covered with a metal ring to gradually form a slender and weak neck

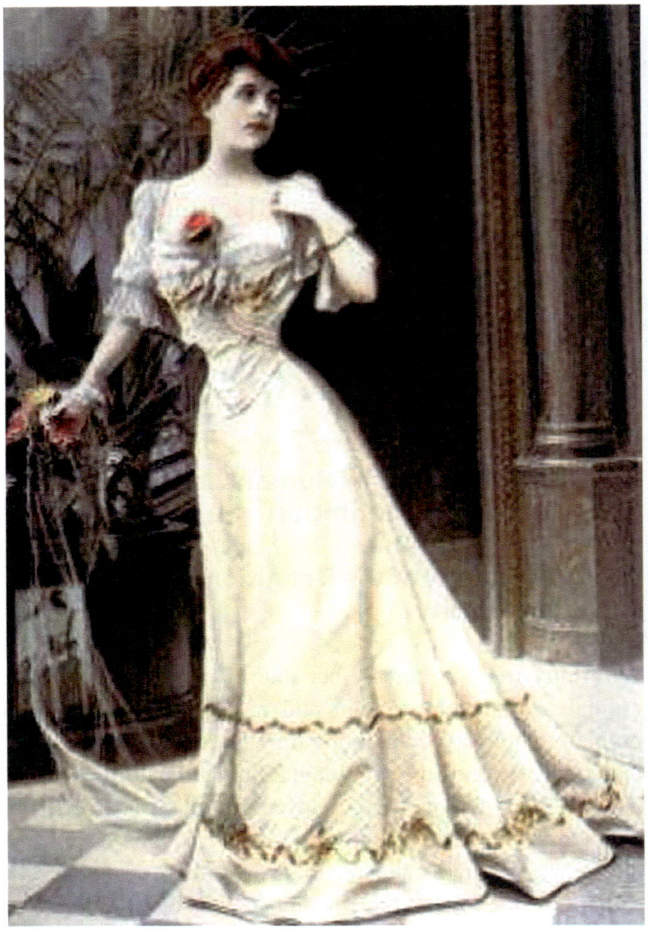

Fig. 1.3 A beautiful woman with a slender waist after removing the 11th and 12th ribs

Egyptian tombs (Fig. 1.5). The mummy of Pharaoh Siptah also shows deformities of the left leg and foot (Fig. 1.6), and the stone carving clearly shows deformities of the lower leg like polio. These evidence suggest that this skeletal metabolic disorder and the poliovirus that infects humans may have existed 3000 years ago (Fig. 1.7).

1.1.3 Limb Deformity and Correction from the Perspective of Biological Evolution and Development

The cognition and intervention of limb deformities in medicine began with Hippocrates. As early as the fifth century BC, Hippocrates discovered scoliosis. He believed that scoliosis was caused by the dislocation of the vertebral body. He invented the Hippocratic Dislocation Treatment Bed to treat scoliosis. Until the sixteenth century, the Hippocratic Treatment Bed was still considered an effective treatment. After the Renaissance, with the progress of anatomy, the cognize of limb deformities has been deepened. John Hunter (1728–1793), the father of British experimental surgery, began to think about the relationship between limb development and species evolution from a scientific point of view, which greatly changed the thinking of surgeons and even orthopedic surgeons. Darwin's good friend Dr. John Struthes (1823–1899), a pioneer of comparative and evolutionary anatomy, was the first to point out that the evolution of the upper limbs of mammals such as humans, birds, whales, and horses was itself homologous. Kaplan (1894–1980), who was born in Ukraine, made great contributions to the development of evolutionary anatomy, made a qualitative leap in the accumulation of knowledge of evolutionary anatomy, and profoundly influenced the understanding of the mechanism of limb deformities. Professor Spinner of the Mayo Clinic and Professor Smith of the Department of Hand and Upper Limbs at the Massachusetts General Hospital of Harvard University have also had a profound impact on the study of evolutionary anatomy. His student Jesse Jupiter observed the elbow bones of different animals at the Natural History Museum of Harvard University and came up with the theory of double

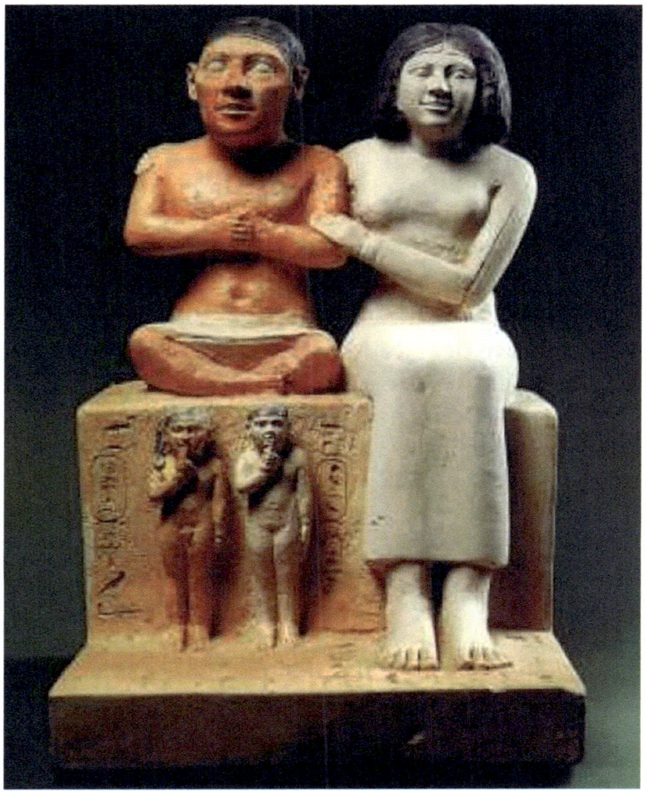

Fig. 1.4 Seneb and his wife Senetis, C. 2500 BC (Cairo Museum)

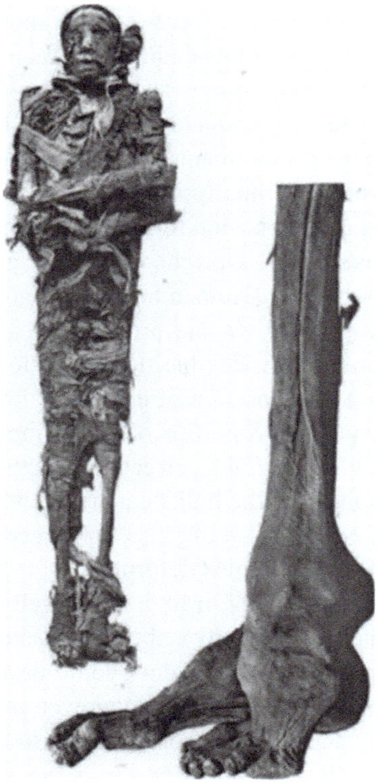

Fig. 1.6 The mummy of Pharaoh Siptah showed deformities of the left leg and foot (Cairo Museum), possibly due to poliomyelitis, equinus deformity, or cerebral palsy

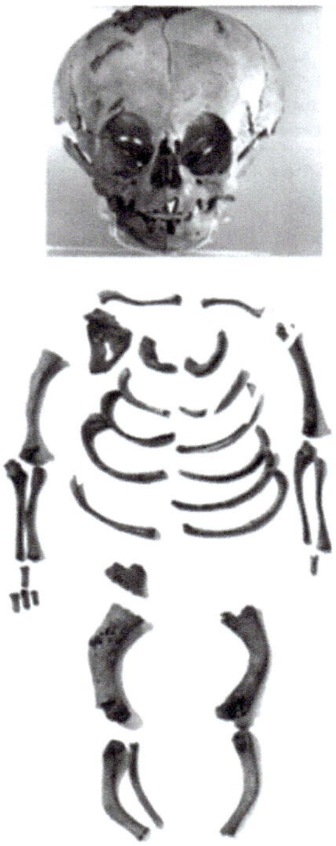

Fig. 1.5 Osteogenesis imperfecta found in Egypt (1000 BC). It consists of a painted coffin and the skeleton of a small child

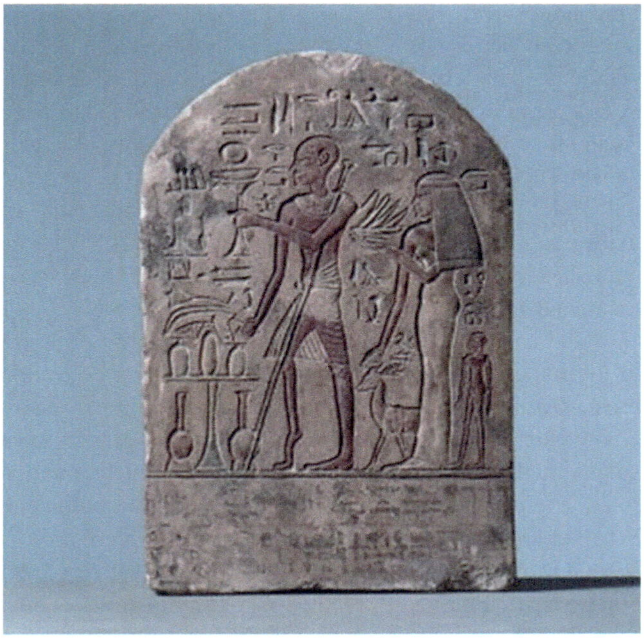

Fig. 1.7 The right lower limb is slender with deformity of foot drop, standing with a crutch. Lower limb deformity characteristics such as poliomyelitis sequelae. His wife and children (1550-1080 BC) are healthy (Cairo Museum artifacts)

columns of elbow joints. It has become a monument in the history of the treatment of distal humeral fractures.

According to evolutionary anatomy, the emergence of Girdle bones in the upper and lower limbs is a key step in the long evolution of species, that is, the emergence of shoulders and pelvis, which eventually separates the limbs from the trunk. Walking upright is vital for impact in terms of the evolution of human bones. Upright walking is a very energy-saving way of exercise. Human beings can go out of Africa and explore the world. In the process of exploration, the upper limbs are mainly flexible, while the lower limbs are mainly stable. The proportion of upper and lower limbs has also changed, and the proportion of upper limbs has become smaller. For a long time, the correction of lower limb deformities has emphasized the holistic concept, whole considering the spine, pelvis, hip joint, knee joint, and ankle, which is very important in complex deformities.

The process of growing from a single cell of a fertilized egg to a complex human body is the condensation of millions of years of evolution. In this embryonic development, the development of the motor system and even the whole body after birth, the main trend is from stiffness to flexibility, and the strength of flexors and extensors is perfectly matched. Once the development process deviates, the limb development moves from flexibility to stiffness, and the flexor muscle strength is too large, trying to lock the joints and body to maintain the most primitive stability for millions of years. This philosophy can basically help understand complex orthopedic surgery. Limb deformities are divided into congenital genetic deformities and acquired secondary deformities. Most congenital malformations have profound genetic background, abnormal gene expression, and familial aggregation, such as the syndactyly caused by HOXD13 gene mutation. The molecular biology research of this kind of malformation is vast, and a large number of papers have been published, but there is still no breakthrough in clinical treatment, and surgical correction is almost the only way.

There is also a secondary limb deformity, which belongs to the imperfect matching of the evolutionary acceleration process after human upright walking, such as excessive elbow carrying angle, acetabular dysplasia, excessive knee valgus angle, flatfoot, toe valgus, and external or internal rotation gait with mild calf torsion during development. Whether these patients need early surgical intervention is still controversial in academia, but the statistical results of hundreds of thousands of outpatient examinations in Qin Sihe and many cases of lower limb deformity surgery in 36,000 show that with the extension of human life, once lower limb deformity occurs, it is appropriate to use early non-surgical or surgical intervention to avoid or reduce the occurrence of osteoarthritis.

A good orthopedic surgeon should have a sense of the overall situation and the spirit of exploring the source, and analyze the occurrence and development of different types of limb deformities based on the basic theory of evolutionary medicine, so as to formulate a correct plan for correcting deformities and reconstructing functions, to benefit the disabled patients with limb deformities.

1.2 Statistical Analysis of Relevant Data of Limb Deformity in China

1.2.1 Statistical Report of 36,664 Cases of Limb Deformity Operation in Qin Sihe Orthopedic Surgery Database (1978.5.25–2021.12.31)

Statistical method: Each patient is counted as one case for each hospitalization operation. If a patient has performed two or three operations during one hospitalization, it is still counted as one case. If a patient has been hospitalized for two or more operations at different times, it is counted as two or more cases.

1.2.1.1 Operation Site

Type of operation	Number of operations	Percentage
Orthopedic and functional reconstruction of lower limb	34,795	94.90
Orthopedic and functional reconstruction of upper limb	622	1.70
Orthopedic and functional reconstruction of neck, spine, etc. *	1247	3.40

*The adventitia of common carotid artery and sympathetic nerve network exfoliation operation was used to treat 983 cases of cerebral palsy, accounting for 78.83% of cervical and spine surgeries

1.2.1.2 Gender

Gender	Number of operations	Percentage
Male	21,294	58.08
Female	15,370	41.92
Male-to-female ratio	1.39: 1	

1.2.1.3 Age at The Time of Operation

Age (years)	Number of operations	Percentage
1–5[a]	2049	5.59
6–10	5449	14.86
11–15	6170	16.83
16–20	7234	19.73
21–25	6445	17.58
26–30	4188	11.42
31–35	2446	6.67
36–40	1211	3.30
41–45	558	1.52

Age (years)	Number of operations	Percentage
46–50	412	1.12
51–60	396	1.08
61–70	94	0.26
71–80	10	0.03
Above 80	2	0.01

[a] The 1-year-old operated case was a congenital clubfoot patient

1.2.1.4 Number of Operations Over the Years

1. Number of operations from 1978 to 2020

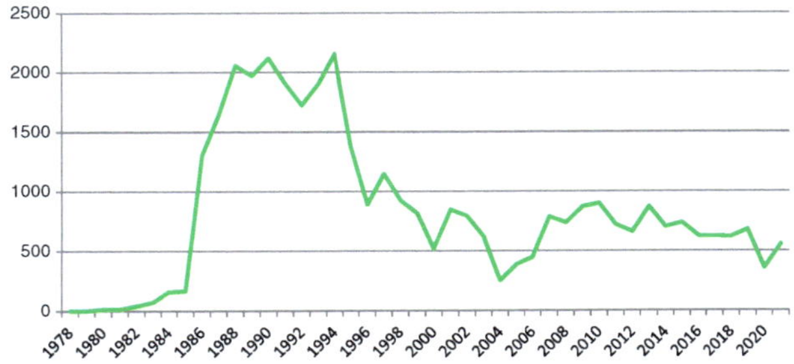

2. The number of operations has decreased in the past 10 years. As the patients treated by Qin Sihe Orthopedic Surgery come from all over the country, the COVID-19 epidemic in 2020 and 2021 has affected patients from other places to come to Beijing for medical treatment and surgery.

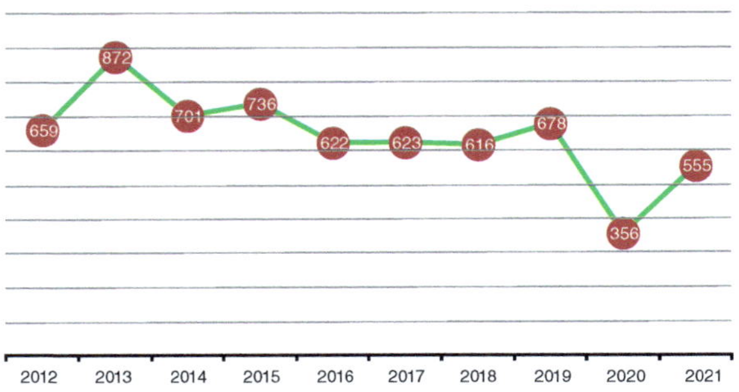

Note: The year with the largest number of operations per year was from 1988 to 1994, when China implemented the salvage surgery for polio sequelae rehabilitation. Qin Sihe also served as the director of two polio sequelae correction centers in Heilongjiang Province and Beijing, and presided over the tasks of polio surgery and correction in Heilongjiang Province and Beijing.

1.2.1.5 Regional Distribution of 36,664 Patients

Chinese patients:

Region	Number of operations	Region	Number of operations	Region	Number of operations
Beijing	1802	Shandong	3143	Guangxi	133
Tianjin	166	Jiangsu	595	Guizhou	206
Shanghai	89	Anhui	1281	Yunnan	170
Chongqing	86	Hubei	3233	Szechwan	361
Heilongjiang *	7511	Hunan	1540	Shaanxi	1541
Jilin	472	Jiangxi	2740	Gansu	1169
Liaoning	520	Zhejiang	595	Ningxia	95
Inner Mongolia	532	Fujian	744	Qinghai	113
Hebei	1764	Guangdong	590	Xinjiang	337
Shanxi	764	Taiwan	2	Tibet	32
Henan	4217	Hainan	89	Hong Kong	1

*Because the author worked in Helongjiang Province for 5 years, there were as many as 7511 surgical patients in Heilongjiang Province

Thirty-one patients from other countries were operated on, 16 of whom were invited to Russia and India by Qin Sihe for operation demonstration.

country	Number of operations	country	Number of operations
India	11 (Surgery in India)	Russia	5 (Surgery in Russia)
America	2	Mongolia	2
Indonesia	2	Syria	2
Palestine	1	Vietnam	1
Romania	1	Kazakhstan	1
Saudi Arabia	1	South Africa	1
Hungary	1		

1.2.1.6 A Total of 36,664 Cases of Limb Deformities (227 Kinds of Causes) Were Collected, of Which 172 Cases of Limb Deformities Had No Clear Cause

Etiology/disease	Totally
Sequela of poliomyelitis	24,067
Cerebral palsy	4902
Traumatic sequelae	1054
Tethered cord sequelae of spina bifida	1045
Congenital clubfoot	762
Congenital/developmental dislocation of the hip, acetabular dysplasia	552
Genua varus	490
Motor neuron disease (Charcot-Marie-Tooth disease)	287
Genu valgum	250

Etiology/disease	Totally
Gluteal muscle contracture	235
Congenital joint contracture	158
Rickets	110
Congenital fibular hemilimb deformity	109
Osteomyelitis	105
Congenital pseudarthrosis of the tibia	98
Guillain-Barre syndrome	86
Iatrogenic limb deformity	79
Encephalitis	76
Hemangioma of lower extremity	68
Muscular torticollis	67
Paralysis of common peroneal nerve	66
Traumatic brain injury	66
Congenital dislocation of patella	58
Osteoarthritis of the knee	53
Sequela of suppurative arthritis	52
Congenital coxa vara	50
Scoliosis	49
Osteogenesis imperfecta	46
Developmental deformity of lower limb caused by epiphyseal injury	42
Congenital shortening of the lower limbs	40
Meningitis	40
Rheumatoid arthritis	38
Bone nonunion	37
Burn and scald sequelae	37
Bone defect	36
Lateral spinal sclerosis	33
Avascular necrosis of the femoral head	31
Diaphyseal aclasis	30
Fibrous dysplasia of bone	26
Hallux valgus	23
Congenital hypoplasia of radius	23
Hydrocephalus	22
Acute myelitis	22
Birth paralysis	21
Hereditary spastic paraplegia	21
Multiple chondrodysplasia	21
Progressive Muscular Dystrophy	21
Endophytic chondroma	21
Multiple epiphyseal dysplasia	20
Congenital heel foot	20
Flatfoot	20
Bone tuberculosis	19
Congenital tibial hemilimb deformity	19
Congenital pterygoid knee joint	18
Injury of common peroneal nerve	18
Familial neurofibromatosis	17
Sciatic nerve injury	16
Blount's disease	16
Scleroderma	16
Gastrocnemius contracture	14
Hand, foot, and mouth disease	14
Congenital vertical talus	13
Kashin-Beck disease	13
Dwarfism	13
Hereditary chondrodysplasia	13
Congenital band syndrome	12

Etiology/disease	Totally
Incomplete paraplegia of spinal cord injury	12
Epidemic encephalitis B	11
Congenital shortening of toes	11
Desmoid tumors	10
Spinal muscular atrophy	9
Melorheostosis	9
Septicemia	7
Poor amputation stump	7
Familial PES cavus	7
Congenital radioulnar synostosis	7
Congenital curvature of the tibia	7
Macromelia	6
Congenital axial absence of proximal femur	6
Congenital foot valgus	6
Gas poisoning	6
Stroke	6
Organophosphorus pesticide poisoning	6
Hemophilia	6
Hyperparathyroidism	5
Hip arthritis	5
Congenital polydactyly	5
TOCP poisoning	5
Vascular embolism	5
Wilson's disease	5
Anhidrosis	5
Nerve injury caused by spinal cord tumor	4
Macrodactyly	4
Ankylosing spondylitis	4
Congenital pseudarthrosis of femur	4
Congenital dysplasia of tibia	4
Congenital dysplasia of ulna	4
Spastic deformity of foot and ankle caused by drug-induced spinal poisoning	4
Lymphangioma	4
Vasculitis	4
Congenital pterygoid elbow joint	4
Osteosarcoma	4
Congenital parasitic fetus	4
Dwarfism	3
Ankle osteoarthritis	3
Spinal nerve injury	3
Progressive muscular atrophy	3
Madelung deformity	3
Sepsis	3
Congenital adduction of thumb	3
Congenital dislocation of radial head	3
Congenital navicular foot	3
Congenital flexion of the fingers	3
Craniopharyngioma	3
Fanconi syndrome	3
Congenital absence of forefoot	3
Mucopolysaccharidosis	3
Marfan syndrome	3
Bone tumor	3
Hip joint synovitis	3
Cerebral hemorrhage	3
Congenital longitudinal absence of ulnar side	3
Congenital longitudinal absence of radial side	3

Etiology/disease	Totally
Dichlorvos poisoning	2
Fibromyositis lateralis femoris	2
Spastic deformity of lower limb due to spinal cord	2
Fascia lata contracture	2
Dermatomyositis	2
Subcutaneous lipodystrophy	2
dysplasia epiphysealis hemimelica	2
Tetanus	2
Knee joint synovitis	2
Congenital ectrodactyly	2
Lower limb deformity due to compression of thoracic spinal cord	2
Bear scratch	2
Lumbar disc herniation	2
Sequelae of intraspinal meningioma	2
Congenital polydactyly	2
Congenital flexion of wrist	2
Congenital fisting deformity	2
Transverse myelitis	2
Brain tuberculosis	2
Femoral periarterial fibroma	2
Spinal cord fibroma	2
Intracranial cyst	2
Congenital dysplasia of talus	2
Lumbar tuberculosis	2
Cerebral vasculitis	2
Toxic encephalopathy	2
Nonossifying fibroma	2
Cerebral vascular malformation	2
Congenital hemihypertrophy	2
Cerebral infarction	1
Arterial calcification	1
Venomous snake bite	1
Residual deformity after replantation of severed limb	1
Malignant peripheral nerve sheath tumor	1
Sequelae of gastrocnemius infection	1
Osteitis of calcaneus tuberosity	1
Humeral tenosynovitis	1
Ossifying fibroma	1
Popliteal artery embolism	1
Synovial tuberculosis	1
Steroid-induced multiple osteonecrosis	1
Nerve injury after operation of spinal meningeal carcinoma	1
Spinal cord glioma	1
Spinal cord hemangioma	1
Cervical Myeloma	1
Spinal arachnoiditis	1
Hemilimb atrophy	1
Myositis ossificans progressiva	1
Ossification of posterior longitudinal ligament of cervical spine	1
Gigantism	1
Osteoarthritis of talonavicular joint	1
Hallux varus	1
Parkinson	1
Lead poisoning	1

Etiology/disease	Totally
Chondritis	1
Typhoid fever	1
Hypoxic-ischemic encephalopathy due to pulmonary embolism	1
Nephrotic syndrome	1
Fetal injection injury	1
Down's syndrome	1
Charcot's arthropathy	1
Congenital syndactyly	1
Congenital absence of femoral head	1
Congenital external dislocation of talus	1
Congenital hypertrophy of great toe	1
Congenital forefoot adduction	1
Congenital axial defect of lower leg	1
Congenital metatarsal adduction deformity	1
Congenital claw toe	1
Thoracic disc herniation	1
Toxic bacillary dysentery	1
Trifunctional protein deficiency	1
Congenital extensional contracture of the hip	1
Dorsal contracture of the wrist	1
Congenital crossed deformity of radius and ulna	1
Congenital scapular elevation	1
Congenital absence of thumb	1
Congenital shortening of the upper limb	1
Dupuytren's contracture	1
Subarachnoid hemorrhage	1
Renal osteopathy	1
Congenital spinal stiffness	1
Poisoning sequela of moldy sugarcane	1
Germ tumor of the brain	1
Cerebral spongiform degeneration	1
Cerebrochoroiditis	1
Cerebral angioma	1
Cerebral thrombosis	1
Cerebral arachnoiditis	1
Epileptic sequelae	1
Dysfunctional peripheral neuropathy	1
Sequelae of femoral artery embolism	1
Acanthosis nigricans	1
Methylmalonic acidemia	1
Pseudorheumatoid	1
Congenital flexion of the knee	1
Congenital absence of elbow flexor muscle	1
Congenital hypertrophy of lower limb	1
Congenital absence of toe	1
Giant cell tumor of bone	1
Desmoid fibroma	1
Gangliocytoma	1
Congenital hypoplasia of fibula	1
Cerebral infarction	1
Other neurogenic deformity of lower limb	3
Other congenital deformity of lower limb	78
Other infective deformity of lower limb	73
Other congenital deformity of upper limb	7
The cause is unknown	172

1.2.1.7 Statistics of the Names of Qin Sihe's Surgical Methods and the Most Frequently Used Surgical Methods

There are 291 kinds of surgical methods used in Qin Sihe Orthopedic Surgery, and the following are the top 40 surgical methods used most frequently (the surgical methods listed in the following tables are all derived from this table, so they are omitted).

Surgical method	Number of times used	Frequency of use [a]
Achilles tendon lengthening	8161	22.26
Femoral supracondylar osteotomy	7575	20.66
Calcanotalar joint fusion	6699	18.27
Osteotomy of tibia and fibula	4526	12.34
Release of plantar aponeurosis	3791	10.34
Achilles tendon replaced by peroneus longus muscle	2636	7.19
Gluteus medius replaced by external oblique transposition	2406	6.56
Hip flexion release	2442	6.66
Triple arthrodesis of foot	2422	6.61
Partial division and release of adductor femoris muscle at origin of pubis	2052	5.60
Posterior tibial tendon lengthening	1980	5.40
Treatment of knee flexion contracture deformity by extensive knee flexion release	1794	4.89
Basal osteotomy of first metatarsal bon	1484	4.05
Subcutaneous distal tenotomy of gracilis tendon	1237	3.37
Osteotomy and lengthening of tibia and fibula	1182	3.22
Peroneus brevis muscle transfer for Achilles tendon replacement	1047	2.86
Tibialis posterior muscle exteriorization	1071	2.92
Common carotid artery adventitia sympathetic plexus decollement	985	2.69
Musculus sacrospinalis instead of gluteus	885	2.41
Iliotibial band release	971	2.65
Iliopubic double osteotomy lengthening	860	2.35
Posterior tibial muscle transfer to replace Achilles tendon	902	2.46
Foot joint fusion	846	2.31
Transfer of peroneus longus muscle to replace tibialis anterior muscle	779	2.12
Tendon transfer to replace extensor malleolus, extensor hallucis and extensor digitorum muscle	710	1.94
Femoral osteotomy orthopedic	728	1.99
Amputation of obturator nerve (total or anterior branch)	673	1.84
Correction of Qin Sihe supine thumb deformity (modified JONES)	584	1.59
Tibialis anterior muscle transfer to replace Achilles tendon	584	1.59
Achilles tendon shortening	542	1.48
Fusion of talonavicular joint	570	1.55
Calcaneocuboid joint fusion	526	1.43
Interphalangeal arthrodesis of great toe	572	1.56
Acetabular shelf operation	503	1.37
Osteotomy of calcaneus	561	1.53
Release of contracture of gluteal muscle fascia	501	1.37
Ankle fusion	560	1.53
Semitendinosus transfer instead of quadriceps femoris	447	1.22
Lengthening of gastrocnemius aponeurosis	361	0.98
Reduction of congenital (developmental) dislocation of hip	298	0.81

[a] Frequency of use: refers to the number of times the method is used per 100 operations

1.2.1.8 Orthopedic Operation Combined with External Fixation in 10,235 Cases

	Number of application cases	Proportion of total cases (%)
Ilizarov external fixation	4537	12.37
Hybrid external fixation	5698	15.54

1.2.2 Statistical Analysis of 22,062 Cases of Foot and Ankle Deformity in Qin Sihe Orthopedic Surgery (1978.5.25–2020.12.31)

1.2.2.1 Gender Ratio

Gender of the patient	Number of operations	Percentage (%)
Male	13,046	59.13
Female	9016	40.87

1.2.2.2 Age Statistics of 22,062 Cases

Age	Number of operations	Percentage (%)
1–5 years old	1137	5.15
6–10 years old	3084	13.98
11–15 years old	3645	16.52
16–20 years old	4341	19.68
21–25 years	4010	18.18
26–30 years	2627	11.91
31–35 years	1560	7.07
36–40 years	759	3.44
41–45 years	349	1.58
46–50 years	264	1.20
51–55 years	149	0.68
56–60 years	83	0.38
61–70 years	48	0.22
Over 70 years old	6	0.03

Among the 22,062 cases, the age group of the most cases of operation was from 16 to 25 years old, with a total of 8351 cases, accounting for 37.85%. 286 cases (1.3%) were over 50 years old.

1.2.2.3 Disease Cause of Foot and Ankle Deformities

Name of disease	Number of operations	Name of disease	Number of operations
Sequela of poliomyelitis	15,661	Dermatomyositis	2
Cerebral palsy	2682	Tetanus	2
Spina bifida and tethered spinal cord	942	Congenital dislocation of patella	2
Congenital clubfoot	731	Congenital shortening of the toes	3
Traumatic sequelae	487	Torticollis	2
Charcot-Marie-Tooth disease	261	Bear scratch	2
Guillain-Barre syndrome	77	Hemophilia	3
Congenital polyarticular contracture	80	Osteogenesis imperfecta	1
Paralysis of common peroneal nerve	79	Venomous snake bite	1
Congenital fibular hemilimb deformity	66	Residual deformity after replantation of severed limb	1
Sequelae of traumatic brain injury	52	Multiple epiphyseal dysplasia	1
Hemangioma	46	Sequelae of gastrocnemius infection	1
Iatrogenic deformity of lower limb	49	Osteitis of calcaneus tuberosity	1
Sequelae of encephalitis	39	Fibrous dysplasia of bone	1
Lateral spinal sclerosis	29	Popliteal artery embolism	1
Congenital pseudarthrosis of the tibia	30	Transverse myelitis	1
Hallux valgus	23	Nerve injury after operation of spinal meningeal carcinoma	1
Chronic osteomyelitis	22	Spinal cord glioma	1
Burn and scald sequelae	24	Spinal cord fibroma	2
Sequelae of meningitis	21	Spinal cord hemangioma	1
Flatfoot	19	Spinal arachnoiditis	1
Congenital heel foot	20	Incomplete spinal cord injury caused by ossification of the posterior longitudinal ligament of the cervical spine	1
Sciatic nerve injury	16	Osteoarthritis of talonavicular joint	1
Ankle deformity secondary to genu varum	17	Lymphangioma	3
Gastrocnemius contracture	14	Intracranial cyst	2
Bone defect	14	Vasculitis	1
Hereditary spastic paraplegia	14	Poisoning sequela of moldy sugarcane	1
Acute myelitis	13	Toe Varus	1
Progressive Muscular Dystrophy	17	Germ tumor of the brain	1
Rheumatoid arthritis	12	Cerebral vasculitis	2
Hydrocephalus	13	Cerebral vascular malformation	1
Gluteal muscle contracture	12	脑出血 Cerebral hemorrhage	2
Congenital developmental dislocation of hip	11	Cerebral arachnoiditis	1
Congenital vertical talus	12	Sepsis	1
Bone nonunion	9	Parkinson	1
Scleroderma	12	Lead poisoning	1
Sequela of suppurative arthritis	8	Typhoid fever	1
Spinal muscular atrophy	8	Renal osteopathy	1
Familial neurofibromatosis	8	Fetal injury	1
Congenital shortening of toes	8	Congenital syndactyly	1
Congenital band syndrome	7	Congenital hypoplasia of tibia	1
Developmental deformity of lower limb caused by epiphyseal injury	6	Congenital dysplasia of talus	2
Familial PES cavus	7	Congenital external dislocation of talus	1
Congenital foot valgus	6	Congenital coxa vara	1
TOCP poisoning	5	Congenital adduction of toes	1
Diaphyseal aclasis	6	Congenital hypertrophy of great toe	1
Scoliosis	7	Congenital forefoot adduction	1
Macromelia	5	Congenital absence of forefoot	2
Melorheostosis	7	Congenital ectrodactyly	1

Name of disease	Number of operations	Name of disease	Number of operations
Hand, foot and mouth disease	10	Congenital hypoplasia of radius	1
Congenital shortening of the lower limbs	5	Congenital claw toe	1
Incomplete paraplegia of spinal cord injury	9	Congenital metatarsal adduction deformity	1
Nerve injury caused by spinal cord tumor	4	Lower limb deformity due to compression of thoracic spinal cord	1
Macrodactyly	4	Thoracic disc herniation	1
Epidemic encephalitis B	4	Lumbar tuberculosis	2
Congenital polydactyly	4	Dwarfism with ankle deformity	2
Congenital tibial hemimelia	7	Sequelae of intraspinal meningioma	1
Desmoid fibromatosis	4	Peripheral nerve paralysis	1
Organophosphorus pesticide poisoning	6	Drug poisoning	1
Hypophosphatemic rickets	5	Congenital absence of toe	1
Ankle osteoarthritis	3	Congenital pterygoid knee joint	1
Poor amputation stump	3	Congenital parasitic syndactyly	1
Gas poisoning	3	Congenital hypoplasia of fibula	1
Stroke	5	Endophytic chondroma	1
Ankle deformity secondary to genu valgum	5	Cerebral infarction	1
Congenital navicular foot	3	Methylmalonic acidemia	1
Vascular embolism of lower limb	3	Acanthosis nigricans	1
Drug-induced spinal poisoning	3	Giant cell tumor of bone	1
Septicemia	2	Sequelae of femoral artery embolism	1
Chondrodysplasia multiplex	3	Epileptic sequelae	1
Wilson's disease	3	Toxic encephalopathy	2
Avascular necrosis of the femoral head	2	Marfan syndrome	2
Bone tuberculosis	2	Neurogenic deformity of lower limb	2
Spinal nerve injury	2	Injury of common peroneal nerve	1
Spastic deformity of lower limb due to spinal cord	2	Other congenital deformities of lower limb	43
Progressive muscular atrophy	2	Other infective deformity of lower limb	18
Craniopharyngioma	3	Foot and ankle deformity of unknown etiology	78
Brain tuberculosis	2		

In 22,062 patients, there were 154 causes of foot and ankle deformities, and 78 cases of foot and ankle deformities could not be identified.

1.2.2.4 Statistics of Foot and Ankle Deformities

Deformity category	Number of cases
Varus deformity of foot	5200
Equinus deformity	8518
Valgus deformity of foot	3547
talipes calcaneus	3054
talipes equinus	1248
pes cavus	97
Claw toe	310
Flail foot (Charcot's disease)	1848
Totally	23,822

a Note: The top four types of foot and ankle deformities are equinus, varus, valgus, and calcaneus. Some patients have two or more malformations at the same time, so the number of malformations is more than the total number of operations

1.2.2.5 Statistics of 6675 Cases of Foot and Ankle Surgery Combined with External Bone Fixation

Category of external fixation	Number of cases used
Hybird external fixation	3966
Ilizarov external fixation	2709
Totally	6675[a]

[a] Prior to the introduction of the external fixation/Ilizarov technique, postoperative fixation at Qin Sihe Orthopedic Surgery was dominated by plaster immobilization

1.2.2.6 11,561 of Simultaneous Hip, Knee, and Leg Operations for Correction of Foot and Ankle Deformity

In this group of cases, most of the foot and ankle deformities were caused by neurogenic causes, so most of them were combined with deformities from hip, knee to ankle. 11,561 cases of correction of foot and ankle deformities were operated on hip, knee, and leg at the same time, accounting for 52.4% of the total. Among them, supracondylar osteotomy of femur, lengthening of lower leg osteotomy, knee flexion release, and quadriceps replacement were the main surgical methods.

1.2.3 Statistics of 2094 Cases of Congenital Limb Deformities in Qin Sihe Orthopedic Surgery

Congenital limb deformity is defined as the presence of a deformity in one or more parts of the limb at birth, including deformity of the limb during development, such as dislocation of the hip and multiple joint contractures. According to the records of Qin Sihe Orthopedic Surgery Database, there were 2094 cases of congenital limb deformity correction and functional reconstruction, accounting for 0.58% of the total number of limb deformity surgery cases in the same period. The statistical results are as follows.

1.2.3.1 Overview

Comprehensive situation			
Total cases	2094	Total etiology	67
Gender			
Male	1108	Female	986
Age			
1–7 years old	716	8–14 years old	623
15–30 years old	640	Over 30 years old	115
Overview of the year of operation			
2011–2020	694	2001–2010	548
1991–2000	489	1980–1990	363

1.2.3.2 Congenital Talipes Equinovarus (744 Cases)

Gender

Gender	Number of operations
Male	487
Female	257

Age

Age	Number of operations
1–7 years old	311
8–14 years old	165
15–30 years old	204
Over 30 years old	64

Year of Operation

Year of surgery	Number of operations
2011–2020	195
2001–2010	203
1991–2000	216
1981–1990	130

Deformity Side

Deformity side	Number of operations
Left side	214
Right side	219
Bilateral	311

1.2.3.3 Statistics of 496 Cases of Congenital or Developmental Dislocation of the Hip (CDH or DDH)

Gender

Gender	Number of operations
Male	113
Female	383

Age

Age	Number of operations
1–7 years old	158
8–14 years old	188
15–30 years old	129
Over 30 years old	21

Age of Operation

Year of surgery	Number of operations
2011–2020	57
2001.–2010	111
1991–2000	173
1981–1990	155

Deformity Side

Deformity side	Number of operations
Left side	192
Right side	163
Bilateral	141

1.2.3.4 Congenital Polyarticular Contracture (155 Cases)

Gender

Gender	Number of operations
Male	96
Female	59

Age

Age	Number of operations
1–7 years old	68
8–14 years old	39
15–30 years old	45
Over 30 years old	3

Year of Operation

Year of surgery	Number of operations
2011–2020	79
2001–2010	42
1991–2000	23
1981–1990	11

Deformity Side

Deformity side	Number of operations
Left side	19
Right side	25
Bilateral	111

1.2.3.5 Congenital Fibular Hemimelia Deformity (107 Cases)

Gender

Gender	Number of operations
Male	78
Female	29

Age

Age	Number of operations
1–7 years old	38
8–14 years old	42
15–30 years old	26
Over 30 years old	1

Year of Operation

Year of surgery	Number of operations
2011–2020	63
2001–2010	37
1991–2000	6
1981–1990	1

Deformity Side

Deformity side	Number of operations
Left side	43
Right side	62
Bilateral	2

1.2.3.6 Congenital Pseudarthrosis of the Tibia (92 Cases)

Male	47		Female	45		
0–14 years old	55		Over 14 years old	37		
2011–2020	58		2001–2010	30		
1991–2000	4		1990 and earlier	0		
Left side	54	Right side	36	Bilateral	2	

1.2.3.7 Congenital Dislocation of Patella (56 Cases)

Male	30		Female	26	
0–14 years old	26		Over 14 years old	30	
2011–2020	34		2001–2010	9	
1991–2000	7		1990 and earlier	6	
Left side	15	Right side	13	Bilateral	28

1.2.3.8 Congenital Coxa Vara (49 Cases)

Male	32		Female	17	
0–14 years old	19		Over 14 years old	30	
2011–2020	5		2001–2010	9	
1991–2000	15		1990 and earlier	20	
Left side	20	Right side	27	Bilateral	2

1.2.3.9 Congenital Unequal Length of Lower Limbs (39 Cases)

Male	23		Female	16	
0–14 years old	24		Over 14 years old	15	
2011–2020	30		2001–2010	6	
1991–2000	2		1990 and earlier	1	
Left side	18	Right side	11	Bilateral	10

1.2.3.10 Congenital Radial Hypoplasia (23 Cases)

Male	18		Female	5	
0–14 years old	19		Over 14 years old	4	
2011–2020	18		2001–2010	4	
1991–2000	1		1990 and earlier	0	
Left side	11	Right side	5	Bilateral	7

1.2.3.11 Achondroplasia (Dwarfism) (34 Cases)

Male	10		Female	24	
0–14 years old	12		Over 14 years old	22	
2011–2020	18		2001–2010	5	
1991–2000	3		Before 1990	8	
Left side	3	Right side	2	Bilateral	29
Note	Achondroplasia is a total limb deformity, but five patients in this group were operated on one side of the lower limb deformity in Qin Sihe Orthopedic Surgery, and the other side of the lower limb could be operated on in other hospitals.				

1.2.3.12 Congenital Heel Foot (20 Cases)

Male	15		Female	5	
0–14 years old	14		Over 14 years old	6	
2011–2020	9		2001–2010	8	
1991–2000	2		1990 and earlier	1	
Left side	8	Right side	3	Bilateral	9

1.2.3.13 Multiple Metaphyseal Dysplasia (18 Cases)

Male	5		Female	13	
0–14 years old	8		Over 14 years old	10	
2011–2020	10		2001–2010	7	
1991–2000	0		1990 and earlier	1	
Left side	0	Right side	0	Bilateral	18

1.2.3.14 Congenital Pterygoid Knee Joint (18 Cases)

Male	10		Female	8	
0–14岁 0–14 years old	9		Over 14 years old	9	
2011–2020	7		2001–2010	11	
1991–2000	0		1990 and earlier	0	
Left side	17	Right side	0	Bilateral	1

1.2.3.15 Congenital Vertical Talus (16 Cases)

Male	10		Female	6	
0–14 years old	11		Over 14 years old	5	
2011–2020	8		2001–2010	3	
1991–2000	4		1990 and earlier	1	
Left side	4	Right side	2	Bilateral	10

1.2.3.16 Congenital Tibial Hemimelia Deformity (16 Cases)

Male	12		Female	4	
0–14 years old	13		Over 14 years old	3	
2011–2020	14		2001–2010	2	
1991–2000	0		1990 and earlier	0	
Left side	6	Right side	10	Bilateral	0

1.2.3.17 Congenital Toe Shortening (11 Cases)

Male	1		Female	10	
0–14 years old	0		Over 14 years old	11	
2011–2020	5		2001–2010	6	
1991–2000	0		1990 and earlier	0	
Left side	2	Right side	3	Bilateral	6

1.2.3.18 Congenital Band Syndrome (10 Cases)

Male	4		Female	6	
0–14 years old	10		Over 14 years old	0	
2011–2020	5		2001–2010	3	
1991–2000	0		1990 and earlier	2	
Left side	4	Right side	5	Bilateral	1

1.2.3.19 Congenital Radioulnar Synostosis (7 Cases)

Male	7		Female	0	
0–14 years old	6		Over 14 years old	1	
2011–2020	4		2001–2010	0	
1991–2000	2		1990 and earlier	1	
Left side	3	Right side	0	Bilateral	4

1.2.3.20 Congenital Foot Valgus (7 Cases)

Male	6		Female	1	
0–14 years old	6		Over 14 years old	1	
2011–2020	0		2001–2010	2	
1991–2000	5		1990 and earlier	0	
Left side	2	Right side	4	Bilateral	1

1.2.3.21 Congenital Axial Absence of Proximal Femur (6 Cases)

Male	6		Female	0	
0–14 years old	5		Over 14 years old	1	
2011–2020	6		2001–2010	0	
1991–2000	0		1990 and earlier	0	
Left side	1	Right side	5	Bilateral	0

1.2.3.22 Macromelia (6 Cases)

Male	1		Female	5	
0–14 years old	0		Over 14 years old	6	
2011–2020	1		2001–2010	4	
1991–2000	1		1990 and earlier	0	
Left side	3	Right side	3	Bilateral	0

1.2.3.23 Congenital Tibial Curvature (6 Cases)

Male	3		Female	3	
0–14 years old	5		Over 14 years old	1	
2011–2020	4		2001–2010	1	
1991–2000	0		1990 and earlier	1	
Left side	2	Right side	4	Bilateral	0

1.2.3.24 Congenital Polydactyly (5 Cases)

Male	0		Female	5	
0–14 years old	3		Over 14 years old	2	
2011–2020	0		2001–2010	3	
1991–2000	0		1990 and earlier	2	
Left side	1	Right side	2	Bilateral	2

In this group, there were less than five cases of congenital limb deformities, with a total of 44 etiological types. Including: Macrodactyly (4 cases), Congenital ulnar dysplasia (4 cases), Congenital femoral pseudarthrosis (4 cases), Madelung's malformation (3 cases), Marfan's syndrome (3 cases), Congenital tarsal navicular (3 cases), Congenital thumb adduction (3 cases), Congenital digital flexion (3 cases), Congenital dislocation of the radial head (3 cases), Congenital pterygoid elbow joint (3 cases), Congenital absence of ulnar longitudinal column (2 cases), Congenital dislocation of the radial head (3cases). Congenital polydactyly (3cases); Congenital flexion of wrist (2 cases), Congenital ectrodactyly (2 cases), Congenital radial longitudinal agenesis (2 cases), Congenital clenching of fist (2 case).

The other etiological types were all 1 case, such as Gigantism, Hemi limb dysplasia, Down's syndrome, Congenital absence of proximal femur, Congenital radioulnar chiasma deformity, Congenital right acetabular invagination, and Congenital joint laxity.

1.2.4 Statistical Analysis of 1012 Cases of Lower Limb Deformity of Spina Bifida Sequelae (1986.10–2020.12.31)

1.2.4.1 Gender

Gender	Number of operations	Percentage (%)
Male	457	45.16
Female	555	54.84

1.2.4.2 Age

Age	Number of operations	Percentage (%)
Under 15 years old	367	36.26
15–30 years old	538	53.16
31–45 years	101	9.98
Over 45 years old	6	0.59

1.2.4.3 Deformity Side

Deformity side	Number of operations	Percentage (%)
Left side	174	17.19
Right side	186	18.38
Bilateral	652	64.43

1.2.4.4 Operative Site

Operative site	Number of operations
Hip joint	83
Knee joint	97
Ankle joint	969

[a] Some patients underwent two or three sites of surgery at the same time, so the sum of the above statistics is more than 1012 cases

1.2.4.5 Use of Surgery Combined with External Fixation

Type of external fixation	Number of operations	Usage ratio (%)
Ilizarov external fixation	442	43.68
Hybird external fixation	315	31.13
Internal fixation	66	6.52

1.2.4.6 Number of Operations Over the Years

Year of surgery	Number of operations
1980s	44
1990s	136
2000s	176
2010s	619
2020s	37

1.2.4.7 Complications were Recorded in 554 of 1012 Cases of Spina Bifida

1. There were 111 cases (20%) with ulcer in the weight-bearing area of the foot and 85 cases (15.34%) with hair on the waist.
2. Dysfunction of defecation

Defecation	Number of cases	Percentage (%)
Basically normal	128	23.10
Partial control	187	33.75
Basically out of control	49	8.84
Completely out of control	29	5.23
Not recorded	161	29.06

3. Spina bifida lower limb deformity with sensory disturbance.

Sensory disturbance plane	Number of cases	Percentage (%)
Plantar	107	19.31
Ankle	202	36.46
Knee	56	10.11
Unknown	189	34.12

1.2.5 Statistical Analysis of 837 Cases of Traumatic Lower Limb Deformity in Qin Sihe Orthopedic Surgery 1978.5.25–2020.12.31

1.2.5.1 Gender

Gender	Number of operations	Proportion
Male	551	65.8%
Female	286	34.2%

1.2.5.2 Age

Age	Number of operations	Proportion
Under 16 years old	172	20.55%
16–30 years old	374	44.68%
31 –45 years	185	22.10%
46–60 years	86	10.27%
Over 60 years old	20	2.39%
Maximum age	84 years old	
Minimum age	3 years old	
Average age	27.6 years old	

1.2.5.3 Year of Operation

Year of surgery	Number of operations
1978–1982	2
1983–1987	13
1988–1992	61
1993–1997	47
1998–2002	69
2003–2007	64
2008–2012	194
2013–2017	250
2018–2020	137

1.2.5.4 Deformity Side

Deformity side	Number of operations	Percentage
Left side	394	47.07%
Right side	376	44.92%
Bilateral	67	8.00%

1.2.5.5 1048 Deformity Sites

Deformity site	Total number
Hip joint	41
Thigh	86
Knee joint	254
Shank	160
Ankle, foot, toe	507

Because some patients had malformations in two parts at the same time, there were 1048 malformations in this group, more than 837 cases.

1.2.5.6 624 Cases Were Treated with External Fixation

Type of external fixation	Number of operations	Percentage
Hybrid external fixation	157	18.75%
Ilizarov external fixation	467	55.79%

1.2.6 Statistical Analysis of 567 Cases of Upper Limb Deformity

According to the database analysis of Qin Sihe Orthopedic Surgery Database, Professor Qin Sihe recorded the first upper limb operation on June 18, 1985. As of June 15, 2020, a total of 567 upper limb operations had been performed. Among them, male patients were significantly more than female patients, mainly adolescents aged 10–25 years old, and most of them were upper limb deformities or functional disorders caused by cerebral palsy and trauma, followed by poliomyelitis and various congenital upper limb deformities. The surgical patients came from 27 provinces, autonomous regions, and municipalities directly under the Central Surgical procedures include soft tissue release, muscle balance, osteotomy, upper limb lengthening, and other categories, and about 34% of the patients were treated with extraosseous bindings. The following is the detailed statistics.

1.2.6.1 Gender

Gender	Number of operations	Percentage (%)
Male	420	74.07
Female	147	25.93

1.2.6.2 Age

Age	Number of operations
0–5 years old	35
6–10 years old	84
11–15 years old	119
16–20 years old	148
21–25 years	95
26–30 years	51
31–40 years	18
41–50 years	9
Over 50 years old	8

1.2.6.3 Statistics of 567 Cases of Upper Limb Deformity

Disease type	Number of operations
Cerebral palsy	212
Sequela of poliomyelitis	50
Trauma	154
Osteomyelitis sequela	5
Sequelae of lateral sclerosis	3
Congenital multiple joint contracture	7
Scleroderma	2
Poisoning by drugs or pesticides	3
Neuritis	4
Hemangioma	1
Enchondroma	6
Madelung deformity	1
Diaphyseal aclasis	3
Various congenital malformations of the upper extremities	74
Others	42

1.2.6.4 External Fixation was Used in 192 Cases, Accounting for 33.86% of 567 Cases

Type of external fixation	Number of cases used	Utilization rate per 100 cases (%)
Ilizarov external fixation	107	18.87
Hybrid external fixation	85	14.99

1.2.7 Statistical Analysis of Surgical Cases of Lower Limb Deformity in Qinghai and Tibet Plateau Areas (131 Cases as of December 2018)

From 1986 to the end of December 2018, among the patients with limb deformity and disability in Qin Sihe Orthopedic surgery, a total of 131 patients lived in the Qinghai-Tibet Plateau above 3000 meters above sea level, including 27 cases in Tibet and 104 cases in Qinghai. Due to different diseases and disease characteristics from patients living in low-altitude areas, the statistics are pretended.

1.2.7.1 Gender

Gender	Number of operations	Proportion
Male	65	49.6
Female	66	50.4

1.2.7.2 Age

Age (years)	Number of operations	Proportion
1–5	17	12.98
6–10	20	15.27
11–15	31	23.66
16–20	18	13.74
21–30	22	16.79
31–40	16	12.21
41–50	1	0.76
51–60	3	2.29
60+	3	2.29

1.2.7.3 Nationality

Nation	Number of operations	Proportion
Tibetans	46	35.11
Han	43	32.82
Hui	21	16.03
Salar	3	2.29
Dong	1	0.76
Mongolian	1	0.76
Unrecorded	16	12.21

1.2.7.4 Year of Operation

Year of surgery	Number of operations
1986–1989	6
1990–1999	21
2000–2009	7
2010–2018	97

1.2.7.5 Statistics of 131 Cases of Limb Deformities in the Qinghai-Tibet Plateau

No.	Etiology and disease	Number of operations
1	Sequela of poliomyelitis	44
2	Cerebral palsy	13
3	Traumatic sequelae	13
4	Congenital dislocation of hip	8
5	Congenital clubfoot	6
6	Congenital joint contracture	6
7	Spina bifida sequelae	4
8	Congenital dislocation of patella	4
9	Hereditary motor neuron disease	3
10	Guillain-Barre sequelae	3
11	Avascular necrosis of the femoral head	2
12	Osteomyelitis	2
13	Osteoarthritis of the knee	2
14	Genu valgum	2
15	Paralysis of common peroneal nerve	1
16	Injury of common peroneal nerve	1
17	Femoral artery fibroma	1
18	Femoral periarterial fibroma	1
19	Progressive Muscular Dystrophy	1
20	Iatrogenic deformity of lower extremity	1
21	Sciatic nerve injury	1
22	Muscular torticollis	1
23	Kashin-Beck disease	7
24	Unclear	4

1.2.8 Statistical Analysis of 3547 Cases of Severe Deformity and Disability of Lower Limbs

Statistics from January 2000 to December 2019, Qin Sihe Orthopedic Surgery Database, with the degree of lower limb dysfunction recorded in preoperative cases as the evaluation criteria, starting from bare-handed severe claudication, followed by hand-pressed leg (upper limb supporting the affected lower limb) walking, crutch walking or loss of standing walking function, as the evaluation criteria for severe deformity disability of lower limbs. A total of 3547 cases were counted.

1.2.8.1 Gender

Gender	Number of operations	Proportion
Male	1987	56.02%
Female	1560	43.98%

1.2.8.2 Age

Age (years)	Number of operations	Proportion
1–5	126	3.55%
6–10	241	6.79%
11–15	573	16.15%
16–20	623	17.56%
21–25	680	19.17%
26–30	507	14.29%
31–35	279	7.87%
36–40	181	5.10%
41–45	112	3.16%
46–50	101	2.85%
51–60	100	2.82%
61–70	21	0.59%
70+	3	0.08%
Maximum age	84 years old	
Latest age	1 year old	
Average age	25.28 years old	

This group of data shows that most of the patients with severe lower limb deformities and disabilities are young adults.

1.2.8.3 Causes of Severe Lower Limb Deformities and Disabilities (92 Kinds)

Etiology	Number of operations
Sequela of poliomyelitis	2089
Cerebral palsy	532
Spina bifida sequelae	206
Traumatic sequelae	163
Congenital joint contracture	55
Motor neuron disease	40
Congenital pseudarthrosis of the tibia	33
Congenital clubfoot	31
Congenital fibular hemilimb deformity	23
Bone defect	21
Osteomyelitis	21
Bone nonunion	18
Hemangioma	18
Osteogenesis imperfecta	16
Rheumatoid arthritis	15
Traumatic brain injury	14
Congenital pterygoid knee joint	14
Scoliosis	12
Fibrous dysplasia of bone	11
Guillain-Barre	10
Congenital dislocation of patella	9
Iatrogenic deformity of lower extremity	9
Sequela of suppurative arthritis	7
Acute myelitis	6
Congenital tibial hemimelia	6
Multiple epiphyseal dysplasia	5
Developmental deformity of lower limb caused by epiphyseal injury	5
Encephalitis	5
Developmental dislocation of the hip	4
Bone tuberculosis	4
Spinal muscular atrophy	4

Etiology	Number of operations
Incomplete paraplegia of spinal cord injury	4
Gluteal muscle contracture	4
Hereditary spastic paraplegia	4
Septicemia	3
Chondrodysplasia multiplex	3
Diaphyseal aclasis	3
Lateral spinal sclerosis	3
Poor amputation stump	3
Hydrocephalus	3
Burns and scalds	3
Genu valgum	3
Organophosphorus pesticide poisoning	3
TOCP poisoning	2
Paralysis of common peroneal nerve	2
Wilson's disease	2
Osteosarcoma	2
Spinal nerve injury	2
Familial neurofibromatosis	2
Progressive Muscular Dystrophy	2
Meningitis	2
Congenital pseudarthrosis of femur	2
Congenital coxa vara	2
Congenital shortening of the lower limbs	2
Vascular embolism	2
Drug poisoning	2
Scleroderma	2
Sequelae of intraspinal meningioma	2
Gollop-wolfgang complex	1
Epileptic sequelae	1
Fanconi syndrome	1
Injury of common peroneal nerve	1
Dysfunctional peripheral neuropathy	1
Rickets	1
Avascular necrosis of the femoral head	1
Popliteal artery embolism	1
Transverse myelitis	1
Steroid-induced multiple osteonecrosis	1
Spinal cord fibroma	1
Nerve injury caused by spinal cord tumor	1
Osteoarthritis of hip	1
Hip joint synovitis	1
Melorheostosis	1
Lymphangioma	1
Intracranial cyst	1
Marfan syndrome	1
Vasculitis	1
Cerebral arachnoiditis	1
Stroke	1
Endophytic chondroma	1
Parkinson	1
Lead poisoning	1
Hand, foot, and mouth disease	1
Osteoarthritis of the knee	1
Charcot arthropathy	1
Congenital heel foot	1
Congenital dysplasia of talus	1
Congenital flexion of the knee	1
Congenital axial defect of lower leg	1
Thoracic disc herniation	1
Hemophilia	1
Mucopolysaccharidosis	1
Infective lower limb deformity	12
Other congenital deformities of lower limb	11
Unknown	15

1.2.8.4 Degree of Dysfunction of Severe Lower Limb Deformity (Pathological Gait) Classified by Qin Sihe

Gait classification	Number of operations	Proportion
Severe claudication	884	24.92%
Walk with hands on legs	364	10.26%
Use single crutch/stick/bench	909	25.63%
Use double crutch/walking aid	873	24.61%
Crawl/Squat/Crouch/Kneel	187	5.27%
Unable to walk/Use wheelchair	330	9.30%

Note; Of 3547 patients, 517 (14.6%) lost the ability of standing and walking, and could only crawl on the ground, move in squatting position or rely on wheelchair before operation

1.3 Characteristics and Etiological Classification Methods of Limb Deformity in China

1.3.1 Characteristics of Limb Deformity and Disability in China

1.3.1.1 Neurogenic Causes of Limb Deformities Account for a Relatively High Proportion

Neurogenic limb deformity disability is the most common type of motor system deformities. Only Qin Sihe Orthopedic Surgery has treated 24,065 cases of polio sequelae, 4902 cases of cerebral palsy and 1045 cases of lower limb deformity after spina bifida (tethered spinal cord), often accompanied by muscle paralysis, spasm and deformity. It is characterized by childhood onset, accompanied by lifelong, and often cannot be completely cured. However, the relatively developed medical and health systems in European and American countries with small population make complex and severe physical disabilities such as those left to the adult stage relatively rare, and almost no one studies the surgical treatment of polio sequelae. It proves that the causes, diseases and degree of disability of patients with limb deformities in China are quite different from those in Western countries.

1.3.1.2 Limb Deformities that Develop to Adulthood After Delayed Treatment Are Defined As New Diseases

Some limb deformities with delayed treatment are introduced as independent diseases. Congenital talipes equinovarus in adulthood; Congenital dislocation of patella in adulthood; Delayed treatment of developmental dislocation of the hip in adulthood. The reason why Qin Sihe named a deformity as two diseases is that a congenital limb deformity develops from childhood to adulthood, from pathology, deformity category and nature, patient's constitution, degree of dysfunction and surgical reconstruction principle, although it is a person, it is two deformity categories.

1.3.1.3 Limb Deformities Caused by Rare Diseases Are Not Uncommon in China

Osteogenesis imperfecta (brittle bone disease) is a rare disease in Western countries. In China, Dr. Ren Xiuzhi in Tianjin alone has operated on more than 2000 patients. It is obviously not uncommon for Qin Sihe to correct 287 cases of peroneal muscular atrophy and 109 cases of fibular hemimelia deformity. Congenital pterygoid knee deformity is an extremely rare case, and Qin Sihe's team has operated on 18 cases. The book also includes rare causes rarely reported in the literature, such as knee stiffness caused by umbilical cord infection and septicemia in infants, severe scar contracture caused by injection infection in the buttocks of infants, and moldy sugarcane poisoning.

1.3.2 Selection Method and Macro Classification Basis of Limb Deformity

1.3.2.1 Disease Selection and Inclusion Method

This book contains 284 etiological categories, which are divided into congenital and non-congenital categories. The selected criteria are all patients who have been clinically diagnosed and treated by the author, and almost every disease is based on real limb deformity pictures, which can achieve the effect of recognizing diseases by looking at pictures.

1.3.2.2 Classification Basis of Diseases

According to the causes and locations of limb deformities, it can be divided into 13 categories, including spine, pelvis, limbs, hands, and feet. The causes range from congenital, genetic, immune, traumatic to acquired teratogenic diseases. Diseases run through more than a dozen disciplines besides orthopedics, such as congenital, genetic, immune, vascular, neurological, endocrine, skin, cancer, and so on. This classification, to a certain extent, reveals the disease spectrum and disease characteristics that lead to limb deformities in China, and opens up a new research field for subsequent scholars.

1.3.2.3 Naming of New Diseases-Based on Clinical Diagnosis and Treatment

There are also some diseases whose names are based on the diseases treated by Qin Sihe orthopedic surgery, such as congenital cervical hyperextension deformity; Stress genu recurvatum deformity; Ankle deformity after organophosphorus pesticide poisoning; Developmental subluxation of the hip due to hip adductor spasm. The introduction of iatrogenic limb deformity is intended to remind medical staff to pay attention to the prevention and avoidance of serious complications in clinical work! Whether the author's classification method of etiology and disease is reasonable, and whether the naming and analysis of new diseases are appropriate, we hope to get the objection and correction of colleagues.

China has a long history, with more than 1.4 billion people of 56 ethnic groups, living in areas ranging from the Qinghai-Tibet Plateau, which is more than 4500 m above sea level, to the Turpan Basin, which is more than 100 m below sea level. Different regions, different nationalities, different cultural customs, different economic conditions, different types of work, life patterns, marriage and reproductive habits, genetic genes, and so on are different, resulting in different causes and diseases of limb deformities. There are also some endemic diseases that can produce developmental disorders and limb deformities related to the living environment. This group of cases shows that the incidence rate in northern China is higher than that in southern China, and that in western mountainous areas is higher than that in eastern plain areas. With the development of social and economic level, congenital malformations are generally declining, and the proportion of malformations caused by chronic diseases, tumors, systemic diseases, and bone and joint degeneration in the elderly will increase.

Suggested Reading

1. Qin S, Guo B, Zang J, et al. Statistical analysis of 35,075 cases of surgical treatment for limb deformities in disabled patients (Qin Sihe Orthopedics, May 25, 1978, to December 31, 2018). Chin J Reparative Reconstr Surg. 2019;33(11):1333–9. https://doi.org/10.7507/1002-1892.201907108.
2. Qin S, Guo B, Wang Y, et al. Preliminary analysis of the characteristics of 1,012 patients with secondary lower limb deformities in spina bifida (Qin Sihe Orthopedics Database, October 12, 1986, to December 31, 2020). Chin J Reparative Reconstr Surg. 2021;35(11):1380–3.

2 Congenital Deformity of Lower Limbs

Sihe Qin, Lei Shi, Baofeng Guo, Shaofeng Jiao, and Jiancheng Zang

2.1 The Pelvis, Hip, and Femur

2.1.1 Congenital Dislocation of Hip

2.1.1.1 Etiology

Congenital dislocation of the hip (CDH) is also called developmental dislocation of the hip (DDH). Scholars at home and abroad recognize that it is related to many factors, including (1) congenital factors, such as heredity, fetal position, ligament relaxation, etc. (2) Acquired factors, such as child-rearing methods, countries and nationalities accustomed to carrying their children on their backs, have a low incidence of congenital dislocation of the hip, but a high incidence of tying and wrapping the legs of the newborn together. (3) Gender difference, researchers found that the ratio of female to male is 6:1, the incidence ratio of male and female is very different. In addition, the relaxin in female fetus is more than that in male fetus. It has also been reported that the female fetus has a greater anteversion of the femoral neck than the male fetus and is prone to dislocation. (4) Left and right differences, it is showed that the total number of cases was divided into 4, while the bilateral incidence was 1, the left incidence was 2, and the right incidence was 1. That is to say, the incidence of unilateral disease is three times that of bilateral disease. The incidence on the left side was twice that on the right side.

2.1.1.2 Clinical Manifestation

1. The hip on the affected side is widened, the groin crease and the posterior hip crease are asymmetric, the crease on the affected side is deep, the position is high, or the number is increased. The affected limb is short, and the tip of the foot is often turned outward.
2. Ortolani, Barlow, Galeazzi (Allis) and Trendelenburg test are positive.
3. In adults, the femoral head bends out of the acetabulum and rests on the iliac wing, forming a false acetabulum. Dislocation of the hip is suggested by any of the following conditions in children: (1) The epiphyseal nucleus of the femoral head is located outside the lower quadrant of Perkin's square; (2) increase in acetabular index; (3) Shenton's line and calves line are discontinuous; (4) the CE angle (center edge angle) decreases; (5) sharp angle increased (Fig. 2.1).

2.1.1.3 Treatment Principle

The treatment of congenital dislocation of the hip in children is different in different age groups. From birth to one and a half years old, conservative treatment, that is, non-surgical treatment, can be adopted. From one and a half to 3 years old, either conservative treatment or surgical treatment can be adopted. For 3- to 6-year-old patients, surgical reduction; repositioning surgery is contraindicated for patients older than 12 years of age, and Ilizarov pelvic support osteotomy may be performed to improve gait.

2.1.2 Congenital Acetabular Dysplasia

2.1.2.1 Etiology

Congenital subluxation of the hip, spina bifida, cerebral palsy, multiple joint contractures, aseptic necrosis of the femoral head, and hereditary sensorimotor neuropathy can be associated with congenital acetabular dysplasia.

S. Qin (✉)
Department of Orthopaedics, Rehabilitation Hospital of the National Research Center for Rehabilitation Technical Aids, Beijing, China

L. Shi · S. Jiao
Department of Orthopaedics, Rehabilitation Hospital, National Research Center for Rehabilitation, Beijing, China

B. Guo
Department of Orthopedics, Chuiyangliu Hospital affiliated to Tsinghua University, Beijing, China

J. Zang
Department of Hand and Foot Surgery, Beijing University of Chinese Medicine Third Affiliated Hospital, Beijing, China

S. Qin et al. (eds.), *Atlas of Limb Deformity*, https://doi.org/10.1007/978-981-97-0999-1_2

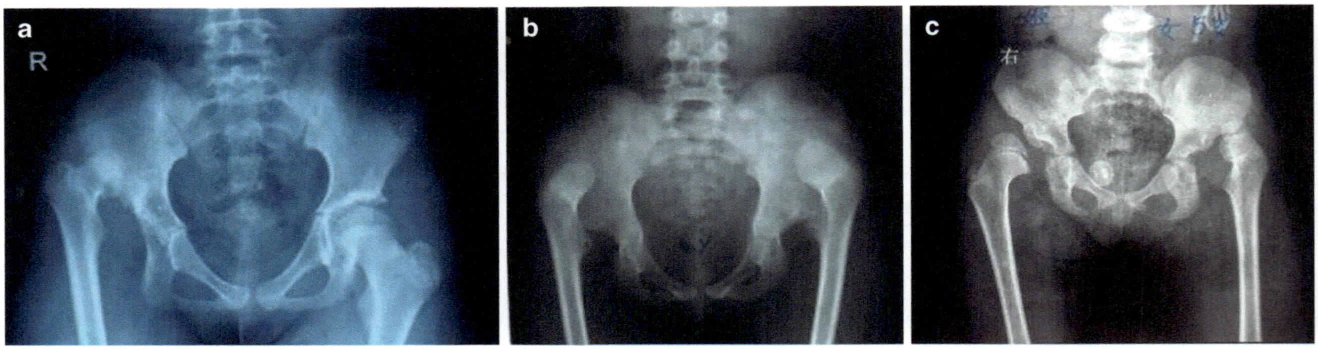

Fig. 2.1 Congenital dislocation of hip. (**a**) Unilateral congenital dislocation of the hip; (**b**) bilateral congenital dislocation of the hip; (**c**) congenital dislocation of the hip in children

2.1.2.2 Clinical Manifestation

The early symptoms of congenital acetabular dysplasia are gait instability, claudication, and then walking limb fatigue, joint pain, and other symptoms. Unilateral acetabular dysplasia can lead to unequal lengths of the lower limbs. The acetabular index was increased, the CE angle was decreased, and the coverage of femoral head was decreased. CT three-dimensional reconstruction showed that the acetabulum became shallow and the anteversion angle increased. Arthrography may show dysplasia of the articular capsule, labrum, and round ligament (Fig. 2.2).

2.1.2.3 Treatment Principle

Early detection, early treatment. Within 3 years old, conservative treatment is available; over 3 years old, X-ray films should be reexamined every year to determine whether surgical treatment is needed and the timing of surgery should be determined according to the degree of acetabular development.

2.1.3 Otto's Disease

Otto's disease is also known as acetabular pelvic protrusion and Otto pelvis. It is characterized by chronic progressive protrusion of the femoral head into the acetabulum and pelvis.

2.1.3.1 Etiology

The disease may be associated with osteomalacia or rheumatoid arthritis.

2.1.3.2 Clinical Manifestation

Most of them are unilateral onset, manifested as limb shortening, limited hip joint movement, and pain in secondary arthritis. X-ray and CT showed that the acetabulum was depressed and protruded into the pelvis (Fig. 2.3).

2.1.3.3 Treatment Principle

1. If there is no obvious pain and dysfunction in the hip joint, limb lengthening is feasible to improve the unequal length of the limbs.
2. Artificial joint replacement can be considered for patients with hip pain and dysfunction.

2.1.4 Congenital and Developmental Coxa Vara

2.1.4.1 Etiology

The etiology of congenital and developmental coxa vara is unknown, but many diseases can cause developmental coxa vara, such as osteogenesis imperfecta, hypophosphatemic rickets, fibrous dysplasia of bone, epiphyseal chondrodysplasia, and so on.

2.1.4.2 Clinical Manifestation

In infancy, the disease has no obvious signs and is not easy to be found. After learning to walk, unstable walking and swaying gait may gradually increase. Physical examination showed that the hip was wide and Trendelenburg's sign was positive. X-ray film showed that the femoral neck-shaft angle was reduced, the greater trochanter was high, and the femoral neck was short (Fig. 2.4).

2.1.4.3 Classification

It can be divided into congenital and developmental. Congenital is born with coxa vara, often accompanied by other deformities, unilateral more common; with the growth and development of children, the malformation is gradually aggravated.

2.1.4.4 Treatment Principle

Subtrochanteric osteotomy and other operations were performed to change the femoral neck-shaft angle.

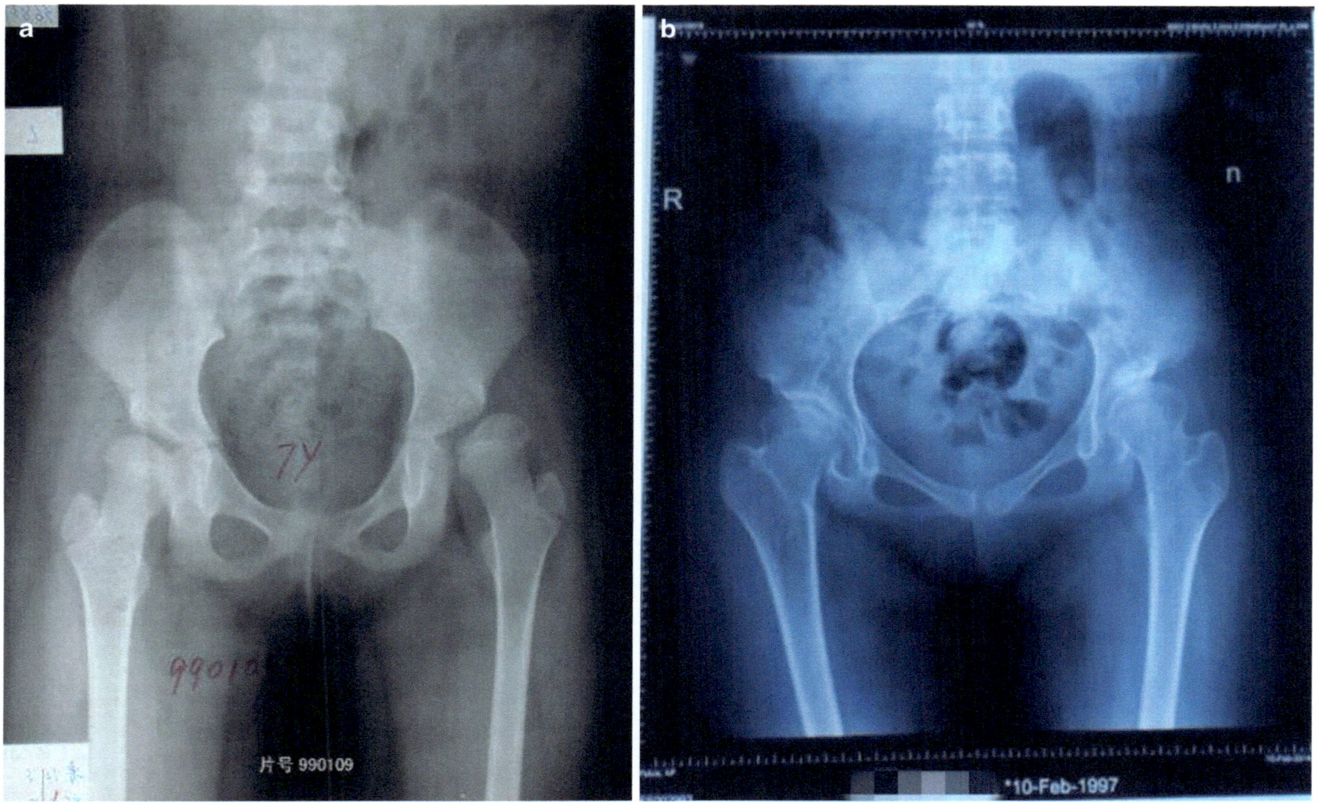

Fig. 2.2 Bilateral congenital acetabular dysplasia: (**a**) Bilateral congenital acetabular dysplasia in childhood; (**b**) Bilateral acetabular dysplasia in adulthood

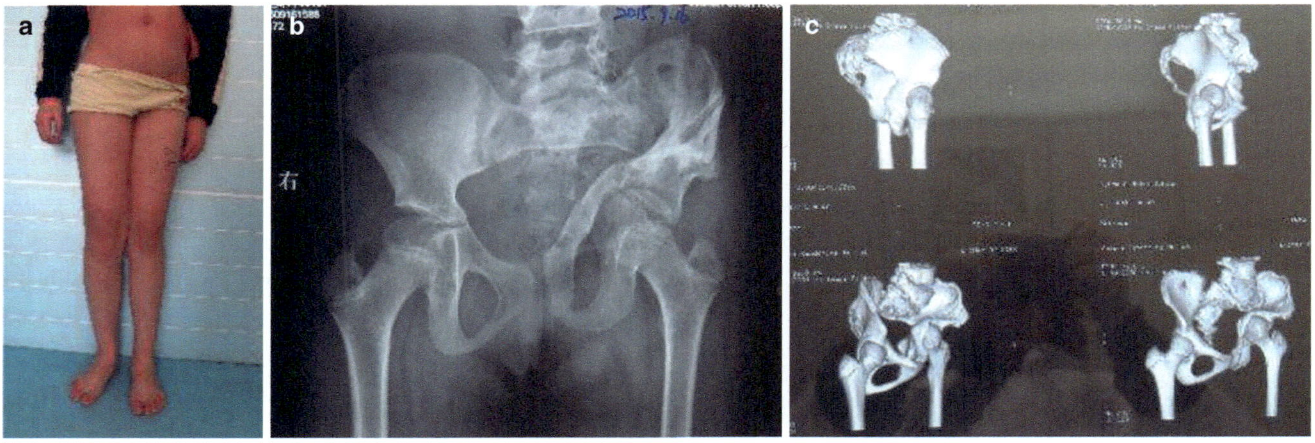

Fig. 2.3 Congenital Otto's disease, female, 14 years old: (**a**) Standing appearance; (**b**) anteroposterior X-ray of pelvis; (**c**) CT three-dimensional reconstruction of pelvis

2.1.5 Congenital Proximal Focal Femoral Deficiency

2.1.5.1 Etiology

Congenital proximal focal femoral deficiency is a congenital malformation without definite etiology, which may be related to maternal diabetes mellitus.

2.1.5.2 Clinical Manifestation

Severe limb shortening, mainly thigh shortening, without normal hip transverse lines and groin lines, hip instability. It may be accompanied by different degrees of deformity of the ipsilateral lower leg and ankle. Imaging findings can be referred to classification.

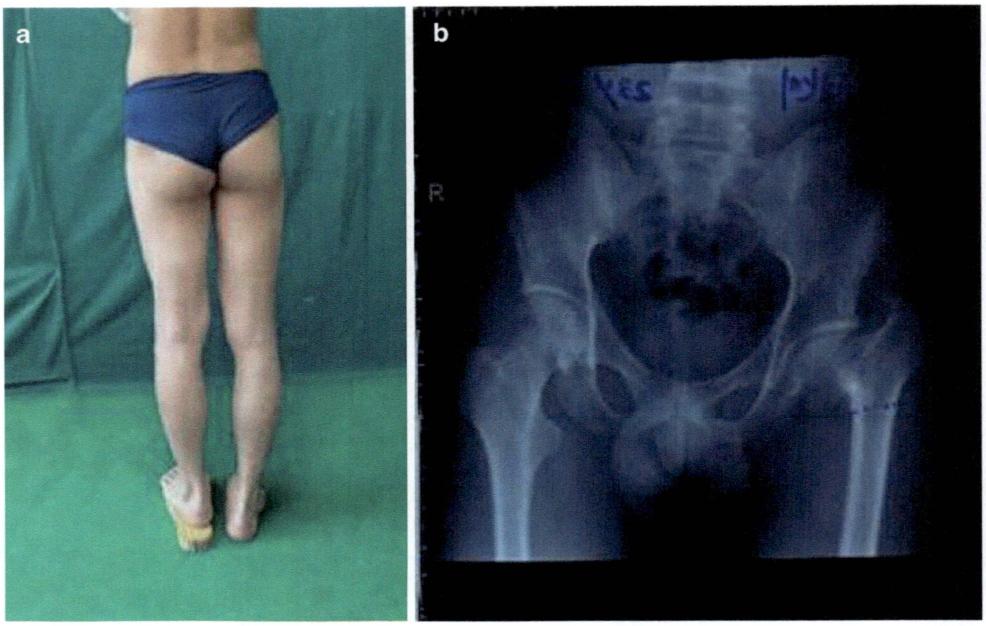

Fig. 2.4 Left coxa vara with limb shortening: (**a**) Observation from standing position; (**b**) pelvic X-ray film showing shortening of the femoral neck on the left with the greater trochanter elevated

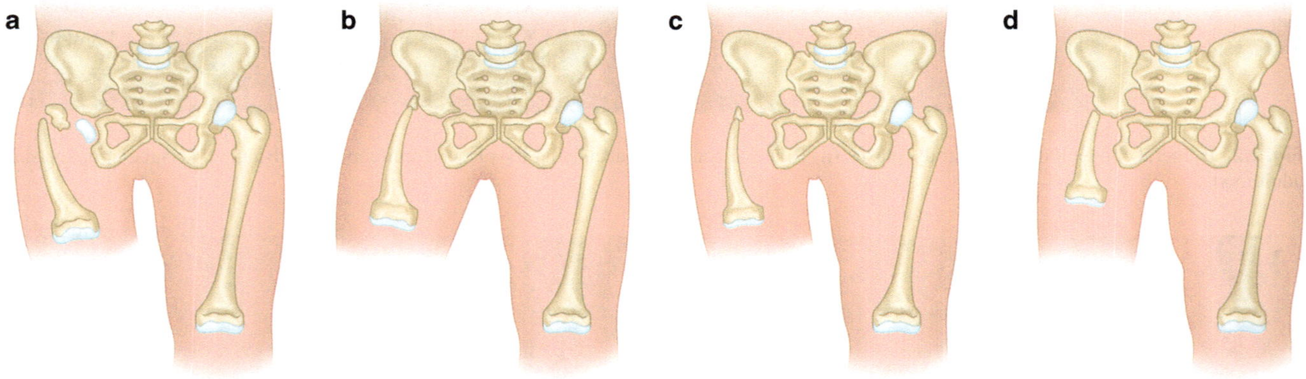

Fig. 2.5 Aitken classification of proximal focal femoral deficiency: (**a**) The hip joint was formed in appearance, but the femoral neck was absent and the femur was shortened in the early X-ray film. (**b**) The femoral head is more primitive, the proximal femoral shaft defect is more obvious, and there is often a pseudarthrosis between the femoral shaft and the femoral head. (**c**) The femoral head is absent, the acetabulum is shallow, and the proximal femur is replaced by a small cluster of bone. (**d**) The femoral head and acetabulum are absent, and the femoral shaft defect is more obvious

2.1.5.3 Classification

1. Aitken four-type classification (Fig. 2.5)
2. Kalamchi's simplified five-type classification

   Type I: femoral shortening deformity with intact hip joint;

   Type II: femoral shortening deformity, coxa vara deformity;

   Type III: femoral shortening deformity with well-developed acetabulum and femoral head;

   Type IV: absence of hip joint and segmental dysplasia of femur;

   Type V: complete absence of the entire femur.

2.1.6 Typical Cases

See Fig. 2.6.

2.1.6.1 Treatment Principle

1. Increase the stability of hip joint and rebuild the function of hip joint.
2. Correction of deformities.
3. Equal-length lower limbs, artificial limbs, or braces to improve walking ability.

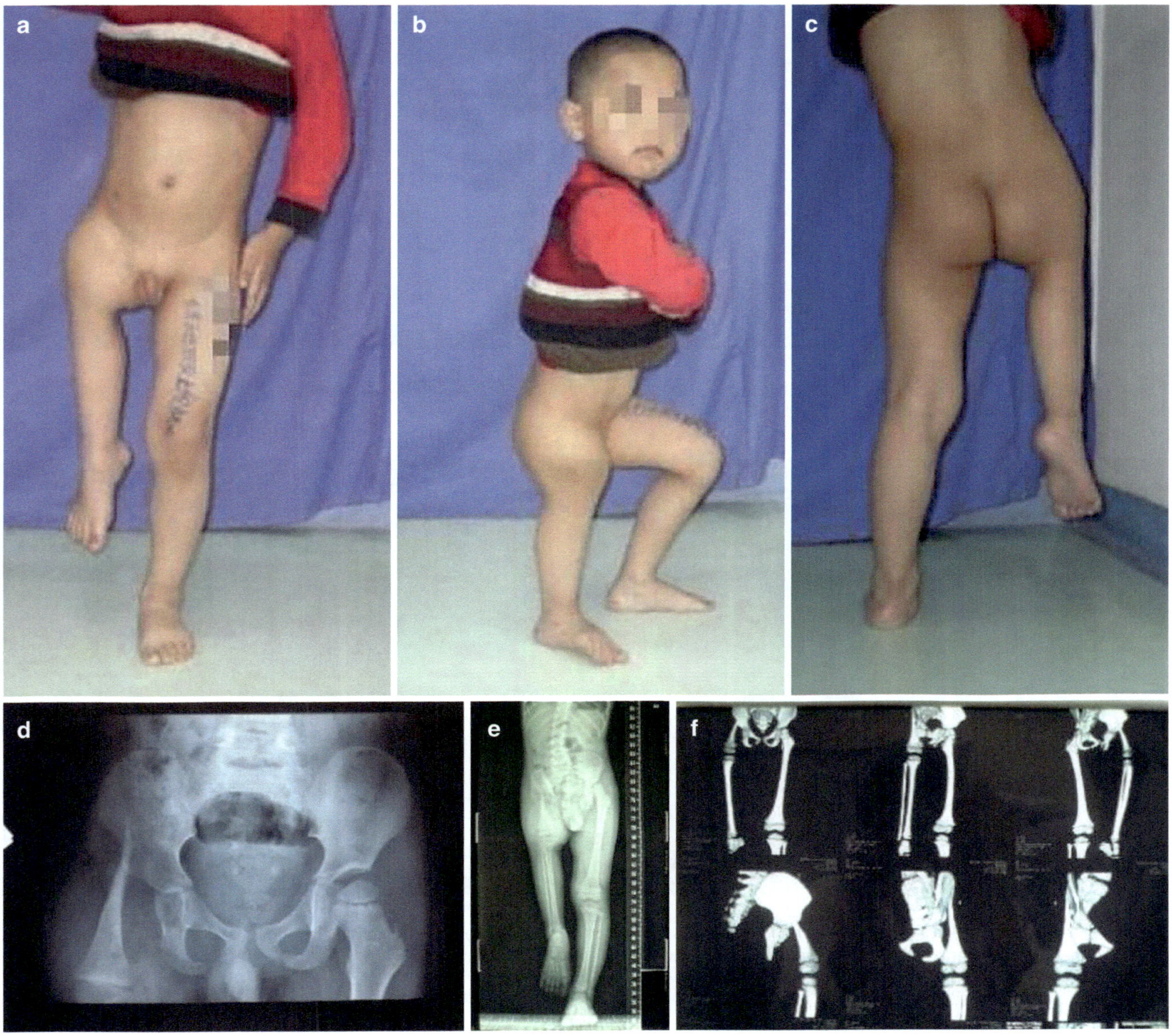

Fig. 2.6 Aitken type D of congenital proximal focal femoral deficiency. Male, 5 years old: (**a**) Standing frontal view; (**b**) side view; (**c**) back view;(**d**) pelvic X-ray; (**e**) lower limb full-length X-ray; (**f**)three-dimensional reconstruction of pelvis and femur

2.1.7 Congenital Proximal Femoral Dysplasia

2.1.7.1 Etiology

The disease is a congenital malformation with unknown etiology.

2.1.7.2 Clinical Manifestation

The clinical manifestations were severe limb shortening, mainly thigh shortening, asymmetric transverse lines of buttocks, instability of hip and knee joints. It may be accompanied by different degrees of deformity of the ipsilateral lower leg and ankle. X-ray of the pelvis showed abnormal morphology of the proximal femur and normal or nearly normal acetabulum.

2.1.7.3 Typical Cases

See Figs. 2.7 and 2.8.

2.1.7.4 Treatment Principle

1. Correction of proximal femoral deformity.
2. Lengthen the femur and equalize the length of both lower limbs.

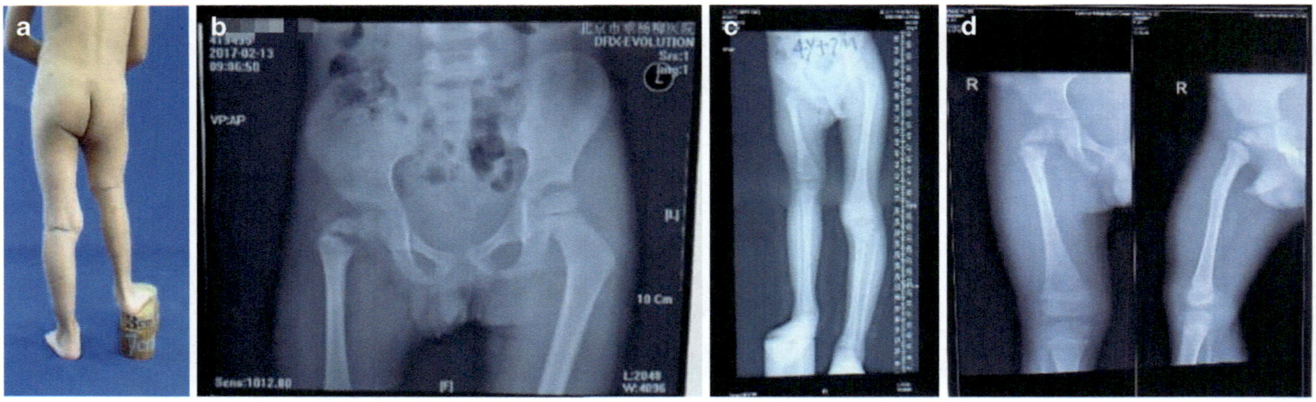

Fig. 2.7 Congenital dysplasia of proximal femur. Male, 4 years and 7 months: (**a**) Standing dorsal view; (**b**) pelvic X-ray; (**c**) lower limb full-length X-ray; (**d**) full-length X-ray film of right femur

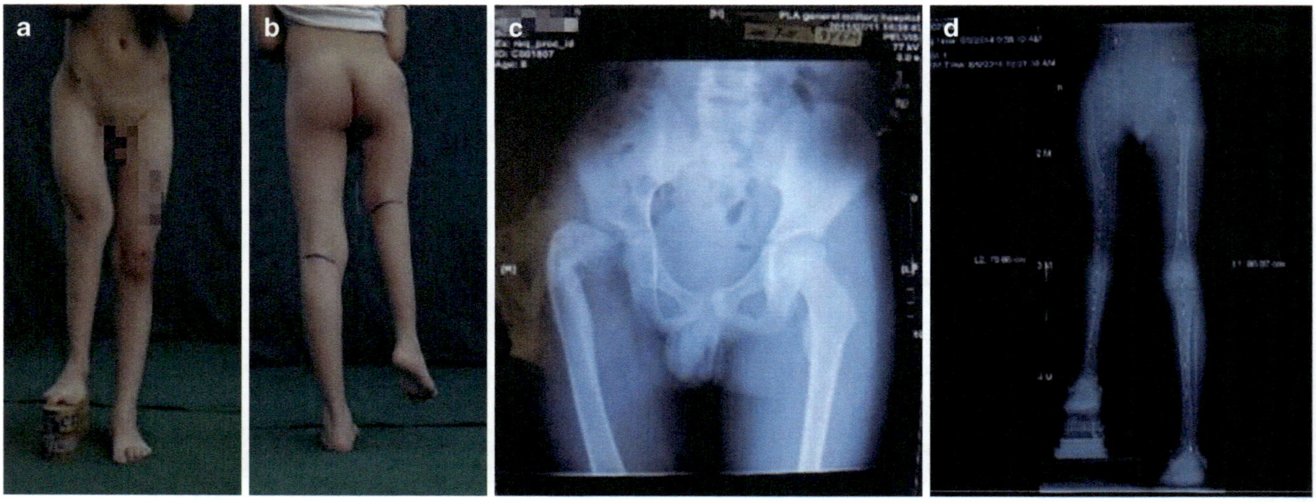

Fig. 2.8 Congenital dysplasia of proximal femur. Male, 12 years old: (**a**) Frontal photograph in standing position; (**b**) dorsal photograph in standing position; (**c**) pelvic X-ray; (**d**) full-length X-ray film of lower limb

2.1.8 Delayed Treatment of Congenital Dislocation of the Hip in Adulthood

2.1.8.1 Etiology

Congenital dislocation of the hip did not be found early, or due to various reasons, cannot be treated timely and effectively, or the failure of surgical treatment, dislocation recurrence and other reasons, resulting in patients to adulthood, there is still dislocation of the hip.

2.1.8.2 Clinical Manifestation

The main manifestations of unilateral dislocation were unequal length of both lower limbs, protrusion and upward displacement of the greater trochanter of the femur at the hip, and compound limping gait. The main manifestations of bilateral dislocation were severe swaying gait (duck gait), protrusion and upward displacement of the greater trochanter of the femur at both hips. X-ray film of the pelvis shows bilateral dislocation of the femoral head, with upward displacement (Fig. 2.9).

2.1.8.3 Treatment Principle

The goal of treatment is to improve gait. If hip pain occurs, joint pain should be relieved at the same time. Ilizarov pelvic support osteotomy (Ilizarov hip reconstruction surgery) can effectively improve walking function, and those who meet the requirements can be treated with artificial hip replacement.

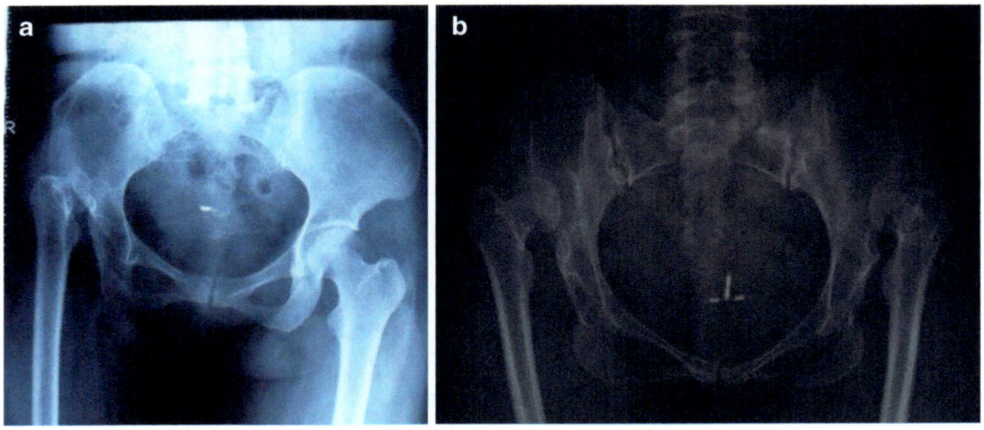

Fig. 2.9 Delayed treatment of adult congenital dislocation of the hip. (**a**) Unilateral dislocation of hip joint; (**b**) bilateral congenital dislocation of the hip

2.2 The Knee and Lower Leg

2.2.1 Congenital Dislocation of Patella

Congenital dislocation of the patella (CDP) is often familial and characterized by bilateral morbidity and is occasionally associated with other abnormalities, such as congenital polyarticular contracture and Down syndrome. Congenital dislocation of the patella is usually stubborn and cannot recover by itself. It is often accompanied by an abnormal knee extension function. The vastus lateralis may be absent or severely contracture. The patella dislocates outward and adheres to the anterior iliotibial band. The patella is usually small, abnormal in shape, and abnormal in position within the quadriceps knee extension function.

2.2.1.1 Etiology

The etiology of this disease is unknown and may be related to heredity.

2.2.1.2 Clinical Manifestation

Congenital dislocation of the patella is difficult to diagnose before the age of 4 because the ossification center of the patella has not yet appeared and there are no obvious symptoms and signs. Some patients were born with knee flexion contracture, genu valgum, tibial external rotation, and foot deformity. Habitual dislocation is mostly adolescent women, knee joint is weak when walking, patella moves to the outside when squatting, and automatic reduction after standing. Physical examination showed knee valgus deformity, and there was a sense of relaxation and instability when touching the patella and knee joint. In the case of unilateral onset, developmental limb shortening of the affected side and unequal length of both lower limbs may occur (Fig. 2.10); bilateral onset, children in the development process gradually appear with knee flexion contracture deformity and gradually lose the ability to walk upright, can only squat or kneel to walk.

2.2.1.3 Classification

It can be divided into stationarity dislocation and reducible (habitual) dislocation. Stationarity dislocation, in which the patella is fixed to the lateral side of the knee joint and cannot be reduced actively or passively; reducible (habitual) dislocations generally involve a reduction of the patella when the knee is extended and a lateral dislocation of the patella when flexed.

2.2.1.4 Treatment Principle

1. Early detection and treatment, perform operation of patellar reduction early, without knee deformity (flexion, varus, valgus), lateral patellar retinaculum release, medial retinaculum tightening, lateral half patellar ligament displaces inward.
2. For children with severe knee flexion deformity and untreated or failed treatment, lateral retinaculum release, iliotibial band release, biceps femoris tendon lengthening, combined with Ilizarov technique, were performed to correct knee flexion deformity slowly in order to avoid neurovascular injury caused by one-time correction of knee flexion deformity. Restore the lower limb to hold the gravity line, restore the ability to walk upright, and do not have to force patella reduction.

2.2.2 Congenital Patellar Dislocation with Delayed Treatment Leads to Lower Limb Flexion Deformity

2.2.2.1 Etiology

Congenital dislocation of the patella, not detected early, or the treatment fails, and the deformity of lower limbs gradually leads to the loss of upright walking function.

2.2.2.2 Clinical Manifestation

Knee flexion contracture, genu valgum, external rotation of tibia, and deformity of foot can be shown. Patients with

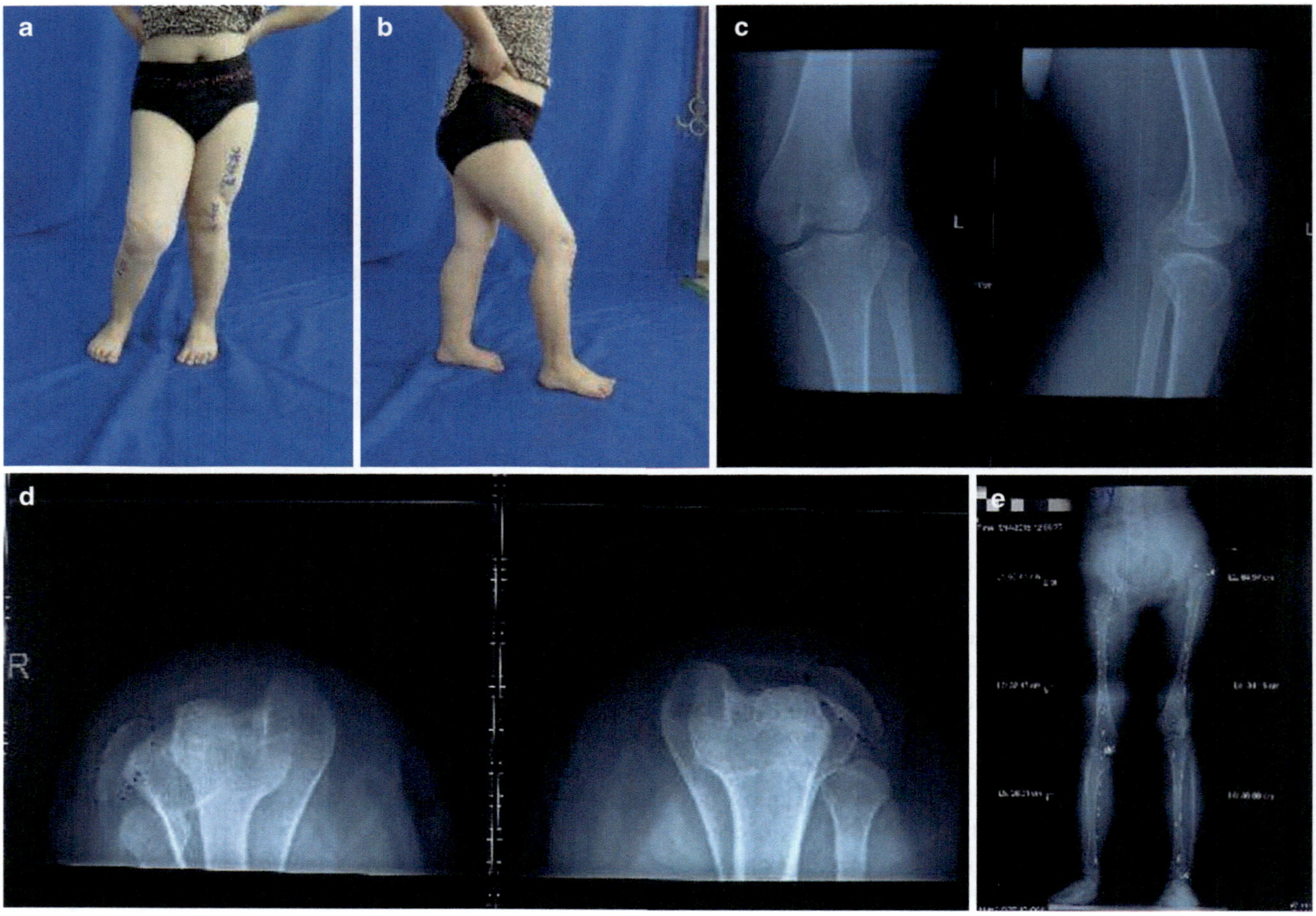

Fig. 2.10 A 21-year-old female presented with bilateral congenital external dislocation of patella. (**a**) Frontal view in standing position; (**b**) lateral view in standing position; (**c**) anteroposterior X-ray film of both knees; (**d**) axial view of both patellae showing the patella lateral to the femoral condyle; (**e**) full-length radiograph of both lower limbs in standing position

unilateral onset may have developmental limb shortening on the affected side and unequal length of both lower limbs. In the case of bilateral onset, the child gradually develops knee flexion contracture deformity during development and gradually loses the ability to walk upright and can only squat, kneel, or rely on a wheelchair instead of walking (Fig. 2.11).

2.2.2.3 Treatment Principle

Release the contracture of soft tissue, correct the deformity of knee flexion, restore the gravity line of lower limbs, restore the ability of upright walking, and do not have to force patella reduction.

2.2.3 Congenital Genu Recurvatum

Congenital genu recurvatum (congenital genu recurvatum), also known as congenital genu hyperextension, is often complicated by other diseases, such as polyarticular contracture, spina bifida, developmental dysplasia of that hip, and foot deformities. Mother of some cases have a history of breech delivery. Pathological changes depend on the severity of the deformity. Cases of knee dislocation often have fibrosis of the quadriceps muscle, absence of the suprapatellar bursa, and valgus deformity of the knee. Other malformations need to be identified during the assessment. Check for acetabular dysplasia or dislocation.

2.2.3.1 Etiology

The cause is unknown or related to the poor position of the fetus in the uterus.

2.2.3.2 Clinical Manifestation

The main manifestation is hyperextension of the knee joint, accompanied by dislocation of the knee joint in severe cases (Fig. 2.12). It may be combined with other deformities, such as talipes equinovarus, dislocation of hip joint, genu varum, and genu valgum.

2.2.3.3 Classification

According to the severity of the deformity and whether it is accompanied by dislocation, it can be divided into three

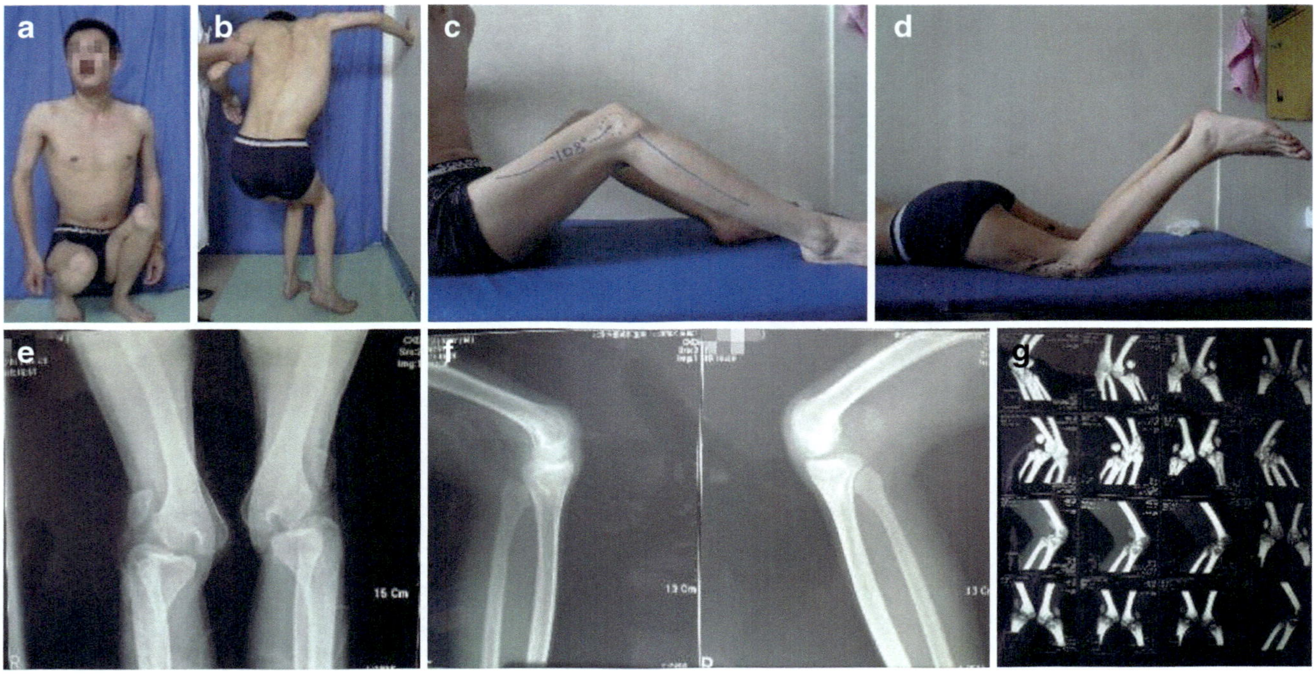

Fig. 2.11 Male, 26 years old, bilateral knee flexion deformity caused by bilateral congenital dislocation of patella. (**a**) Squatting gait before treatment; (**b**) could not stand; (**c**) bilateral knee flexion deformity; (**d**) prone position, bilateral knee flexion deformity; (**e**) anteroposterior X-ray of both knees, bilateral patella located on the lateral side of femoral condyle; (**f**) lateral X-ray of both knees; (**g**) three-dimensional CT reconstruction of bilateral knee joint

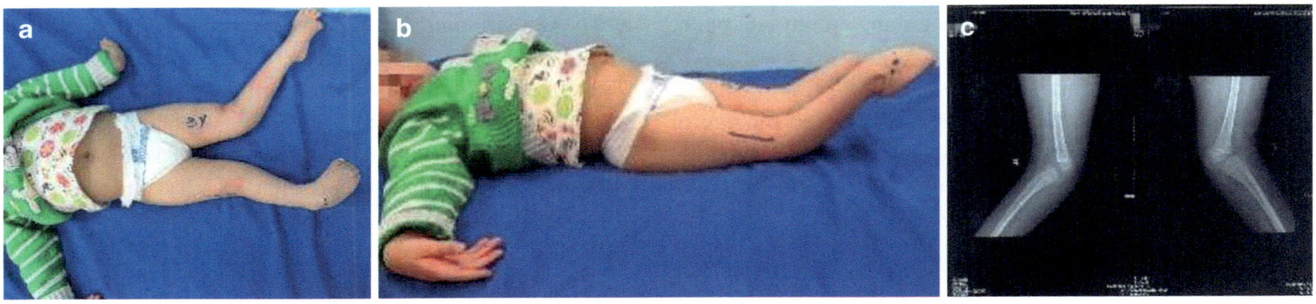

Fig. 2.12 Bilateral congenital genu recurvatum deformity: (**a**) Appearance in supine position, (**b**) bilateral genu stiffness in recurvatum deformity position; (**c**) lateral radiograph of the knee, showing anterior dislocation of the tibial plateau

types: Type I, knee hyperextension without dislocation; type II, knee hyperextension with subluxation; type III, hyperextension of the knee with complete dislocation of the knee.

2.2.3.4 Treatment Principle

Neonates with knee hyperextension can be treated with plaster, to increase the flexion of the knee joint, and children aged 6–18 months can be treated with surgical release of the joint capsule and quadriceps tendon. In children and adults over 3 years of age, knee flexion was increased by surgical release of soft tissue and slow distraction with the Ilizarov technique.

2.2.4 Tibial Varus

2.2.4.1 Etiology

Tibial varus, also known as Blount disease, cause is unknown. Possible due to infection, trauma, ischemic necrosis, or recessive rickets. It may also be a combination of genetic and developmental factors. Premature walking and obesity are associated with the disease.

2.2.4.2 Clinical Manifestation

Tibial varus, internal rotation, and genu recurvatum (Fig. 2.13). Typical radiographic findings include a short,

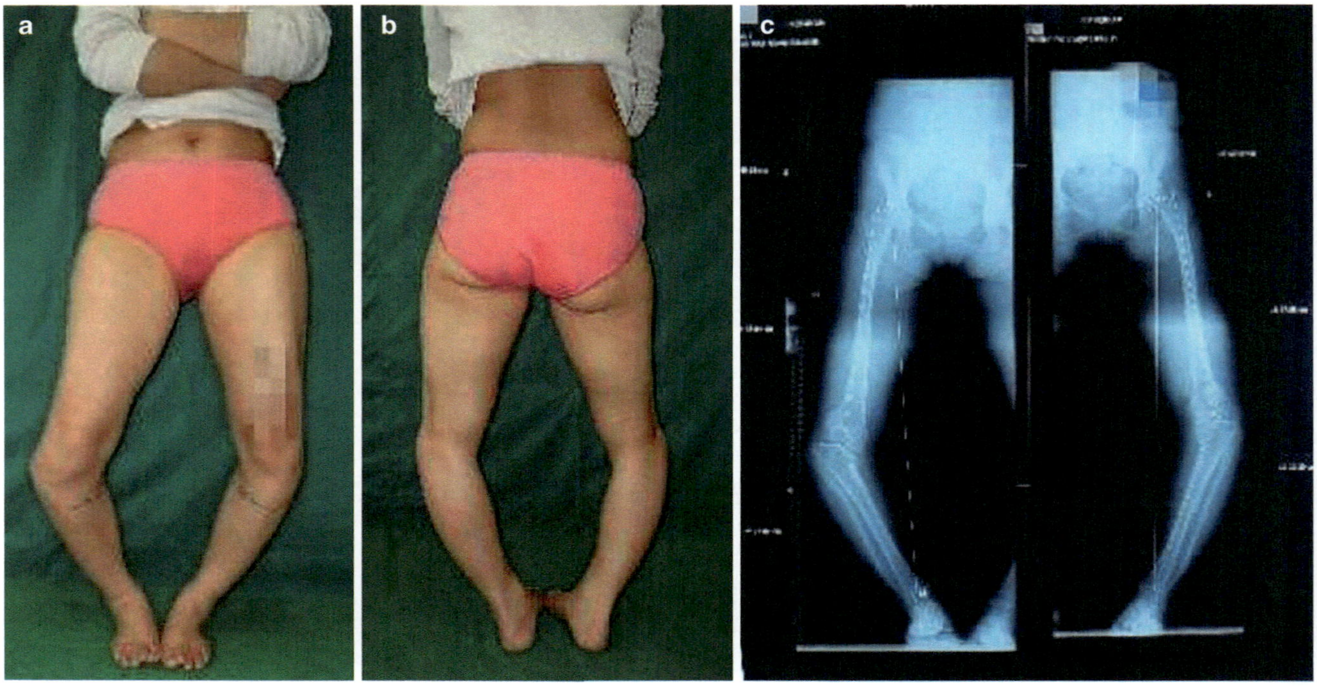

Fig. 2.13 Bilateral tibial varus (Blount's disease) in adulthood. (**a**) Frontal view in standing position; (**b**) dorsal view in standing position; (**c**) full-length X-ray film of both lower limbs in standing position

thin, and wedge-shaped medial half of the proximal tibial epiphysis, and an irregular, inward sloping epiphyseal plate.

2.2.4.3 Classification

Blount classifies it into two types according to the age of onset: 1. Infant type, onset before 8 years old; 2. Juvenile type, onset after 8 years of age and before skeletal maturity.

2.2.4.4 Treatment Principle

Proximal tibiofibular osteotomy corrects varus and internal rotation deformity while lengthening and restoring limb length.

2.2.5 Congenital Tibial Curvature

Congenital tibial curvature is also known as congenital angular deformity of lower leg.

2.2.5.1 Etiology

The cause of the disease is unknown.

2.2.5.2 Clinical Manifestation

The lower leg is bent and may be accompanied by shortening. Radiographs show that the tibia and fibula are angulated anteriorly or posteriorly, or bent laterally, with increased bone density at the bend (Fig. 2.14 and 2.15).

2.2.5.3 Classification

1. The tibia is angulated posteriorly, which can be gradually improved with age and can also be accompanied by unequal length of both lower limbs.
2. The tibia is angulated anteriorly, which is potentially associated with congenital pseudarthrosis of the tibia, especially with narrow medullary cavity, and should be vigilant for the development of pseudarthrosis of the tibia.

2.2.5.4 Treatment Principle

1. If the tibia is angulated posteriorly, the development of the disease should be closely observed. Generally, it will improve by itself. If the length of both lower limbs is unequal, limb lengthening can be performed after maturity.
2. If the tibia is angulated anteriorly, it should be fixed with a brace to prevent fracture until the bone is mature.

2.2.6 Congenital Fibular Hemimelia

2.2.6.1 Etiology

The cause of the disease is unknown.

2.2.6.2 Clinical Manifestation

The clinical manifestations of congenital fibular hemimelia depend on the specific type and associated deformities.

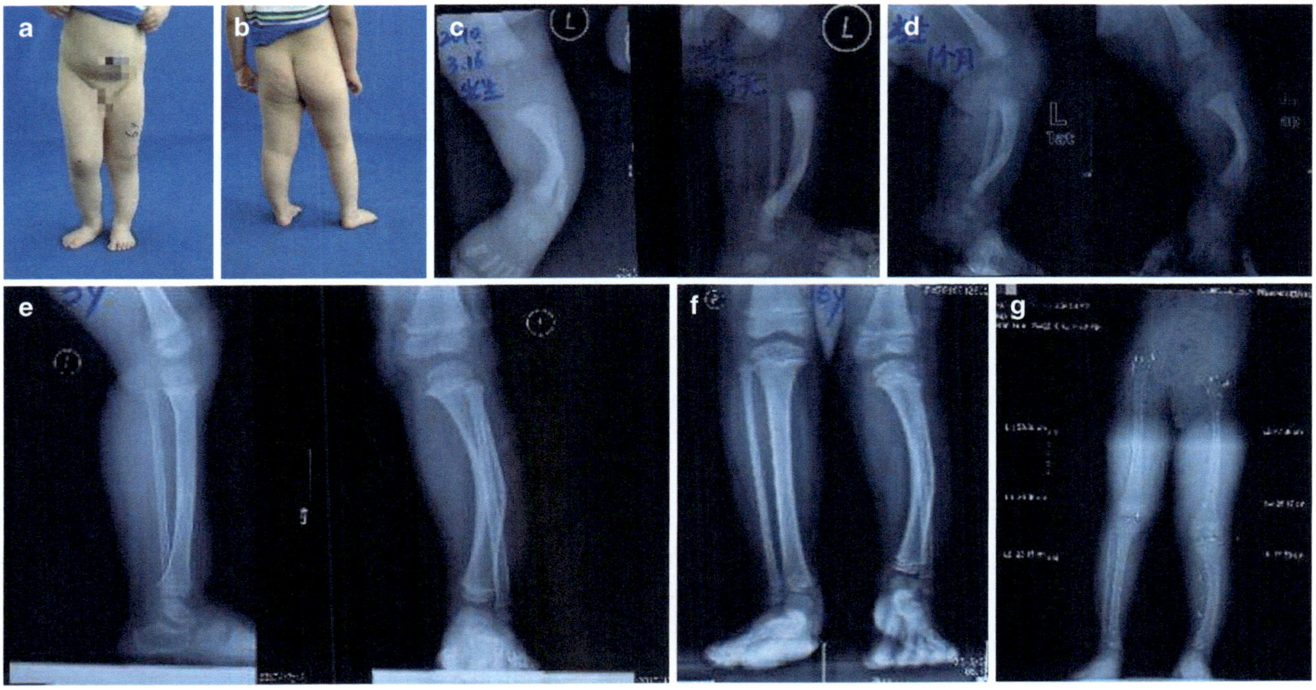

Fig. 2.14 Congenital left tibial curvature. (**a**) Frontal view in standing position; (**b**) dorsal view in standing position; (**c**) X-ray film of left leg at birth; (**d**) X-ray film of left leg at 1 month after birth; (**e**) X-ray of left leg at 3 years old; (**f**) X-ray of left calf at 6 years old; (**g**) Full-length standing radiographs of both lower extremities at 6 years of age

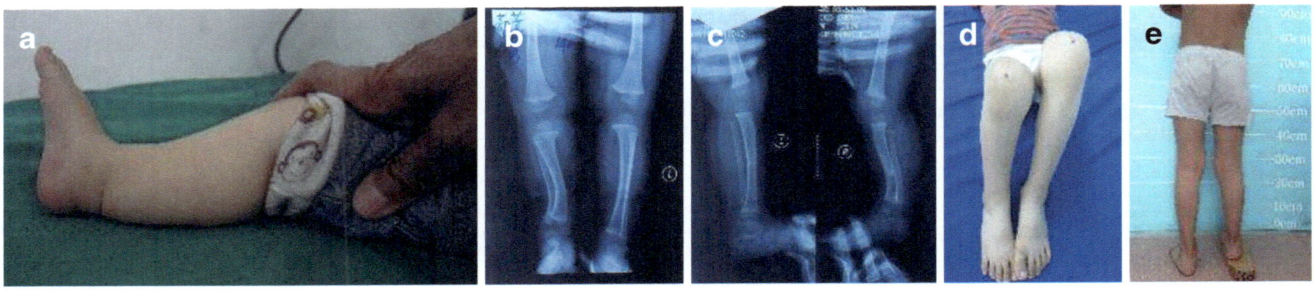

Fig. 2.15 Congenital posteromedial curvature of right tibia. (**a**) Appearance of the left lower leg at 14 months of age; (**b**) anteroposterior radiographs of both lower legs at 14 months of age; (**c**) lateral radiographs of both lower legs at 14 months; (**d**) appearance of both legs at 6 years of age; at the age of 6 years, (**e**) the natural correction of standing tibial bending deformity resulted in lower limb shortening

Usually, congenital absence of fibula is manifested by unequal length of both lower limbs, talipes valgus, absence of 2–3 metatarsal rows on the lateral side of the foot, and stiffness of the hind foot (Fig. 2.16). Although talipes valgus is the most common deformity, talipes equinovarus can also occur (Fig. 2.17). Sometimes it can also be accompanied by knee flexion contracture, femoral shortening, knee and ankle instability.

2.2.6.3 Classification and X-Ray Characteristics

Achterman and Kalamchi classified fibular hemimelia as type 1 (hypoplasia of fibula) and type 2 (complete absence of fibula), and type 1 was subdivided into type 1A and type 1B (Fig. 2.18). In type 1A, the proximal fibular epiphysis is lower than the proximal tibial epiphysis, and the distal fibular epiphysis is proximal to the trochlea of the talus. The fibular defect of type 1B is more serious, the length of the defect is more than 30–50%, and there is no end support for the ankle joint. In type 2 deformity, the fibula is completely absent, and there is a tense fibrous band or fibrocartilaginous tissue band in the absence of the fibula, which starts from the lateral edge of the proximal tibia and extends downward to the posterolateral side of the calcaneus, like a bowstring, causing foot drop, eversion, and forward bending of the tibia into an arch.

The main X-ray features of type 1A were that the affected tibia was shorter than the healthy side, arched to the anterolateral side, the inferior joint of tibia was

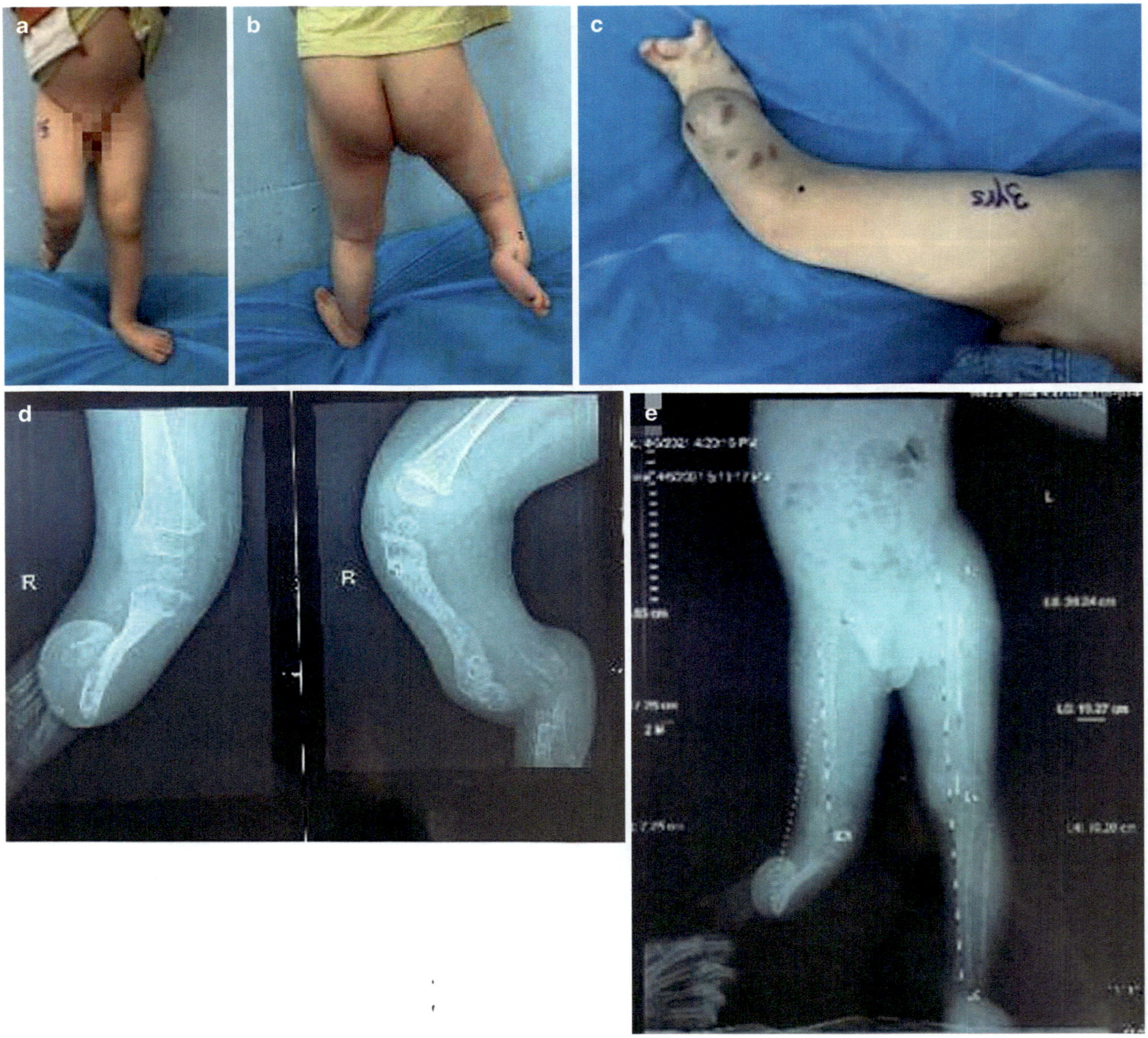

Fig. 2.16 A 3-year-old male presented with congenital right fibular hemimelia. (**a**) Standing position and positive view; (**b**) back view in standing position; (**c**) appearance of right lower limb; (**d**) X-ray film of right leg and foot; E. full-length radiographs of both lower limbs

inclined to the lateral side, the fibula was shorter and the proximal fibular head (or epiphysis) was distally oriented, the tip of the lateral malleolus (or distal fibular epiphysis) was retracted above the level of the inferior articular surface of the tibia, and the ankle-foot joint was valgus. The structure of 1–2 lateral metatarsal row joints is dysplastic or absent (Fig. 2.19); in Type 1B, except for the shortening and bending of the tibia, the defect of the fibula is more serious, the length of the defect is more than 30–50%, there is no terminal support for the ankle joint, the ankle and foot joints are everted, and the structure of 1–2 lateral metatarsal row joints is absent (Fig. 2.20). In type 2 malformation, fibula is completely absent, the tibia bends heavily anterolateral, mostly located in the middle and lower 1/3 of the tibia, the ankle and foot bone joints are equinus valgus deformity, a few are equinus varus deformity, the calcaneus and talus are congenitally fused, and 1–2 lateral metatarsal bone joint structures are absent (Fig. 2.21).

2.2.6.4 Treatment Principle

The goal of treatment of congenital absence of fibula is to restore the length of the affected limb and correct the deformity of the foot and ankle, so as to improve the walking function of patients and reduce dysfunction and claudication.

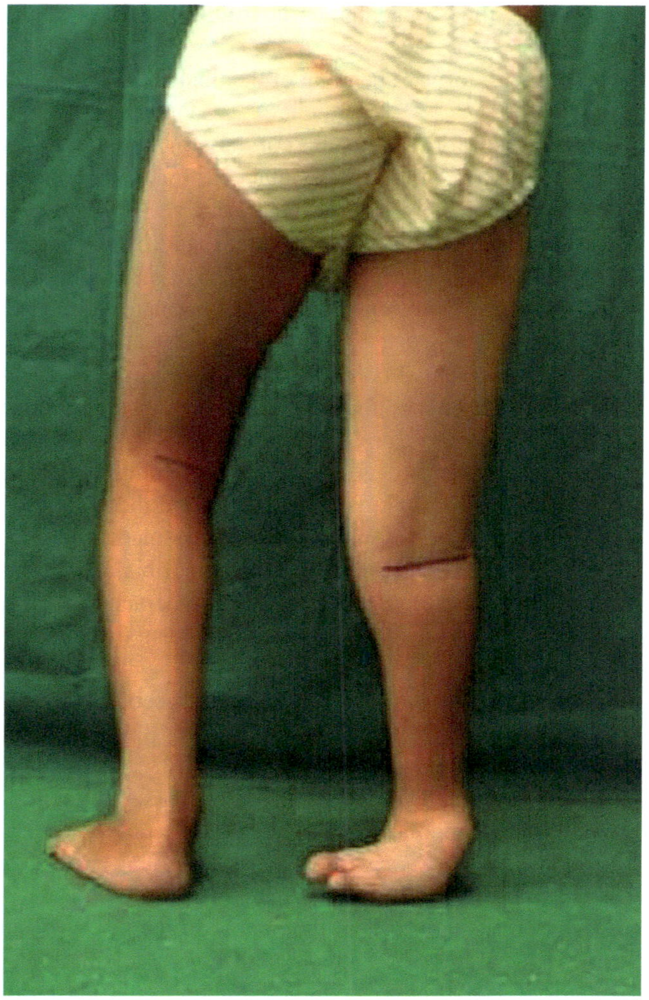

Fig. 2.17 Congenital absence of fibula on the right side, unequal length of both lower limbs, absence of right clubfoot and the fourth and fifth toes

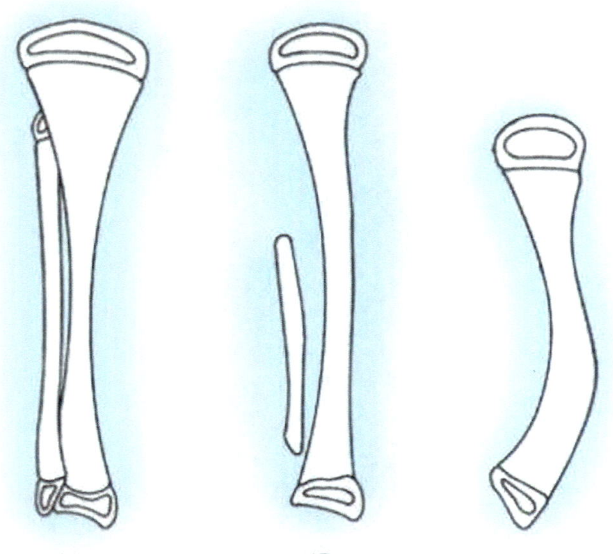

Fig. 2.18 Achterman and Kalamchi fibular hemimelia. Type 1A: The proximal fibular epiphysis is distally biased and the distal fibular epiphysis is proximally biased compared to normal; Type 1B: more severe fibular shortening and loss of lateral ankle support; Type 2: complete absence of fibula with curvature and shortening of tibia

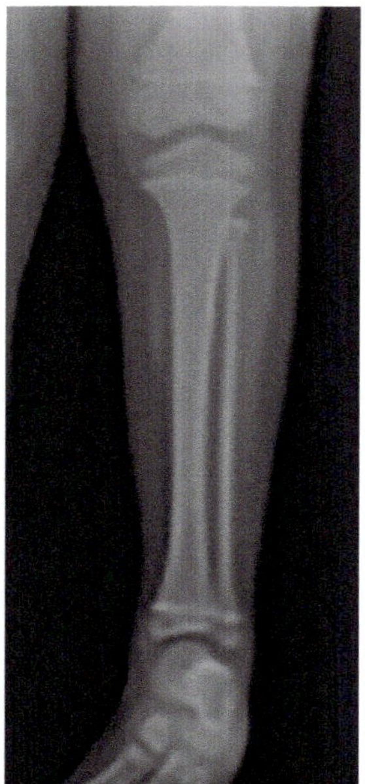

Fig. 2.19 Type 1A absence of fibula: The affected tibia is shorter than the healthy side, the inferior tibial joint is inclined laterally, the fibula is shortened and the proximal fibular head is distally biased, the tip of the lateral malleolus is retracted to the level above the inferior tibial articular surface, and the two lateral metatarsal joint structures are absent

2.2.7 Congenital Pseudarthrosis of the Tibia

2.2.7.1 Etiology

The etiology of congenital pseudarthrosis of the tibia is unknown, and the incidence of congenital pseudarthrosis of the tibia is significantly increased in patients with neurofibromatosis. Neurofibromatosis has a distinct genetic predisposition.

2.2.7.2 Classification and Clinical Manifestation

The most common manifestations are the formation of pseudarthrosis in the middle and lower part of the tibia or tibia and fibula, severe shortening of the leg, forward angular deformity of the pseudarthrosis, and dorsal extension of the ankle joint (Fig. 2.22). Some patients were accompanied by skin cafe au lait spots scattered all over the body (Fig. 2.23). In patients with neurofibromatosis, scattered cutaneous neurofibroma masses of varying sizes can be seen (Fig. 2.24).

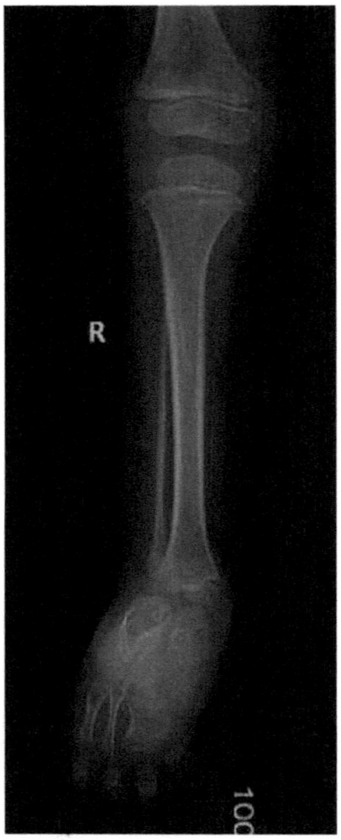

Fig. 2.20 Absence of fibula in Type 1B, shortening of the affected tibia compared with the healthy side, absence of more than 30% of the proximal fibula, upward displacement of the lateral malleolus, congenital fusion deformity of calcaneus and talus, and absence of joint structures of two lateral metatarsal bones

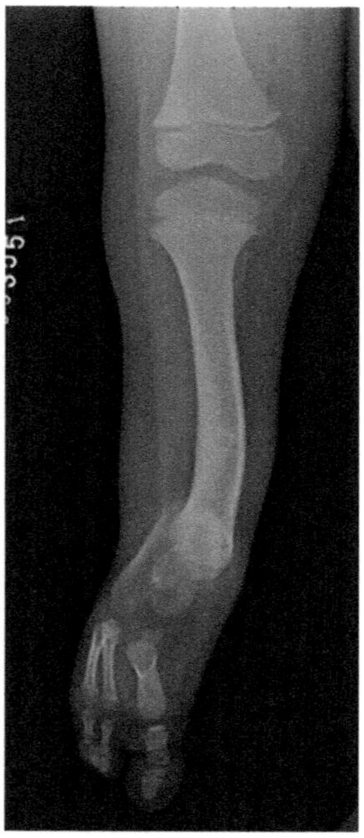

Fig. 2.21 Type 2 fibula is completely absent. The affected tibia was shorter than the healthy side, the middle and lower part of the tibia was arched anterolateral, the ankle and foot joints were everted, the calcaneus and talus were congenitally fused, and the two lateral metatarsal joints were absent

Boyd classified congenital pseudarthrosis of the tibia into six types:

Type I, with forward bending of the tibia and tibial defect at birth;

Type II, with forward bending of the tibia with hourglass narrowing at birth, often with spontaneous fractures or minor post-traumatic fractures before the age of 2 years. That is, the high-risk tibia, the tibia becomes thin, round, and sclerotic, and the medullary cavity disappears. This type is the most common, usually associated with neurofibromatosis, and has a poor prognosis.

Type III, congenital bone cyst at the junction of the middle and lower 1/3 of the tibia, and the forward bending of the tibia may occur before or after the fracture.

Type IV, pseudarthrosis occurs in the sclerotic segment of the typical site, the tibia is not thinned, and the medullary cavity is partially or completely lost. An "incomplete" or "stress" fracture occurs in the cortex of the tibia and gradually extends into sclerotic bone. If a complete fracture occurs, it will not heal and the fracture line will widen, thus becoming a pseudarthrosis.

Type V, pseudarthrosis of the tibia is accompanied by fibular dysplasia, and pseudarthrosis of the tibia or fibular pseudarthrosis, or both, may occur.

Type VI is a rare type caused by intraosseous neurofibroma or schwannoma.

2.2.7.3 Treatment Principle

Congenital pseudarthrosis of the tibia is difficult to treat and has a high failure rate. Patients with high-risk tibia under 5 years old should be treated conservatively, and plaster or brace can be used to prevent fracture. For those who already have pseudarthrosis of the tibia, prevent the aggravation of the deformity of the pseudarthrosis. Patients older than 5 years old can be treated with pseudarthrosis resection, tibial intramedullary nail through ankle joint fixation to maintain the tibial axis, autogenous iliac bone graft, and Ilizarov technique, which can significantly improve the cure rate of one operation.

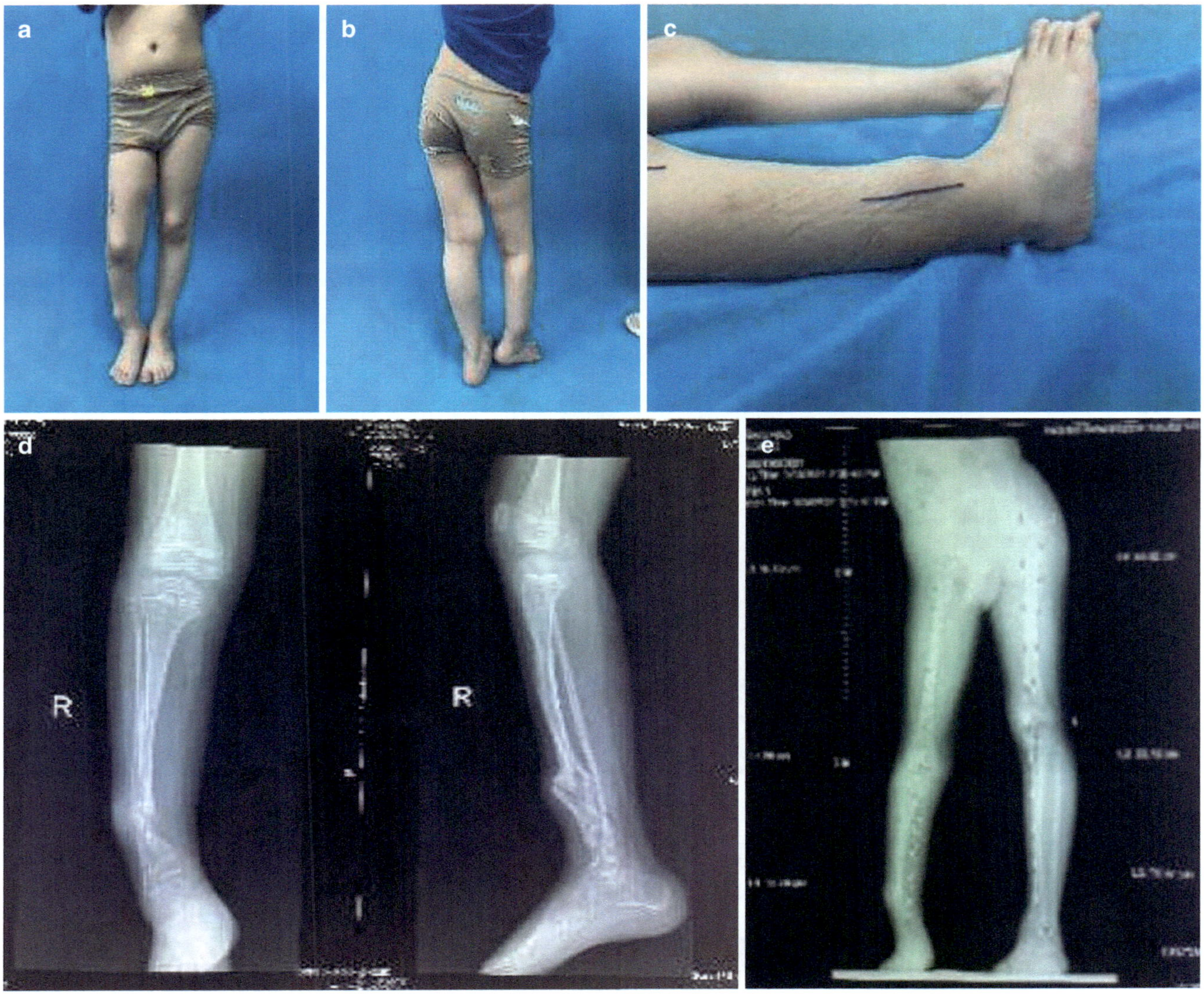

Fig. 2.22 A 7-year-old male presented with congenital pseudarthrosis of the right tibia. (**a**) Frontal view in standing position; (**b**) dorsal view in standing position; (**c**) appearance of right lower leg; (**d**) X-ray film of right lower leg; E. full-length radiograph of both lower limbs in standing position

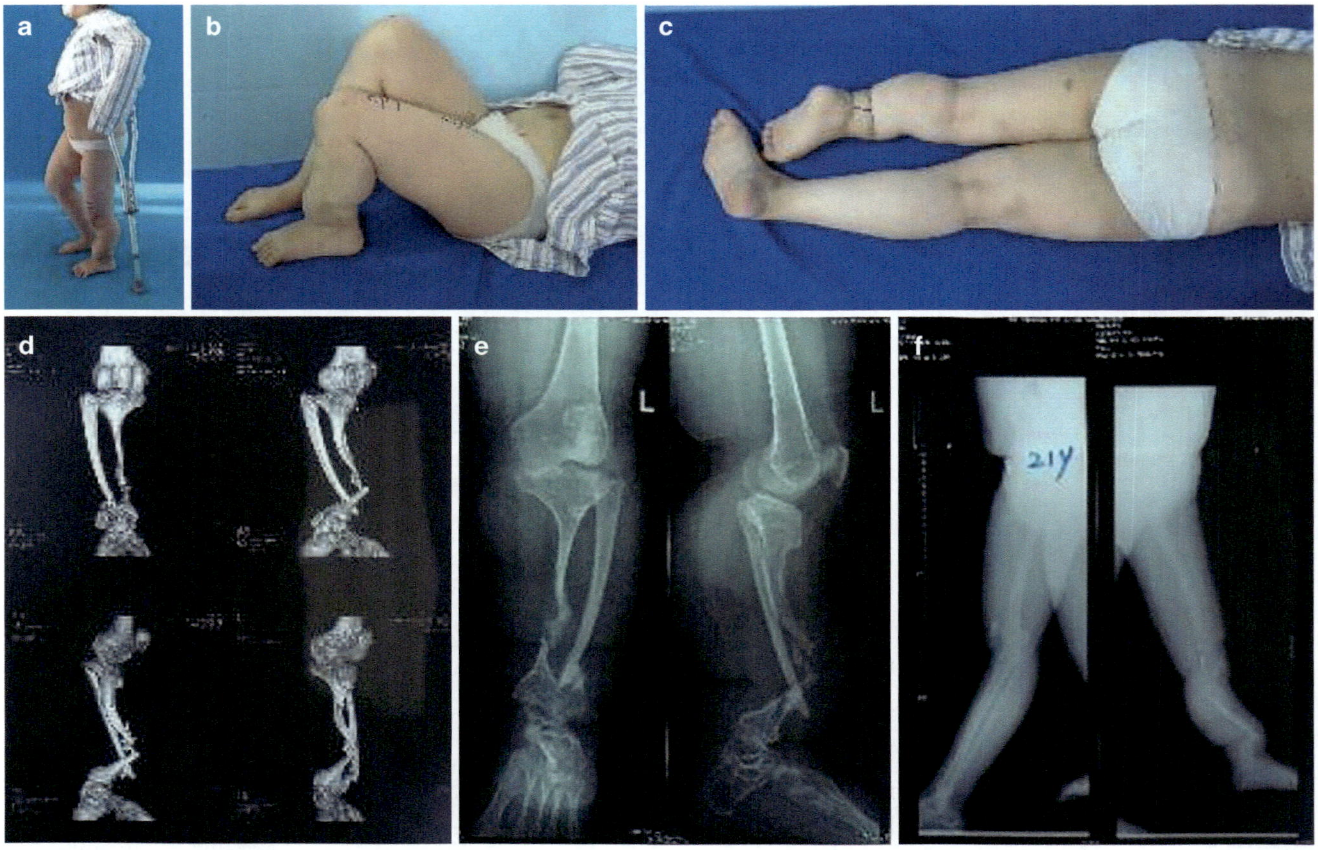

Fig. 2.23 A 21-year-old female presented with congenital pseudarthrosis of the left tibia. (**a**) Lateral view of standing position, severe shortening of the left leg, angulation of the middle and lower 1/3; (**b**) lateral view of the left lower limb; (**c**) dorsal view of both lower limbs, multiple scattered skin cafe au lait spots on the back and leg skin; (**d**) three-dimensional CT reconstruction of the left tibia and fibula; (**e**) X-ray film of left leg; (**f**) lateral full-length radiograph of both lower extremities

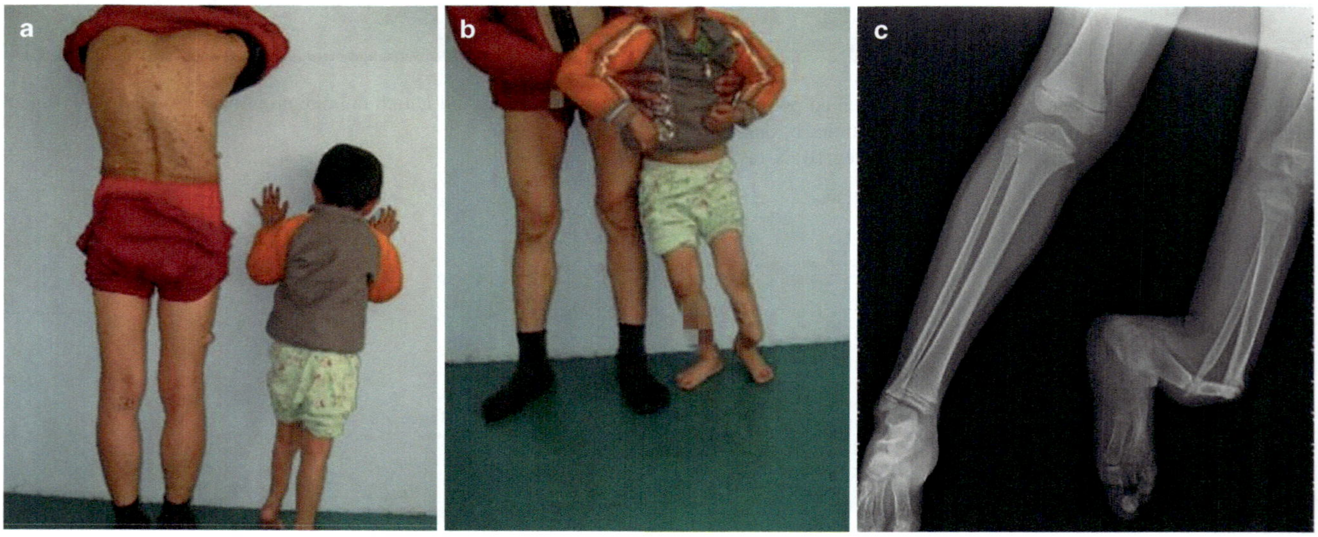

Fig. 2.24 Neurofibromatosis. The picture shows a father and son. The son has a pseudarthrosis of the left tibia. (**a**) From the back of the standing position, the father had multiple skin masses on his back and both lower limbs, and the son's left leg was shortened and deformed; (**b**) from the front, the son's left leg was shortened, and the lower pseudarthrosis was angulated forward, so he could not stand with weight; (**c**) X-ray film of both legs of son, right tibiofibular pseudarthrosis

2.3 The Ankle and Foot

Sihe Qin, Shaofeng Jiao, and Lei Shi

2.3.1 Congenital Equinovarus

The congenital equinovarus is the seventh of all the birth defects, accounting for 85% of the foot deformities. The incidence is about 1‰, and the ratio of male to female is about (2–2.5):1. Prevalence rates varied by ethnicity, ranging from 0.39‰ for Chinese, 7‰ for Hawaiians and Maori, about 1.2‰ for Caucasians, and about 6.8‰ for Polynesians.

2.3.1.1 Etiology

The exact cause of this disease is still unknown, but it is believed to be related to neuromuscular lesions, skeletal dysplasia, soft tissue contracture, vascular abnormalities, and genetic factors. Most scholars support the theory of neuromuscular disease and the theory of skeletal abnormalities. Studies have found that the peroneal muscle strength of congenital talipes equinovarus patients is generally weakened, and the muscle contracture in the inner and rear of the calf causes muscle imbalance. The contracture of bone, joint, and soft tissue is secondary to the adaptive change of muscle imbalance, and the change of muscle strength is based on nerve abnormalities. Some scholars used immunohistochemical method to study the calcaneal bone of congenital talipes equinovarus and found that the chondrocytes were small, undifferentiated, and immature, the extracellular mucin was reduced, the growth cartilage was similar to articular cartilage, and the abnormal ossification of ossification center could lead to skeletal deformity. Recent studies suggest that congenital talipes equinovarus is related to Hox gene, DTDST gene, PITX1 gene, COL9A1 gene, and other mutations.

2.3.1.2 Clinical Manifestation

The initial manifestations of congenital talipes equinovarus are soft tissue abnormalities, contracture of medial foot muscles, increased tension, thickening and shortening of joint capsule, ligaments, and aponeurosis (Fig. 2.25). With the increase in age, the deformity is becoming more and more serious. Achilles tendon, tibialis posterior tendon, flexor digitorum longus tendon, flexor hallux longus tendon, and plantar aponeurosis are extremely contracted, with strong elastic resistance. The lateral soft tissue and muscle of the foot are continuously pulled and extended. The abduction function of

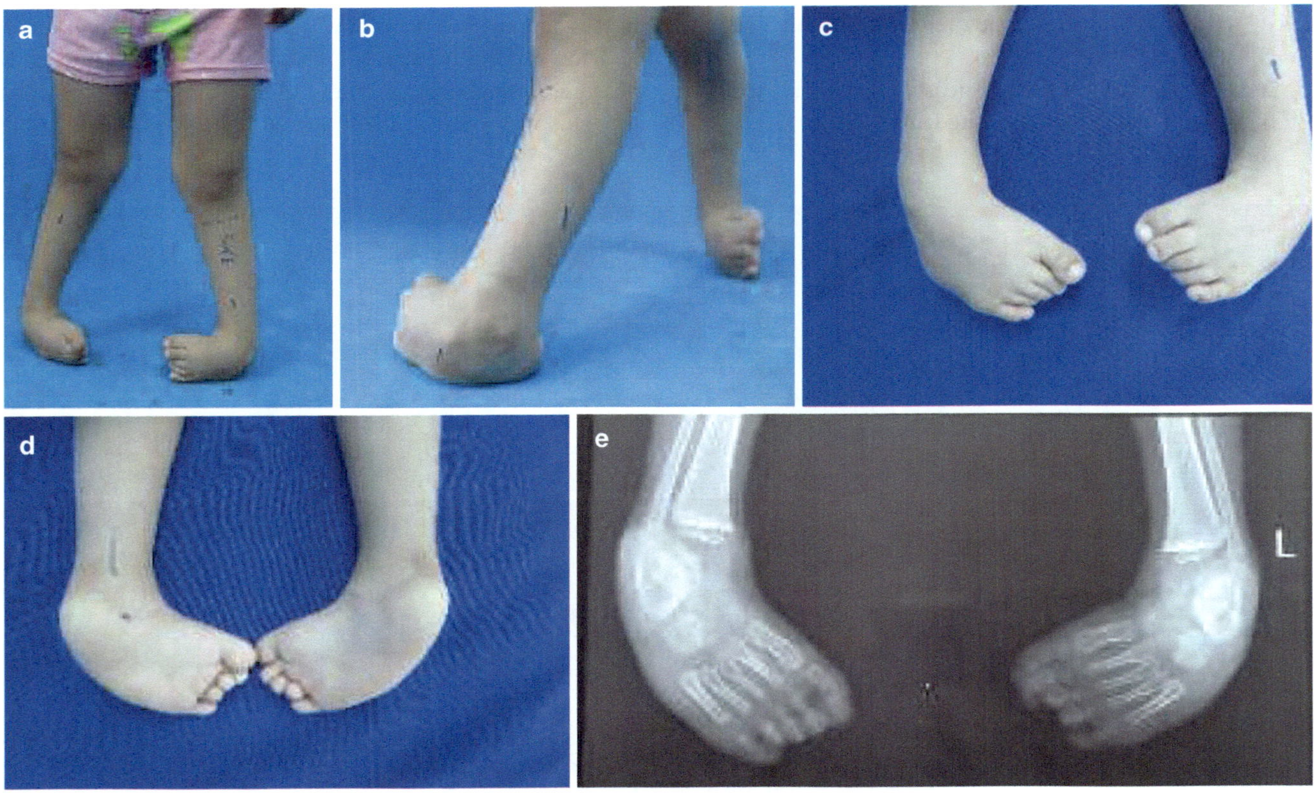

Fig. 2.25 Female, 3 years old, bilateral congenital clubfoot. (**a**) Front view in standing position, with the lateral edge of both feet touching the ground; (**b**) side view in standing position; (**c**) front view of both feet; (**d**) back view of both feet; (**e**) anteroposterior X-ray film of both feet and ankles

the foot is basically lost, but the muscle nerve function is intact and the myoelectric excitability still exists. If the deformity is corrected at this time, the muscle function can be restored, on the contrary, skeletal deformity can gradually occur, the tarsal bone is arranged abnormally, the calcaneus is in a varus position, the tibia is biased to the medial and metatarsal sides, in severe cases, its articular surface is on the lateral side of the ankle cave, the scaphoid bone becomes smaller and moves inward and rotates, so that the medial and lower parts of the talus head form pseudarthrosis, and the talus head forms subcutaneous protuberance. The cuboid bone is abnormally large and connected with the medial non-articular surface of the distal calcaneus. In addition, the metatarsal bone is deformed and may deviate from the tarsometatarsal joint, or the joint is normal and the metatarsal shaft is adducted.

2.3.1.3 Classification

According to the manipulative reduction of ankle deformity, it can be divided into soft type and rigid type. Soft type ankle and hindfoot intertarsal joints have a greater range of motion, and manipulation can partially correct the deformity. Rigid type ankle and hindfoot intertarsal joints are stiff and cannot be corrected by manipulation.

2.3.1.4 Treatment Principle

1. Infants were treated with Ponseti technique.
2. In childhood, soft tissue release, muscle strength balance.
3. In adolescence, soft tissue release, muscle balance combined with osteotomy or limited arthrodesis.
4. Soft tissue release and muscle strength balance combined with arthrodesis in adulthood. Severe malformations were corrected slowly with the Ilizarov technique.

2.3.2 Congenital Vertical Talus

2.3.2.1 Etiology

The exact cause of this disease is unknown, but many studies have shown that it is related to gene mutation.

2.3.2.2 Clinical Manifestation

Typical congenital vertical talus (CVT) patients are born with obvious rocking chair deformity of both feet, that is, the medial round bulge of the vola, the top of the bulge can touch the talus head, the forefoot is dorsiflexion and abduction, and the calcaneus is equinus deformity caused by Achilles tendon contracture. When standing, the affected foot is obviously everted, with the vola touching the ground, and there is a thick callus in the vola. With the increase in age and weight-bearing, the tarsus of the foot will undergo adaptive changes, that is, severe eversion and external rotation of the forefoot, tension of peroneal tendon and anterior tibial tendon, and obvious limitation of ankle joint and subtalar joint movement, resulting in clumsy gait when walking (Fig. 2.26). The disease has four major features: (1) plantar protrusion; (2) heel is equinus; (3) the foot was severely stiff and deformed, and the deformity was not changed by position, weight-bearing, or massage; (4) X-ray film of the foot showed that the talus was vertical, the scaphoid bone was located at the

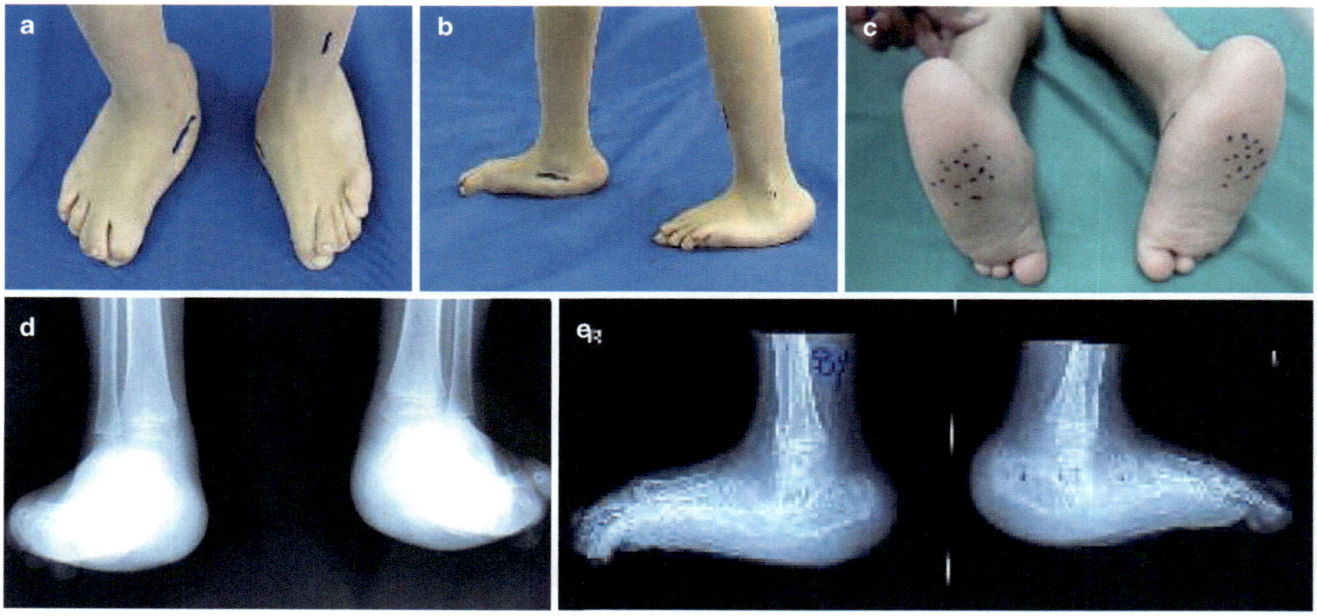

Fig. 2.26 Male, 8 years old, bilateral congenital vertical talus. (**a**) Bipedal appearance in standing position; (**b**) bipedal lateral view; (**c**) bipedal plantar view; (**d**) bipedal anteroposterior X-ray film; (**e**) lateral X-ray film of both feet

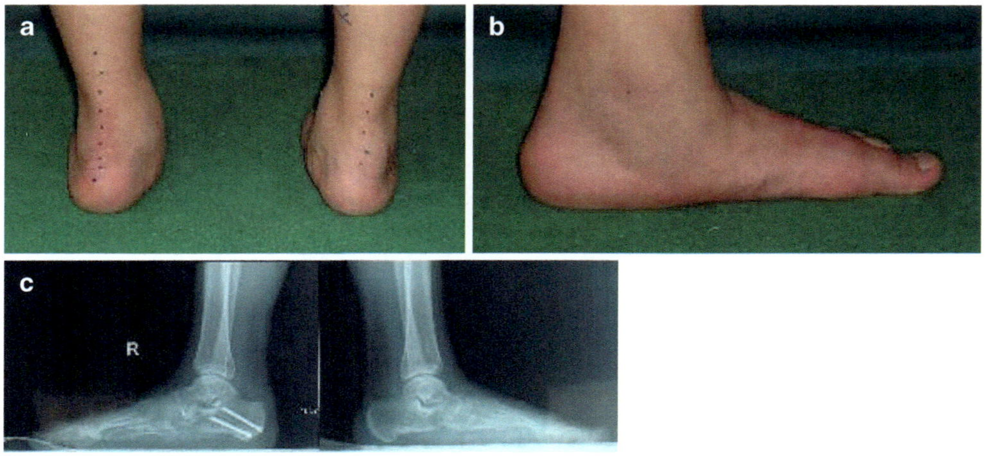

Fig. 2.27 Male, 22 years old, bilateral congenital flatfoot: (**a**) Valgus of the left hindfoot, valgus of the right foot was corrected by surgery; (**b**) from the side view, the medial longitudinal arch of the foot disappeared; (**c**) lateral X-ray film of both feet with weight-bearing showed that the angle of the longitudinal arch of the foot increased

dorsal side of the talus head, the long axis of the first metatarsal bone was located at the dorsal side of the long axis of the talus, and the calcaneus was plantar flexion.

2.3.2.3 Treatment Principle

Restore the anatomical relationship of talus, navicular bone, calcaneus, and cuboid bone, as well as rebuild the weight-bearing capacity and restore the plantar function of the foot.

2.3.3 Congenital Flatfoot

2.3.3.1 Etiology

Flatfoot can be congenital or acquired. Children's arches often begin to form at the age of 4–6. Most children and adolescents have congenital flat feet, and adult flat feet can be the continuation of children's flat feet. Symptomatic secondary flatfoot in adults is called adult acquired flatfoot.

2.3.3.2 Clinical Manifestation

The main manifestation of this disease is the collapse of the foot arch (Fig. 2.27). Arch collapse can cause the following structural changes in the foot: (1) Achilles tendon contracture: After the collapse of the medial longitudinal arch, the moment of the Achilles tendon acting on the ankle joint decreases, and the traction force of the Achilles tendon cannot be effectively transmitted to the forefoot through the hard arch. (2) Midfoot relaxation: So that the middle tarsal joint cannot be locked. (3) Forefoot displacement: The forefoot and midfoot were displaced dorsally and laterally around the talus. (4) The stress of the posterior tibial tendon was increased, and the strain of the posterior tibial tendon was easy to occur. In severe cases, the medial ligament of the foot may be injured. (5) Pronation of subtalar joint and eversion of calcaneus. (6) The instability of the midfoot makes the subtalar joint and talonavicular joint in an abnormal position for a long time. Over time, these joints degenerate and become fixed deformities.

2.3.3.3 Treatment Principle

1. Asymptomatic flatfoot cannot be treated.
2. If pain and other symptoms occur, conservative treatment should be carried out first, such as arch pad, heel lifting training, etc.
3. When conservative treatment is ineffective and pain and other symptoms affect walking function, surgical treatment is used.

2.3.4 Congenital Metatarsal Adduction

2.3.4.1 Etiology

Congenital metatarsal adduction is caused by genetic factors, and some scholars believe that it is caused by the malposition of the fetus in the uterus. Malformations are not necessarily evident at birth. It may exist independently or occur simultaneously with congenital talipes equinovarus.

2.3.4.2 Clinical Manifestation

It is characterized by varus and adduction of the forefoot at the joint of the lower foot (Fig. 2.28). The appearance of the foot is arched outward. The deformity is completely in front of the ankle joint, while the heel and leg still maintain a normal relationship.

2.3.4.3 Classification

Bleck classified the metatarsal adduction into three types: mild, moderate, and severe. Light: The forefoot may be abducted to the midline of the foot and may exceed the midline; Medium: The forefoot has some flexibility, allowing the forefoot to be abducted to the midline but usually not beyond the midline; Severe: The forefoot is stiff, unable to abduct, with transverse skin folds visible at the inner edge of the foot, or the web space between the toe and the second toe is enlarged (Fig. 2.29).

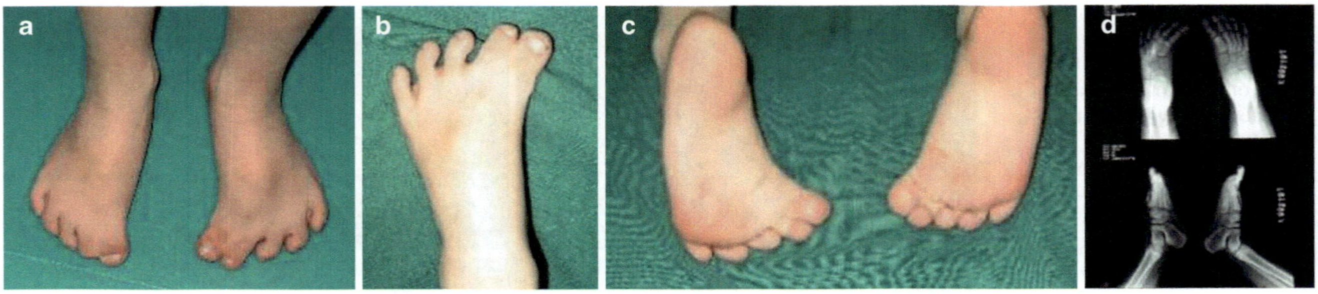

Fig. 2.28 Congenital adduction of bilateral metatarsals with syndactyly 1 and 2. (**a**) Front view of both feet; (**b**) appearance of left foot; (**c**) appearance of both feet; (**d**) anteroposterior and lateral radiographs of both feet

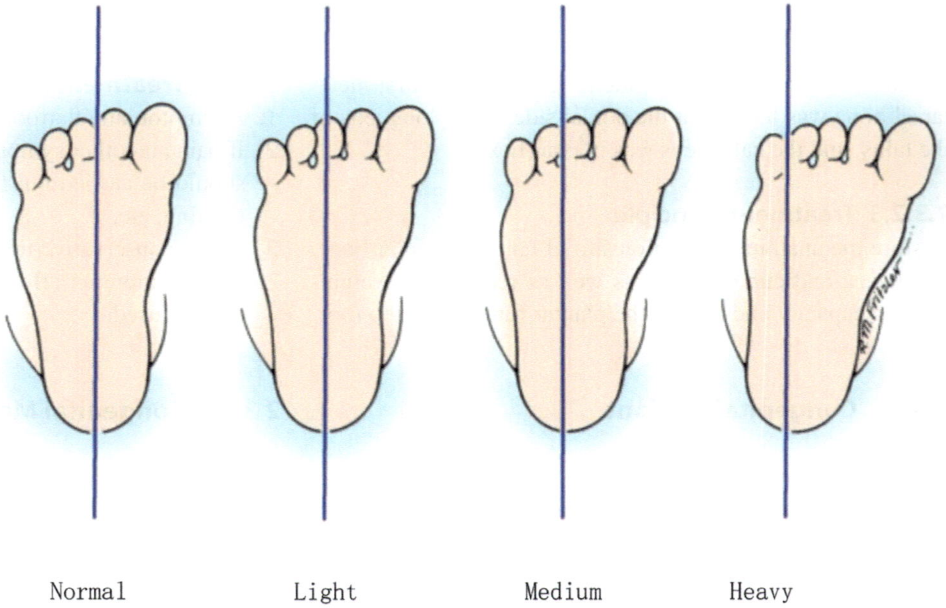

Fig. 2.29 Classification of congenital bilateral metatarsal adduction (Modified from Bleck EE: Metatarsus adductus: classification and relationship to outcomes of treatment. J Pediatr Orthop 3:2–9, 1983)

2.3.4.4 Treatment Principle

Mild cases generally do not require treatment and may heal spontaneously with growth and development. Moderate and severe infants were corrected by manipulation and series of plaster. After the age of 12, those who could not be corrected by conservative treatment were corrected by surgery.

2.3.5 Congenital Hallux Varus

2.3.5.1 Etiology

The cause of the disease is unknown.

2.3.5.2 Clinical Manifestation

Congenital hallux varus is characterized by a deformity of the great toe of the foot that angles medially at the metatarsophalangeal joint (Fig. 2.30), which is usually unilateral and associated with one or more of the following deformities: (1) The first metatarsal is short and thick. (2) Redundant bones or toes. (3) One or more of the four lateral metatarsals had varus deformity. (4) There is a hard fibrous band extending from the medial side of the great toe to the base of the first metatarsal bone. X-ray film showed that the first metatarsophalangeal joint was angulated medially, the angle between the first and second metatarsals was enlarged, and the first metatarsal bone was short and thick.

2.3.5.3 Treatment Principle

Excess bone or toes were removed to correct hallux deformities.

2.3.6 Congenital Brachymetatarsia

Congenital brachymetatarsia, also known as short metatarsus, commonly known as brachydactyly, is a relatively rare deformity of metatarsal development. The disease has an obvious genetic tendency, with an incidence of 0.02–0.05%. Metatarsal shortness has an ugly appearance, which often causes patients to bear a serious psychological burden.

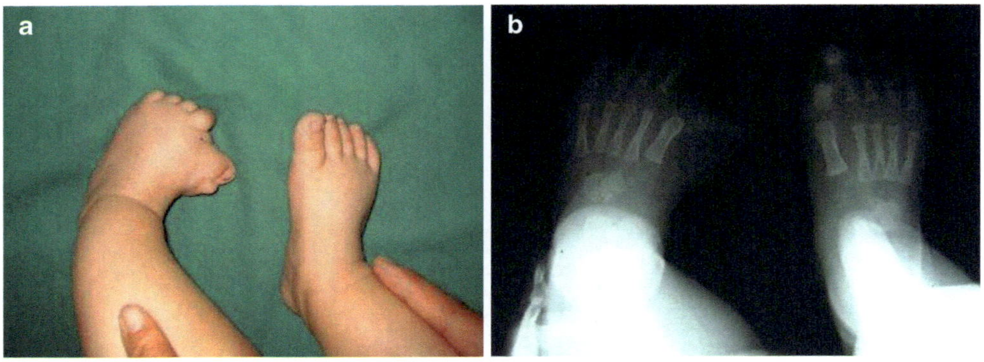

Fig. 2.30 Congenital hallux varus deformity of left side, male, 6 months old. (**a**) Appearance of both feet, left adduction deformity of the thumb; (**b**) anteroposterior X-ray film of both feet

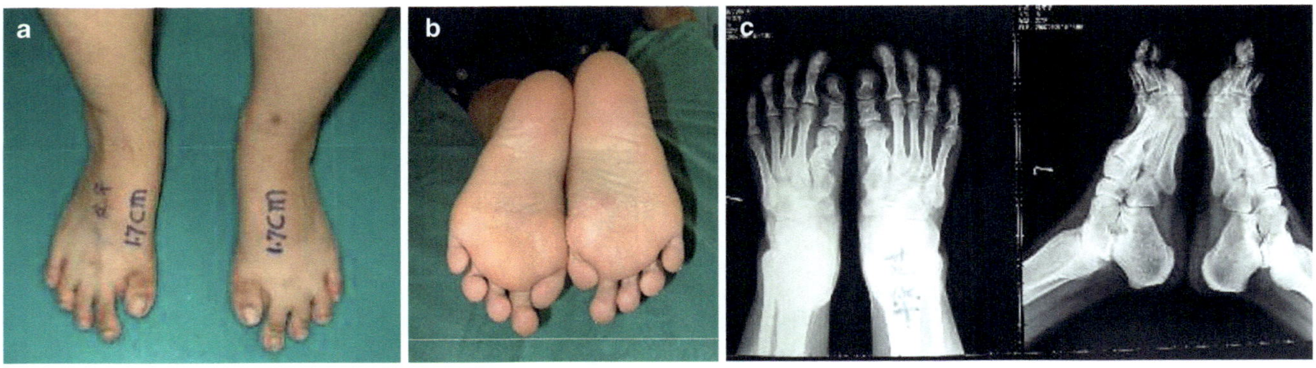

Fig. 2.31 Female, 22 years old, bilateral congenital shortening of the first metatarsal: (**a**) Appearance of both feet; (**b**) plantar view of appearance; (**c**) anteroposterior and lateral radiographs of both feet

Shortened metatarsal bones can also affect the overall weight-bearing function of the affected foot. It is easy to form painful callosity locally, and the upturned short toes hinder the wearing of shoes.

2.3.6.1 Etiology

The cause is unknown.

2.3.6.2 Clinical Manifestation

It is common in the first and fourth metatarsals (Figs. 2.31, 2.32 and 2.33). It is manifested as shortening of the hallux and (or) the fourth metatarsal, metatarsalgia when walking, plantar callus, and upward tilting of the short toe that affects shoe wearing; Normal toes will deviate from their original position to fill the gap caused by the short adjacent metatarsal bones, resulting in valgus deformity of the toes located on the medial side of the short toes and varus deformity of the toes located on the lateral side of the short toes. The X-ray film showed that the first metatarsal and/or the fourth metatarsal was obviously shortened and could not maintain the normal arc line of the metatarsals.

2.3.6.3 Treatment Principle

If toe shortening affects the appearance of the foot or causes foot pain, shortened metatarsal lengthening is feasible to restore the length of the metatarsal bone.

2.3.7 Congenital Macrodactylia

2.3.7.1 Etiology

Congenital macrodactylia is a rare congenital malformation characterized by hypertrophy of the foot and toes, including hypertrophy of skin, subcutaneous tissue, tendons, blood vessels, nerves, bones, and nails. At present, the etiology is not clear, chromosome examination has not found abnormalities, most of them occur in one side, male slightly more than female, non-familial. Brooks and Lehman proposed in 1924 that macrodactyly is associated with generalized neurofibromatosis.

2.3.7.2 Clinical Manifestation

Macrodactyly usually occurs after birth, and one or more toes are significantly enlarged, while the other toes are normal. Not all toes are involved (Fig. 2.34). Macrodactyly grows up gradually with the growth and development of children, and its speed is different. Macrodactyly is primarily an accumulation of fibrofatty tissue, often on the lateral or plantar surface, with asymmetric hypertrophy leading to scoliosis. Although acromegaly is a prominent feature, forefoot involvement is often overlooked, making the inclusion of metatarsals in the disease controversial. However, the most recent views still tend to include metatarsal hypertrophy in

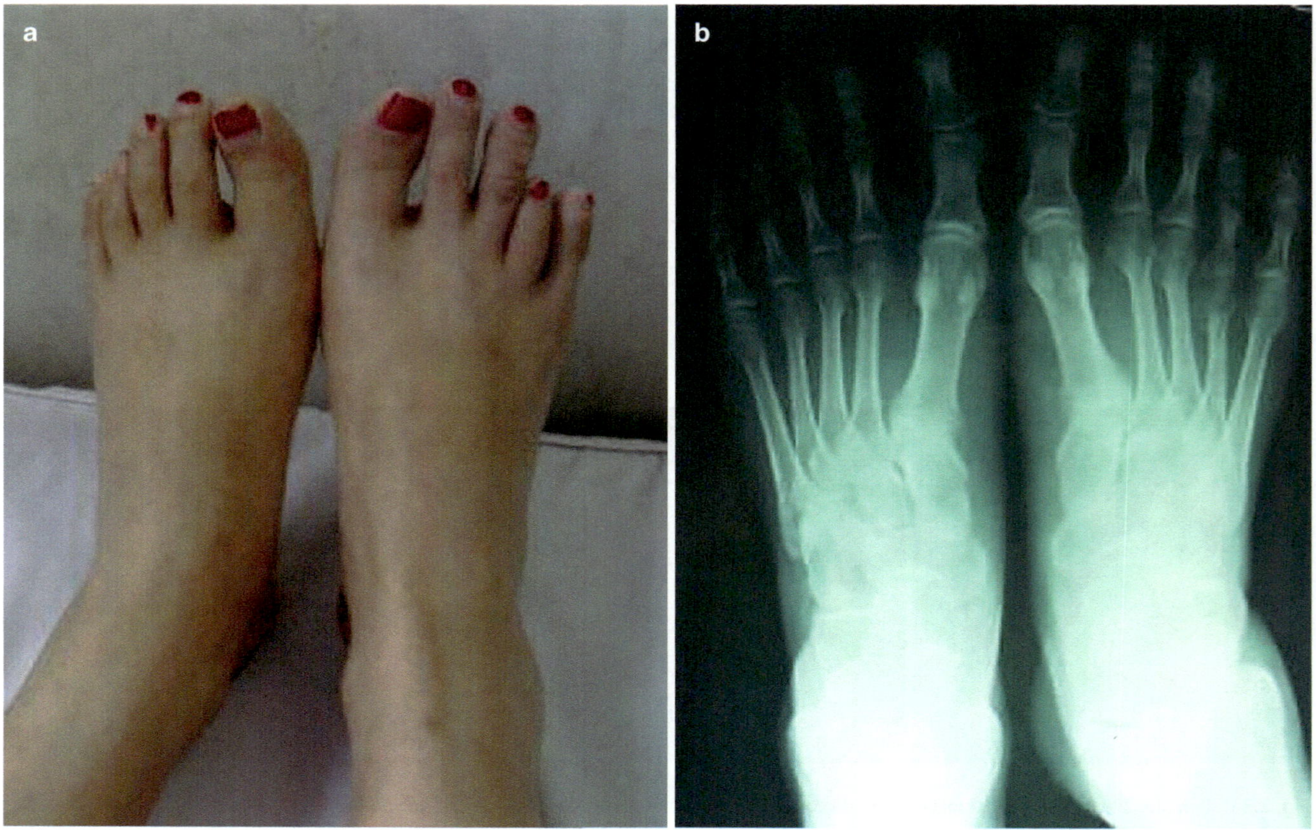

Fig. 2.32 Congenital fourth metatarsal shortening

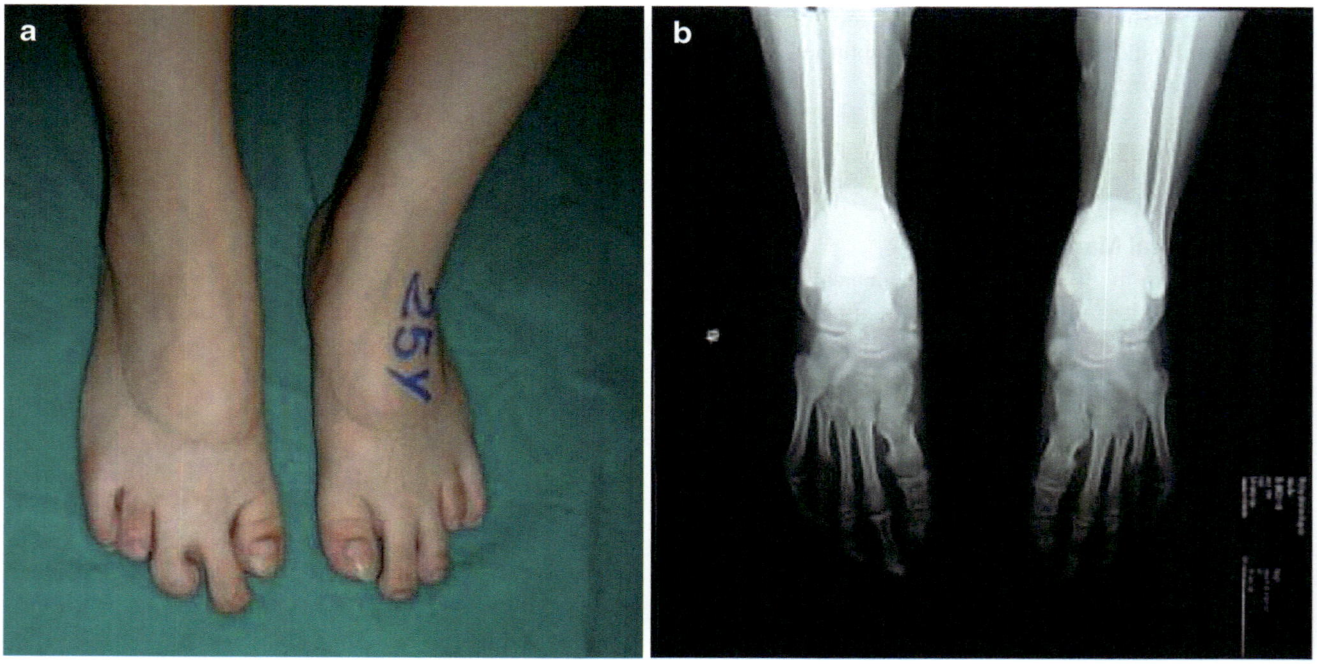

Fig. 2.33 Congenital shortening of the first and fourth metatarsals

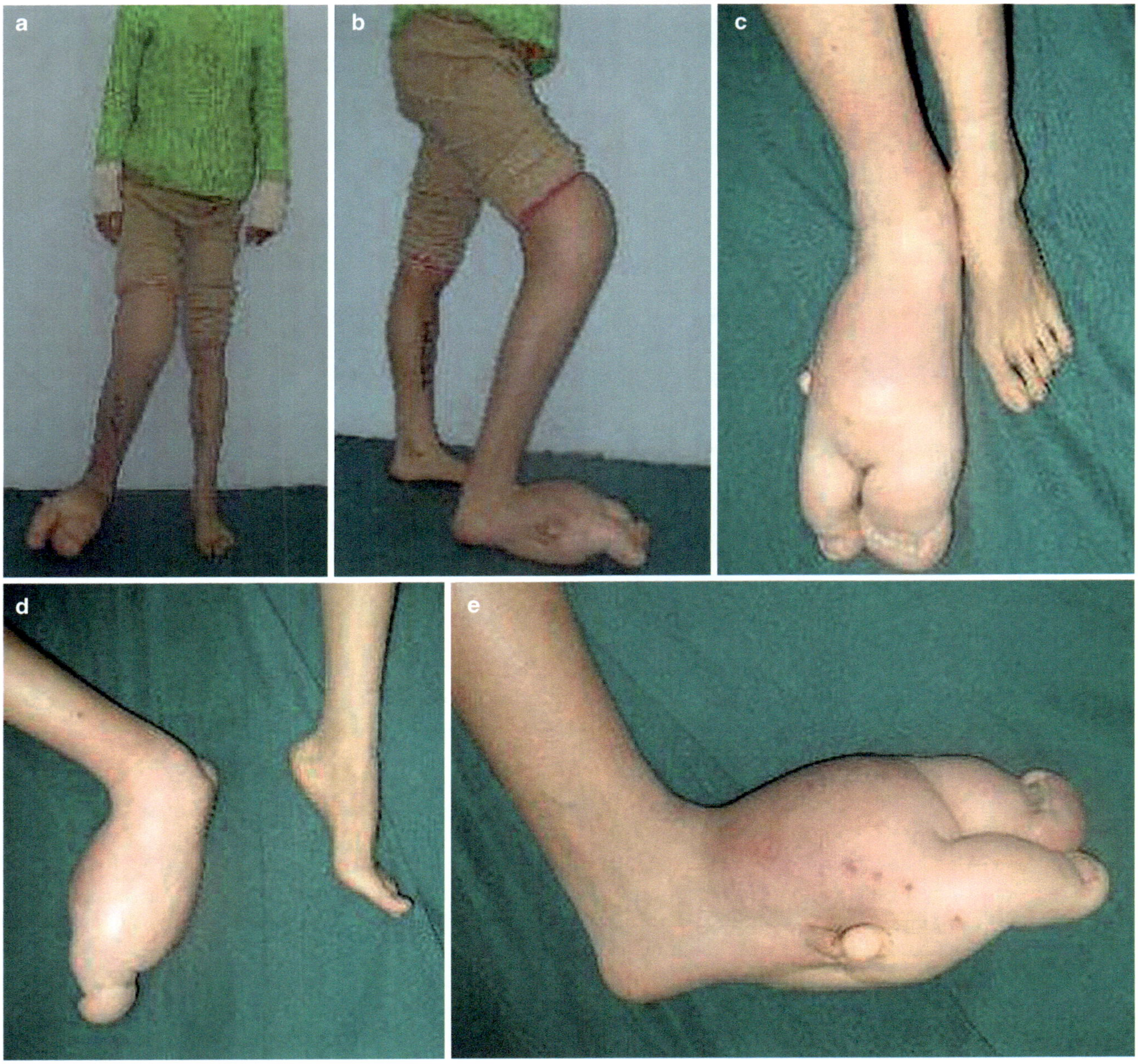

Fig. 2.34 A 14-year-old female with congenital macrodactylia on the right side. (**a**) Standing appearance; (**b**) lateral view of right lower limb; (**c**) appearance of both feet; (**d**) medial view of both feet; (**e**) lateral surface of right foot

macrodactyly. The fibrous tissue extends from the toe to the forefoot, resulting in lateral expansion. Soft tissue hypertrophy on the dorsum of the foot is rare, and more hypertrophy occurs on the plantar surface. X-ray showed that the length and width of the affected phalanges were increased, and the metatarsals of some patients were also enlarged to varying degrees.

2.3.7.3 Classification

Flatt divided the disease into four types according to the pathology: type I-lipofibromatosis, type II-neurofibromatosis, type III-hyperostosis, and type IV-mixed.

2.3.7.4 Treatment Principle

The purpose of treatment is to make the foot convenient to wear shoes through orthopedics, cut the foot to fit the shoes, and try to preserve the function of the foot.

2.3.8 Congenital Polydactyly

2.3.8.1 Etiology

The etiology of hyperdactyly is unknown, and 30–39% of cases are inherited in families. This suggests that polydac-

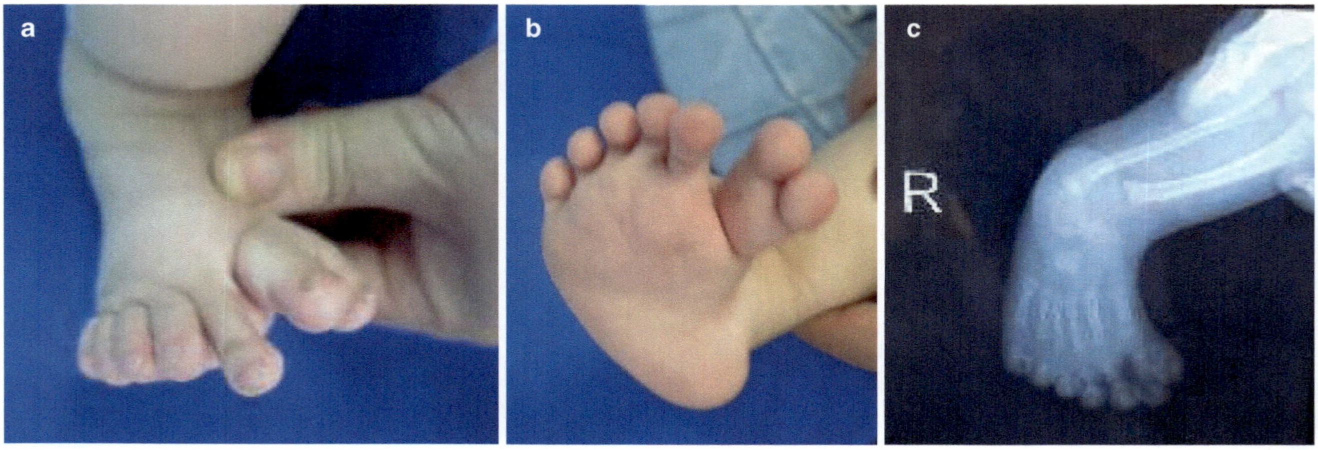

Fig. 2.35 A 2-year-old boy with congenital right polydactyly. (**a**) Appearance of the right foot, with one excrescent toe on the medial and one excrescent toe on the lateral side; (**b**) appearance of the right sole; (**c**) X-ray film of right foot

tyly may be an autosomal dominant disorder, the incidence of which is influenced by differences in gene expression diversity and penetrance.

2.3.8.2 Clinical Manifestation

One or more supernumerary toes are found at birth. The supernumerary toes may be located on the medial side of the toe, the lateral side of the little toe, or the middle toe. Most of them are accompanied by corresponding increased metatarsals (Fig. 2.35).

2.3.8.3 Classification

Temtamy and McKusick classified polydactyly into three types according to the anatomical location of the vegetated toes: preaxial (toe side), central, and postaxial (little toe side). Postaxial type is the most common polydactyly, accounting for about 77–87% of the total. The preaxial type accounts for about 8–15%; The central type is about 6%.

2.3.8.4 Treatment Principle

The main purpose of surgical correction of polydactyly is to correct the shape of the foot as much as possible without affecting walking and standing. Excision of the supernumerary toe and reconstruction of the shape and function of the foot are the main treatment methods.

2.3.9 Congenital Absence of Digits or Thumb

2.3.9.1 Etiology

The etiology of congenital absence of digits or thumb is unknown or related to congenital amniotic band or complicated by congenital axial hemimelia (see Sect. 2.5 of this chapter) (Fig. 2.36).

2.3.9.2 Clinical Manifestation

At birth, it is accompanied by partial or complete absence of one or both toes and normal or partial shortening of the metatarsals.

2.3.9.3 Treatment Principle

Correct foot deformity and increase the stability of foot weight-bearing walking.

2.3.10 Congenital Talipes Calcaneus

2.3.10.1 Etiology

Congenital talipes calcaneus, the specific cause is unknown, which may be related to the abnormal position of the fetus in the uterus.

2.3.10.2 Clinical Manifestation

The disease can be unilateral or bilateral. Dorsiflexion deformity of the affected ankle joint can be found immediately after birth. In severe cases, the dorsum of the foot can contact with the skin in front of the tibia. At the same time, plantar flexion of the foot is limited due to soft tissue and skin contracture on the dorsum of the foot. The disease is difficult to treat, the deformity is easy to recur, after learning to walk, only the heel touches the ground to walk, the forefoot cannot touch the ground, the heel is enlarged for a long time, and the length of the foot is shorter than that of the contralateral development. The extensor dorsi muscles of the foot contracted, and the range of motion of the ankle joint was reduced (Fig. 2.37).

2.3.10.3 Treatment Principle

Increase the plantar flexion angle of the ankle joint, restore the plantar line foot, and increase the weight-bearing area of the foot.

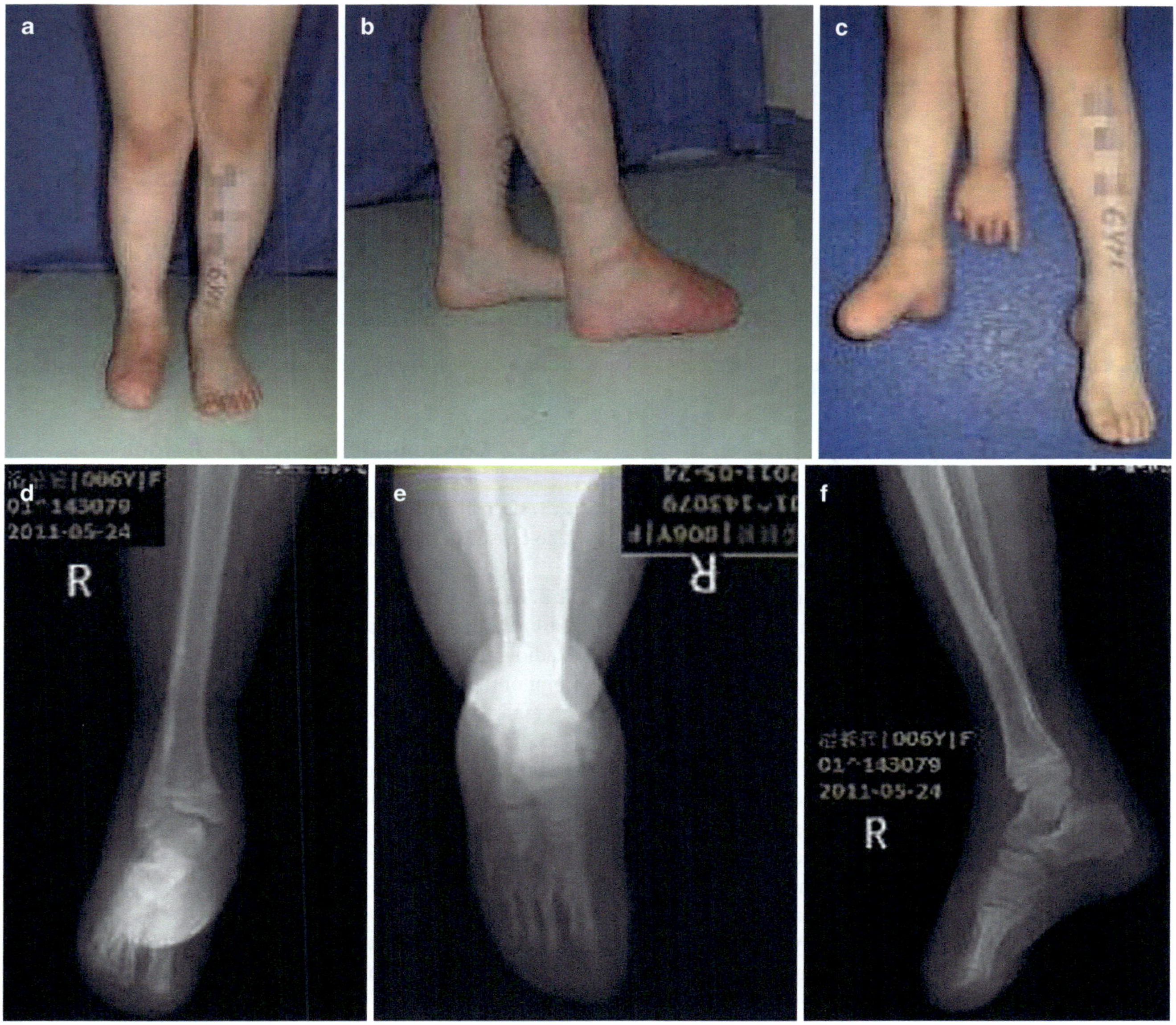

Fig. 2.36 A 6-year-old female with congenital absence of the right toe. (**a**) Appearance of both feet, all five toes of the right foot were absent; (**b**) lateral view of the right foot; (**c**) combined with congenital partial absence of the left toe; (**d**) right ankle anteroposterior X-ray film; (**e**) right foot anteroposterior X-ray film; (**f**) lateral radiograph of right foot

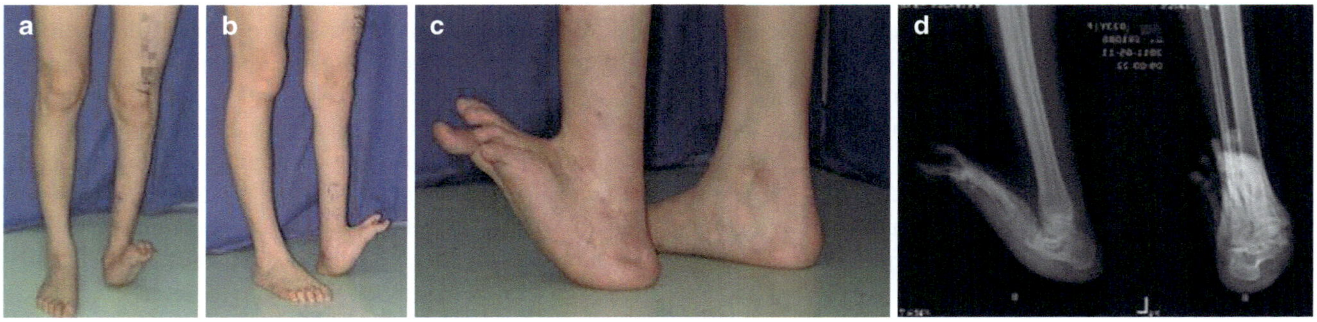

Fig. 2.37 A 24-year-old female presented with congenital talipes calcaneus deformity on the left side. (**a**) Frontal view in standing position; (**b**) medial view; (**c**) lateral view; (**d**) ankle and foot anteroposterior and lateral radiographs

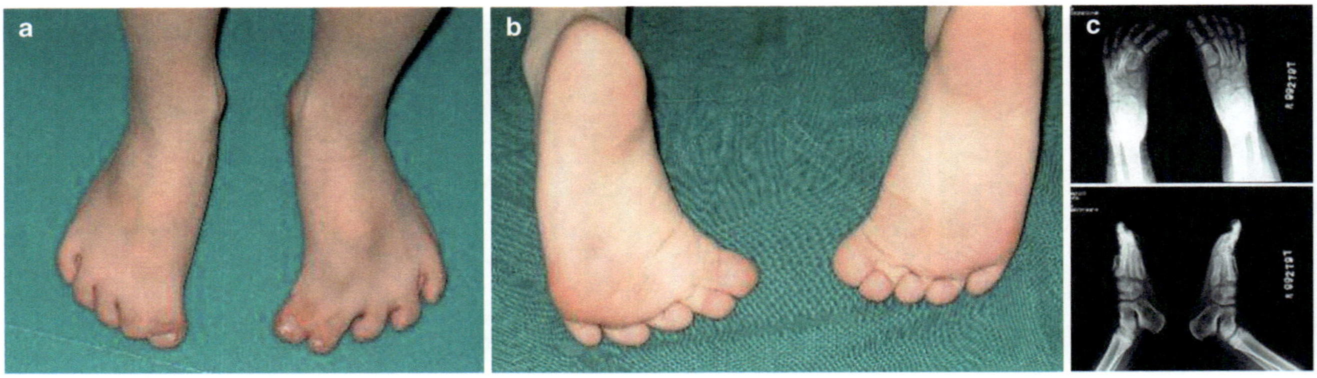

Fig. 2.38 Male, 6 years old, congenital syndactyly. (**a**) Frontal view of both feet, bilateral syndactyly of the first and second toes; (**b**) plantar view; (**c**) anteroposterior and lateral radiographs of both feet

2.3.11 Congenital Syndactyly

2.3.11.1 Etiology

Syndactyly is one of the most common congenital foot deformities, and its incidence in male is three times higher than that in female. The outline of the toes began to appear at the end of the lower limb bud at the fourth week, and the toes differentiated clearly at the eighth week. At 7–8 weeks, syndactyly occurs if the embryo has a local pause in differentiation (caused by a palmar plate differentiation disorder).

2.3.11.2 Clinical Manifestation

The type of expression is varied, often two toes are connected, but also three or four toes are connected. It is characterized by the connection of skin and soft tissue or bony fusion (Fig. 2.38). X-ray examination: The anteroposterior and lateral radiographs of the foot can be used to examine whether there is bony connection between the toes, the relationship with the surrounding tissues, and the development of metatarsal bones, phalanges, and metatarsophalangeal joints.

2.3.11.3 Classification

According to the degree of syndactyly, it can be divided into complete syndactyly and incomplete syndactyly. According to the structure of parallel tissue, it can be divided into simple syndactyly and complex syndactyly. The former only has parallel skin and soft tissue, while the latter has interphalangeal fusion.

2.3.11.4 Treatment Principle

Surgical treatment of toe separation can restore the normal appearance and function of the normal foot as far as possible.

2.3.12 Congenital Absence of Forefoot

2.3.12.1 Etiology

The cause is unknown.

2.3.12.2 Clinical Manifestation

At birth, the child was found with absence of forefoot sole. Radiographs showed absence of the distal tarsometatarsal joint of the foot (Fig. 2.39).

2.3.12.3 Treatment Principle

Before adulthood, walking function can be improved by artificial limbs. In adulthood, the Ilizarov technique can be used to lengthen the tarsus of the foot to increase the length and weight-bearing area of the foot.

2.3.13 Congenital Longitudinal Defect of Forefoot

2.3.13.1 Etiology

Its etiology is unknown, and it is common in congenital fibular hemimelia.

2.3.13.2 Clinical Manifestation

The foot is short, the forefoot is narrow, the third, fourth, and fifth metatarsals of the foot together with the corresponding third, fourth, and fifth toes are absent (Fig. 2.40), or only the fourth and fifth toes together with the corresponding metatarsals are absent, which may be combined with syndactyly, accompanied by shortening of the lower leg and unequal length of both lower limbs. X-ray examination showed that the tarsals of the foot were fused and part of the metatarsals together with the corresponding toes was absent.

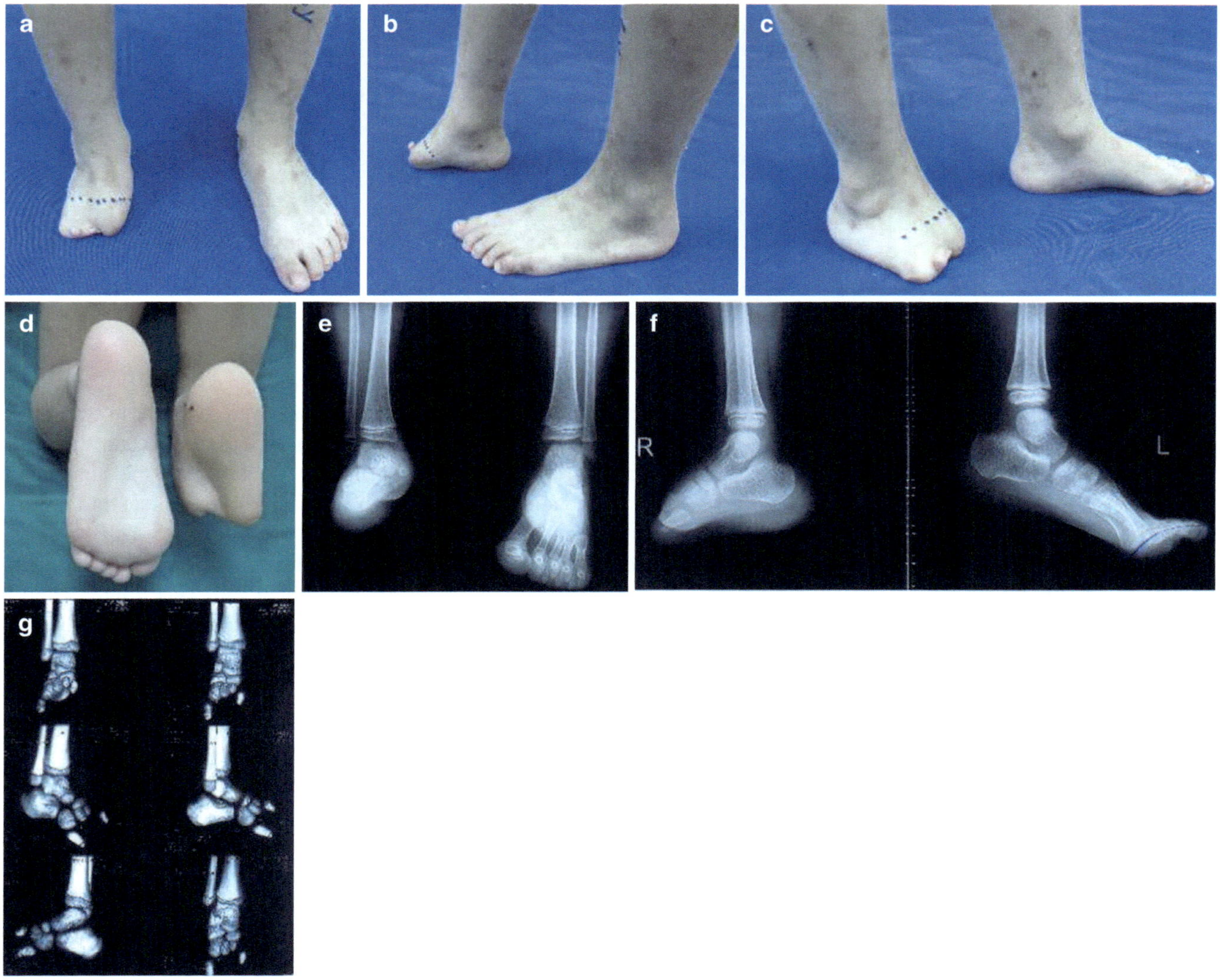

Fig. 2.39 Male, 6 years old, congenital absence of toes on the right side. (**a**) Appearance of both feet, all five toes of the right foot are absent; (**b**) medial view of the right foot; (**c**) lateral view of the right feet; (**d**) plantar view of both feet; (**e**) anteroposterior X-ray film of both feet; (**f**) lateral X-ray film of both foot; (**g**) CT three-dimensional reconstruction of right foot

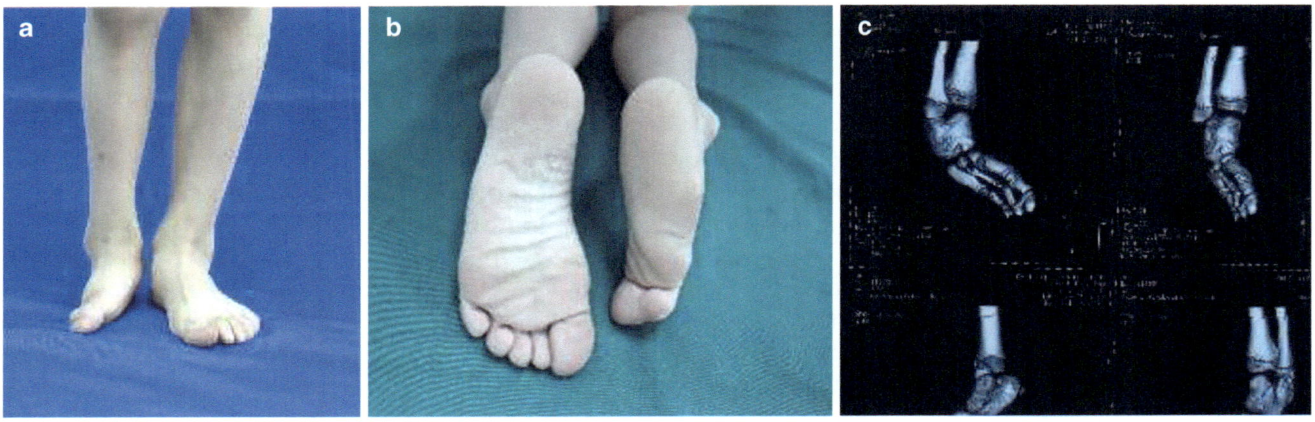

Fig. 2.40 A 7-year-old male presented with a congenital longitudinal cleft defect of the right foot. (**a**) Standing view; (**b**) plantar view; (**c**) CT three-dimensional reconstruction of right foot

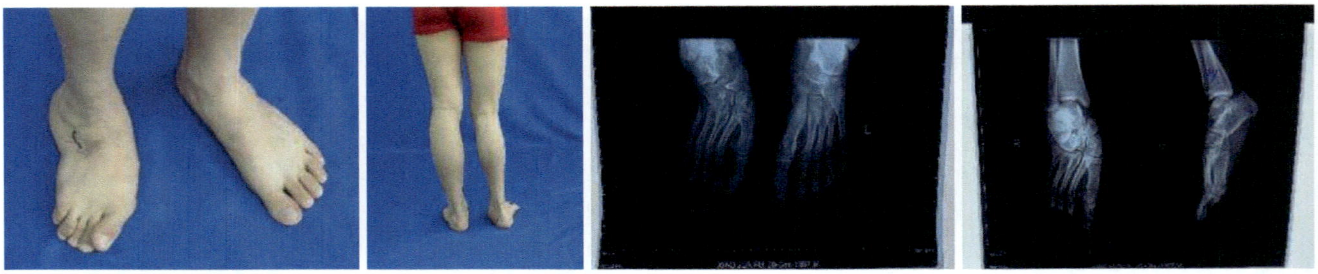

Fig. 2.41 Male, 17 years old, right congenital foot valgus deformity: (**a**) Appearance of both feet; (**b**) posterior view of both feet in standing position; (**c**) anteroposterior X-ray of both feet; (**d**) right foot anteroposterior and lateral X-ray film

2.3.13.3 Treatment Principle

Lengthen the calf, equal-length lower limbs, improve walking function.

2.3.14 Congenital Foot Valgus

2.3.14.1 Etiology

The cause of the disease is unknown.

2.3.14.2 Clinical Manifestation

Patients are born with congenital foot valgus deformity, which is gradually aggravated with growth and development. The deformity is rigid and cannot be corrected artificially (Fig. 2.41). Radiographs showed disappearance of the tarsal sinus, a short lateral calcaneal column, a small cuboid, and a valgus deformity of the calcaneus.

2.3.14.3 Treatment Principle

Correction of foot valgus deformity and restoration of foot longitudinal arch.

2.3.15 Congenital Cleft Foot

2.3.15.1 Etiology

The cause is unknown.

2.3.15.2 Clinical Manifestation

A cleft foot, also known as a lobster foot, is a foot deformity in which a single cleft extends proximally, sometimes to the midfoot. In general, one or more of the toes and their metatarsals are partially absent, and the tarsals are often abnormal (Fig. 2.42). Although the degree and type of cleft foot deformity vary, it is more common in the first and fifth phalangeal rows.

2.3.15.3 Classification

Blauth and Borisch divided them into six types according to the number of metatarsals based on the results of their study of the radiographic features of 173 cases of cleft foot (128 cases reported in the literature). Types I and II had a mild cleft foot and all five metatarsals were present. In type I, the metatarsals were all normal, in type II, the metatarsals were partially hypoplastic, and in types III–VI, the number of metatarsus decreased in turn, with 4 metatarsus in type III, 3 in type IV, 2 in type V, and 1 in type VI.

Abraham et al. introduced a simplified clinical classification based on the method of treatment. Type I has a central phalangeal laceration or absence (usually absent in the second or third phalangeal row or both) up to the level of the middle tarsal bone without involvement of the medial or lateral rows. For this type of cleft foot, they recommend soft tissue correction of partial hallux valgus deformity if surgery is needed. Type II has a deep pedal cleft extending from the forefoot to the tarsal bone. For this type of cleft foot, they recommend soft tissue correction of syndactyly with an osteotomy of the first phalangeal row before the age of 5 if surgery is required. Type III is a complete absence of the first to third or fourth phalangeal rows. For this type of cleft foot, they suggest that surgery is not required.

2.3.15.4 Treatment Principle

Any operation for the treatment of cleft foot should be aimed at improving function and appearance. When the cleft foot extends proximally between the two metatarsals, the corresponding skin on the surface of the cleft should be removed, but the dorsal and plantar flaps should be retained so that the two flaps can be sutured together when the incision is closed.

2.3.16 Congenital Talipes Equinovarus in Adult

2.3.16.1 Etiology

Congenital talipes equinovarus is not treated in time in infancy or recurs after treatment.

2.3.16.2 Clinical Manifestation

When congenital talipes equinovarus develops into adulthood, it is characterized by severe ankle-stiffness talipes equinovarus deformity, muscle atrophy of the calf, weight on

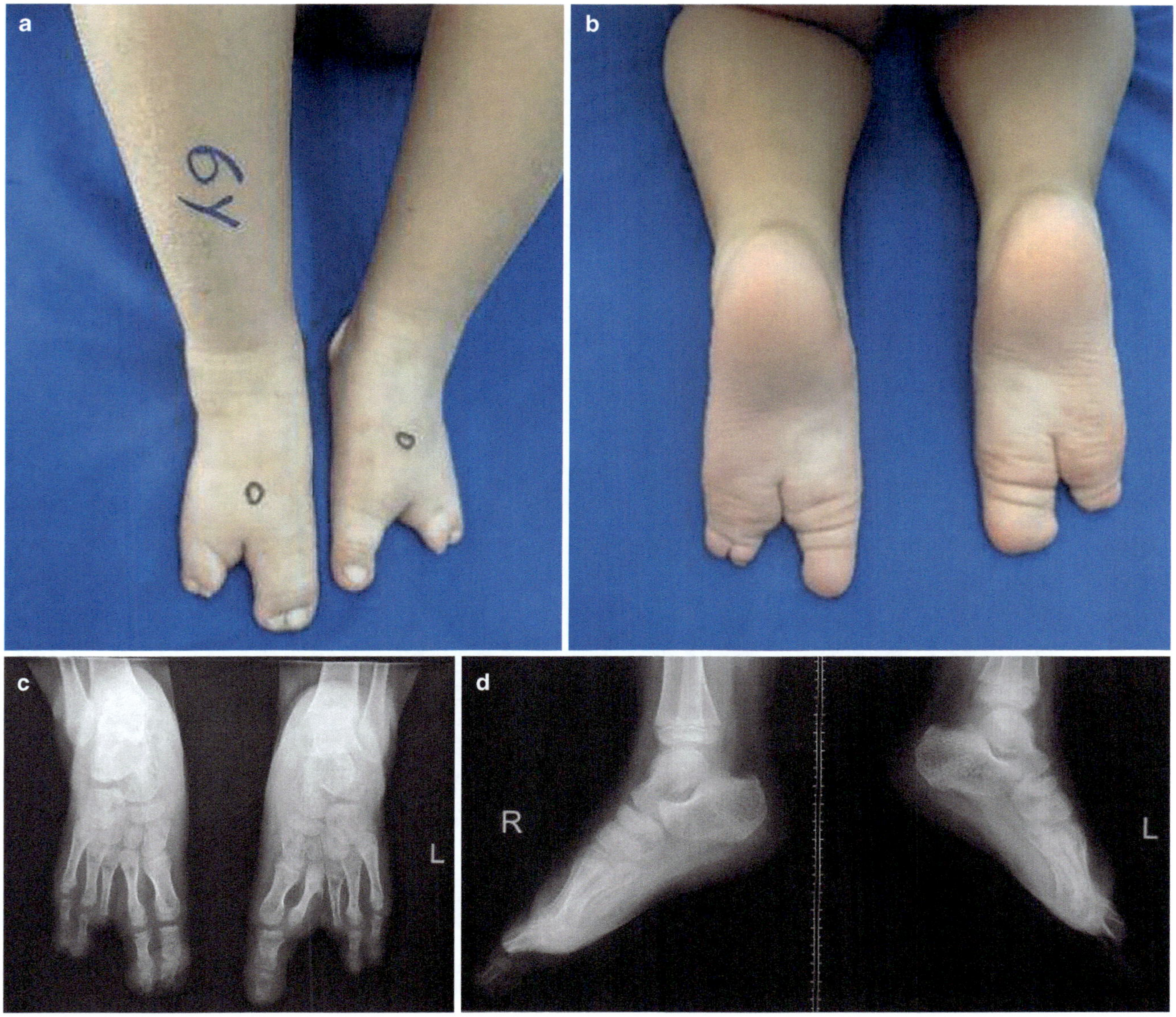

Fig. 2.42 Male, 6 years old, congenital bilateral cleft foot. (**a**) Dorsal view of both feet; (**b**) plantar view of both feet; (**c**) anteroposterior X-ray film of both ankles; (**d**) lateral X-ray film of both ankles and feet

dorsum of the foot, sole of the foot facing backward, and toe facing medial (Fig. 2.43).

2.3.16.3 Treatment Principle

Soft tissue release, three-joint of foot osteotomy, and Ilizarov technique were used to correct the ankle deformity slowly.

2.3.17 Children's Deputy Scaphoid of Foot

2.3.17.1 Etiology

The deputy scaphoid of the foot is a congenital anomaly located in the center of the second ossification of the tuberosity of the scaphoid bone, resulting in the formation of an independent deputy bone at the tuberosity of the scaphoid bone.

2.3.17.2 Clinical Manifestations

The deputy scaphoid of foot is usually bilateral and can be divided into three types. Type I is round and has no contact with the scaphoid. It grows on the posterior tibial tendon and its bottom is a cartilage surface composed of hyaline cartilage, sliding in the canal along the course of the posterior tibial tendon generally does not produce clinical symptoms. Type II is round or triangular and is part of the scaphoid but is separated from the tubercle of the scaphoid by fibrocartilage and is more prone to symptoms. In type III, the deputy scaphoid has fused with the scaphoid, resulting in an enlarged tuberosity of the scaphoid, which may rub against the vamp and cause pain (Fig. 2.44).

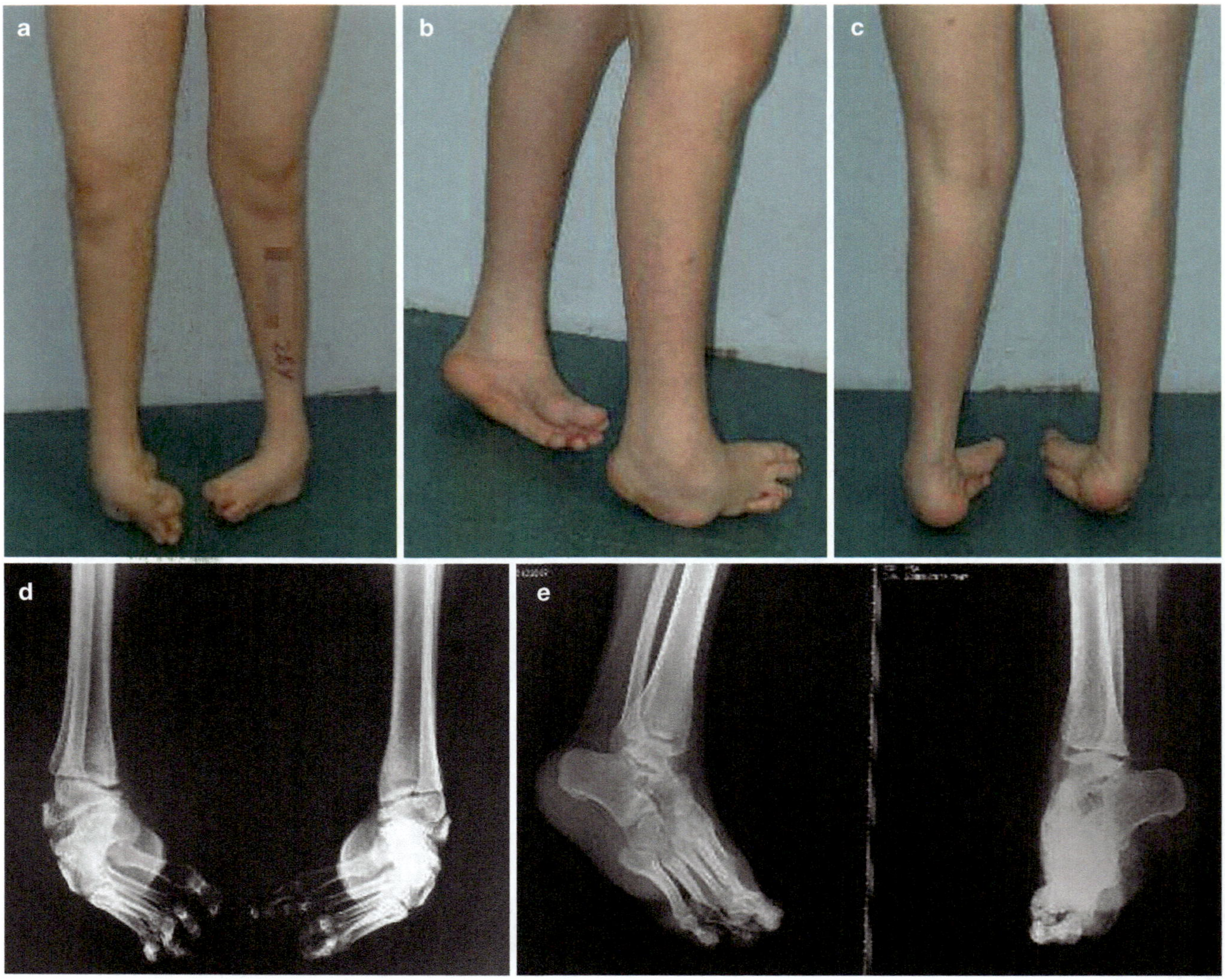

Fig. 2.43 Female, 26 years old, bilateral congenital talipes equinovarus. (**a**) Frontal view in standing position, with the lateral edge of both feet touching the ground; (**b**) lateral view in standing position; (**c**) dorsal view in standing; (**d**) anteroposterior X-ray film of both ankles; (**e**) lateral radiographs of both ankles

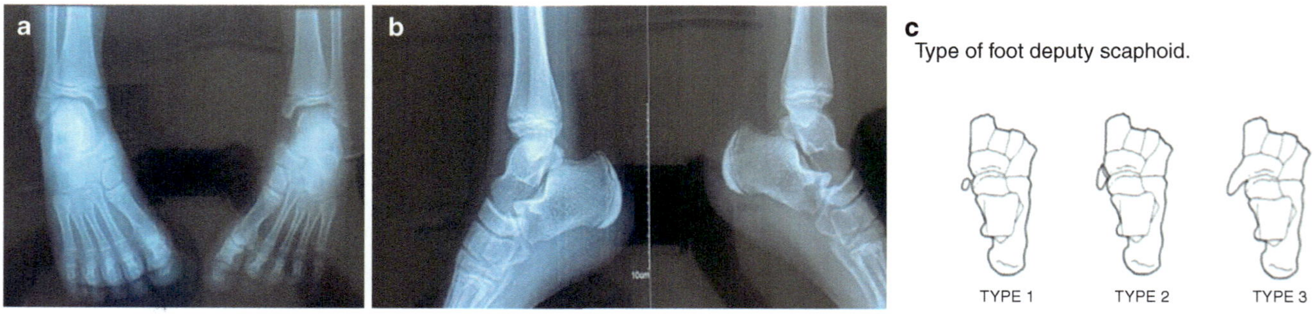

Fig. 2.44 Children's bilateral type III foot deputy scaphoid. (**a**) Anteroposterior radiograph of both feet; (**b**) lateral radiograph of both feet; (**c**) type of foot deputy scaphoid

2.3.17.3 Treatment Principle

Type I generally does not produce clinical symptoms and may not be treated. Type II and III can be treated with symptomatic treatment when they have clinical symptoms and can be resected when the symptoms are difficult to control.

2.4 Rare Congenital Deformities of the Lower Limbs

2.4.1 Parasite and Sirenomelus

Parasite is a rare congenital disease, also known as "fetus in fetus" in genetics, with an incidence of 1/500000. It refers to one or more incomplete fetal bodies parasitizing a part of the complete fetal body, which is extremely rare in China.

2.4.1.1 Etiology

Twins are divided into true twins and false twins. Dizygotic twins are false twins; identical twins are true twins. Parasite embryos usually occur in true twin embryos, which are divided into two groups of cells by the inner cell group of the embryo, forming two developmental centers. If the cell masses of the two inner cell populations are the same size and continue to be normal, they will develop into twins. If one of the two cell clusters is large and the other is small, and the small cell cluster is dysplastic, it may be enclosed into the fetus developed by the inner cell cluster of the other cluster and become an enclosed parasitic fetus, also known as "fetus in fetus."

2.4.1.2 Clinical Manifestation

Parasite vary greatly in their degree of development and have different types. If the separation of the two twins is incomplete, a conjoined fetus is formed; if the small fetus is parasitic in the body of the large fetus, this kind of parasitic fetus is called "fetus in fetus," mostly parasitic in the abdominal cavity, some of which are similar to the fetus in shape, and some of which have incomplete organ development. Parasite is a small fetus wrapped in normal fetus, which often has human characteristics such as organs, tissues, hair, and so on. Moreover, the parasitic fetus is small and difficult to detect when it is wrapped in the body of the fetus. Some children were not unexpectedly discovered until they were several years old or even adults when they went to the hospital for treatment because of illness (Fig. 2.45).

2.4.1.3 Classification

Parasite can be divided into monozygotic parasitism and dizygotic parasitism according to the source of egg cells. In monozygotic parasitism, the two are genetically identical. Monozygotic parasitism accounts for the vast majority, while dizygotic parasitism has only been reported sporadically in the world. For example, Nigeria has reported a case of a 6-month-old girl with a male parasite on her waist and back, with testicles.

They were classified according to the development degree of parasitic fetus.

1. If the separation of two twins is incomplete, a conjoined fetus is formed.
2. If the small fetus is parasitic in the body of the large fetus, this kind of parasitic fetus is called "fetus in fetus," mostly parasitic in the abdominal cavity, some of which are similar to the fetus in shape, and some of which have incomplete organ development. Parasitic fetus is actually a small fetus that is not fully developed by the normal fetus wrapped in the body.

2.4.1.4 Treatment Principle

According to different types, the parasite was removed or separated by surgery to preserve the patient's life. The remaining limb deformities can be corrected according to the patient's condition to improve the quality of life of patients.

2.4.2 Gollop-Wolfgang Syndrome

Gollop-Wolfgang syndrome is a rare congenital limb deformity characterized by distal femoral bifurcation, hypoplasia of the tibia, and ectrodactyly of the hands and feet, which is the loss or absence of one or more middle phalanges of the hands or feet. It is called hand crack or foot crack. In 1980, Gollop et al. reported that two brothers had unilateral distal femoral bifurcation, bilateral tibial absence and single toe deformity. In 1986, Lurie and Ilyina named the disease Gollop-Wolfgang syndrome. The disease may also be associated with malformations of the heart, digestive and urinary systems, or hypoplasia of the sacrococcygeal vertebrae.

2.4.2.1 Etiology

The etiology of this disease is unknown, which may be related to heredity and gene mutation.

2.4.2.2 Clinical Manifestation

At birth, it was accompanied by complex deformities of knee joint, lower leg and ankle, wide knee joint (Fig. 2.46), knee flexion deformity, abnormal activity trajectory of flexion and extension, shortening of lower leg, bending deformity, talipes equinovarus, and polydactyly. X-ray showed bifurcation of the distal femur, hypoplasia or absence of the tibia and fibula, and abnormal bone and joint structure of the foot and ankle.

2.4.2.3 Treatment Principle

The malformation of this disease is complex and requires multiple operations throughout the development period to reconstruct the shape and function of the limbs. Correct the deformity of knee, ankle, and foot, restore the gravity line of lower limbs, and equal-length lower limbs.

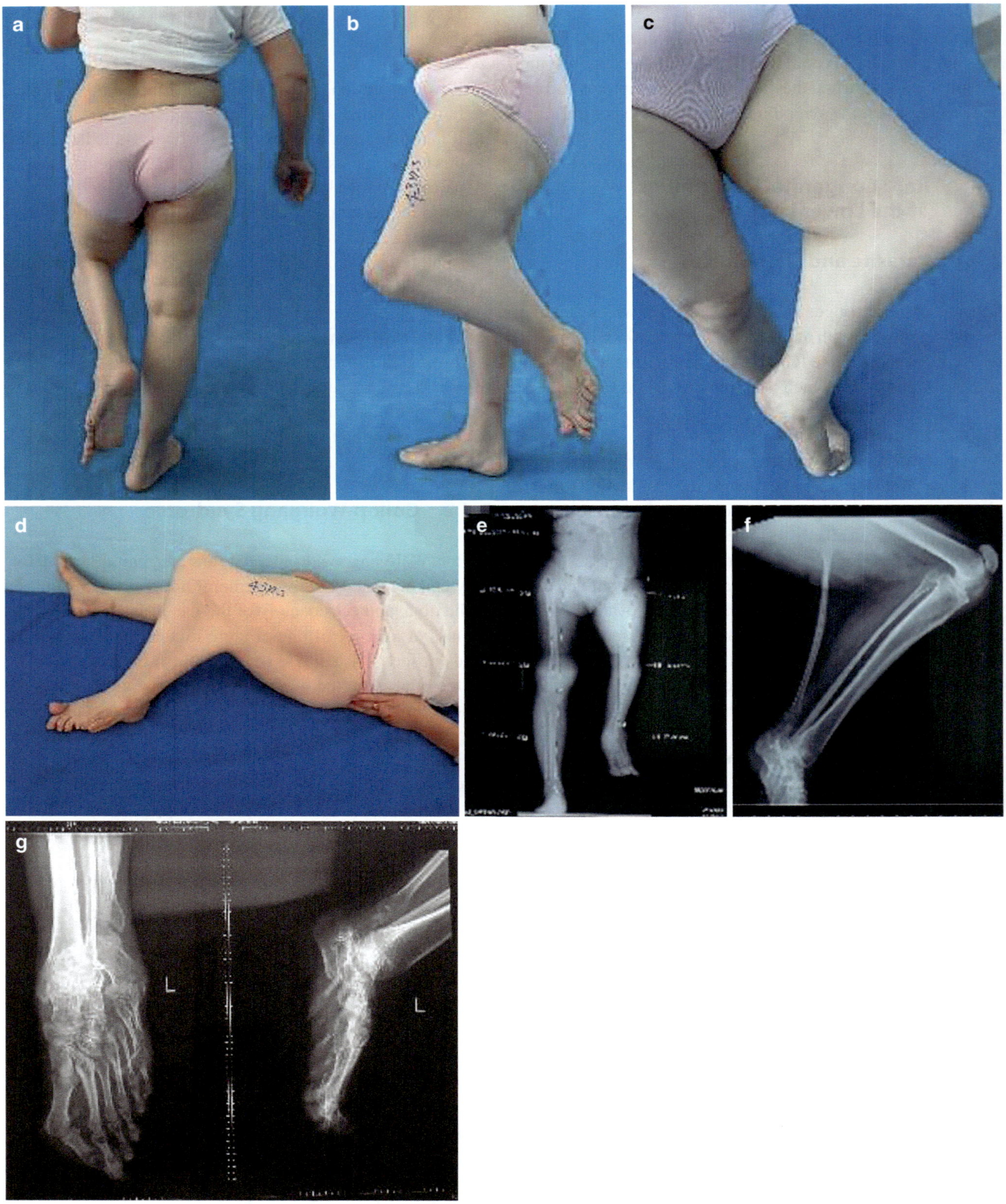

Fig. 2.45 A 43-year-old female presented with pterygoid knee deformity caused by a parasite on her left lower limb. (**a**) Dorsal view in standing position; (**b**) lateral view; (**c**) medial view; (**d**) lateral view in supine position; (**e**) full-length X-ray of both lower limbs in standing position; (**f**) lateral X-ray of left lower limb; (**g**) anteroposterior and lateral radiograph of left ankle

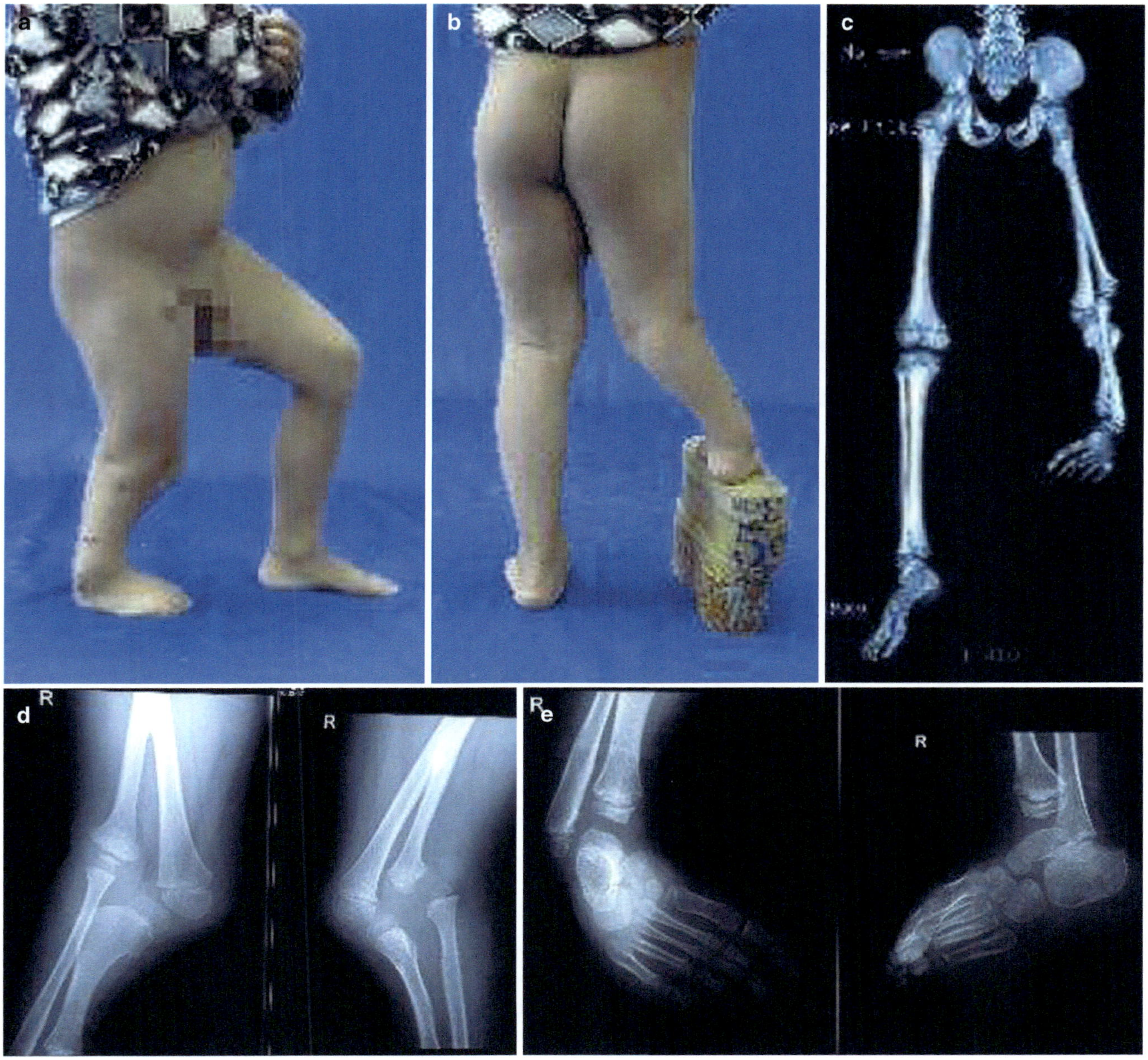

Fig. 2.46 Male, 7 years old, Gollop-Wolfgang syndrome, right lower limb deformity. (**a**) Standing appearance, right lower leg short, knee joint widened, talipes equinovarus; (**b**) standing dorsal view; (**c**) CT three-dimensional reconstruction of both lower limbs, bifurcation of the lower femur, shortening of the tibia, fibula longer than the tibia; (**d**) anteroposterior and lateral X-ray of the right knee joint; (**e**) anteroposterior and lateral X-ray film of right ankle

2.4.3 Congenital Tibial Hemimelia

2.4.3.1 Etiology

The cause of the disease is unknown.

2.4.3.2 Clinical Manifestation

When the patient was born, there was obvious shortening of the affected limb, bending of the knee joint and lower leg, and the proximal displaced fibular head could be touched in the lower thigh. The fibula was relatively intact, and the patient's general development could not be affected (Fig. 2.47). Absence of the tibia can cause serious defects, often accompanied by knee instability, limb shortening, severe deformity of the foot, such as varus plantar flexion, adduction, etc. The inside of the foot is absent to varying degrees, often with stiffness of the hindfoot. In older children, the proximal tibia is not visible on radiographs, but the proximal tibial anlage is palpable. Usually, the knee joint has flexion deformity. When the flexion deformity is more serious, the quadriceps femoris hypoplasia lacks the function of extending the knee joint.

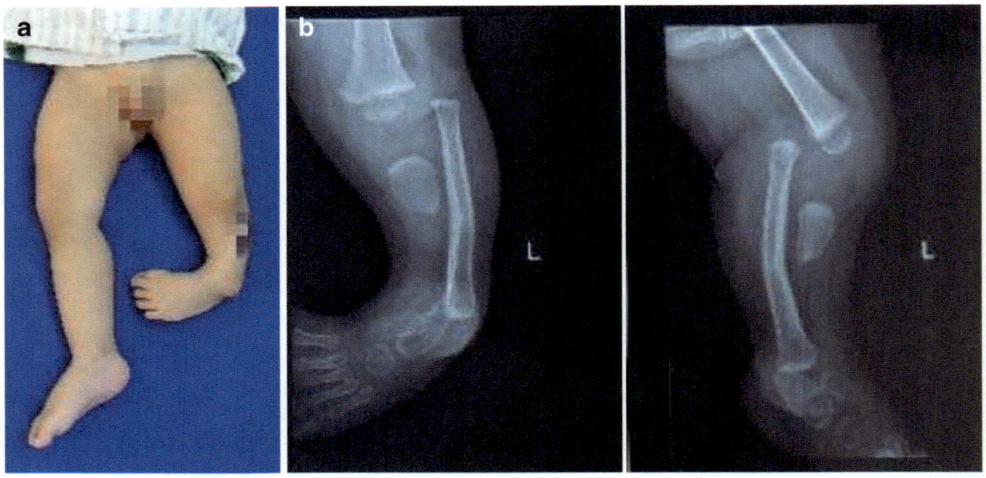

Fig. 2.47 A 15-month-old boy with congenital left tibial hemimelia. (**a**) Lower limb appearance, left leg shortening and varus; (**b**) anteroposterior and lateral X-ray film of the left leg, with short left tibia

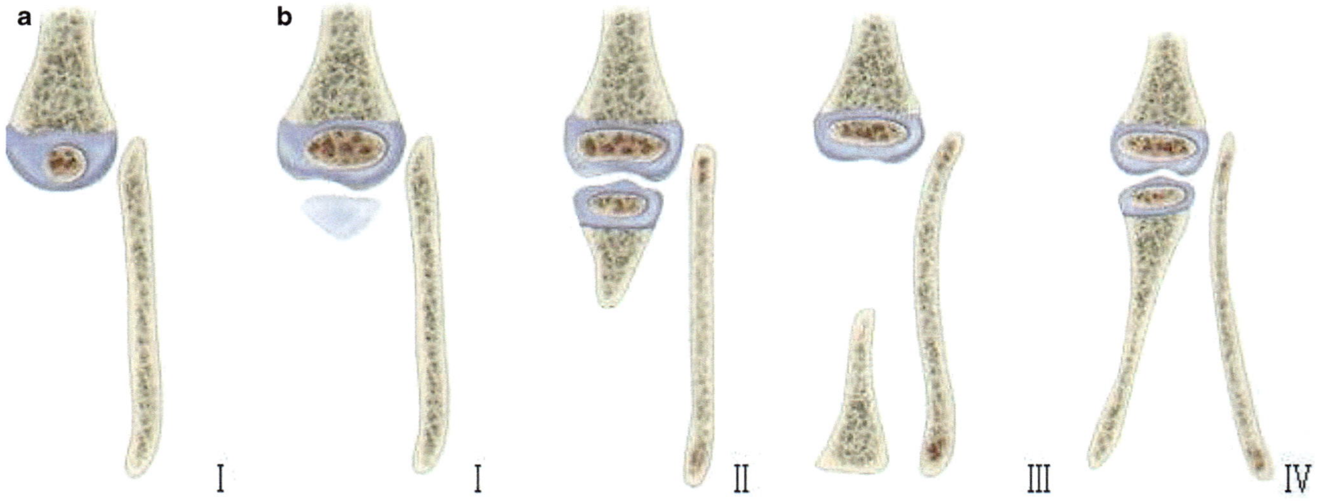

Fig. 2.48 Classification of congenital absence of tibia

2.4.3.3 Classification

Congenital absence of the tibia is usually classified by Jones. According to the clinical and X-ray findings, it can be divided into four types: Type Ia: Complete absence of the tibia and dysplasia of the distal femoral epiphysis. Type Ib: The distal tibia is completely absent, but the shape and size of the distal femoral epiphysis are closer to normal. Type II: The size of the proximal tibia is different at birth, while the fibula is mostly normal, and the fibular head is displaced proximally. Type III: Rare, the proximal tibia is absent, and there is a high density area in the cartilage matrix of the distal tibia due to diffuse calcification. The distal femur is usually well developed, but the upper end of the fibula is displaced proximally, and the knee joint is often unstable. Type IV: Rare, shortening of the tibia with upward displacement of the proximal fibula and separation of the distal tibia and fibula (Fig. 2.48). Among them, type I is the most common.

2.4.3.4 Treatment Principle

The goal of treatment is to obtain a limb with the same length as the normal limb and weight-bearing function, so the principle of treatment is to correct the deformity of knee joint and ankle foot, stabilize the knee and ankle joints, tibialization of the fibula, partially equal-length lower limbs through Ilizarov limb lengthening, and some types of artificial limbs can be installed after amputation.

2.4.4 Congenital Tibial Hemimelia with Contralateral Dissociate Toe

2.4.4.1 Etiology

The cause of the disease is unknown.

2.4.4.2 Clinical Manifestation

At birth, there were obvious shortening of the right leg, talipes equinovarus deformity of the right foot, and abnormal movement of the right ankle joint. The left toe is curled to the lateral side of the dorsum of the foot, and the toe web space is proximal (Fig. 2.49).

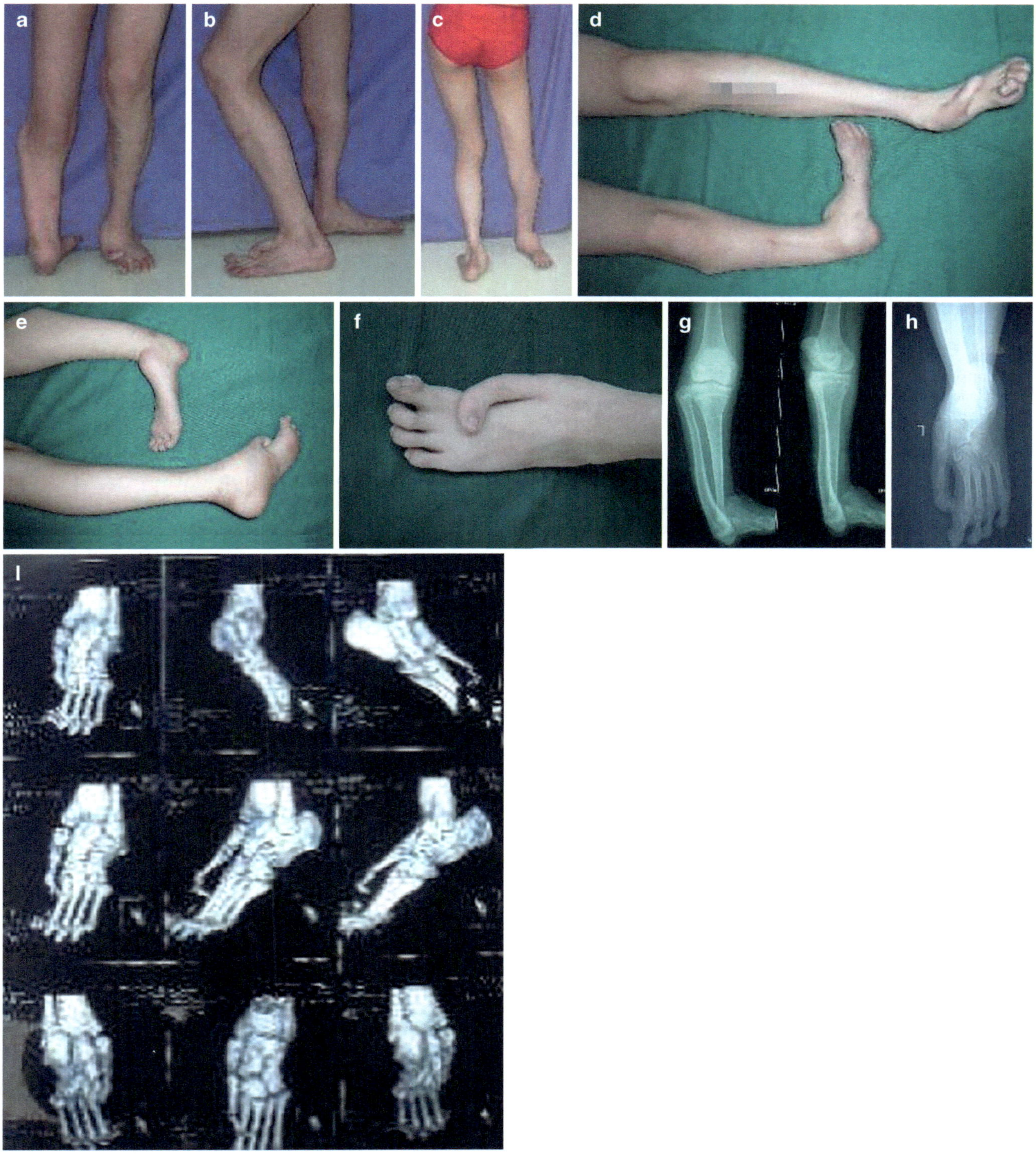

Fig. 2.49 A 14-year-old female presented with congenital tibial hemimelia on the right side combined with left split foot malformation. (**a**) Front view of standing position, right lower leg shortening, clubfoot, lower segment of the fibula touched the ground and walked; (**b**) side view of standing position; (**c**) back view of standing; (**d**) appearance of both legs in sitting position; (**e**) appearance of both legs in prone position; (**f**) appearance of left foot; (**g**) X-ray film of right leg, lower fibula thickening, distal tibia thinning, abnormal anatomical relationship of ankle joint; (**h**) anteroposterior X-ray film of the left foot, with the first metatarsal row displaced proximally; (**i**) CT three-dimensional reconstruction of left foot

2.4.4.3 Treatment Principle

The goal of treatment is to obtain a limb with the same length as the normal limb and weight-bearing function, so the principle of treatment is to correct the deformity of knee joint and ankle foot and stabilize the knee and ankle joints, through Ilizarov limb lengthening technique to equal-length limb.

2.5 Congenital Limb Compound Deformity

2.5.1 Congenital Polyarticular Contracture

2.5.1.1 Etiology

The cause of the disease is unknown.

2.5.1.2 Clinical Manifestation

The typical congenital polyarticular contracture is usually accompanied by different degrees of limitation of movement of the six major joints of the limbs at birth: shoulder joint adduction and internal rotation, elbow joint extension contracture, wrist joint flexion and ulnar deviation, hip joint flexion, and knee joint flexion, talipes equinovarus, disappearance of joint texture of the six major joints, and atrophy of limb muscles to varying degrees (Fig. 2.50). Atypical cases of joint contracture may occur only in a few joints, but often bilaterally symmetrical, such as double knee flexion contracture with double talipes equinovarus deformity.

2.5.1.3 Classification

According to the limitation of joint flexion and extension, it can be divided into flexion joint contracture and extension joint contracture. Flexion joint contracture is characterized by joint flexion deformity and limitation of extension. Extension-type joint contracture is characterized by deformity of joint extension or retroflexion and limitation of flexion.

2.5.1.4 Treatment Principle

Correct joint deformity and improve function. The upper limbs were mainly used to correct the wrist drop and improve the function of wrist and hand. The goal of the lower limb is to correct the deformity of hip flexion, knee flexion, and equinus and to restore the negative gravity line of the lower limb.

2.5.2 Congenital Pterygoid Joint

2.5.2.1 Etiology

Congenital pterygoid joint is a rare malformation of unknown etiology.

2.5.2.2 Clinical Manifestation

The main manifestation of congenital pterygoid knee joint is knee flexion contracture, accompanied by the formation of a pterygoid soft tissue from the buttocks to the calcaneus on the posterior side of the knee joint. The traction of webbed tissue leads to knee flexion contracture with equinus deformity. The function of knee flexion is generally not affected, but the extension of the knee is severely limited, resulting in patients unable to walk upright. The morphology and function of the patient's lower extremities were seriously affected (Fig. 2.51).

2.5.2.3 Treatment Principle

Avoid performing extensive soft tissue release; the Ilizarov technique was used to correct knee flexion and equinus deformity and restore upright walking function.

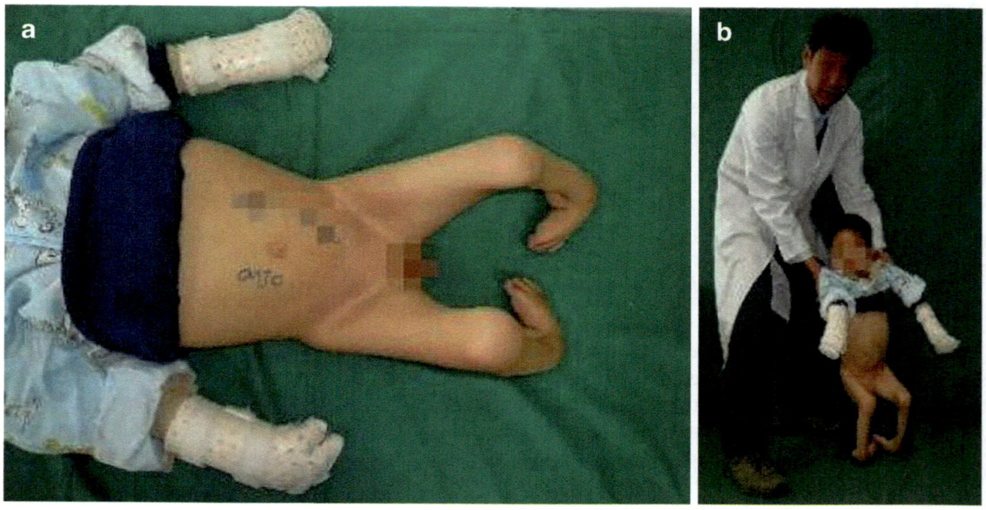

Fig. 2.50 Male, 7 years old, congenital polyarticular contracture: (**a**) Bilateral elbow, wrist, hip, knee flexion deformity, talipes equinovarus deformity; (**b**) unable to stand independently, can stand reluctantly under the support

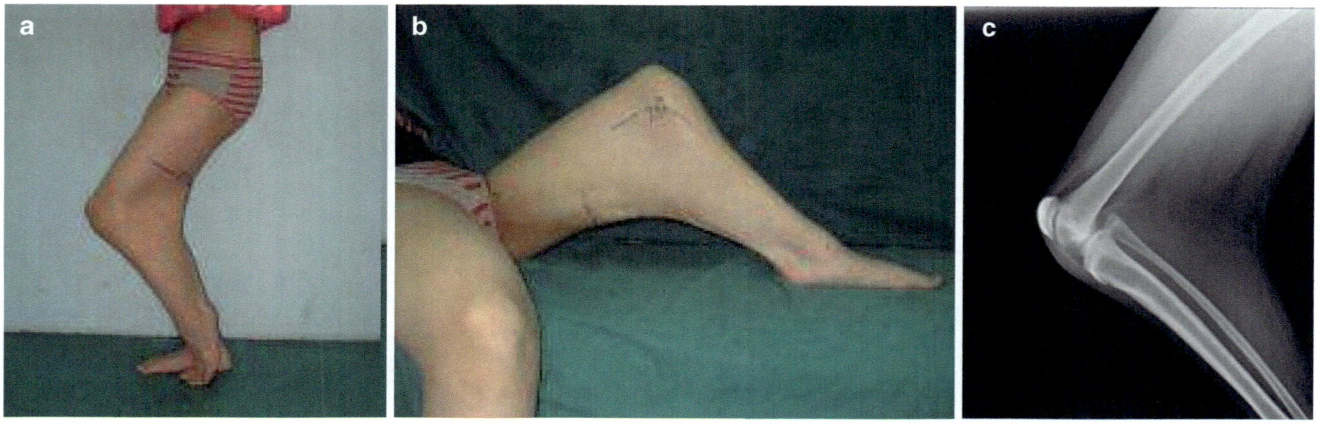

Fig. 2.51 Left congenital pterygoid knee joint. (**a**) Standing position, left knee flexion, equinus deformity, pterygoid tissue from hip to heel; (**b**) the supine position shows the pterygoid tissue on the posterior side of the left knee joint. (**c**) X-ray of the knee showed flexion deformity with an enlarged proximal tibial condylar angle

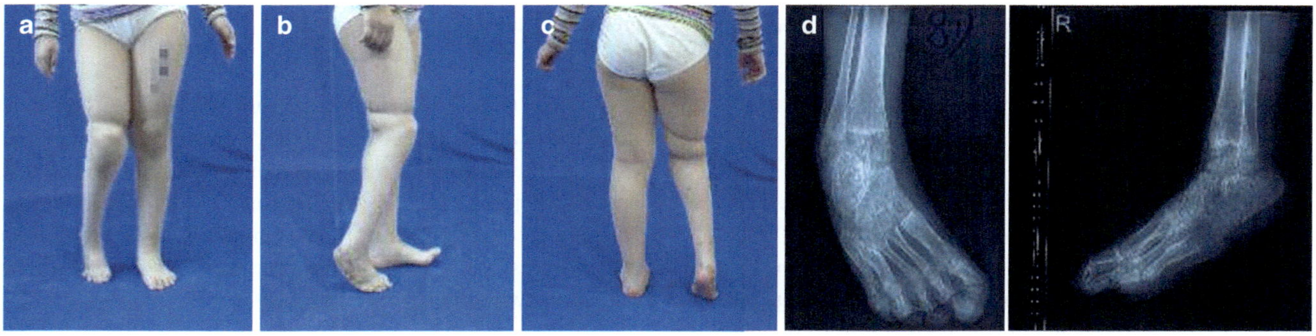

Fig. 2.52 Female, 10 years old, congenital annular band of right lower thigh with talipes equinovarus deformity. (**a**) View from a standing position, annular skin depression can be seen in the lower part of the thigh; (**b**) view from the right side; (**c**) view from back; (**d**) X-ray film of foot and ankle

2.5.3 Congenital Band Syndrome

2.5.3.1 Etiology

Congenital band syndrome is a lipid defect, similar to the formation of cleft lip, which originates from hypodermic mesoderm development. Kino believes that it is caused by excessive contraction of uterine muscle 5–6 weeks after conception, which leads to bleeding in the mesenchymal tissue of the embryo and amniotic membrane adhesion, which is caused by prenatal environment. It is also believed that it is caused by the rupture of amniotic membrane during development.

2.5.3.2 Clinical Manifestation

At birth, there is a complete band-like constriction around the soft tissue of the limb, mostly located far from the middle of the lower leg, usually accompanied by hypertrophic deformity. The constriction ring may be shallow and bandages only the skin and subcutaneous tissue. Deep annular compression bands can reach muscle and bone tissue, which can affect venous and lymphatic return and cause persistent edema and hypertrophy of distal limbs. If the blood circulation is severely blocked, self-amputation can occur in the fetus, that is, the so-called congenital amputation (Figs. 2.52 and 2.53).

2.5.3.3 Classification

Clinically, it is often divided into four degrees: Degree 1: The band is only embedded in the subcutaneous; Degree 2: The band goes deep into the fascia and does not affect the circulation of the distal limb; Degree 3: The band goes deep into the fascia and affects the circulation of the distal limb, with swelling, color change, and nerve injury; Degree 4: Congenital amputation.

2.5.3.4 Treatment Principle

The circular band was resected, the soft tissue was released and shaped, and the tissue compression was relieved. Patients with limb deformities should be corrected at the same time.

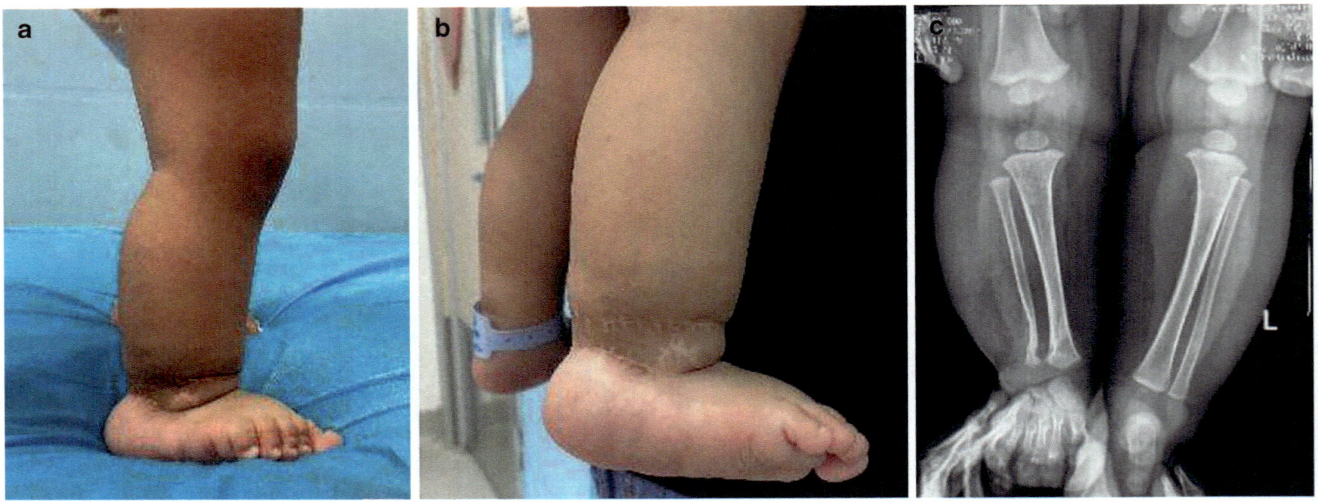

Fig. 2.53 Male, 1 year and 6 months old, with a circular band at the lower end of the right leg. (**a**) Appearance of the right lower limb in standing position; (**b**) skin Z-shaped release plasty has been performed on the annular band of the lower part of the right leg; (**c**) X-ray films of both legs showed that the lower part of the tibia and fibula was compressed and thinned

2.5.4 Congenital Insensitivity to Pain with Anhidrosis

2.5.4.1 Etiology

Congenital insensitivity to pain with anhidrosis (CIPA), also known as hereditary sensory and autonomic neuropathy (HSAN) type IV, is an autosomal recessive genetic disease and a rare disease. It is now believed that CIPA are caused by mutations in the neurotrophin receptor kinase 1 (NTRK1) gene. The NTRK 1 gene in normal humans is located on chromosome 1 (1q21-q22) and encodes a tyrosine receptor that is required for nerve growth factor (NGF). Because of the mutation of NTRK1 gene, the protein encoded by NTRK1 is abnormal, which leads to a series of clinical symptoms.

2.5.4.2 Clinical Manifestation

The main manifestations of this disease are as follows: (1) No sense of pain: It is systemic, 80% of the patients have complete loss of pain, temperature sense is reduced or disappeared, and they are prone to scald, and tactile sensation is fine. Infants and young children have self-mutilation behavior after tooth eruption. (2) No sweat: No sweat all over the body, dry skin, small chaps on the back of the hand and the end of the fingers (toes), especially in winter. Individual patients only sweat on both sides of the nose or back in summer. (3) Fever: Because of perspiration dysfunction, the patient has repeated high fever after birth, manifested as remittent fever or irregular fever, and the body temperature is affected by the ambient temperature. About 20% of the children died of high fever before the age of 3. (4) Mental retardation: Psychomotor retardation, optic atrophy in some children, and inability to see in both eyes. (5) Multiple fractures: Due to the lack of defensive response to pain, fractures are prone to occur. Children with greenstick fractures or epiphyseal injuries are prone to secondary limb deformities (Fig. 2.54). (6) Joint capsule relaxation: The whole body joint capsule is relaxed, the range of motion of each joint exceeds the normal range, joint dislocation often occurs, superficial joint capsule swelling, and so on. (7) Infection: Because frequently biting finger, tongue, lips, etc. can cause infection easily, it may also have a certain relationship with the patient's low immune function.

2.5.4.3 Treatment Principle

Correct limb deformity, restore the gravity line of lower limbs, and improve walking function.

2.5.5 Multiple Synostosis Syndrome

2.5.5.1 Etiology

Multiple synostosis syndromes (SYNS) are a group of rare syndromes of bone dysplasia. This group of diseases mainly involve finger (toe) joints, carpal tarsal joints, elbow joints and so on, resulting in fusion or adhesion of these joints. In addition, it can also affect the auditory ossicles, cervical or lumbar spine, and other joints, resulting in hearing impairment or limited spinal movement. Genetic studies have shown that there is genetic heterogeneity in this group of diseases, but it is mainly related to NOGGIN gene, bone morphogenetic protein gene cluster, and growth differentiation factor 5.

2.5.6 Clinical Manifestation and Classification

Multiple synostosis syndrome type 1 (SYNS1) is an autosomal-dominant genetic disease, which affects the finger/toe joints in the early stage and later affects the hip and

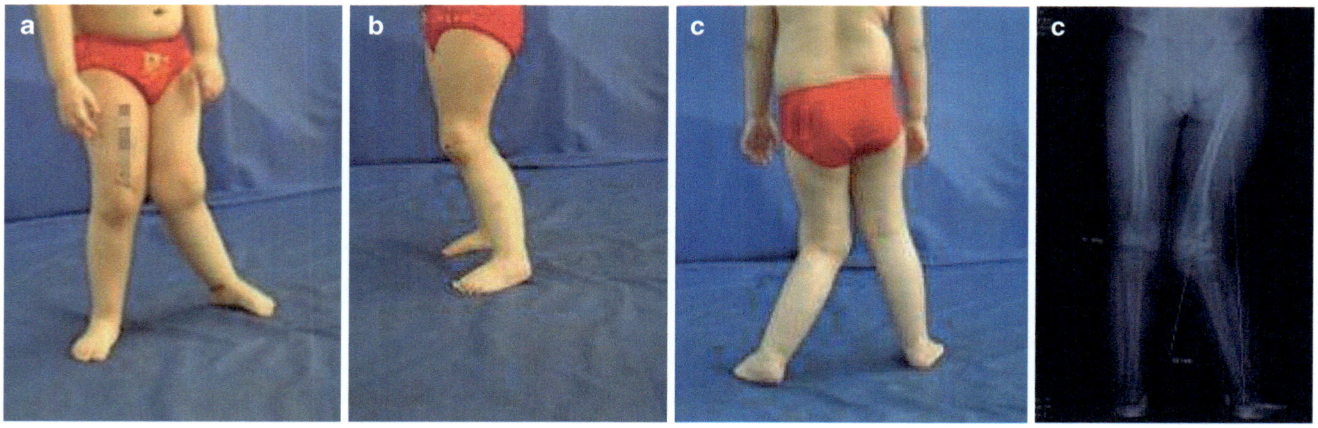

Fig. 2.54 Valgus deformity of left knee caused by CIPA. (**a**) Standing frontal view; (**b**) standing lateral view; (**c**) standing dorsal view; (**d**) full length orthostatic X-ray of both lower limbs

spinal joints. Some patients have hearing impairment due to ossicular fusion.

Multiple synostosis syndrome type 2 (SYNS2) is also an autosomal dominant genetic disease, mainly involving finger joints, wrist joints, and elbow joints, but the spinal joints and auditory ossicles are generally not involved, and there is no hearing impairment.

Proximal symphalangism (SYM1) is mainly characterized by proximal interphalangeal adhesion, tarsal and carpal fusion, conductive deafness, and radial head dislocation and humeroradial joint fusion in a few patients.

Tarsal-carpal coalition syndrome (TCC) is characterized by tarsal and carpal bone fusion, accompanied by finger/toe joint fusion, humeroradial joint fusion, and first metacarpal bone shortening (Fig. 2.55).

2.5.6.1 Treatment Principle

Correct limb deformity, restore the gravity line of lower limbs, and improve walking function.

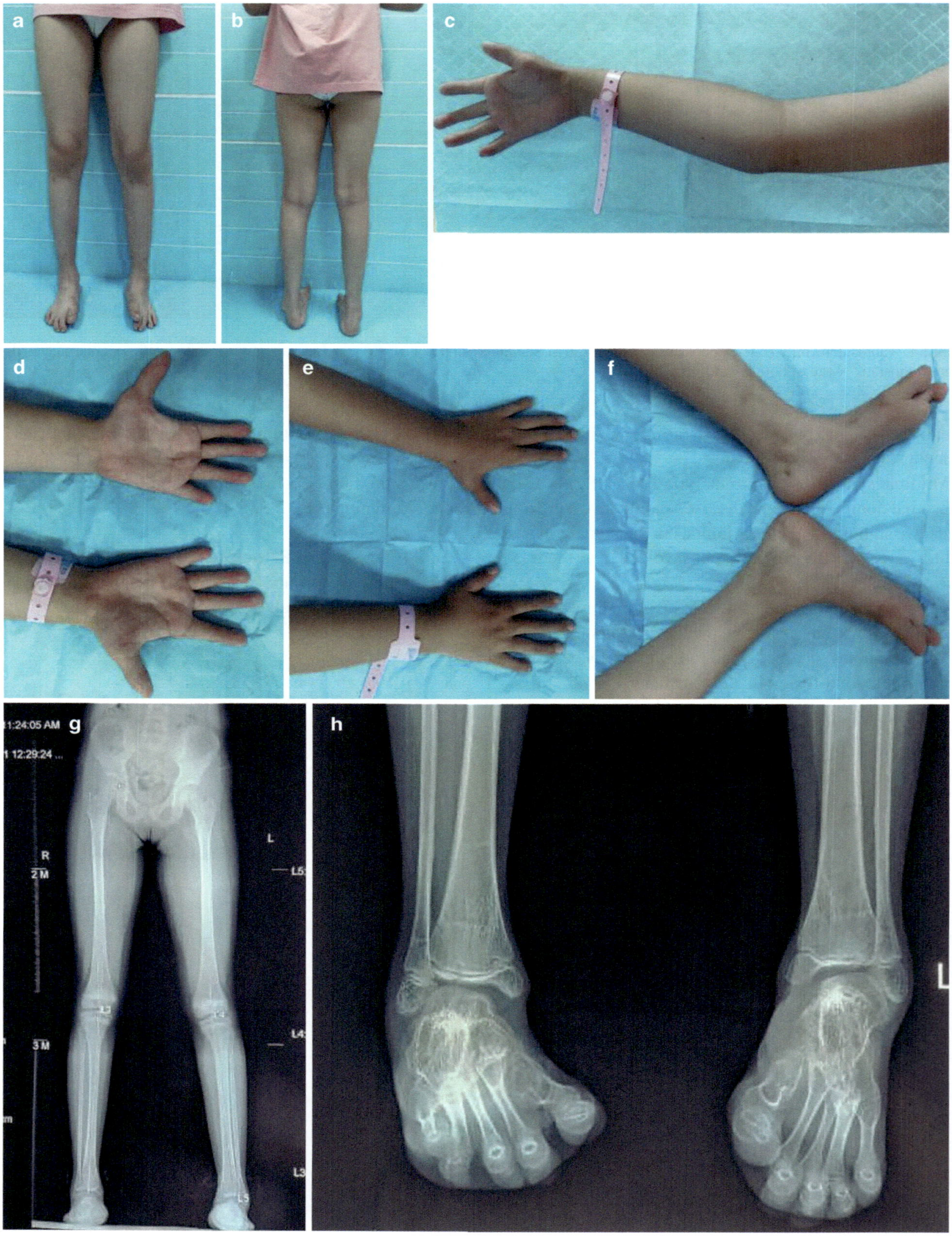

Fig. 2.55 Multiple synostosis syndrome: interphalangeal fusion. Bilateral tarsal and intermetatarsal fusion with left foot varus. (**a**) Frontal view in standing position; (**b**) posterior view in standing position; (**c**) elbow joint flexion; (**d**, **e**) no transverse striation between both fingers; (**f**) arch of both feet almost disappeared; (**g**) full-length anteroposterior radiographs of both lower limbs in standing position H: anteroposterior radiographs of both feet

Suggested Reading

1. Qin S, Xia H. Treatment of congenital fibular aplasia with concurrent unequal leg length. Chin J Orthop Surg. 2000;9:908–9.
2. Jiao S, Qin S, Wang Z, et al. Ilizarov technique combined with composite surgery for the treatment of congenital lateral hemimelia of the fibula. Chin J Orthop Surg. 2017;25(004):312–6.
3. Wang J, Mei H. Progress in the adjuvant treatment of congenital tibial pseudoarthrosis in children with bisphosphonates. Chin J Orthop Surg. 2016;37(001):77–80.
4. Qin S, Guo B, Shi L, et al. Ilizarov technique combined with intramedullary nail fixation for the treatment of adult type I neurofibromatosis-related tibial pseudoarthrosis. Chin J Orthop Surg. 2021;41(11):687–93.
5. Qin S, Guo B, Ren L, Zheng X, Jiao S. Limited orthopedic surgery combined with Ilizarov technique for the treatment of adolescent congenital clubfoot. Chin J Orthop Surg. 2012;26(1):31–5.
6. Qin S, Li C, Wu H, et al. Traction treatment of congenital tibial aplasia with severe knee joint flexion deformity: a case report (with literature review). Chin J Orthop Surg. 2005;13(21):1629–33.

3 Heredity and Genetic Defects and Metabolic Disorders Lead to Deformity

Sihe Qin

3.1 The Skeleton and Muscles Disease

3.1.1 Hypophosphatemic Rickets

3.1.1.1 Etiology

Hypophosphatemic rickets (HR), also known as hypophosphatemic vitamin D-resistant rickets, is a disease characterized by low blood phosphorus, bone pain, and limb fatigue. In adults, the disease involves only the bones and is called osteomalacia. In children, the disease also occurs in the growth plate and cartilage to be mineralized, resulting in characteristic skeletal deformities. The disease is mainly related to heredity. Hereditary hypophosphatemic rickets can be divided into X-linked dominant hypophosphatemic rickets (XLH), autosomal dominant hypophosphorous rickets (ADHR), autosomal recessive hypophosphorous rickets (ARHR), hypophosphatic rickets with hyperparathyroidism (HRHPT), McCune-Albright syndrome (MAS), osteoglophonic dysplasia (OGD), etc.

3.1.1.2 Clinical Manifestation

Skeletal deformities are mostly manifested as deformities of long bones of lower limbs, including severe O-shaped legs, X-shaped legs, K-shaped legs, and blowing deformities of both lower limbs (Fig. 3.1), accompanied by mild obesity and short stature.

According to the Qin Sihe case database statistics (time: 1978.05.25–2018.12.31; Total number of cases: 35075 cases), a total of 75 patients with rickets were treated, including 31 male patients and 44 female patients, with an average age of 20.14 years. The main manifestations are: severe rickets in infancy, with different degrees of residual skeletal deformities, such as O-shaped legs, X-shaped legs, lower limb bending deformities and chicken breast deformities.

S. Qin (✉)
Department of Orthopaedics, Rehabilitation Hospital of the National Research Center for Rehabilitation Technical Aids, Beijing, China

3.1.1.3 Treatment Principle

1. High phosphorus diet, oral phosphate mixture to supplement blood phosphorus.
2. Osteotomy of lower limb deformity to restore the normal mechanical axis and joint line of lower limb.

3.1.2 Osteogenesis Imperfecta

3.1.2.1 Etiology

Osteogenesis imperfecta is also called brittle bone disease. Primary Brittle bone disease and Periosteum Dysplasia, etc., is due to the hypoplasia of mesenchymal tissue. Congenital hereditary pain caused by the collagen formation of obstacles. The cause is unknown. It is a congenital developmental disorder, which can be divided into congenital type and delayed type. Congenital type refers to the onset of the disease in the uterus, which can be subdivided into the fetus type and baby type, severe illness, mostly death, or death occurred shortly after postpartum, is autosomal recessive heredity; Delayed type is milder and can be divided into childhood type and adult type. Most patients can survive for a long time, is autosomes dominant inheritance. More than 15% of the patients had a family history.

3.1.2.2 Clinical Manifestation

The blue sclera and sclera became thinner, and the transparency increased. Progressive deafness is caused by ossicular sclerosis and sound conduction disorder. The teeth were hypoplastic and sallow, the incisors became thin, and the incisal margin was defective. Triangular-shaped head, wide forehead, prominent cheekbones, and relatively small mandible. There may be scoliosis, flat pelvis, or short stature. Due to increased bone fragility, minor injuries can cause fractures, often manifested as spontaneous fractures, or repeated multiple fractures. The limbs are often bent or angled (Fig. 3.2). After puberty, the probability of fractures gradually decreases.

S. Qin et al. (eds.), *Atlas of Limb Deformity*, https://doi.org/10.1007/978-981-97-0999-1_3

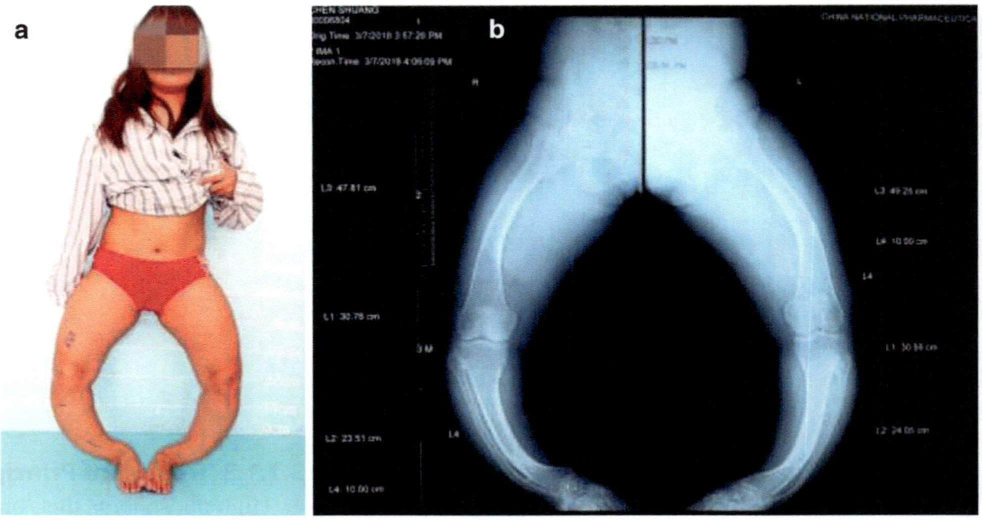

Fig. 3.1 (**a**) Severe genu varum deformity caused by hypophosphatemic rickets. (**b**) X-ray showed bending deformity of both femur and tibia

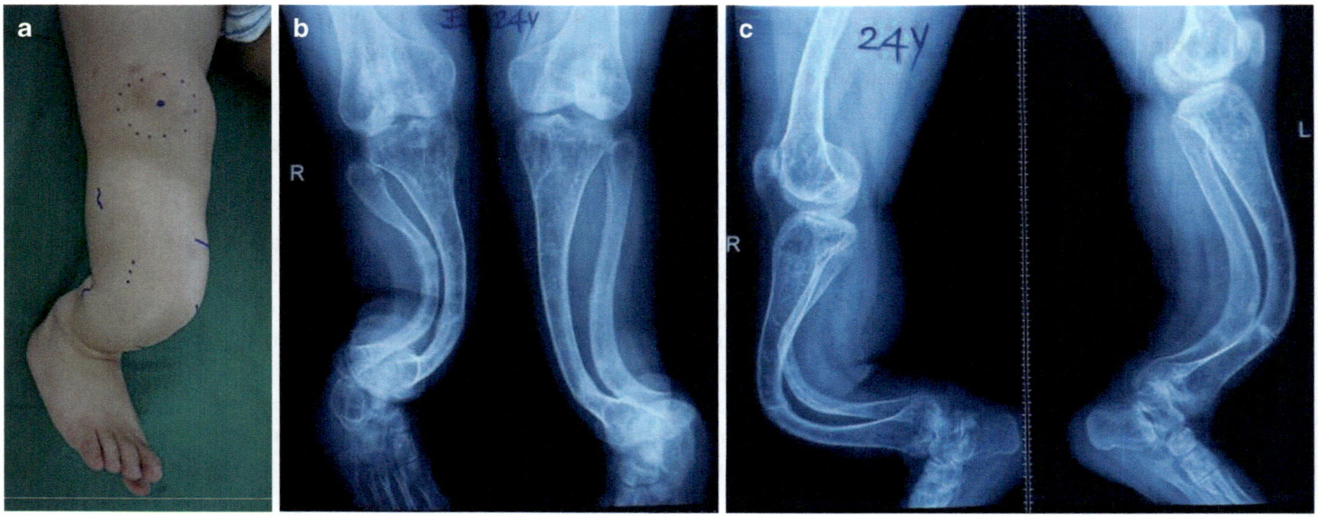

Fig. 3.2 Limb deformity after osteogenesis imperfecta. (**a**) Full-length frontal view of right lower limb, compound deformity; (**b**) Bilateral tibiofibular anteroposterior radiographs; (**c**) Bilateral tibiofibular lateral radiograph: anterior arch of tibiofibula

3.1.2.3 Treatment Principle

1. Patients with no limb deformity or mild deformity should be prevented from fracture and malunion after fracture.
2. For patients with limb deformities that affect their walking function, osteotomy should be performed to improve their walking function and prevent re-fracture.

3.1.3 Progressive Muscular Dystrophy

3.1.3.1 Etiology

Progressive muscular dystrophy (PMD) is a genetic disease of primary striated muscle. The main clinical manifestations were bilateral symmetrical progressive muscle weakness and atrophy starting from the proximal limb, and myocardial involvement was present in some cases. Modern molecular genetics has found that muscular dystrophy is associated with defects in sarcolemma proteins, juxtamembrane proteins, and nuclear membrane proteins. However, the mechanism by which protein defects cause muscle degeneration and necrosis, leading to progressive muscle atrophy, is still unclear.

3.1.3.2 Clinical Manifestation

In the early stage of the disease, the prominent symptoms are the weakness of the pelvic girdle muscles and the hypertrophy of the calf. Duchenne muscular dystrophy (DMD) is a common X-linked recessive fatal muscle disease, which is more common in men and accounts for about 1/3500 live births of male infants. The disease usually occurs at 3–5 years old, mainly manifested as progressive weakness and atrophy of skeletal muscles of the whole body and pseudohypertrophy of calf gastrocnemius muscle, and gradually secondary to lower limb deformity, with talipes equinus being the most common (Fig. 3.3). With the gradual aggravation of the disease, it may lose walking function at about 12 years old and died of respiratory muscle atrophy, weakness, respiratory and heart failure at about 12 years old.

3.1.3.3 Treatment Principle

At present, there is no definite treatment for the cause. Orthopedic treatment is mainly suitable for patients who could walk independently. When the deformity of lower limbs (mainly ankle joint) occurs contracture and affects standing and walking, soft tissue release or bony osteotomy can be used to correct the deformity and restore the gravity line of lower limbs, but the time of lying in bed must be delayed after operation, and early exercise and walking should be carried out.

3.1.4 Hereditary Spastic Paraplegia

3.1.4.1 Etiology

Hereditary spastic paraplegia (HSP) is an inherited neurodegenerative disease caused by the injury of corticospinal tract. It has obvious genetic heterogeneity and various genetic forms.

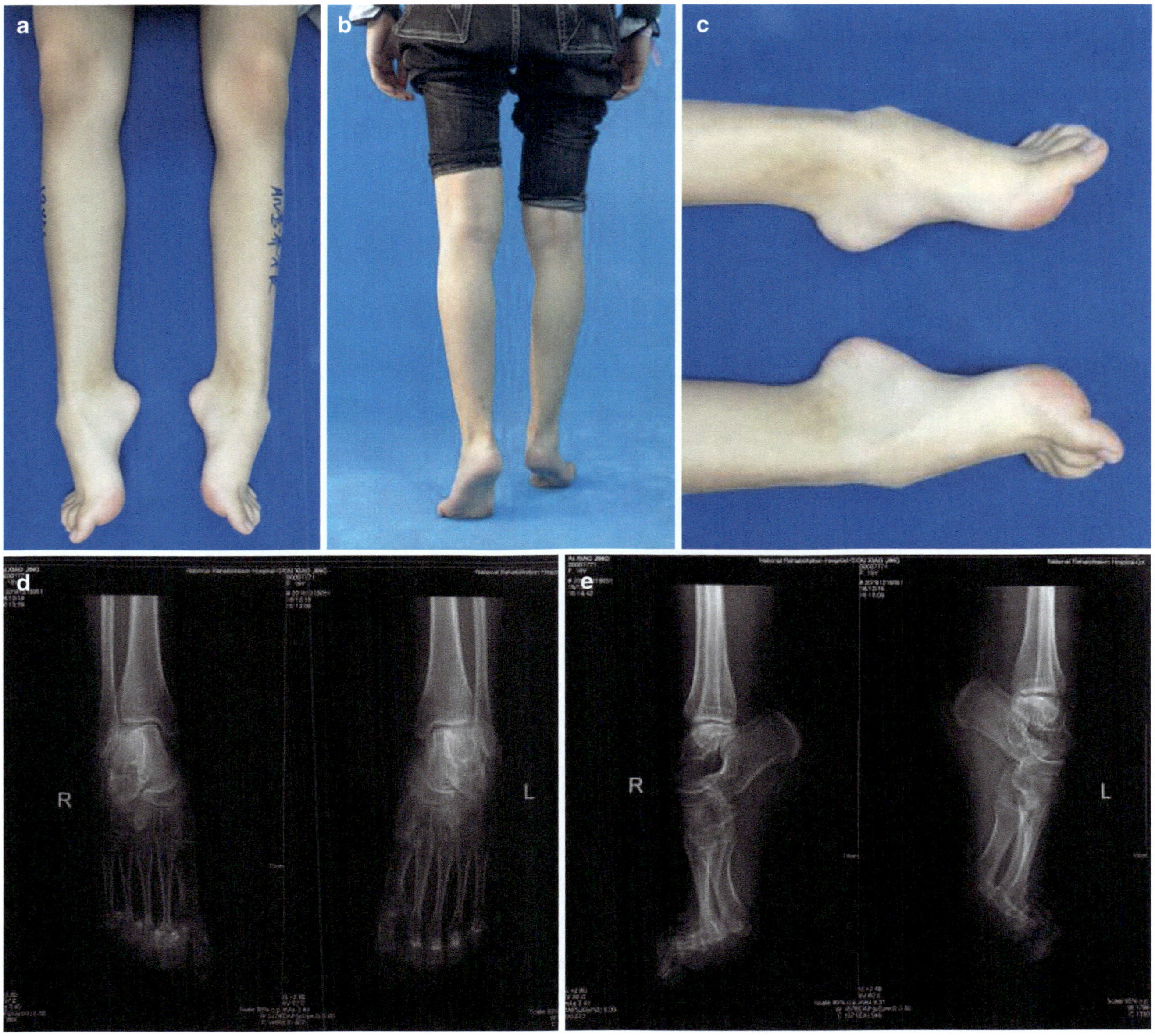

Fig. 3.3 Limb deformity after progressive muscular dystrophy. (**a**) Supine position, full-length frontal view of both lower extremities; (**b**) Posterior view of the full length of both lower limbs, bilateral talipes equinus deformity; (**c**) Bipedal local view; (**d**, **e**). Anteroposterior and lateral radiographs of both ankles, bilateral talipes equinus deformity

3.1.4.2 Clinical Manifestation

The clinical manifestations were slowly progressive spastic muscle weakness of both lower limbs, hypertonia, hyperactive tendon reflexes, knee and ankle clonus, positive pathological signs, scissors gait, talipes equinovarus deformity, etc. (Fig. 3.4). According to the clinical manifestations, it can be divided into simple type and complex type. The simple type only shows spastic paraplegia, while the complex type can also be combined with muscular atrophy, mental retardation, dementia, ataxia, polyneuropathy, optic atrophy, retinitis pigmentosa, deafness, extrapyramidal symptoms, skin lesions, and so on.

3.1.4.3 Treatment Principle

Orthopedic treatment mainly aims at the correction of limb deformities and the improvement of function. Through the release of soft tissues and peripheral nerves, joint fixation relieves spasticity, achieves the dynamic and static balance of limbs, and improves standing and walking function.

3.1.5 Achondroplasia

3.1.5.1 Etiology

Achondroplasia (ACH) is an autosomal dominant genetic disease, which is due to the defect of endochondral ossification affecting the growth and development of long bones. The clinical manifestation is a special type of short stature (adult height < 130 cm), short-limbed dwarfism.

3.1.5.2 Clinical Manifestation

The main manifestations of this disease are skeletal system deformities: characteristic short-limbed dwarfism, short limbs found at birth, limbs out of proportion to the length of the trunk, thick and short fingers, separated like a "trident," elbow joints cannot be straightened, and genu varum may occur in both lower limbs due to joint relaxation (Fig. 3.5). Trunk development is similar to normal, ribs are short, sternum is short and wide, thorax is flat, which can be manifested as mild thoracic vertebra protrusion, lumbar vertebra

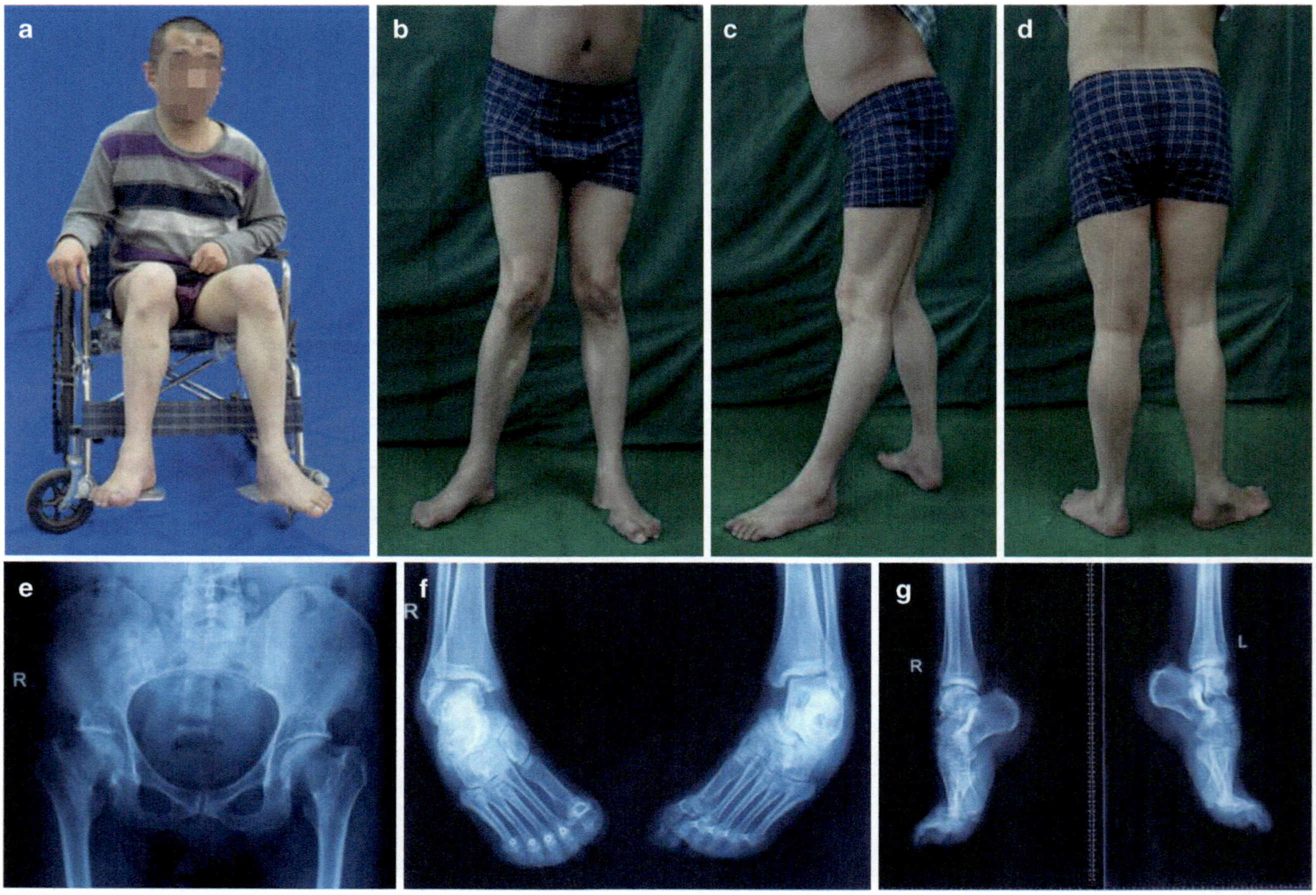

Fig. 3.4 Limb deformity caused by hereditary spastic paraplegia. (**a**) Patients travel in wheelchairs all year round; (**b**) Front view of the whole length of both lower limbs and eversion of both knee joints; (**c**) View of the whole length of both lower limbs in profile, "bending the waist and protruding the buttocks"; (**d**) Full-length posterior view of both lower limbs; (**e**) Plain radiograph of pelvis; (**f**, **g**). Bilateral ankle anteroposterior and lateral radiographs: bilateral talipes equinovarus

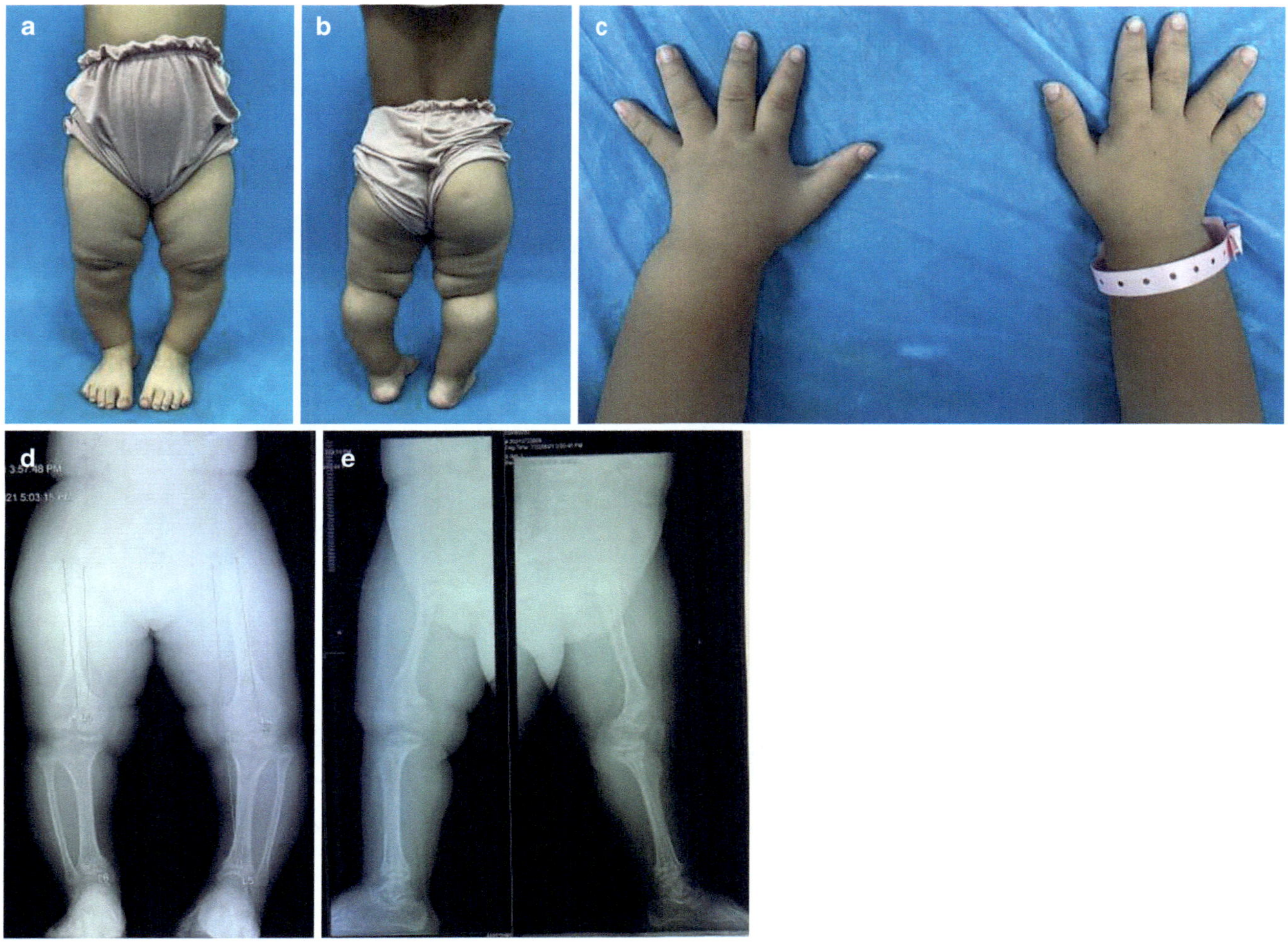

Fig. 3.5 Achondroplasia limb deformity. (**a**) Full length of both lower limbs, frontal view, with both legs turned inside out; (**b**) Total length of both lower limbs, posterior view, "siltation" of knee joint skin; (**c**) The hands are "trident" like; (**d**) Full-length anteroposterior radiographs of both lower extremities; (**e**) Full-length lateral radiograph of both lower extremities

protrusion, lumbosacral angle enlargement, and buttocks are characteristically prominent.

The skull is enlarged, and the anteroposterior diameter is short. The face is broad, the fornix and the forehead are prominent, the saddle-shaped nose bridge, some patients are accompanied by hydrocephalus.

3.1.5.3 Treatment Principle

1. Prevent nervous system complications such as hydrocephalus.
2. Correct limb deformity and moderately lengthen limbs to improve the appearance and function of limbs.

3.1.6 Pseudoachondroplasi

3.1.6.1 Etiology

Pseudoachondroplasia is a specific type of spondyloepiphyseal dysplasia with autosomal dominant and recessive inheritance. It was first reported by Maroteaux and Lamy in 1959. It is characterized by moderate to severe epiphyseal and metaphyseal involvement.

The pathogenesis of pseudoachondroplasia is associated with mutations in the cartilage oligomeric matrix protein (COMP) gene located on chromosome 19. COMP is highly expressed in chondrocytes and synthesized in tendons, ligaments, smooth muscles, synovium, and osteoblasts. Mutations in the COMP gene can lead to two related skeletal diseases, namely pseudoachondroplasia and multiple epiphyseal dysplasia.

3.1.6.2 Clinical Manifestation

Patients usually have abnormal gait since learning to walk, and gradually find short stature, short limbs, short fingers/toes, skeletal deformities (such as scoliosis, bracelet sign, ankle bracelet sign, knee joint deformity, etc.), hip backward and other manifestations. Some patients may have joint pain, and craniofacial and intellectual development are normal (Fig. 3.6).

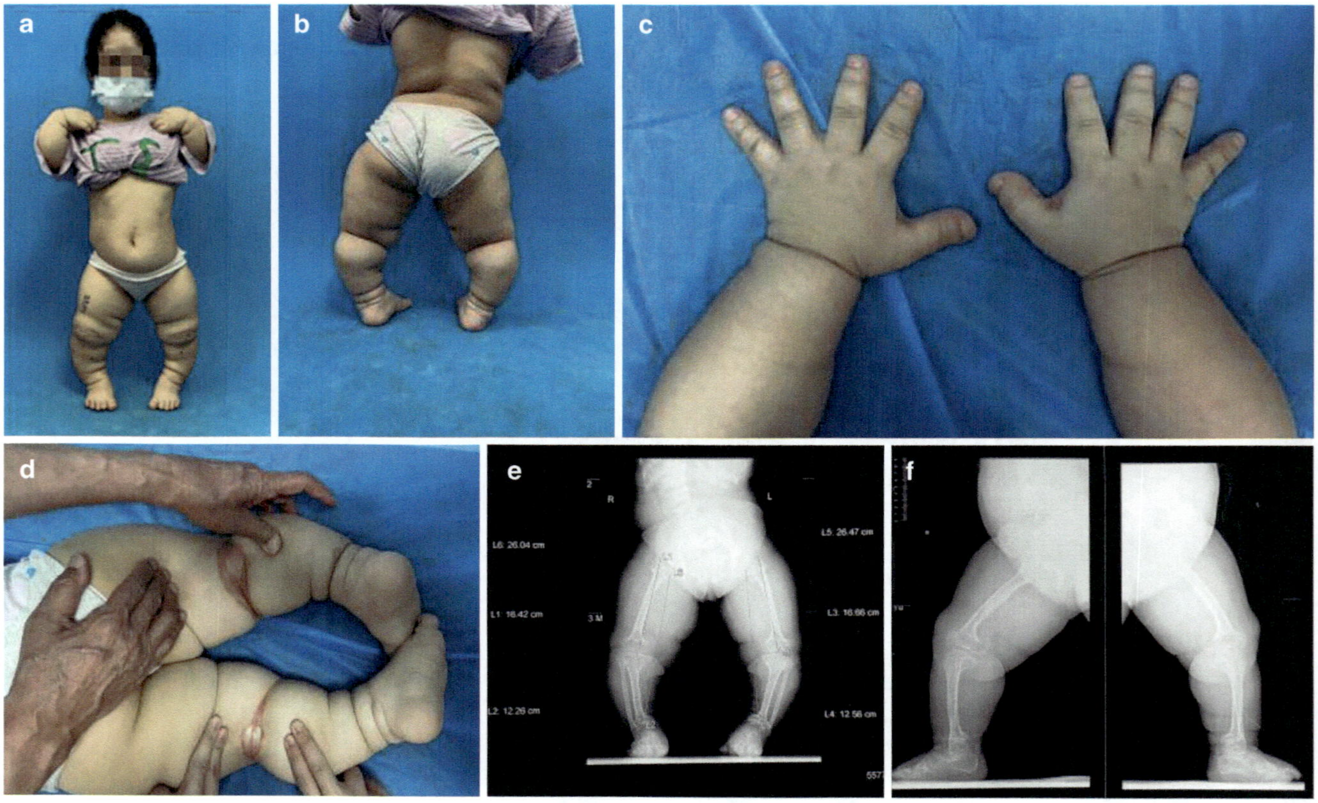

Fig. 3.6 Pseudoachondroplasia is only 110 cm in height in adulthood, with retroflexion and varus of knee joint. (**a**) Front view of full length of both lower limbs, varus of both lower limbs; (**b**) Back view of the full length of both lower limbs; (**c**) Both hands show "trident" changes; (**d**) Multiple skin deposits on both lower extremities; (**e**) Anteroposterior radiographs of both lower extremities, bilateral knee varus; (**f**) Full-length lateral radiographs of both lower extremities with bilateral knee flexion

3.1.6.3 Treatment Principle

1. If the height is less than 130 cm, which seriously affects life, study, and work, limb lengthening should be performed by stages.
2. For patients with lower limb deformity, osteotomy should be performed to correct the deformity of lower limb at the same time, and the lower limb should be extended appropriately to improve walking function.

3.1.7 Multiple Epiphyseal Dysplasia

3.1.7.1 Etiology

Multiple epiphyseal dysplasia (MED) is a rare disease of epiphyseal dysplasia. The etiology of this disease is unknown. It is a rare hereditary developmental abnormality. It is mainly autosomal dominant inheritance with complete dominance, and a few are recessive inheritance. There is a family history, but the mode of inheritance is heterogeneous, even in the same family, the performance is different.

3.1.7.2 Clinical Manifestation

The main manifestations of this disease are pain in hip and knee joints, limitation of movement, difficulty in walking and swaying gait. Shoulder joint movement is also limited. Bone ends are often bulky, and a few patients have joint flexion deformity or joint relaxation. With shorter fingers, thicker fingers and short stature. Because the disease affects the long bones of the limbs more obviously than the spine, it is manifested as a certain degree of short-limbed dwarfism. Besides, there are also genu varum and valgum, unequal lengths of bilateral lower limbs, and kyphosis of the spine, etc (Fig. 3.7).

3.1.7.3 Treatment Principle

1. For the deformity of long bones of lower limbs affecting walking function, before the closure of epiphyseal plate, temporary block of epiphyseal plate or staged osteotomy can be used to restore the normal axis of lower limbs.
2. Osteotomy was used to correct the deformity of long bones and restore the mechanical axis and joint line of lower limbs in patients with closed epiphyseal plate.

3.1.8 Kashin-Beck Disease

3.1.8.1 Etiology

Kashin-Beck disease (KBD) is an endemic, chronic, and deformational osteoarthropathy. It mainly occurs in epiphyseal cartilage, epiphyseal plate cartilage, and articular cartilage of limbs before the closure of epiphysis of tubular

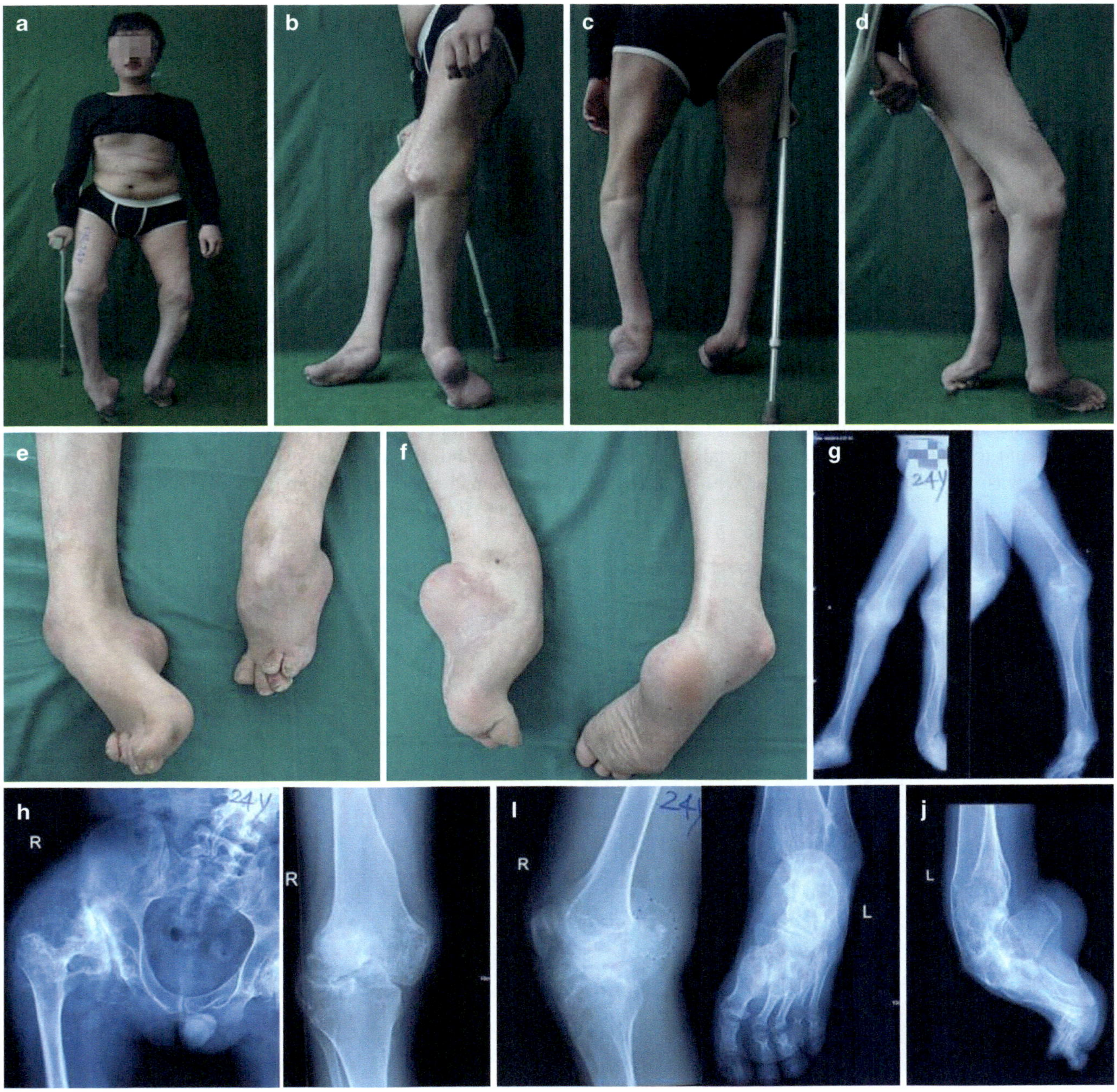

Fig. 3.7 Limb deformity caused by multiple epiphyseal dysplasia. (**a**) Full-length frontal view of both lower limbs, multiple deformities of both lower extremities; (**b**, **d**) Full-length lateral view of both lower limbs; (**c**) Full-length posterior view of both lower limbs; (**e**, **f**) Local view of both feet: severe deformity of both feet. (**g**) Full-length lateral radiographs of both lower extremities: multiple deformities of both lower limbs; (**h**) Abnormal structure of right hip joint; (**i**) Severe deformity of right knee joint; (**j**) Left severe talipes equinovarus

diaphysis in children, resulting in degeneration and deep cell necrosis. It is more common in high altitude areas of Northwest China. At present, there are many studies on the pathogenesis of Kashin-Beck disease, but there is no more perfect theory of the pathogenesis. Selenium deficiency and grain contamination are the main environmental risk factors for KBD, and multiple environmental and genetic factors interact to contribute to the etiology of KBD.

3.1.8.2 Clinical Manifestation

The clinical manifestations of Kashin-Beck disease are multiple and symmetrical joint involvement. Most patients have finger, toe, and adjacent joint deformities at the age of 5 or even earlier, and even leg deformities and osteoarthritis-like symptoms. The pathological changes caused by the disease are systemic, including joints, limbs, spine, and so on. Compared with normal people, the articular cartilage of patients with KBD is severely damaged, and the necrotic area is composed of a large number of necrotic chondrocyte clusters, resulting in focal necrosis of epiphyseal growth plate and inhibition of longitudinal growth of tubular bone, resulting in skeletal dysplasia, short stature, and large bone end swelling in patients with KBD (Fig. 3.8). The disease is mainly distributed in high altitude, humid, and cold valley areas in Northeast China, Northwest China, and Inner Mongolia.

3.1.8.3 Treatment Principle

1. Because there is no specific treatment at present, symptomatic treatment should be given to those who have no obvious limb deformity.
2. Orthopedic surgery was performed to correct the deformity and improve walking function in patients with bone and joint deformities, and artificial joint replacement was performed in patients with severe joint damage.

3.1.9 Melorheostosis

3.1.9.1 Etiology

Melorheostosis is a rare osteosclerotic disease that usually affects unilateral limb. So far, the etiology of melorheostosis has not been determined. Because the hyperplastic bone flows downward from top to bottom along the diaphysis, it looks like wax tears on the surface of a candle, so it is called melorheostosis.

3.1.9.2 Clinical Manifestation

The inchoate that comes on does not have apparent symptom commonly, as the development of the disease can have: 1. Pain, which is the common chief complaint of this disease, local pain, and limitation of limb movement, with different degrees of performance, symptoms alleviated or disappeared at rest, and aggravated at activity; 2. Stiffness of joints; 3. Segmental or complete limb asymmetry; 4. Muscle emaciation; 5. If there is nerve compression, there may be sensory

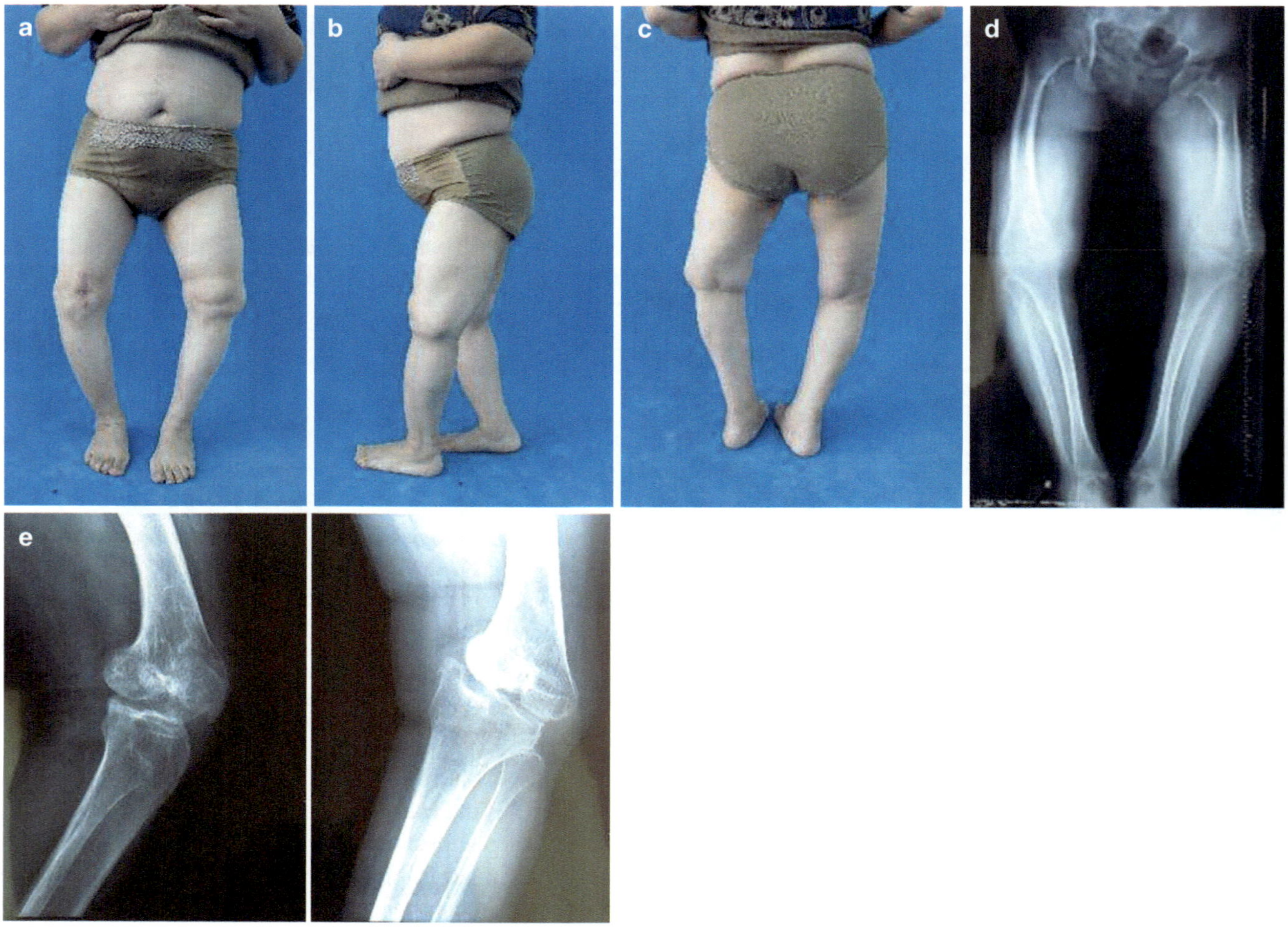

Fig. 3.8 Deformity of both lower limbs caused by Kashin-Beck disease. (**a**) In the frontal view of standing position, varus deformity of both knees; (**b**) Lateral view in standing position; (**c**) dorsal view in standing position; (**d**) X-ray film of full length of both lower limbs in standing position. (**e**) Anteroposterior and lateral X-ray film of left knee joint

disturbance, compression of blood vessels causing soft tissue edema, skin tightness, shiny or erythema.

The typical X-ray findings were as follows: in the long tubular bone cortex, there were continuous or intermittent sclerotic bone strips or plaques, extending from the proximal side to the distal side, mostly confined to one side of the bone cortex, or surrounding the whole bone cortex; The surface of the bone is uneven, like melted and dripping wax, and the density is as high as ivory bone (Fig. 3.9).

3.1.9.3 Treatment Principle

Wax tear bone disease itself does not require treatment, mainly for secondary bone and joint deformities for surgical correction, through soft tissue release and osteotomy to correct bone and joint deformities, improve walking function. However, abnormal bone sclerosis osteotomy orthopedic surgery is extremely difficult.

3.1.10 Gout

3.1.10.1 Etiology

Gout is a crystal-related arthropathy caused by the deposition of monosodium urate (MSU), which is directly related to hyperuricemia caused by the disorder of purine metabolism and (or) the decrease of uric acid excretion, and belongs to the category of metabolic rheumatism. Hyperuricemia is the basis of gout, which occurs when the level of blood uric acid exceeds the saturation of joint monosodium urate and precipitates in peripheral joints and surrounding tissues.

3.1.10.2 Clinical Manifestation

Gout patients often have tophus, which can be seen under the skin around the auricle, joints, tendons, and soft tissues. Tophus are yellowish or white protuberances or excrescence of different sizes, hard in texture and similar to stones. The formation of tophi in various parts of the body, especially in

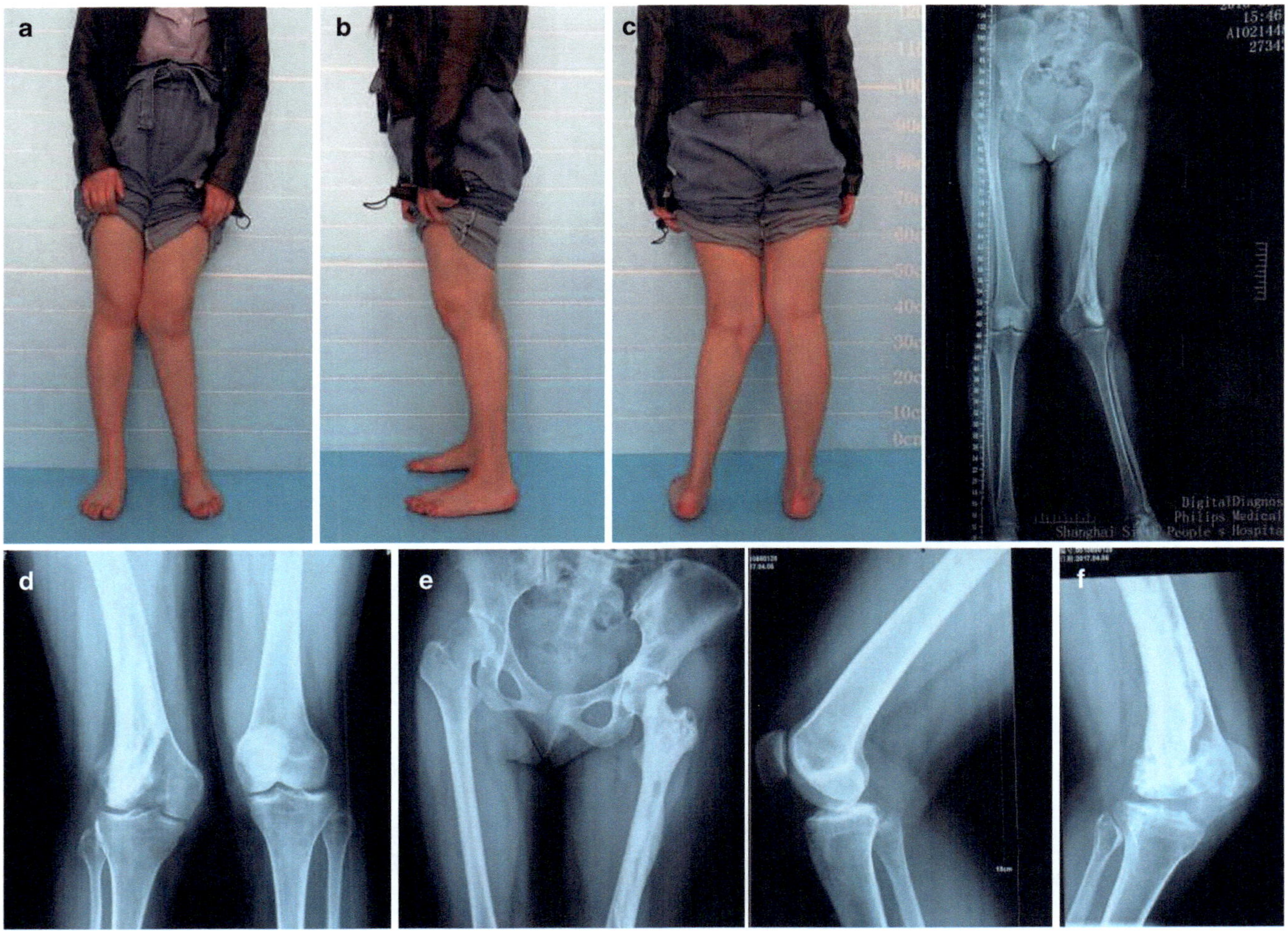

Fig. 3.9 Limb deformity caused by Melorheostosis (**a**) Full-length frontal view of both lower extremities, left knee valgus; (**b**) Full-length profile view of both lower limbs; (**c**) Back view of full length of both lower limbs, left knee valgus, left foot valgus; (**d**) Full-length antero-posterior radiograph of both lower limbs: extensive sclerosis of the left femur; (**e**) Lateral position of both knee joints: the lesion has invaded the knee joint. (**f**) The pelvis tilted to the diseased side; (**g**) Lateral posterior calcification of the left distal femur

the limbs, not only leads to joint deformity, dysfunction, nerve compression, skin ulceration, sinus tract not healing for a long time, but also limb necrosis and the risk of amputation (Fig. 3.10).

3.1.10.3 Treatment Principle

1. Control diet to prevent hyperuricemia;
2. Drug therapy to reduce the content of uric acid in blood;
3. Surgical clearance of tophus, secondary deformities, orthopedic surgery.

3.1.11 Osteopathia Striata

3.1.11.1 Etiology

Osteopathia striata is a rare developmental malformation of bone characterized by bilateral symmetrical longitudinal striations of increased bone density. Genetic and family factors may have an impact on this disease. Voorhoeve believes that it may be related to Achondroplasia and Osteopoikilosis.

3.1.11.2 Clinical Manifestation

Patients have no normal clinical manifestations, generally have no skeletal symptoms, and occasionally have limb deformities. There were no clinical and laboratory abnormalities. X-ray showed that the bones of the whole body were involved in varying degrees except the skull and clavicle. The tubular bones of the extremities were the predilection sites, which were bilateral lesions. The longitudinal striated dense shadows were most obvious in the metaphysis, and gradually faded and disappeared in the middle of the diaphysis. Generally, there are several parallel textures with different widths (Fig. 3.11). The part that grows fast has longer stripes, and the bone between the stripes may be loose.

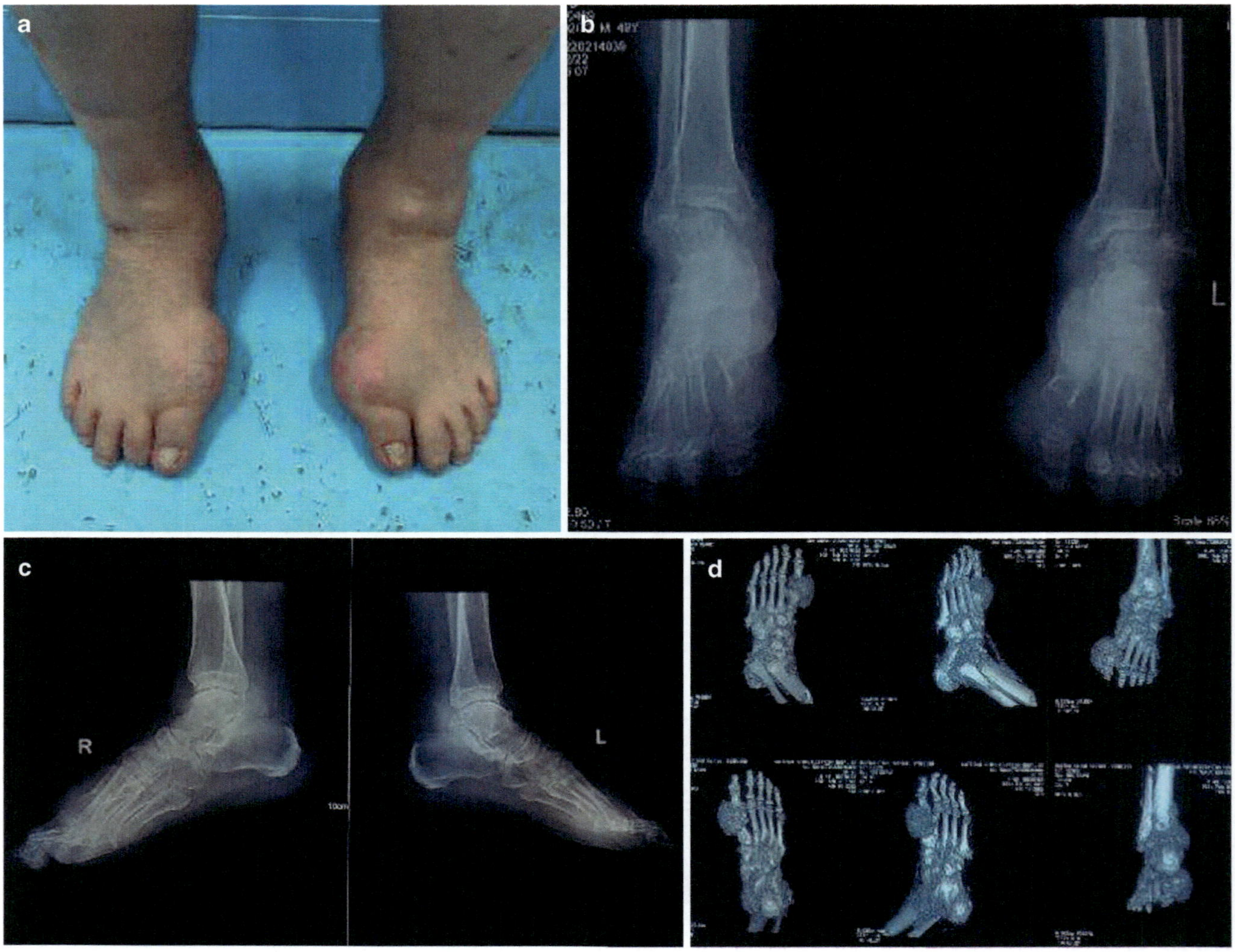

Fig. 3.10 Male, 49 years old, gout. (**a**) appearance photograph of both feet, bilateral first metatarsophalangeal joints, ankle joints, multiple gout masses can be seen; (**b**) anteroposterior X-ray of both feet, bilateral first metatarsophalangeal joints bone destruction can be seen; (**c**) lateral X-ray of both feet; (**d**) CT three-dimensional reconstruction of ankle and foot showed a large number of tophus in ankle joint and first metatarsophalangeal joint

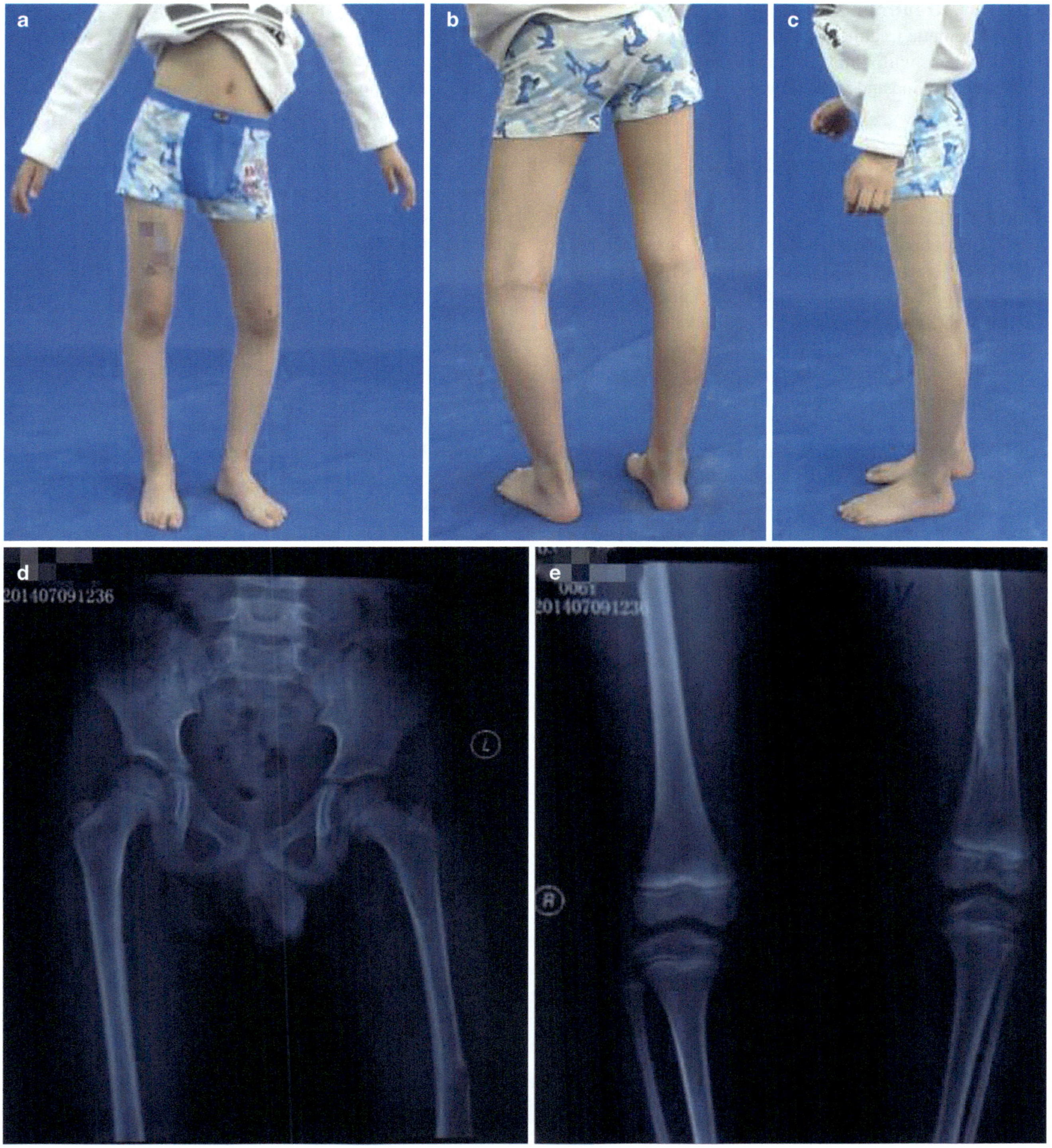

Fig. 3.11 Limb deformity after osteopathia striata of left femur. (**a**) Full-length frontal view of both lower limbs, left knee joint varus; (**b**) Full-length posterior view of both lower limbs; (**c**) Full-length profile view of both lower limbs; (**d**) Bilateral hip joint anteroposterior film: pelvic obliquity; E. The left femur was partially sclerotic with "striated" changes

3.1.11.3 Treatment Principle

1. Symptomatic treatment;
2. For patients with limb deformities, osteotomy can restore the gravity line and improve walking function.

3.1.12 Albers-Schonberg Disease

3.1.12.1 Etiology

Albers-Schonberg disease is also known as marble bone, primary brittle osteosclerosis, sclerosing hyperplastic osteopathy, and chalk-like bone. It is a rare disorder of bone development, which was first discovered by Albers-Schonberg (1904). The etiology is unknown and may be related to genetic factors, which may be a significant lack of normal osteoclasts or functional defects.

3.1.12.2 Clinical Manifestation

It is prone to fracture, mostly located in the bone shaft, and its healing is delayed. Because medullary antrum is narrow, causes progressive anemia, compensatory enlargement of extramedullary hematopoietic organs was observed; fluorosis severe cases showed different degrees of trunk joint pain, limited movement, and dental fluorosis were the most common signs.

X-ray findings showed that the bone density was widely and evenly increased, the bone trabecula became thick and blurred, the cortex was thickened, and the medullary cavity was narrowed or even disappeared, especially in the limbs, ribs, and pelvis (Fig. 3.12).

3.1.12.3 Treatment Principle

1. Symptomatic treatment to prevent fracture;
2. For patients with severe bone and joint deformities, osteotomy is performed, but the bones of these patients are extremely hard, osteotomy is extremely difficult, and there is a possibility of nonunion or delayed healing after operation.

3.1.13 Marfan Syndrome

3.1.13.1 Etiology

Marfan syndrome is autosomal dominant inheritance. Dietz et al. (1991) mapped the disease gene to the 15q15-q 21.3 by family linkage analysis. Chondroitin sulfate A or C and other mucopolysaccharides accumulate in many tissues of the human body, such as endocardium, heart valves, large blood vessels, bones, and so on, thus affecting the structure and function of elastic fibers and other connective tissue fibers, resulting in dysplasia and dysfunction of the corresponding organs.

3.1.13.2 Clinical Manifestation

1. Musculoskeletal system: The main parts are slender limbs, spider fingers (toes), the distance between the fingers of both arms is longer than the body length, the hands hang down over the knees, and the upper body is longer than the lower body; Long head deformity, narrow face, high palatal arch, large and low ear; Laxation of ligaments, tendons, and joint capsules leads to bone and joint deformity (Fig. 3.13); Pectus excavatum, pectus carinatum, kyphosis, scoliosis, and spina bifida are sometimes seen (Fig. 3.13).
2. Eyes mainly include lens dislocation or subluxation, high myopia, cataract, retinal detachment, iris tremor, etc.
3. About 80% of patients have congenital cardiovascular malformations.

3.1.13.3 Treatment Principle

1. Cardiovascular system and eye diseases are treated by corresponding specialties.
2. Soft tissue balance and osteotomy should be performed to improve the shape and motor function of limbs.

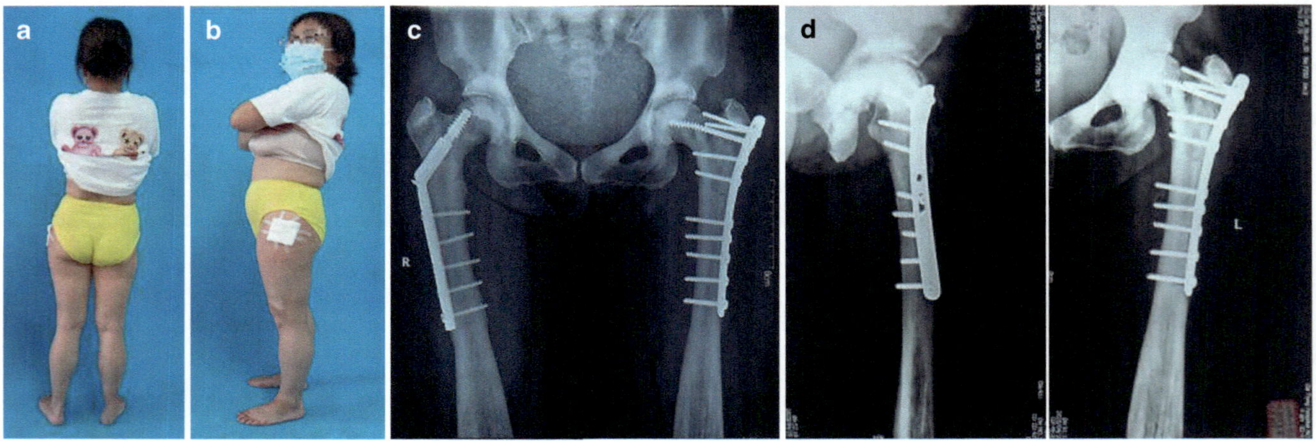

Fig. 3.12 Postoperative deformity of both lower limbs caused by Albers-Schonberg disease. (**a**) Standing position, view from the back of the lower limbs; (**b**) Standing position, lateral view of lower limbs; (**c**) Changes after internal fixation of both lower extremities with pelvis plain film; (**d**) The X-ray film of the left hip joint showed that the bone density was widely and evenly increased, the cortex was thickened, and the medullary cavity was narrowed

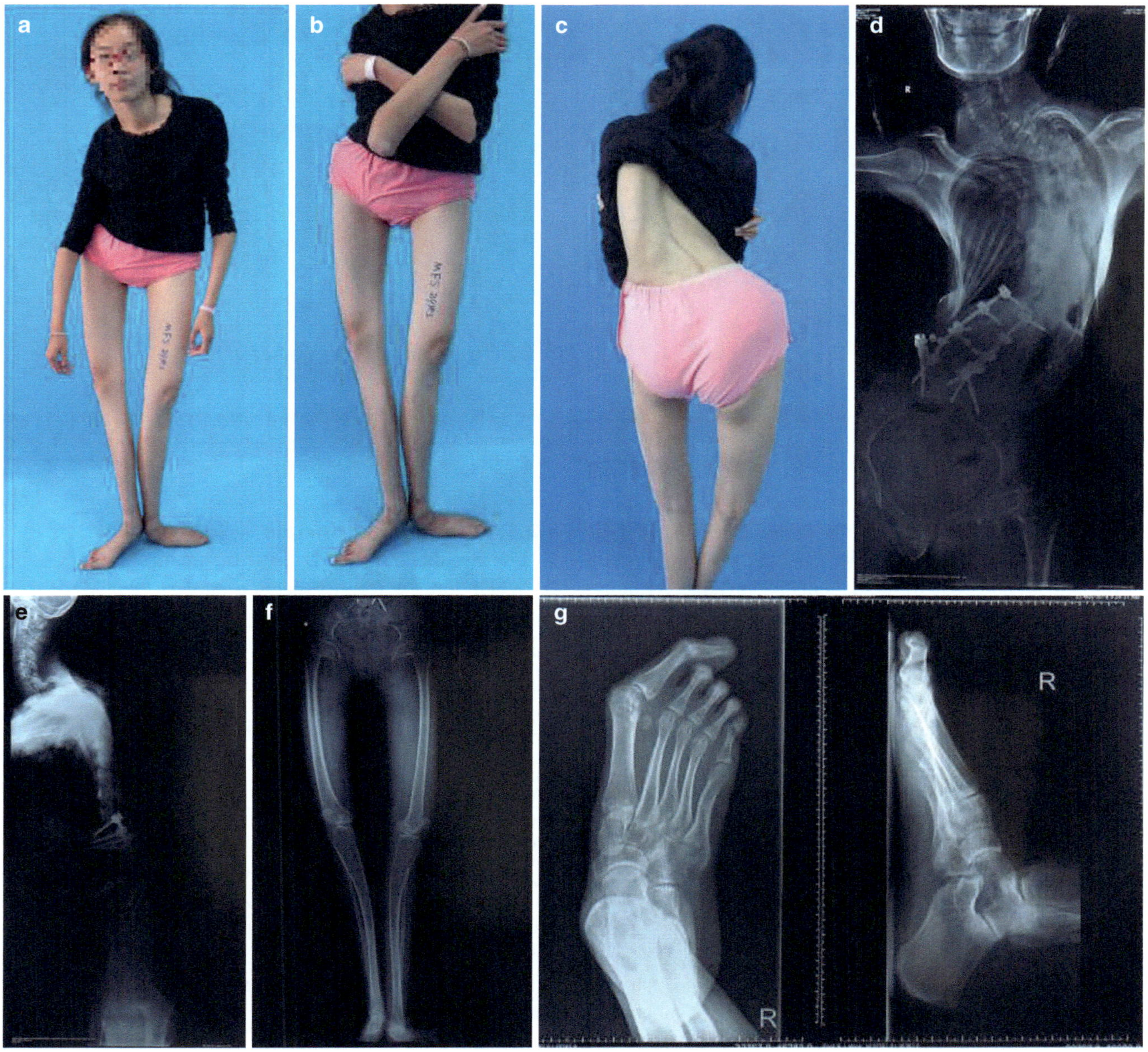

Fig. 3.13 Severe malformation of Marfan syndrome. (**a**) Whole body frontal view, scoliosis, slender limbs, (**b**) Front view of both lower limbs, both lower limbs are slender and deformed; (**c**) Back view of the whole body, severe deformity of the spine; (**d**) Full-length spinal anteroposterior film: spinal deformity, after lumbar internal fixation; (**e**) Full-length lateral radiograph of spine; (**f**) Full-length anteroposterior radiographs of both lower extremities: multiple deformities of both lower extremities; (**g**) Anteroposterior and lateral radiographs of the right foot: right foot valgus, valgus

3.1.14 Congenital Hemihypertrophy

3.1.14.1 Etiology

Hemihypertrophy can be caused by many reasons, such as endocrine abnormalities, vascular abnormalities, lymphatic abnormalities, autonomic nervous dysfunction, embryonic developmental abnormalities, genetic factors, but the real cause of the disease is still unknown.

3.1.14.2 Clinical Manifestation

Patients often show that one side of the whole body is enlarged and deformed, the trunk is asymmetric on both sides, the circumference of the affected side is larger than that of the healthy side, and the development of bones and ossification centers is faster (Fig. 3.14). The upper and lower limbs and external genitalia are asymmetric on both sides, and the internal organs on the same side are enlarged, but the

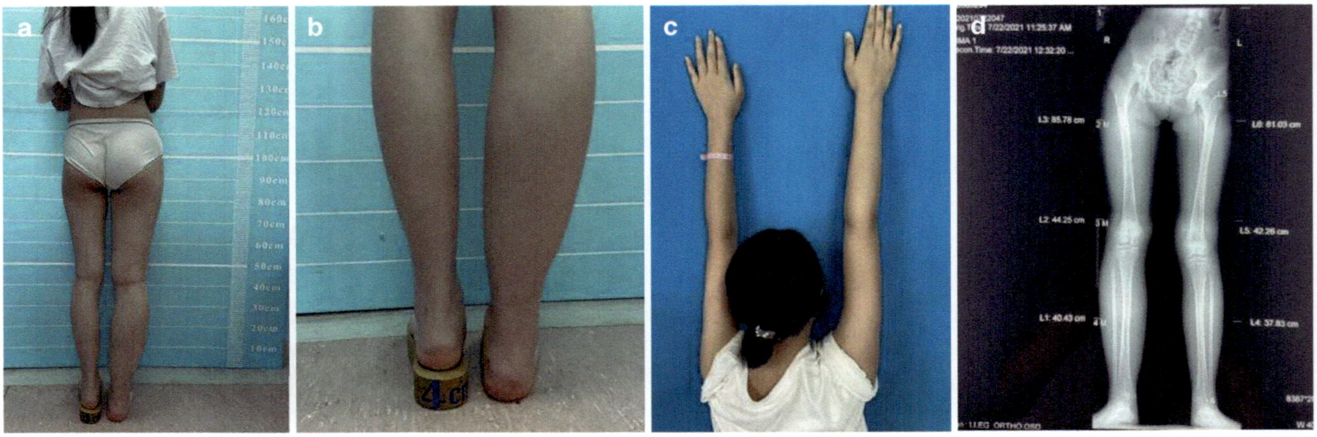

Fig. 3.14 Congenital right hypertrophy. (**a**) Posterior view of the total length of both lower limbs: the left lower limb is small and short; (**b**) Local appearance of both lower limbs, left lower limb shortened by 4 cm; (**c**) From the back of both upper limbs, the left upper limb is small and short; (**d**) Full-length anteroposterior radiographs of both lower extremities, unequal pelvic obliquity of both lower extremities

structure of tissues and organs on each side of the body is normal. Nearly 10–15% of the patients had poor intellectual development, and 50% of the patients had syndactyly, polydactyly, hyperthelia, congenital heart disease, etc.

3.1.14.3 Treatment Principle

Ilizarov limb lengthening was performed on the short limb side or shortening on the long limb side to equalize the length of both lower limbs and improve walking function.

3.2 Endocrine and Metabolic Disorders

3.2.1 Lipodystrophy

3.2.1.1 Etiology

Lipoatrophy, also known as lipoatrophy syndrome, is a very rare disease, which is characterized by the lack of subcutaneous adipose tissue, including extensive involvement and local involvement, with or without abnormal accumulation of adipose tissue in non-atrophic sites. It is often combined with insulin resistance, abnormal blood sugar metabolism, abnormal blood lipid metabolism, hypertension, fatty liver, and other metabolic disorders. The specific pathogenesis is unknown, and the compound heterozygous mutation of zinc metalloproteinase STE24 (ZMPSTE24) in some patients can lead to bone and joint deformities.

3.2.1.2 Clinical Manifestation

Local, half-body or systemic subcutaneous fat deficiency, muscle contour and subcutaneous veins are clearly visible, skin elasticity is weakened, unilateral subcutaneous fat atrophy patients may be accompanied by limb shortening, deformity changes, manifested as unequal length of both lower limbs, joint contracture, genu varum, etc. (Fig. 3.15).

3.2.1.3 Treatment Principle

1. Improve diet and symptomatic treatment.
2. When limb deformity occurs, surgery should be performed to correct the deformity and improve the limb function.

3.2.2 Lower Limb Deformity Secondary to Nephrotic Syndrome

3.2.2.1 Etiology

The nephrotic syndrome (NS) can be caused by a variety of etiological factors. It is a group of clinical symptoms characterized by increased glomerular basement membrane permeability, massive proteinuria, hypoproteinemia, severe edema and hyperlipidemia. Limb deformities caused by NS may be related to chronic metabolic abnormalities.

3.2.2.2 Clinical Manifestation

The most basic features of nephrotic syndrome are massive proteinuria, hypoproteinemia, (high) edema, and hyperlipidemia, the so-called three high and one low, and a group of clinical syndromes characterized by other metabolic disorders. Long-term metabolic disorders of nephrotic syndrome can be secondary to bone and joint deformities of lower limbs, affecting walking function (Fig. 3.16).

3.2.2.3 Treatment Principle

1. Treatment of primary diseases, symptomatic treatment, and correction of metabolic abnormalities;
2. For secondary limb deformities, soft tissue release and osteotomy were performed to restore the gravity line of limbs and improve walking function.

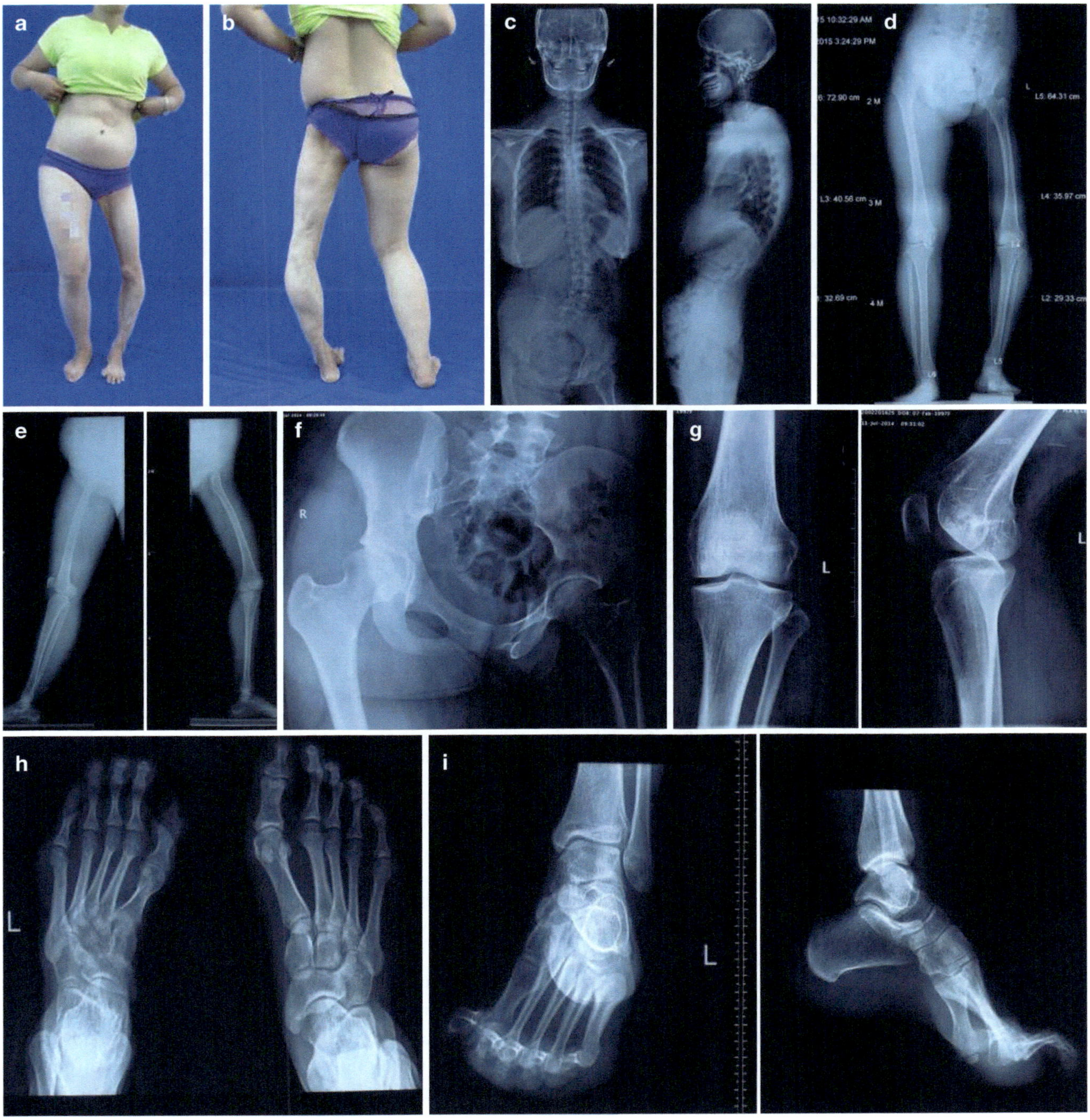

Fig. 3.15 Subcutaneous lipodystrophy of left lower extremity. (**a**) Front view of the whole length of both lower limbs, left lower limb varus, thinning; (**b**) The full length of both lower limbs viewed from the back, left lower limb varus, left foot varus, thinning; (**c**) Full-length spinal anteroposterior and lateral radiographs, scoliosis; (**d**) Full-length anteroposterior radiographs of both lower extremities, with the left lower extremity shortened and varus; (**e**) Full-length lateral view of both lower extremities, left femoral anterior arch deformity; (**f**) Pelvic plain film, left hip dysplasia; (**g**) Anteroposterior and lateral radiograph of left knee joint; (**h**, **i**) Anteroposterior and lateral radiographs of both feet, left varus high arch foot

3.2.3 Limb Deformity Secondary to Hyperparathyroidism

3.2.3.1 Etiology

Hyperparathyroidism (HPT) is a disorder of calcium and phosphorus metabolism caused by excessive parathyroid hormone (PTH) secretion by the parathyroid gland. There are three causes: the pathological changes of the parathyroid gland itself, secondary to other diseases, or neoplastic changes of the parathyroid gland on the basis of long-term secondary hyperthyroidism. In hyperparathyroidism, bone resorption is exacerbated and occurs osteoporosis. It can even produce pathological fractures, which can cause paralysis when they occur in the spine.

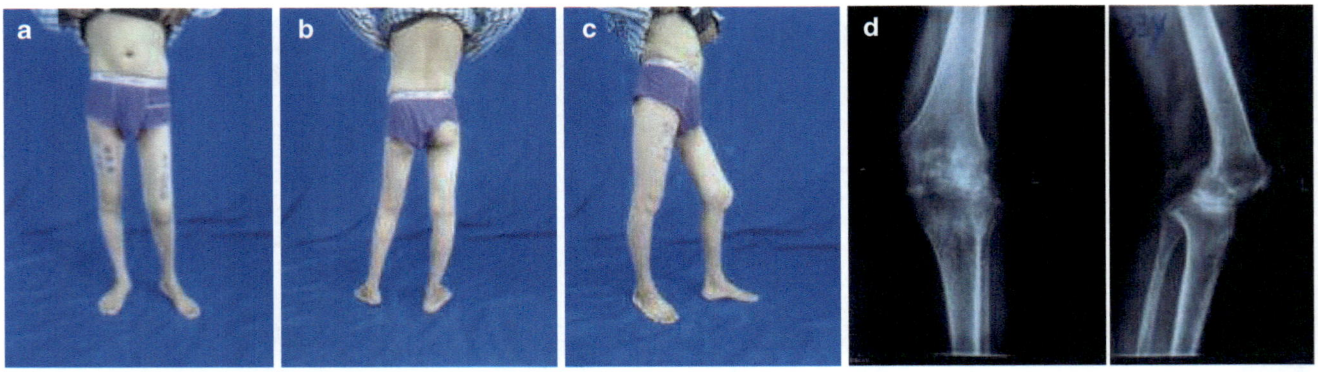

Fig. 3.16 Left lower limb deformity secondary to nephrotic syndrome. (**a**) Full-length frontal view of the lower limb; (**b**) Full-length posterior view of lower limbs; (**c**) Lateral view of the whole length of the lower limb; (**d**) Anteroposterior and lateral radiograph of knee joint

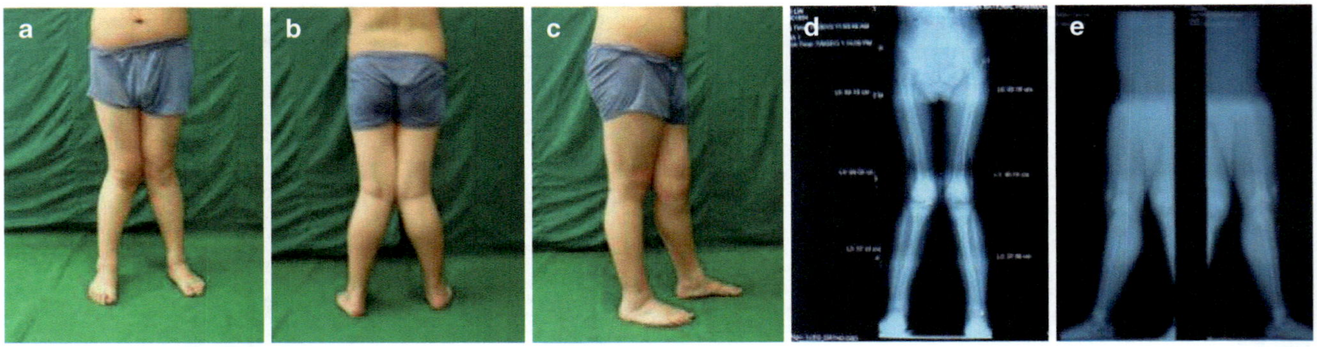

Fig. 3.17 Valgus deformity of both knees caused by hyperparathyroidism. (**a**) Full-length frontal view of both lower extremities, bilateral knee valgus; (**b**) Full-length posterior view of both lower extremities; (**c**) Full-length profile view of both lower limbs; (**d**) Full-length anteroposterior radiographs of both lower extremities, bilateral knee valgus; (**e**) Full-length lateral radiograph of both lower extremities

3.2.3.2 Clinical Manifestation

Skeletal symptoms begin with bone pain, which can be located in the back, spine, hip, chest ribs or limbs, accompanied by tenderness. The lower limbs are unable to support weight and have difficulty in walking. They are often misdiagnosed as arthritis or muscle disease. After a long period of illness, skeletal deformities gradually appear. Some patients still have bone capsule manifestations such as local bone bulge (Fig. 3.17). Sometimes pathological fractures occur, and even bedridden.

3.2.3.3 Treatment Principle

1. Determine the cause and treat the primary disease.
2. Osteotomy can correct deformity and improve limb function.

3.2.4 Gigantism

3.2.4.1 Etiology

The incidence of this disease is mainly caused by pituitary factors, while factors outside the pituitary gland, such as excessive secretion of growth hormone (GH) by the adenohypophysis, can also lead to it.

3.2.4.2 Clinical Manifestation

Adolescents with unclosed epiphyses develop gigantism. After puberty, when the epiphyses have fused, acromegaly forms. A small number of patients develop gigantism from puberty to adulthood (Fig. 3.18). In the early stage of the disease, the general hypertrophy of physique and viscera and the hyperfunction of anterior pituitary were found. In the late stage (declining stage), physical strength declines and secondary anterior pituitary hypofunction occurs. Pituitary gigantism is characterized by excessive growth in childhood, tall stature, and rapid growth of limbs. Excessive appetite and arm strength.

3.2.4.3 Treatment Principle

1. Clear the cause and treat the cause.
2. If deformity of lower limbs occurs, osteotomy should be performed to restore the gravity line and improve walking function.

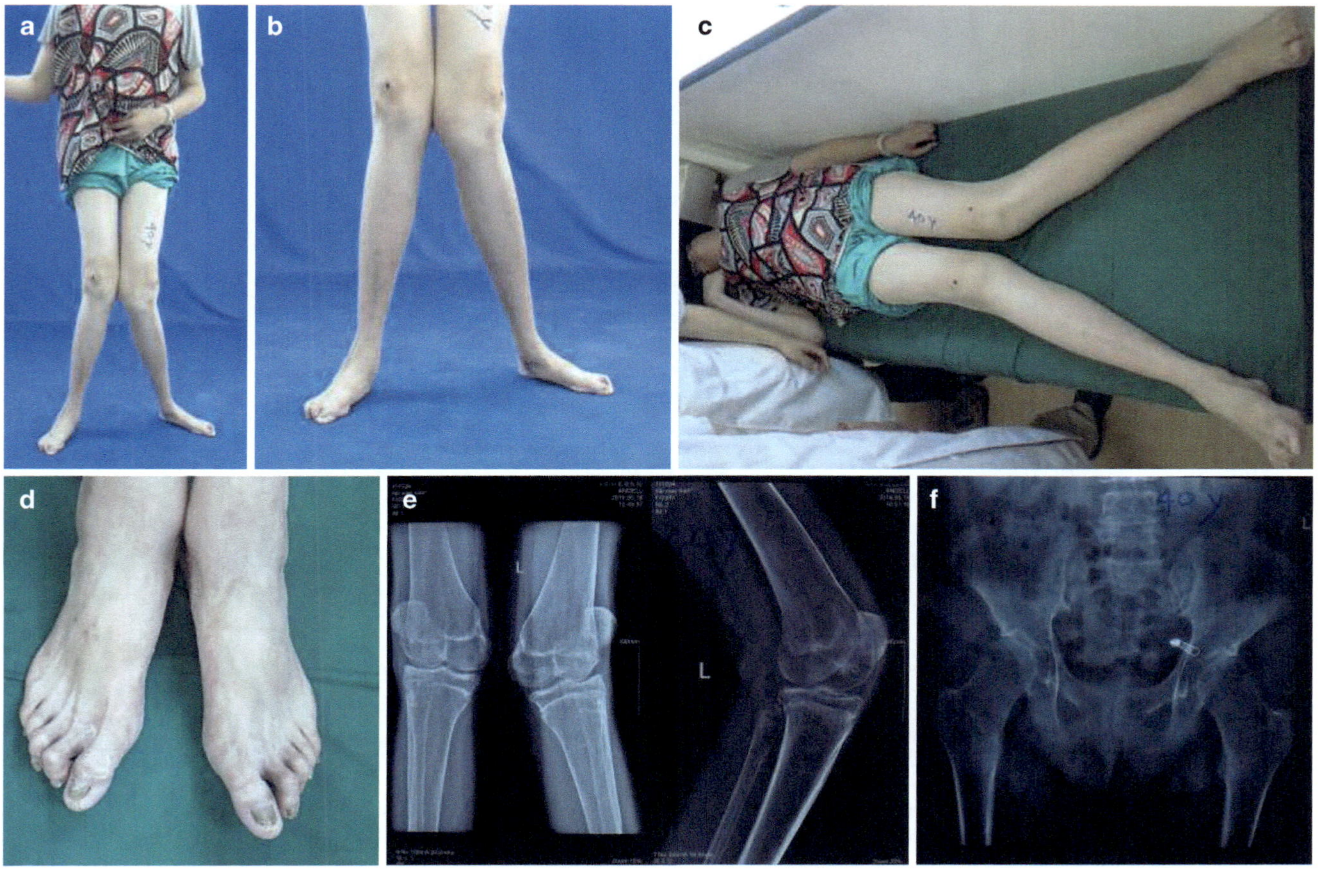

Fig. 3.18 Female, 40 years old, with gigantism. (**a**) Full-length frontal view of both lower limbs, bilateral knee valgus; (**b**) Double genu valgum; bilateral flatfoot valgus; (**c**) Supine position with both knees everted; (**d**) Bipedal local view; (**e**) The patient was 40 years old, but the epiphysis of the knee was not completely closed. (**f**) Plain radiograph of pelvis

3.2.5 Mucopolysaccharidosis

3.2.5.1 Etiology

Mucopolysaccharidosis (MPS) is a complex group of lysosomal diseases with progressive multisystem involvement, resulting from a deficiency of enzymes that degrade glycosaminoglycans (GAGs). Mucopolysaccharides that cannot be completely degraded are stored in lysosomes, which can cause facial abnormalities, nervous system involvement, skeletal deformities, liver and spleen enlargement, heart disease, corneal opacity, and so on.

3.2.5.2 Clinical Manifestation

The clinical manifestations included: (1) physical development disorder: large head, ugly face, prominent forehead and cheeks, much hair and low hairline, small eye fissure, wide eye distance, low and flat nose bridge, large nostril, small mandible and thick lips; Most of the patients showed growth retardation, short stature, and progressive joint distortion after 1 year old (Fig. 3.19). Kyphosis or scoliosis, common genu valgus, claw hand, and other changes. (2) Mental retardation. (3) Ocular lesions.

Skeletal X-ray examination showed that the skull was enlarged and the sella turcica was shallow and long. Kyphosis or scoliosis; the vertebral bodies were wedge-shaped, and the anterior and inferior edges of the thoracic and lumbar vertebral bodies protruded forward like fish lips. The vertebral end of the ribs is small and the sternal end is wide and stream-like; the ulna and radius are thick and short, the base of the metacarpus is pointed, and the distal end of the phalanx is narrow and round.

3.2.5.3 Treatment Principle

1. There is no radical cure for this disease, and symptomatic treatment occurs when symptoms occur.
2. Orthopedic treatment mainly includes the correction of limb deformities. The goal of deformity correction is to restore the gravity line of lower limbs, stabilize joints, improve the function of standing and walking, increase the range of motion of joints, reduce pain and other discomforts, and facilitate self-care in daily life.

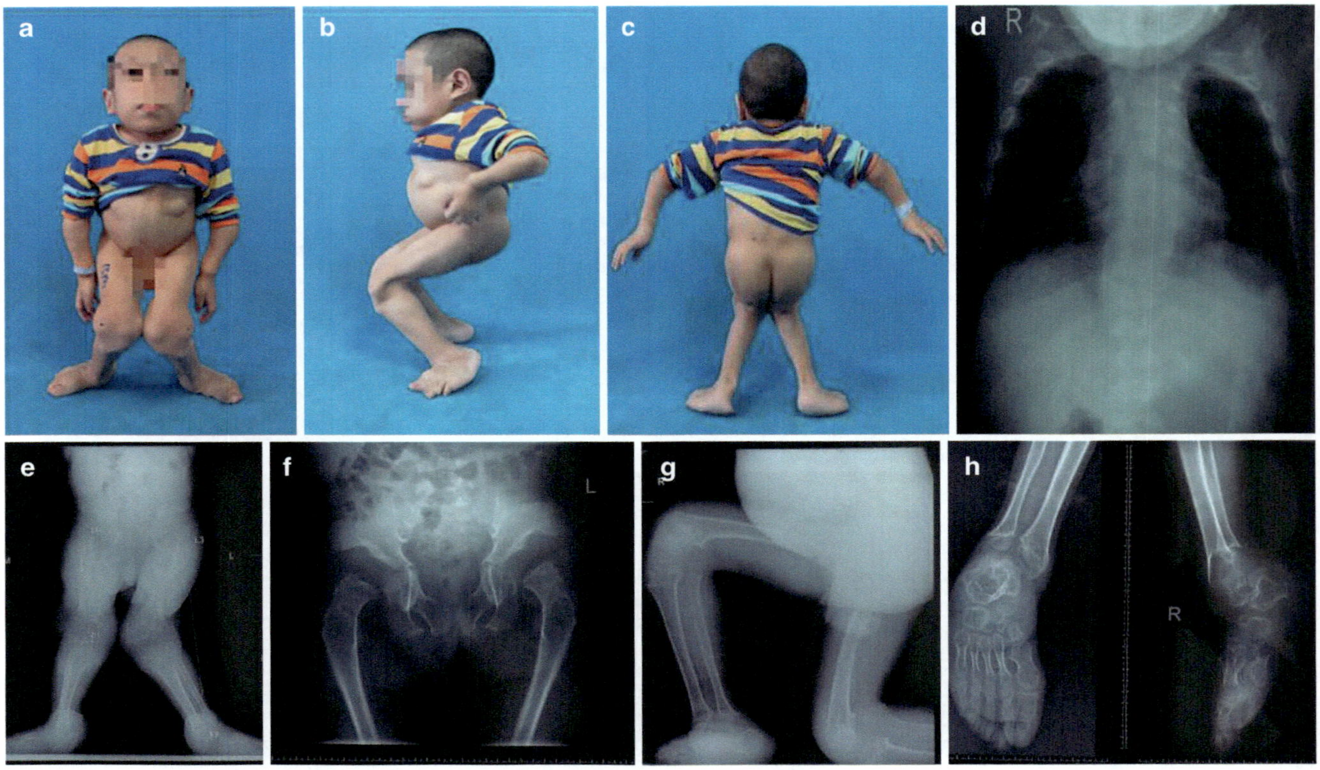

Fig. 3.19 Bilateral knee flexion and varus deformity caused by mucopolysaccharidosis. (**a**) Full-length frontal view of both lower extremities, severe hip flexion and knee flexion; (**b**) Full-length profile view of both lower extremities; (**c**) Full-length posterior view of both lower limbs; (**d**) Full-length spinal anteroposterior radiograph; (**e**) Full-length anteroposterior radiographs of both lower extremities, severe deformity of both lower extremities; (**f**) Anteroposterior radiograph of bilateral hip joint; (**g**) Lateral film of right knee joint, severe deformity of knee joint; (**h**) Anteroposterior and lateral radiograph of right ankle joint

3.2.6 Vitamin D-Dependent Rickets

3.2.6.1 Etiology

Vitamin D-dependent rickets is a rare autosomal recessive inheritance, which can be divided into type I and type II vitamin D-dependent rickets according to the etiology.

3.2.6.2 Clinical Manifestations

Similar to vitamin D deficiency rickets, children often suffer from genu varus deformity of lower limbs when they are standing and learning to walk at the age of 1 or so, which is found by their families. With the increase of age, the deformity of lower limbs is aggravated, or symptoms such as bone pain, cramps, and muscle weakness occur. Biochemical examination showed that the blood calcium was low, the phosphorus was normal or high, the response to physiological amount of active vitamin D3 treatment was good, and there was obvious dependence.

If the patient is in childhood and adolescence, without reasonable drug and orthopedic treatment of lower limbs, he will suffer from refractory bone and joint deformity of lower limbs in adulthood, with short stature and severe dysfunction (Fig. 3.20).

3.2.6.3 Treatment Principles

Vitamin D3 and calcium were used intermittently according to the severity of the disease. Those with lower limb deformities were treated with brace in the early stage. Those with obvious bone and joint deformities were treated with limited orthopedic surgery combined with external fixation.

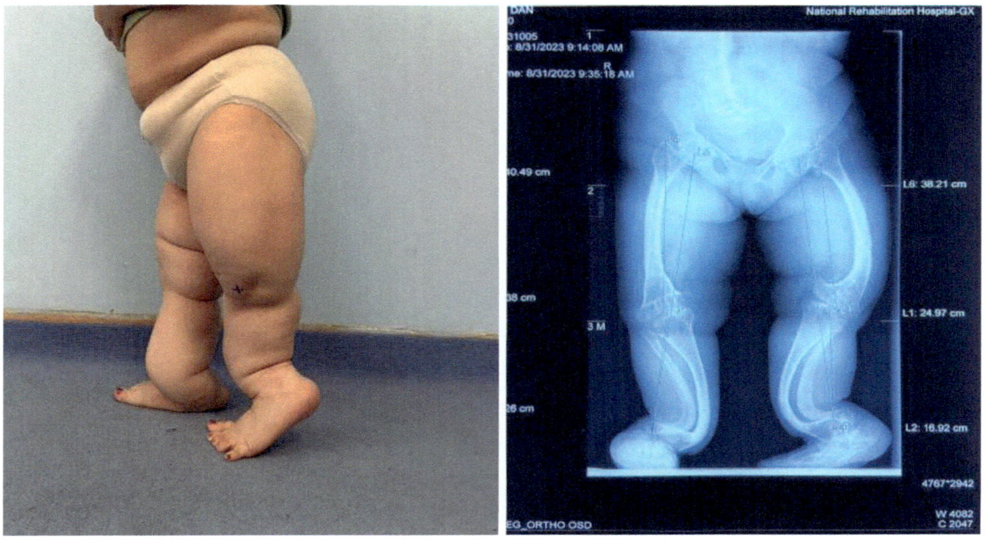

Fig. 3.20 A 27-year-old female with vitamin D-dependent rickets developed severe compound deformity of both legs and ankles under weight-bearing stress due to delayed treatment

4 Developmental Deformity of Lower Limbs

Sihe Qin

4.1 The Hip and Knee Related Diseases

4.1.1 Acetabular Dysplasia in Children and Adolescents

4.1.1.1 Etiology

Acetabular dysplasia in childhood can be caused by congenital sequelae of cerebral palsy, sequelae of brain trauma, spina bifida, poliomyelitis, and other causes.

4.1.1.2 Clinical Manifestation

Most children with acetabular dysplasia have no obvious symptoms of discomfort. Congenital acetabular dysplasia is usually asymptomatic and has no abnormal signs in childhood and is often found on occasional pelvic radiographs. Acetabular dysplasia caused by other reasons, such as cerebral palsy and spina bifida sequelae (Fig. 4.1), may be accompanied by abnormal gait. Radiographs of the pelvis showed poor coverage of the acetabulum with an increased acetabular index; discontinuity in the Shenton and Calve line; CE angle decreases; and Sharp angle increases.

4.1.1.3 Treatment Principle

Periacetabular osteotomy was performed to increase femoral head coverage. Femoral subtrochanteric rotation osteotomy was performed in patients with increased femoral anteversion.

4.1.2 Developmental Subluxation of Hip Joint Caused by Hip Adductor Spasm

4.1.2.1 Etiology

Cerebral palsy sequelae, brain trauma sequelae, tethered cord, and other reasons, leading to adductor spasm, hip joint sustained adduction traction, can cause hip subluxation, acetabular dysplasia.

4.1.2.2 Clinical Manifestation

Spastic paralysis of the lower extremities may be bilateral or unilateral. Scissors gait was found in most of the patients on both sides, and adduction limp gait was found in the patients on one side. Physical examination showed limitation of hip abduction and contracture of adductor femoris. X-ray film of pelvis showed poor coverage of acetabulum and increased acetabular index. Shenton's line and Calve's line are discontinuous; CE angle decreases; Sharp angle increases (Fig. 4.2).

4.1.2.3 Treatment Principle

Femoral adductor release and periacetabular osteotomy were performed to increase femoral head coverage. Femoral subtrochanteric rotation osteotomy was performed in patients with increased femoral anteversion.

4.1.3 Genu Valgum

Bilateral genu valgum is called X-shaped leg, and unilateral genu valgum is called K-shaped leg. It is caused by the valgum of the lower femur or (and) the upper tibia. It means that when the two feet stand side by side, the knee joints on both sides touch together, and the medial malleolus of the two feet cannot close together.

Genu valgum deformity is one of the most common deformities of the lower extremities, which usually occurs bilaterally, accounting for more than 60% of the total incidence of genu valgum.

According to the Qin Sihe Orthopedic Surgery database statistics (From 1978.05.25 to 2018.12.31; Total number of cases: 35075 cases), a total of 245 patients with genu valgum deformity were treated, including 45 male patients and 200 female patients, with an average age of 21 years.

S. Qin (✉)
Department of Orthopaedics, Rehabilitation Hospital of the National Research Center for Rehabilitation Technical Aids, Beijing, China

S. Qin et al. (eds.), *Atlas of Limb Deformity*, https://doi.org/10.1007/978-981-97-0999-1_4

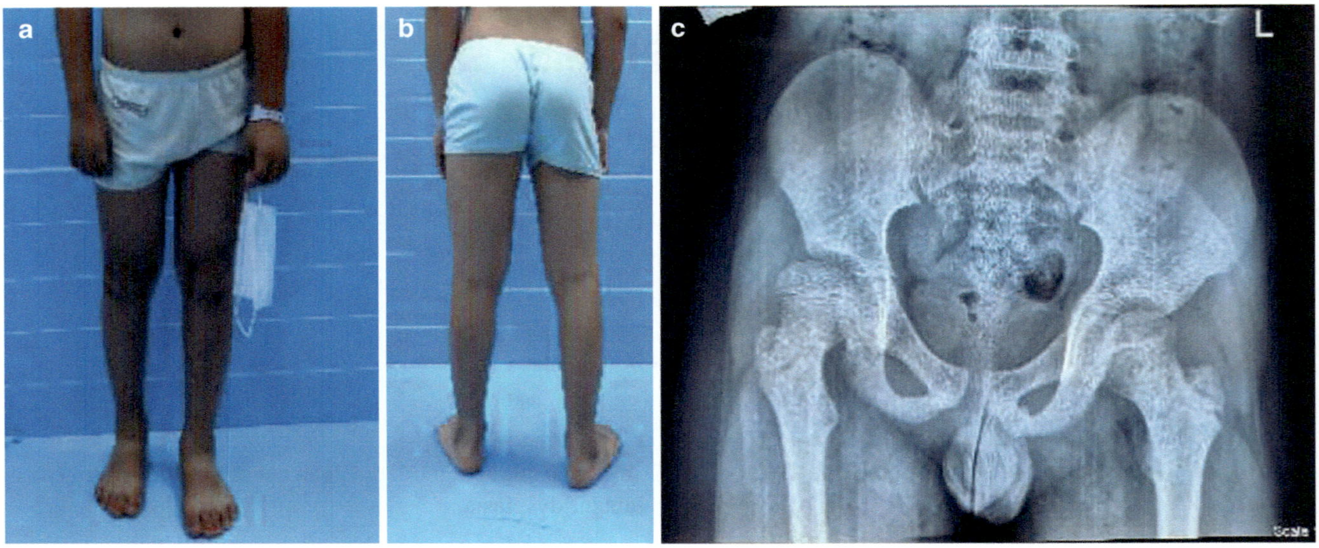

Fig. 4.1 Male, 10 years old, sequelae of brain trauma, spastic paralysis of right lower limb, right acetabular dysplasia. (**a**) View from the front in standing position; (**b**) View from the back in standing position; (**c**) Anteroposterior radiograph of pelvis, right acetabular dysplasia, subluxation of hip joint

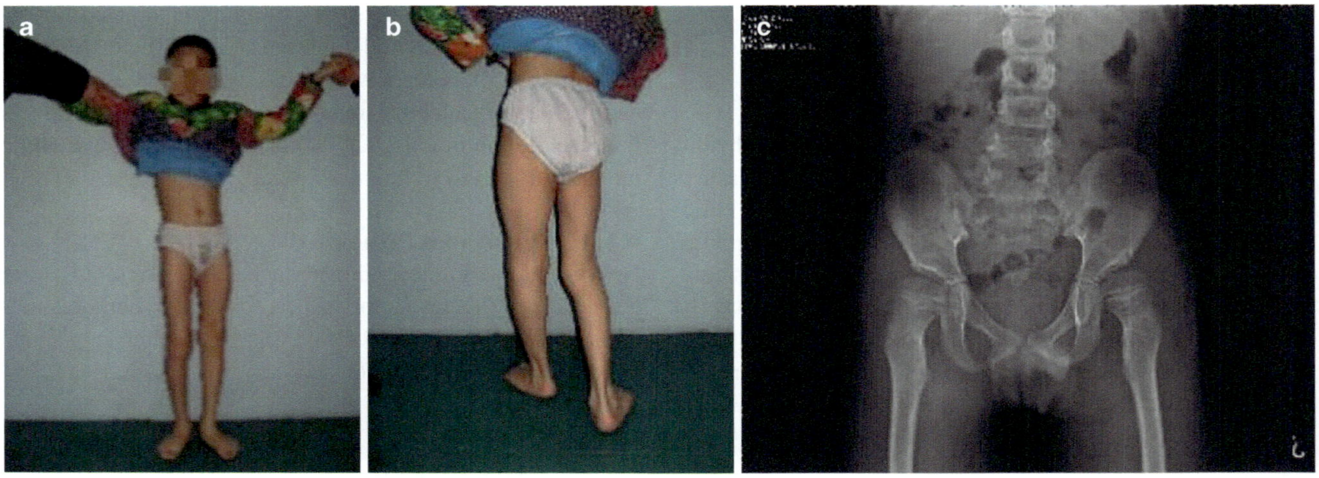

Fig. 4.2 Male, 8 years old, sequela of cerebral palsy, spastic paralysis of both lower limbs, bilateral acetabular dysplasia. (**a**) Patient cannot stand alone but can stand with support; (**b**) Patient can stand with support from the back view; (**c**) Anteroposterior X-ray film of pelvis, bilateral acetabular dysplasia, subluxation of hip joint

4.1.3.1 Etiology

1. Developmental, no clear cause, generally mild deformity, may be related to obesity, obese people are more common;
2. Injury of distal femur or proximal tibia epiphysis caused by juvenile trauma and infection;
3. Metabolic bone diseases such as rickets and osteogenesis imperfecta;
4. Benign tumors of bone or soft tissue, such as osteochondroma and hemangioma;
5. Scar contracture after soft tissue injury around knee joint, such as scar contracture caused by burns, soft tissue contusion and laceration.

4.1.3.2 Clinical Manifestation

The clinical manifestation is the valgus deformity of the knee joint, that is, below the knee joint level, the lower leg deviates from the axis of the lower limb and turns to the lateral side. The X-ray film of the whole length of the lower limb shows that the mechanical axis of the lower leg deviates from the center of the knee joint and is located at the lateral side of the center of the knee. When patients with bilateral genu valgum stand with their knees together, the medial malleolus of both feet cannot be closed, and the shape of the lower limb is similar to the English letter "X," so it is also called X-shaped leg (Fig. 4.3); When patients with unilateral genu valgum stand with their knees together, the shape of

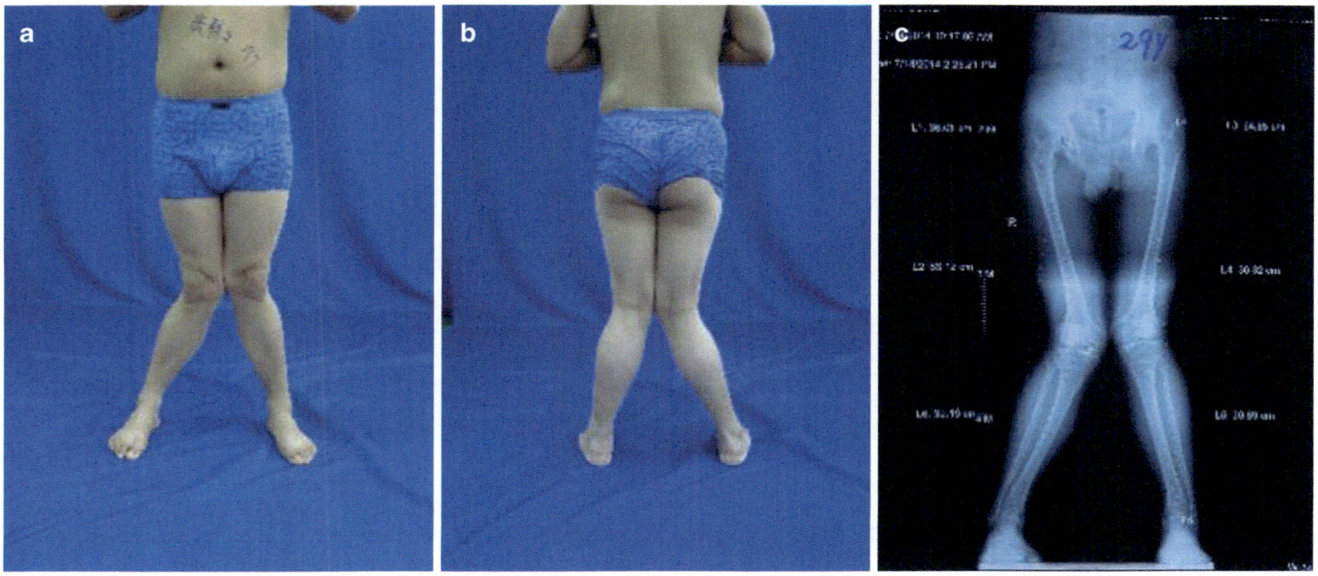

Fig. 4.3 Male, 29 years old, bilateral knee valgus, X-shaped legs. (**a**) frontal view in standing position; (**b**) dorsal view in standing position; (**c**) Full-length anteroposterior radiographs of both lower extremities in standing position

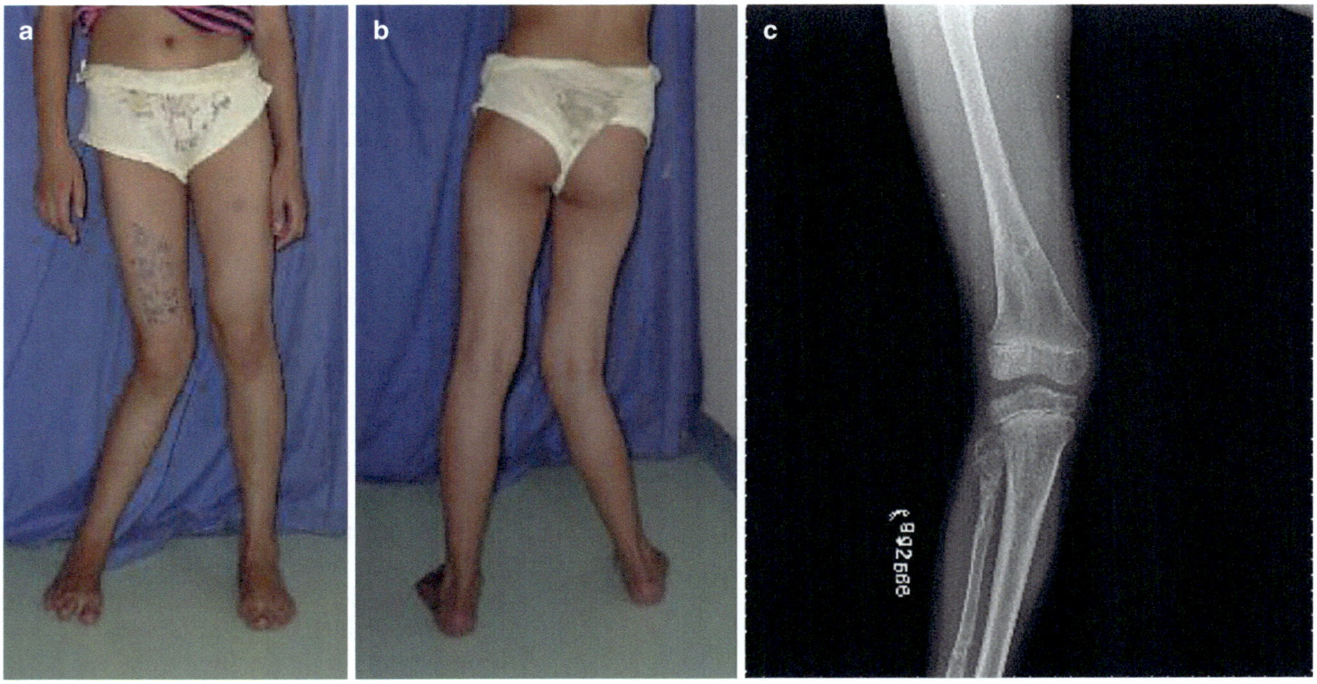

Fig. 4.4 Valgus deformity of right knee, K-shaped leg. (**a**) frontal view in standing position; (**b**) dorsal view in standing position; (**c**) Right knee joint anteroposterior X-ray film

their lower limbs is similar to the English letter "K," also known as K-shaped legs (Fig. 4.4).

4.1.3.3 Classification

Based on the measurement and analysis of the full-length X-ray films of both lower limbs in standing position, Qin Sihe et al. divided the genu valgum into four types (Qin's classification: Fig. 4.5): Type I: genu valgum deformity is caused by the valgus of the distal femur, and the proximal tibia is normal; Type II: genu valgum deformity was caused by valgus of the proximal tibia, normal distal femur; Type III: both the distal femur and the proximal tibia had valgus deformity, which caused valgus deformity of the knee. Type IV: The distal femur and proximal tibia are normal, and the

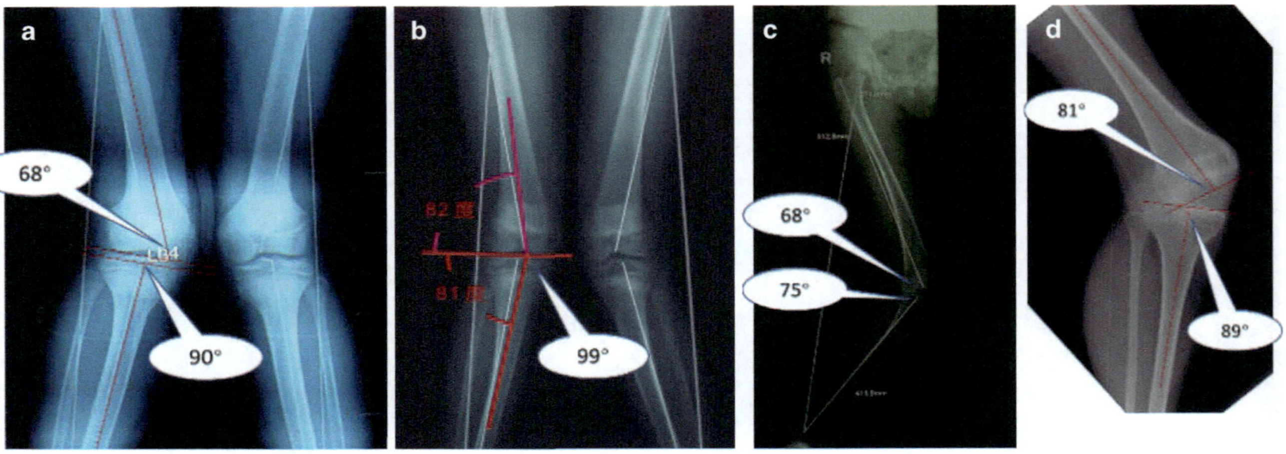

Fig. 4.5 Classification of genu valgum. (**a**) Type I: genu valgum deformity is caused by the eversion of the distal femur, and the proximal tibia is normal (**b**). Type II: genu valgum deformity is caused by valgus of the proximal tibia, normal distal femur; (**c**) Type III: both the distal femur and the proximal tibia had valgus deformity, which caused valgus deformity of the knee. (**d**) Type IV: The distal femur and proximal tibia are normal, and the genu valgum is caused by the relaxation or rupture of the medial collateral ligament of the knee joint

genu valgum is caused by the relaxation or rupture of the medial collateral ligament of the knee joint.

4.1.3.4 Treatment Principle

Patients with bony deformity were treated with osteotomy to restore the mechanical axis and joint line of lower limbs. Reconstruction of the medial collateral ligament in patients with medial collateral ligament laxity or rupture.

4.1.4 Genu Varum

Bilateral genu varus deformity is also called O-shaped leg, and unilateral genu varus deformity is called D-shaped leg. If one leg of the patient is genu varus and the other leg is genu valgus, showing a one-sided deformity, it is called "blowing" deformity. Genu varum is a common deformity of the lower extremities. The intersection of the deformity mostly occurs in the upper tibia. Severe deformity is often accompanied by leg internal rotation deformity.

4.1.4.1 Etiology

Etiology includes: (1) developmental, unknown etiology, genu varus deformity gradually appears in the process of development, because the deformity is mild, it is often ignored. (2) Epiphyseal injury of distal femur or proximal tibia caused by juvenile trauma and infection. (3) Metabolic bone diseases, such as rickets and osteogenesis imperfecta. (4) Tumors of bone or soft tissue, such as osteochondroma and hemangioma. (5) Blount disease, multiple epiphyseal dysplasia, etc. (6) Scar contracture after soft tissue injury around knee joint, such as scar contracture caused by burns, soft tissue contusion, and laceration.

4.1.4.2 Clinical Manifestation

The clinical manifestation is varus deformity of the knee joint, that is, below the knee joint level, the lower leg deviates from the axis of the lower limb and turns to the medial side. The X-ray film of the whole lower limb shows that the mechanical axis of the lower limb deviates from the center of the knee joint and is located at the medial side of the center of the knee. When patients with bilateral genu varum stand with their ankles together, their knees are unable to close together, and the shape of their lower limbs is similar to the English letter O, so they are also called O-shaped legs (Fig. 4.6). When a patient with unilateral genu varum stands with both feet together, the shape of the lower limb is similar to the English letter D, also known as D-shaped leg (Fig. 4.7).

4.1.4.3 Classification

Qin Sihe et al. divided genu varum into four types according to the different parts causing genu varum deformity (Qin's type, Fig. 4.8): Type I: genu varus deformity is caused by varus of the distal femur, and the proximal tibia is normal; Type II: varus deformity of the knee was caused by varus deformity of the proximal tibia, and the distal femur was normal; Type III: varus deformity of the distal femur and proximal tibia, causing varus deformity of the knee. Type IV: The distal femur and proximal tibia are normal, and genu varum is caused by relaxation or rupture of the lateral collateral ligament of the knee joint.

4.1.4.4 Treatment Principle

Patients with bony deformity were treated with osteotomy to restore the mechanical axis and joint line of lower limbs. Patients with laxity or rupture of lateral collateral ligaments need to reconstruct the lateral collateral ligament.

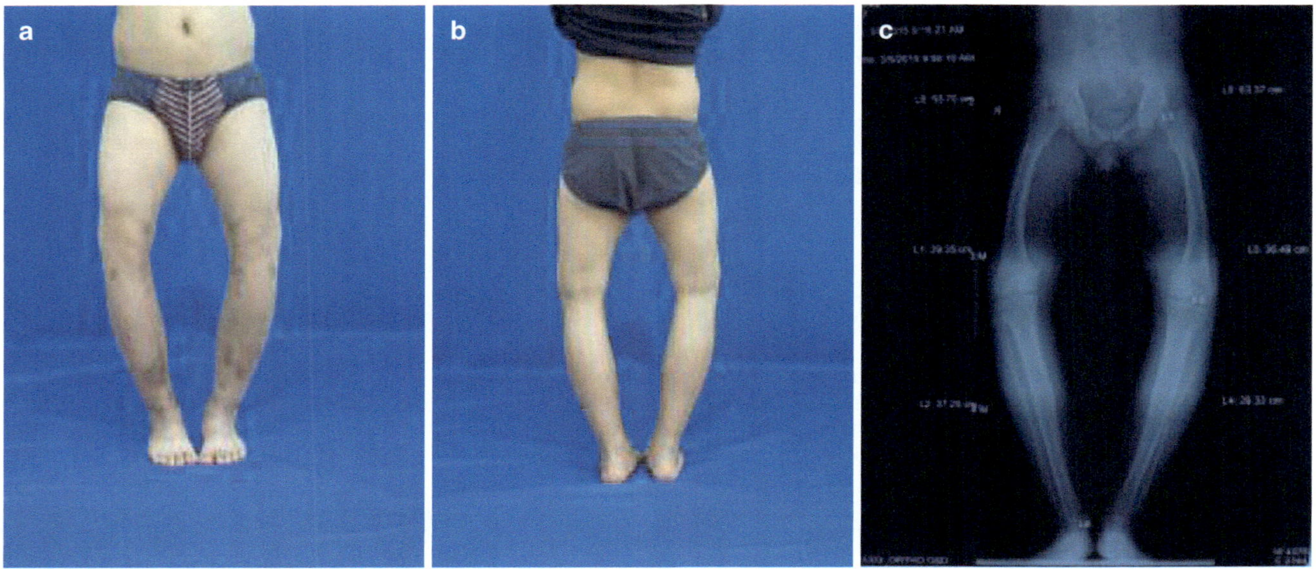

Fig. 4.6 Double genu varus (O-shaped legs) deformity. (**a**) frontal view in standing position; (**b**) dorsal view in standing position; (**c**) full-length anteroposterior X-ray film of both lower limbs in standing position

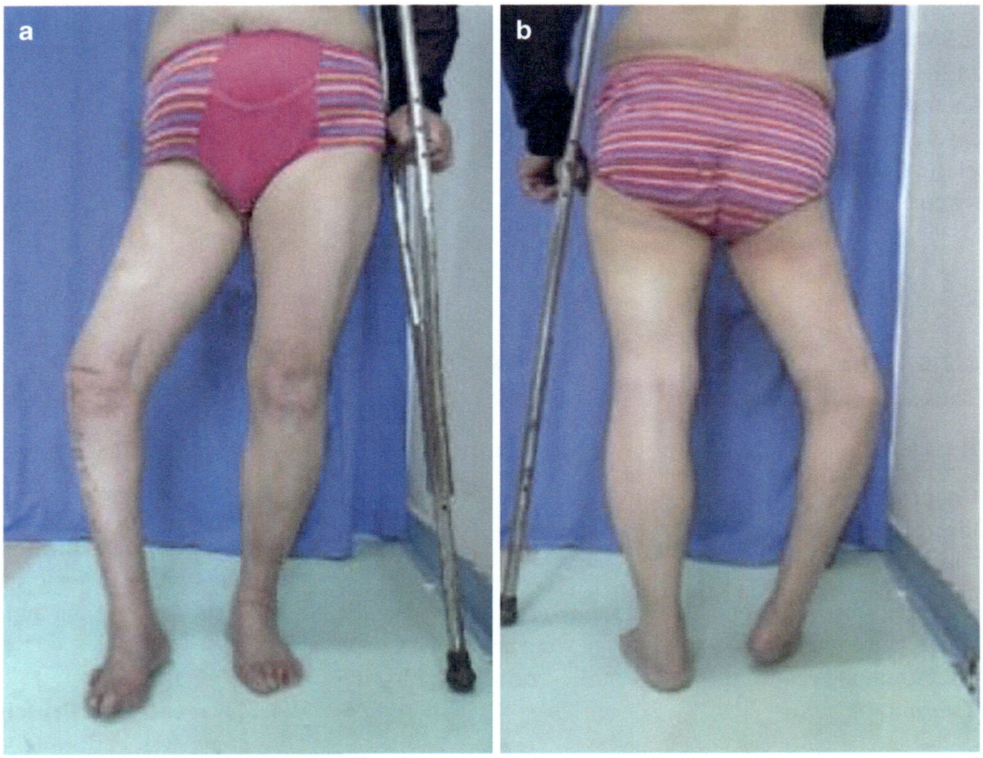

Fig. 4.7 Right genu varus (D-shaped leg) deformity. (**a**) View from the front in standing position; (**b**) View from the back in standing position

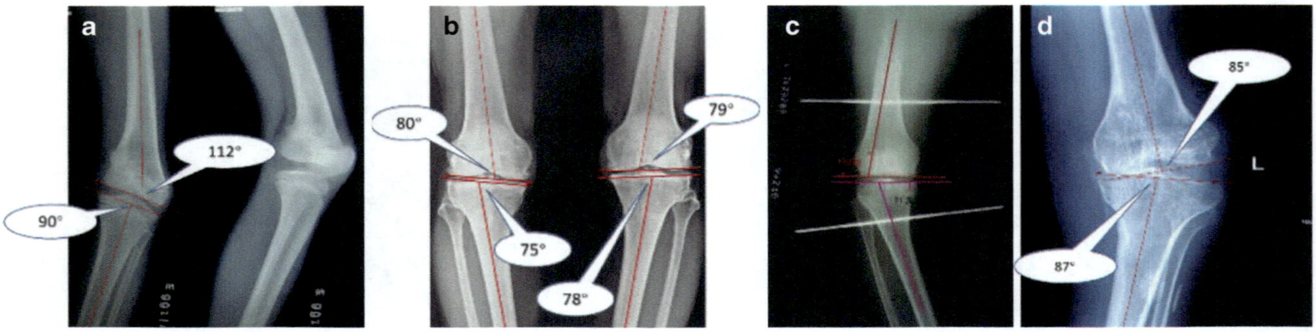

Fig. 4.8 Typing of genu varum. (**a**) Type I: varus deformity of the knee is caused by varus deformity of the distal femur, and the proximal tibia is normal. (**b**) Type II: varus deformity of the knee is caused by varus of the proximal tibia, and the distal femur is normal; (**c**) Type III: varus deformity of the distal femur and proximal tibia, causing varus deformity of the knee. (**d**) Type IV: The distal femur and proximal tibia are normal, and genu varum is caused by relaxation or rupture of the lateral collateral ligament of the knee joint

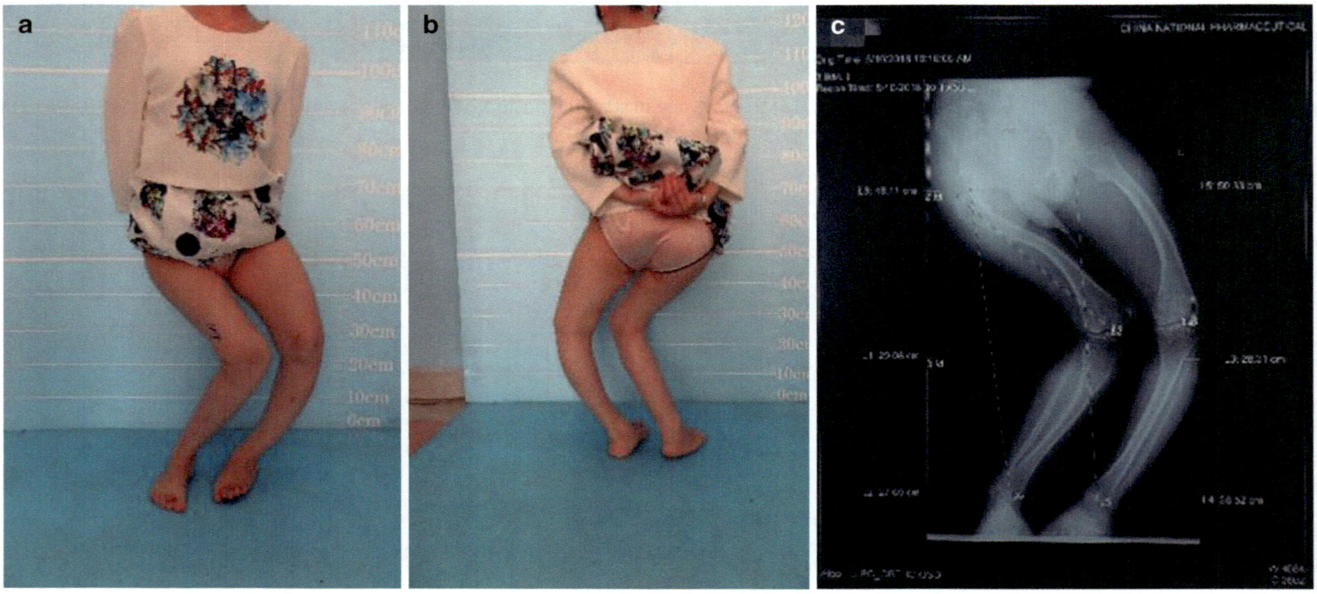

Fig. 4.9 Female, 32 years old, with blowing deformity. (**a**) frontal view in standing position; (**b**) dorsal view in standing position; (**c**) Full-length anteroposterior radiographs of both lower extremities in standing position

4.1.5 Blowing Deformity

Bilateral knee joint, one side is genu varus deformity, one side is genu valgus deformity, like the wind bending the knee joint from one side, the image is described as "blowing deformity."

4.1.5.1 Etiology

The disease is more common in patients with hypophosphatemic rickets.

4.1.5.2 Clinical Manifestation

Valgus deformity of one knee joint, varus deformity of the other knee joint, the angle of genu varus is close to that of the opposite genu valgus, resulting in the knee joint deviating to one side of the body axis; Radiographs of both lower limbs showed valgus and external rotation deformity of the middle and lower femur and the middle and upper tibia on one side, combined with varus and internal rotation deformity of the middle and lower femur and the upper tibia on the other side (Fig. 4.9).

4.1.5.3 Treatment Principle

Osteotomy was performed to correct bilateral femoral and tibial deformities and restore the mechanical axis and joint line of both lower extremities.

4.1.6 Torsion Deformity of Lower Leg

Torsion deformity of the lower leg is a rotation deformity of the lower leg in the frontal plane. When the patella stands in front of it, the toes are not in front of it, but medial (internal rotation) or lateral (external rotation).

4.1.6.1 Etiology

1. Developmental, unknown etiology, some patients with mild genu varum, accompanied by varying degrees of leg internal or external rotation deformity.
2. Metabolic bone diseases, such as rickets and osteogenesis imperfecta.
3. Sequelae of poliomyelitis, paralysis of medial hamstring muscle, lateral hamstring muscle strength above grade 3, due to the traction of iliotibial band and lateral hamstring muscle, secondary leg external rotation deformity, often combined with knee flexion deformity.
4. Patients with spastic lower limb paralysis in cerebral palsy have internal rotation deformity of the leg due to the traction of the medial hamstring muscle.

4.1.6.2 Clinical Manifestation

The main manifestations of leg torsion deformity are: out toeing (external rotation of the leg) or in toeing (internal rotation of the leg); When standing with the patella facing straight ahead, the toes do not face straight ahead, but face medially (internal tibial torsion) (Fig. 4.10) or laterally (external tibial torsion) (Fig. 4.11); In some patients with sequelae of poliomyelitis, severe external rotation deformity of the leg can reach 90 degrees, that is, the knee joint is forward and the toe is lateral, often accompanied by severe flexion deformity.

4.1.6.3 Treatment Principle

Mild leg torsion deformity without other deformities need not be treated. Osteotomy was performed to correct severe leg torsion deformity or accompanied by varus and valgus deformity, which affected the appearance and walking function.

4.1.7 Excessive Growth of Femur after Fracture in Children

4.1.7.1 Etiology

It is caused by femoral fracture of juvenile trauma.

4.1.7.2 Clinical Manifestation

After fracture healing, during the growth and development of the child, the length of both lower limbs was gradually unequal, and the limb on the fracture side was gradually longer than that on the healthy side. When the limbs are unequal and more than 2CM in length, a mild limping gait gradually appeared (Fig. 4.12). The X-ray film showed that the femur of the fractured side was longer than that of the healthy side.

4.1.7.3 Treatment Principle

If the limb length is less than 2 cm and there are no obvious symptoms, it no need to be treated. When limb inequal-

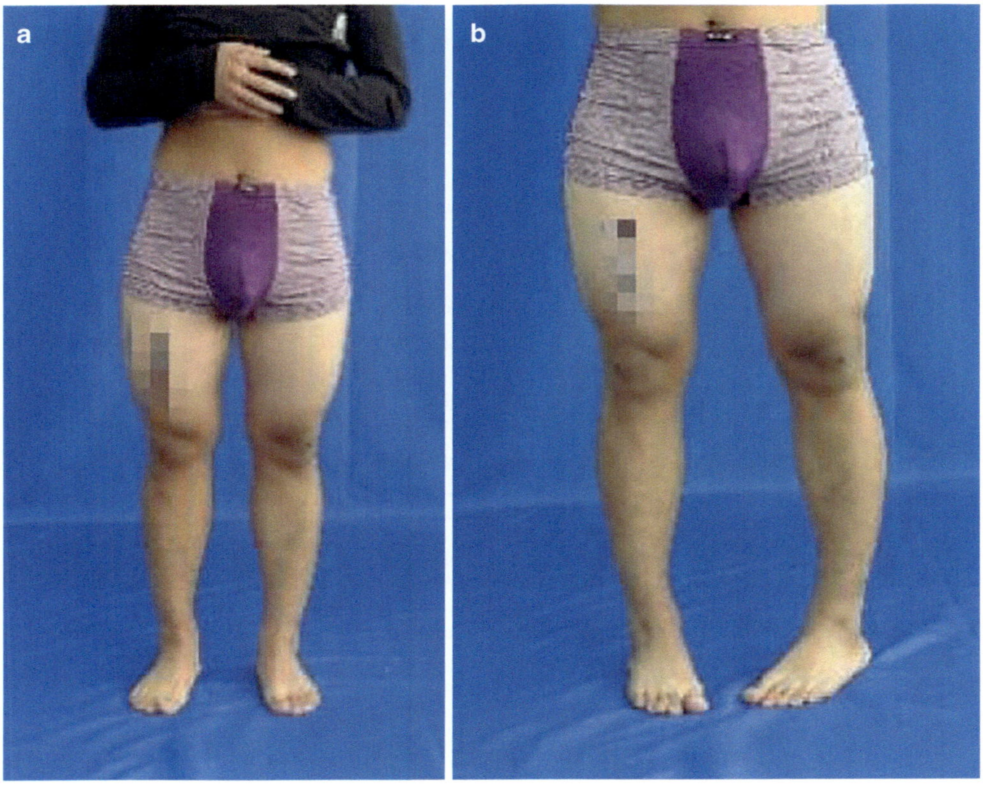

Fig. 4.10 Male, 19 years old, bilateral internal tibial torsion deformity. (**a**) In standing position, when the toes are advanced, the patellas of both sides are facing anterolateral, and the left side is heavier; (**b**) When the patella is facing the front, the toes of both sides are facing the anteromedial side, forming an internal tibial torsion, and the left side is heavier than the right side

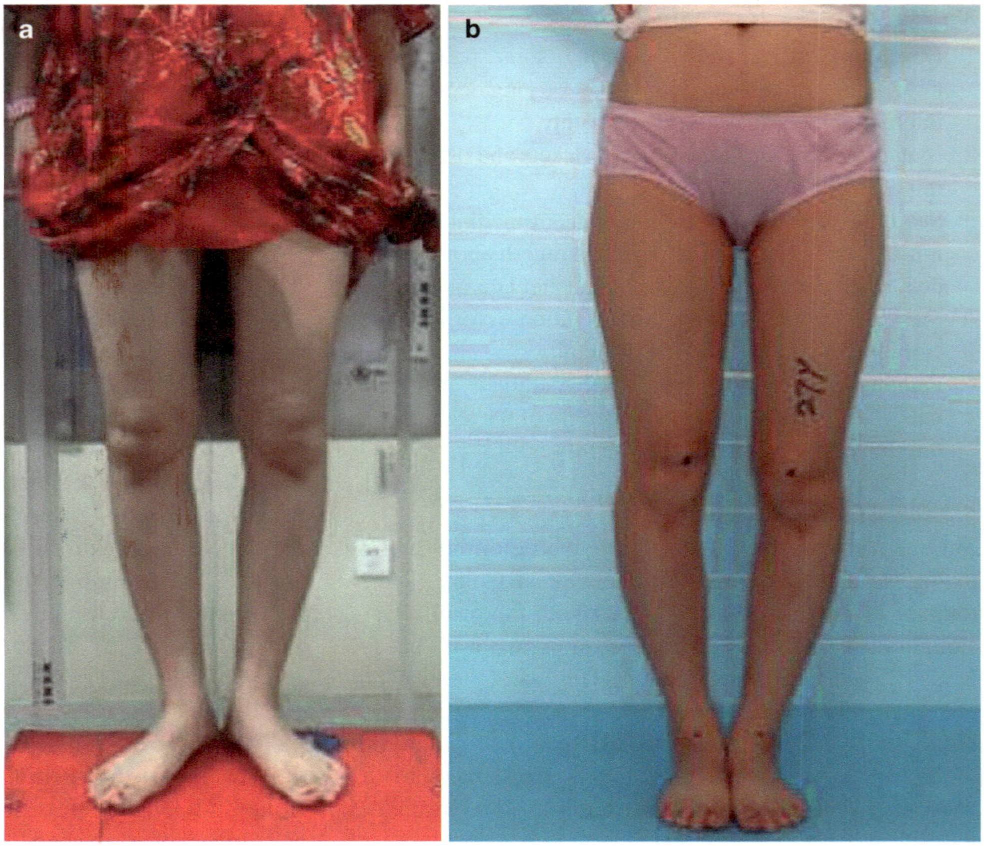

Fig. 4.11 External rotation deformity of both legs. (**a**) When the bilateral patella faces forward, the bilateral toes face anterolateral, forming an external splayed figure; (**b**) When the toes of both sides are forward, the patellas of both sides are anteromedial

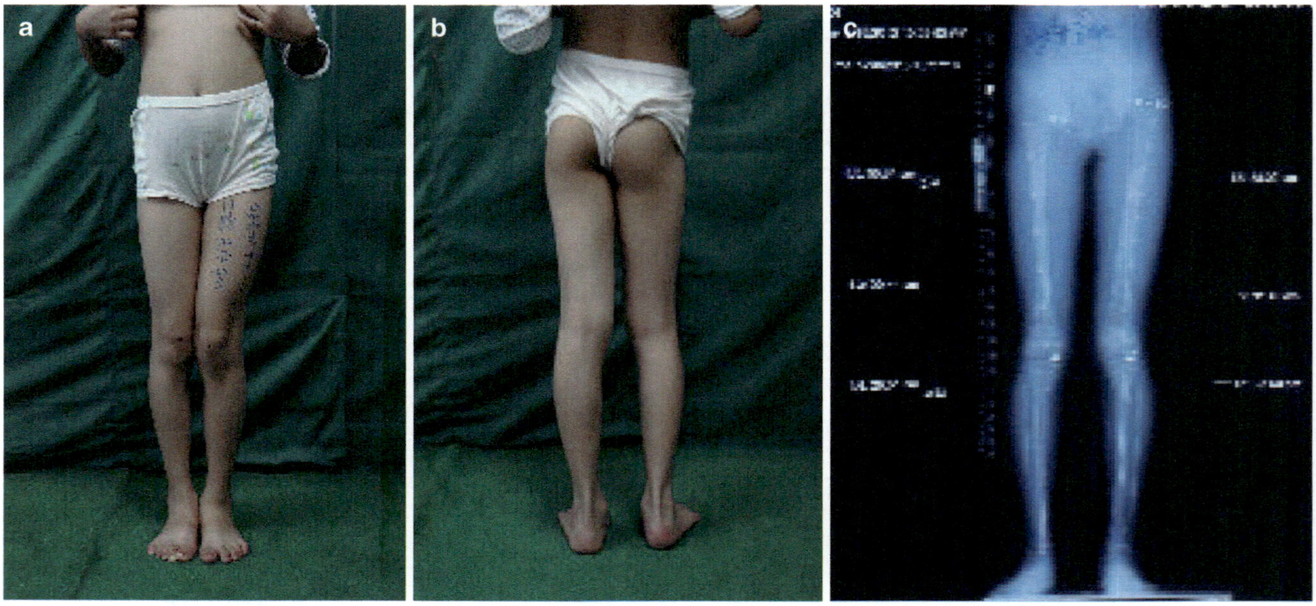

Fig. 4.12 Female, 8 years and 9 months old, fracture of left lower femur at 6 years old, unequal length of lower limbs after 2 and a half years of development

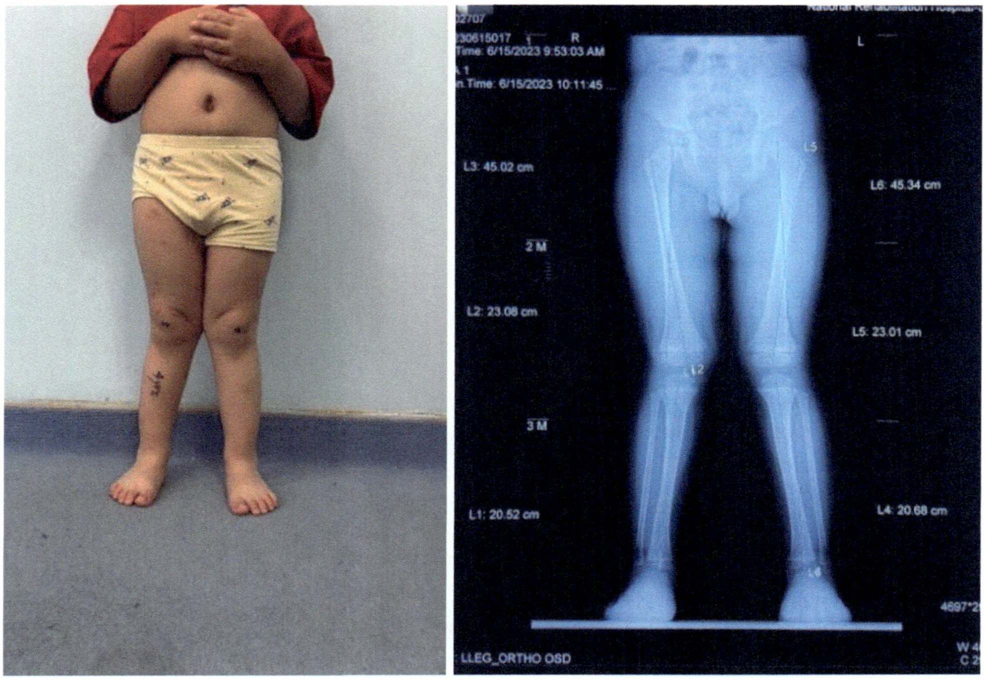

Fig. 4.13 Clinical and X-ray manifestations of a 4-year-old male with developmental double genu valgum

ity exceeds 2 cm and limp gait occurs, surgical treatment should be taken. Distal femoral epiphyseal block on the affected side or limb lengthening on the healthy side is feasible.

4.1.8 Physiological Mild Genu Valgum in Children

4.1.8.1 Etiology

Mild genu valgus in children aged 2–7 is a normal physiological phenomenon, which should not be regarded as a deformity, let alone a disease.

4.1.8.2 Clinical Manifestation

The growth and development of the knee joint in children can be divided into three stages: slight genu varum at the age of 0–2 years; from 2 to 7 years old, mild genu valgum was found (Fig. 4.13).

After 7 years of age, the knee joint gradually returned to normal shape. The X-ray showed that the lateral angle of the distal femur was reduced and the epiphysis was normal. See (Fig. 4.14) for the development of knee joint in preschool standing and walking children.

4.1.8.3 Treatment Principle

Physiological genu valgum does not require treatment and gradually returns to normal with growth and development, but family members are advised that children should not be overweight and should be reexamined regularly.

4.1.9 Developmental Unequal Length of Lower Limbs

4.1.9.1 Etiology

The cause of the disease is unknown.

4.1.9.2 Clinical Manifestation

The child was born with mild inequality in the length of both lower limbs, and the difference in the length of both lower limbs gradually increased with growth and development, resulting in short limb claudication gait. Gradually, the main manifestation was that the femur and tibia of the affected limb were shortened to the healthy side without limb deformity (Fig. 4.15). X-ray film showed that the length of both lower limbs was unequal, and the femur and tibia on the short limb side were evenly shortened compared with the contralateral side, without bone and joint deformities.

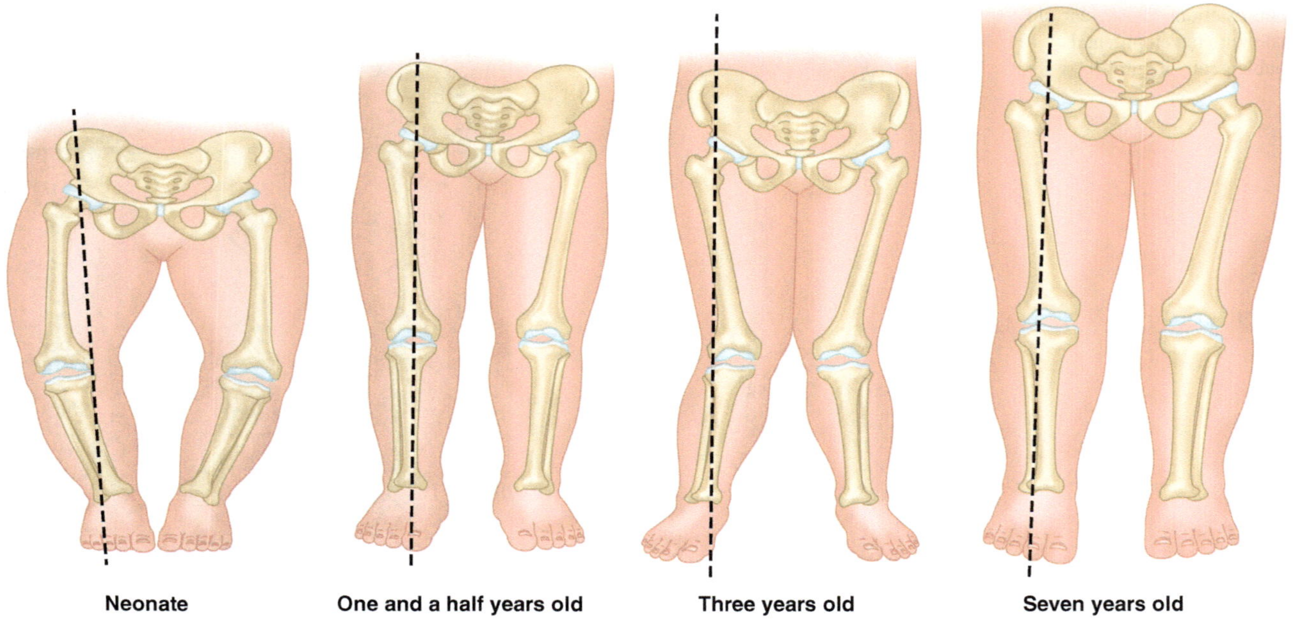

Fig. 4.14 Development of knee joint shape of children after standing and walking

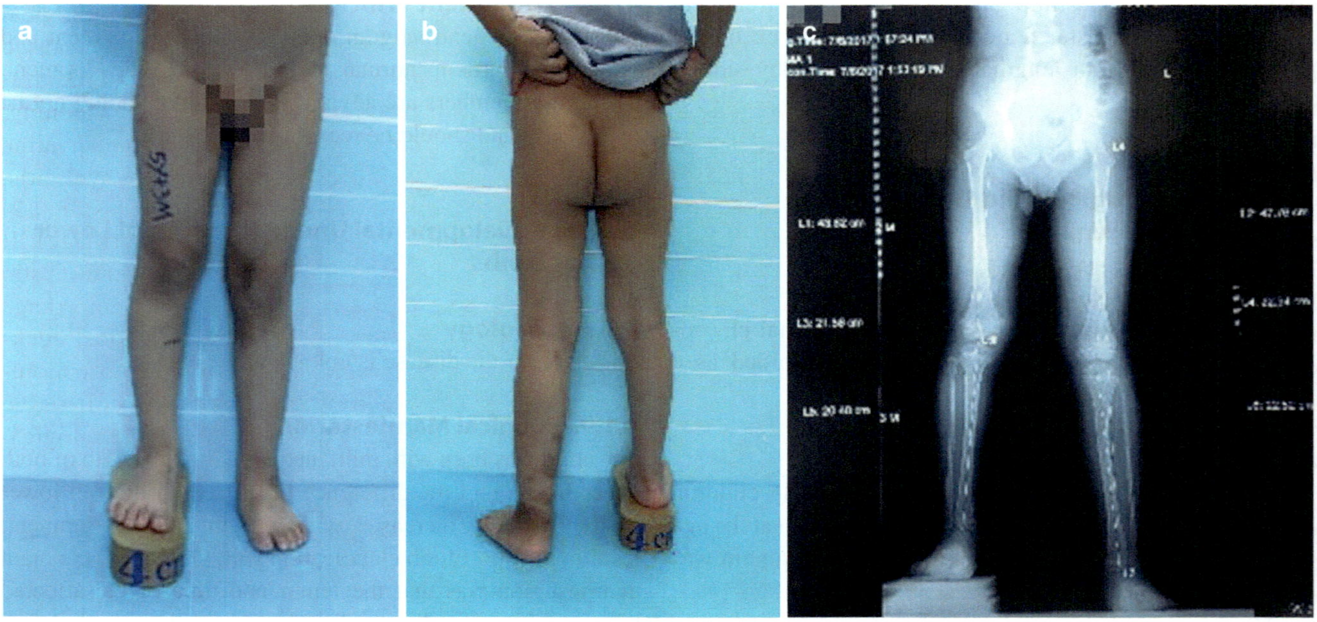

Fig. 4.15 Male, 5 years and 3 months old, unknown cause of developmental shortening of right lower limb. (**a**) appearance in standing position; (**b**) back view in standing position; (**c**) Full-length X-ray film of both lower extremities in standing position

4.1.9.3 Treatment Principle
Limb lengthening on the short limb side was performed.

4.2 The Ankle and Foot Related Diseases

4.2.1 Children's Flatfoot Disease

4.2.1.1 Etiology
Children's foot arch usually begins to form at the age of 4–6. Congenital factors, genetic factors, ligament relaxation, obesity, and other reasons can affect the formation of foot arch, leading to the increase or even disappearance of foot longitudinal arch. Those who cause weakness, pain, and other symptoms of bouncing are called flat feet.

4.2.1.2 Clinical Manifestation
The main manifestations of the patients were that the longitudinal arch of the foot was reduced or even completely disappeared, there was no transverse arch, the whole sole of the foot touched the ground when bearing weight, and the heel was everted. Because of heel collapse, children may have weak jumping ability, foot soreness after exercise, and other symptoms. The X-ray film of the weight-bearing foot showed that the angle of the longitudinal arch of the foot was reduced or even disappeared, the talonavicular joint was subluxated, the tarsal sinus was reduced, and the calcaneus was everted (Fig. 4.16).

4.2.1.3 Treatment Principle
Restore the longitudinal and transverse arches of the foot. First, try conservative treatment with arch pad. If conservative treatment is ineffective, surgical treatment should be considered.

4.2.2 Spastic Hallux Valgus

4.2.2.1 Etiology
Spastic hallux valgus deformity can be caused by central paralysis such as cerebral palsy, sequelae of brain trauma, and tethered spinal cord.

4.2.2.2 Clinical Manifestation
The muscle tension of the lower limbs is increased. It is often associated with hallux pronation deformity and flatfoot or (and) foot valgus deformity; the X-ray film shows that the hallux metatarsophalangeal joint is laterally subluxated and the valgus angle is enlarged (Fig. 4.17).

4.2.2.3 Treatment Principle
Simple hallux valgus deformity without obvious symptoms cannot be treated. Those who cause foot pain or deformity such as foot valgus and horseshoe valgus can be corrected by surgery.

4.2.3 Hypertrophy of the Foot or Macrodactyly

4.2.3.1 Etiology
The cause is unknown, some scholars believe that it is related to neurofibromatosis, and some scholars believe that it is the variation of lipoma. The latest view is that during embryonic development, local growth hormone excess and lack of growth inhibitory factors are the causes of the disease.

4.2.3.2 Clinical Manifestation
Macrodactyly usually occurs after birth, and one or more toes are significantly enlarged, while the other toes are normal, not necessarily all fingers are involved. Macrodactyly grows up gradually with the growth and development of children, and its speed is different. Macrodactyly is primarily an accumulation of fibrofatty tissue, often on the lateral or plantar surface, with asymmetric hypertrophy leading to lateral bending (Fig. 4.18). Although acromegaly is a distinct feature, forefoot involvement is often overlooked, making the inclusion of metacarpals or metatarsals in the disease controversial. However, the most recent views still tend to include metatarsal hypertrophy in macrodactyly. The fibrous tissue extends from the toe to the forefoot, resulting in lateral expansion. Soft tissue hypertrophy on the dorsum of the foot is rare, and more hypertrophy occurs on the plantar surface. Radiographs showed an increase in the length and width of the affected phalanges (Fig. 4.19).

4.2.3.3 Classification
Macrodactyly is divided into two types: one is the static type, that is, it appears at birth and grows in proportion to other toes; the other is the progressive type, which grows much faster than normal toes.

4.2.3.4 Treatment Principle
Congenital macrodactyly is treated according to its size, with soft tissue surgery for mild cases, bone tissue surgery for moderate cases, and amputation for severe cases.

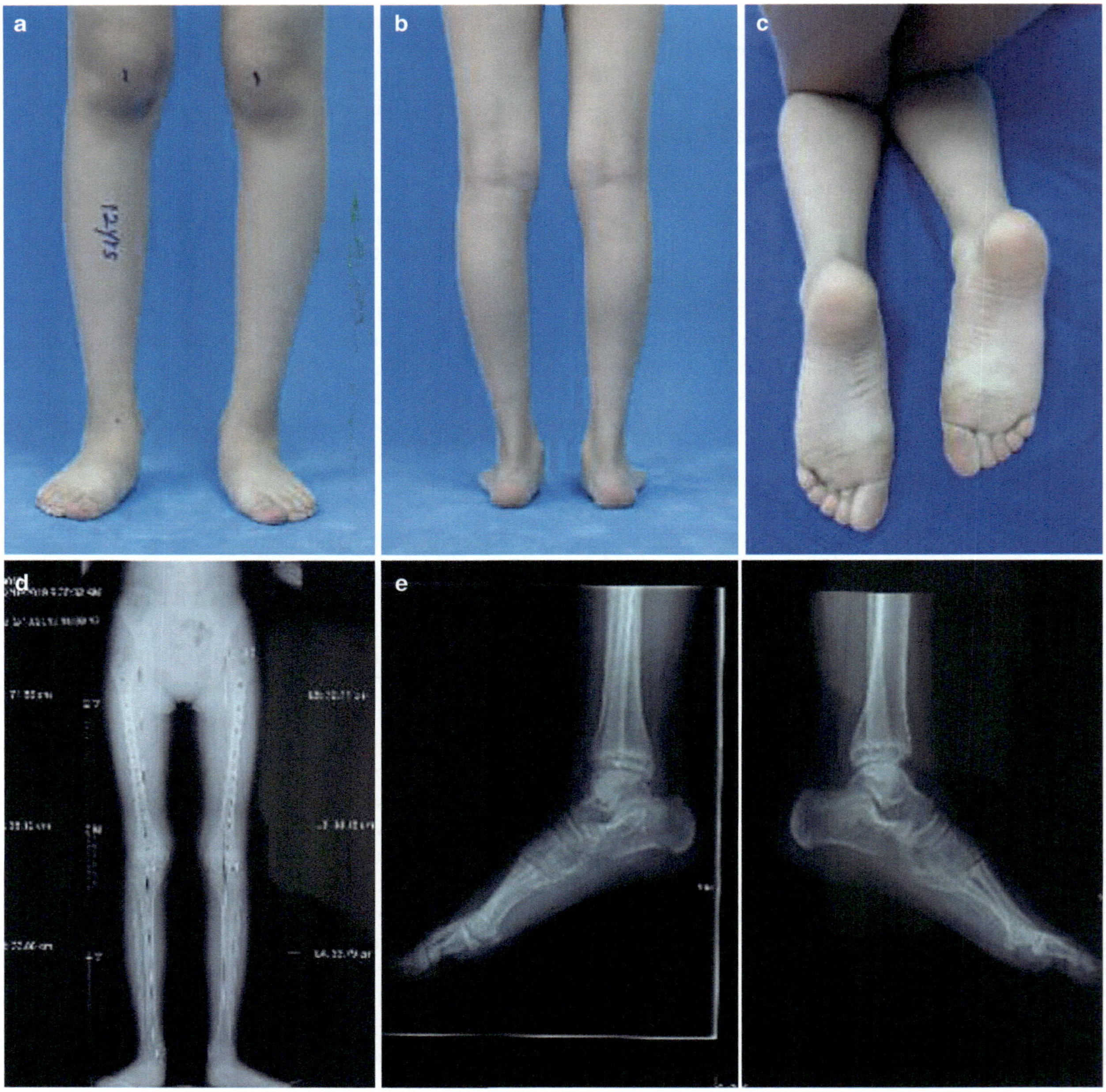

Fig. 4.16 Female, 13 years old, adolescent with flatfeet. (**a**) appearance in standing position, with flat foot and slight torsion of lower leg; (**b**) dorsal view in standing position, with eversion of both feet; (**c**) plantar appearance in kneeling position; (**d**) full-length X-ray of both lower limbs in standing position; (**e**) Lateral X-ray film of both ankles and feet

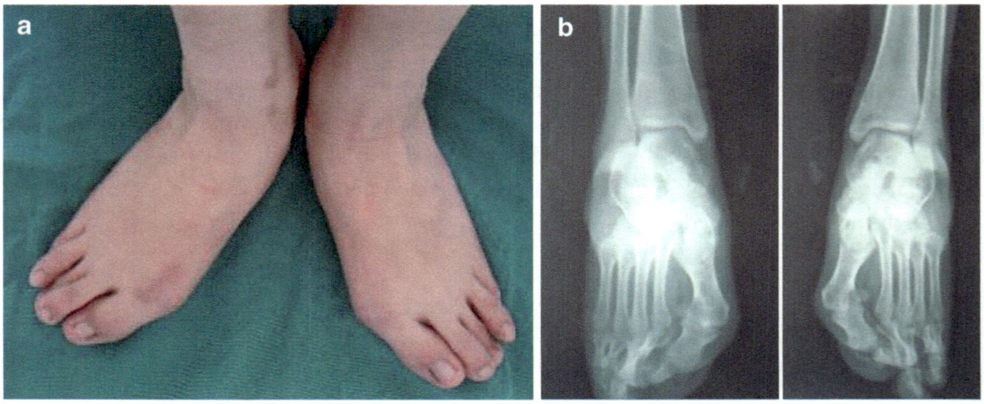

Fig. 4.17 Spastic hallux valgus of cerebral palsy sequelae: (**a**) Bilateral hallux valgus with flatfoot valgus deformity; (**b**) The anteroposterior X-ray film of both feet showed that the bilateral hallux valgus angle was significantly enlarged

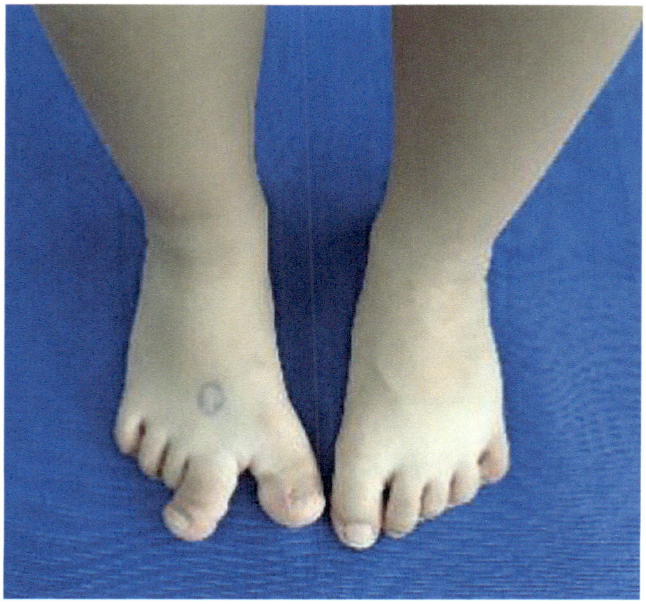

Fig. 4.18 Hypertrophy of right big toe and second toe

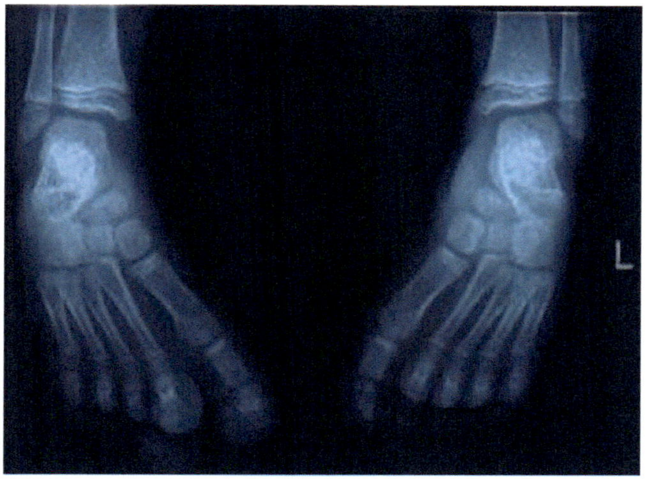

Fig. 4.19 X-ray film of the right foot shows the increase in the length and width of the phalanges of the right big toe and the second toe

5 Rheumatic Immunity and Degenerative Diseases Lead to Deformity

Sihe Qin and Lei Shi

5.1 Rheumatism and Rheumatoid Arthritis

5.1.1 Rheumatic Arthritis

Rheumatic arthritis (RA) is a common acute or chronic inflammation of connective tissue, which is the manifestation of rheumatic fever in joints, so it is not included in the international category of diseases. RA mainly involves large joints, which can be cured without sequelae if properly treated.

5.1.1.1 Etiology

It is related to group a β-hemolytic streptococcal infection, which can be induced by cold, dampness, and other factors.

5.1.1.2 Clinical Manifestation

Clinically, it is characterized by migratory soreness, swelling, and pain of joints and muscles, mainly involving knee and ankle joints, chorea in children, and rheumatic fever involving the heart. It is characterized by prodromal symptoms of streptococcal infection, such as tonsil suppurative infection. The pathological changes in the active stage were edema of the synovial membrane and surrounding tissues, mucinous degeneration, fibrinoid degeneration, and inflammatory cell infiltration in the connective tissue under the synovial membrane. 80% of the patients with rheumatic arthritis have increased anti-O and accelerated erythrocyte sedimentation rate in acute stage. After the active period, the exudate in the joint can be absorbed and generally does not cause adhesion, so there are few sequelae such as joint deformation. The biggest difference with rheumatic arthritis is that there are few joint deformities left after the acute stage.

S. Qin (✉) · L. Shi
Department of Orthopaedics, Rehabilitation Hospital of the National Research Center for Rehabilitation Technical Aids, Beijing, China

Improper treatment in the acute stage, as shown in the figure below, causes joint destruction caused by the application of a large amount of hormones, resulting in hip flexion and knee flexion deformity (Fig. 5.1).

5.1.1.3 Treatment Principle

Drug therapy is the main treatment, including anti-inflammatory treatment and anti-infective treatment, anti-infective drugs for streptococcus, penicillin as the first choice, to adhere to more than 1 year, to avoid damage to the heart, acute attack to use anti-inflammatory analgesics, aspirin as the first choice.

5.1.2 Rheumatoid Arthritis

Rheumatoid arthritis (RA) is a chronic, systemic disease characterized by inflammatory synovitis of unknown etiology. It is characterized by polyarticular, symmetrical and invasive arthritis of the small joints of the hands and feet, often accompanied by involvement of extra-articular organs and positive serum rheumatoid factor. The pathogenesis of RA arthritis may be related to heredity, infection, sex hormones, and so on. Pathology mainly includes synovial lining cell proliferation, interstitial inflammatory cell infiltration, microvascular neogenesis, pannus formation, and cartilage and bone tissue destruction, which can lead to multi-joint deformity and loss of function (Fig. 5.2).

5.1.2.1 Treatment Principle

The main purpose of RA treatment is to reduce the inflammatory reaction of joints, inhibit the development of lesions and irreversible bone destruction, protect the function of joints and muscles as far as possible, and ultimately alleviate the disease and improve limb function.

Patients with severe joint deformity that cannot be controlled by medical treatment can be treated by surgery, including: (1) synovectomy, (2) contracture of fascia and

S. Qin et al. (eds.), *Atlas of Limb Deformity*, https://doi.org/10.1007/978-981-97-0999-1_5

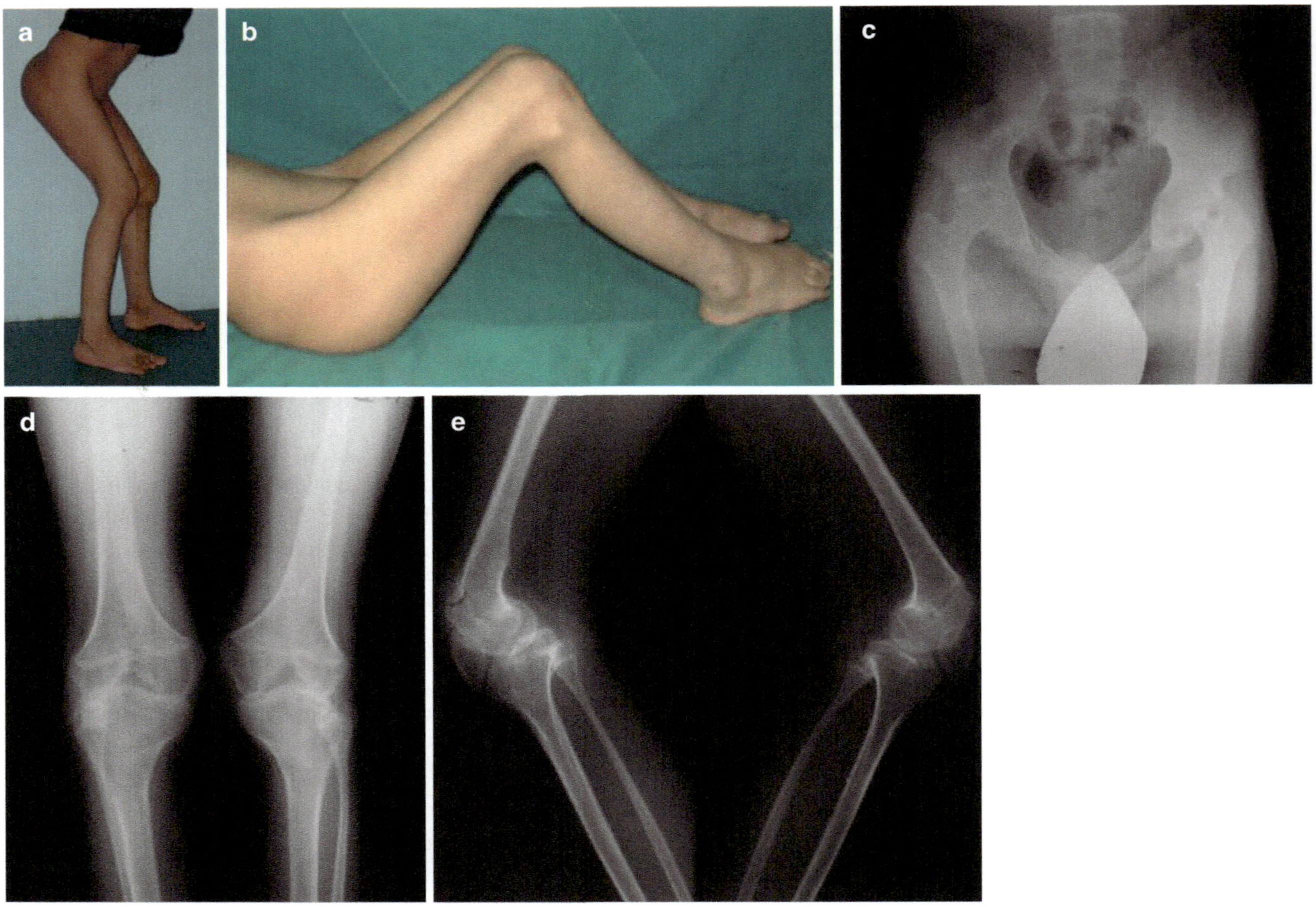

Fig. 5.1 (**a**) Both lower limbs standing side view photo; (**b**) Lateral view of maximum hip and knee extension in lying position; (**c**) Anteroposterior X-ray film of pelvis (bilateral hip joint space nearly disappeared); (**d**, **e**) Bilateral anteroposterior and lateral radiographs of the knees showed flexion contracture

tendon release, (3) joint traction to correct flexion contracture, (4) arthroplasty or fusion, (5) joint replacement.

5.1.3 Juvenile Idiopathic Arthritis

Juvenile idiopathic arthritis (JIA) is a common rheumatic disease in childhood, characterized by chronic synovitis and multiple organ dysfunction. It is an important cause of disability or blindness in childhood (also known as chronic arthritis in children; Juvenile rheumatoid arthritis; Still disease in children; Juvenile chronic polyarthritis, etc.).

5.1.3.1 Etiology

The etiology is not clear and may be caused by the following factors: infectious factors; genetic factors; immunological factors.

5.1.3.2 Clinical Manifestation

1. It is characterized by inflammation of one or more joints, manifested by swelling or effusion of joints and more than two of the following signs: limitation of joint movement, pain or tenderness during movement, and local temperature rise of joints. (Fig. 5.3).
2. The course of the disease is more than 6 weeks.

5.1.3.3 Classification

1. Systemic arthritis fever is flaccid and high fever, and the rash is characterized by the appearance or regression of body temperature. Joint symptoms are mainly arthralgia or arthritis.
2. Polyarticular type, negative rheumatoid factor. The onset of this type can occur at any age, but there are two peaks of onset, namely, 1–3 years old and 8–10 years old. Female is more common. More than five joints were involved, most of which were symmetrical, and both large and small joints were involved. When the temporomandibular joint is involved, it may cause difficulty in opening the mouth and micrognathia. About 10% to 15% of patients eventually develop severe arthritis.
3. Polyarticular type, positive rheumatoid factor. The incidence of this type is also more common in female. The clinical manifestations of this type of RA are basically the same as those of adult RA.

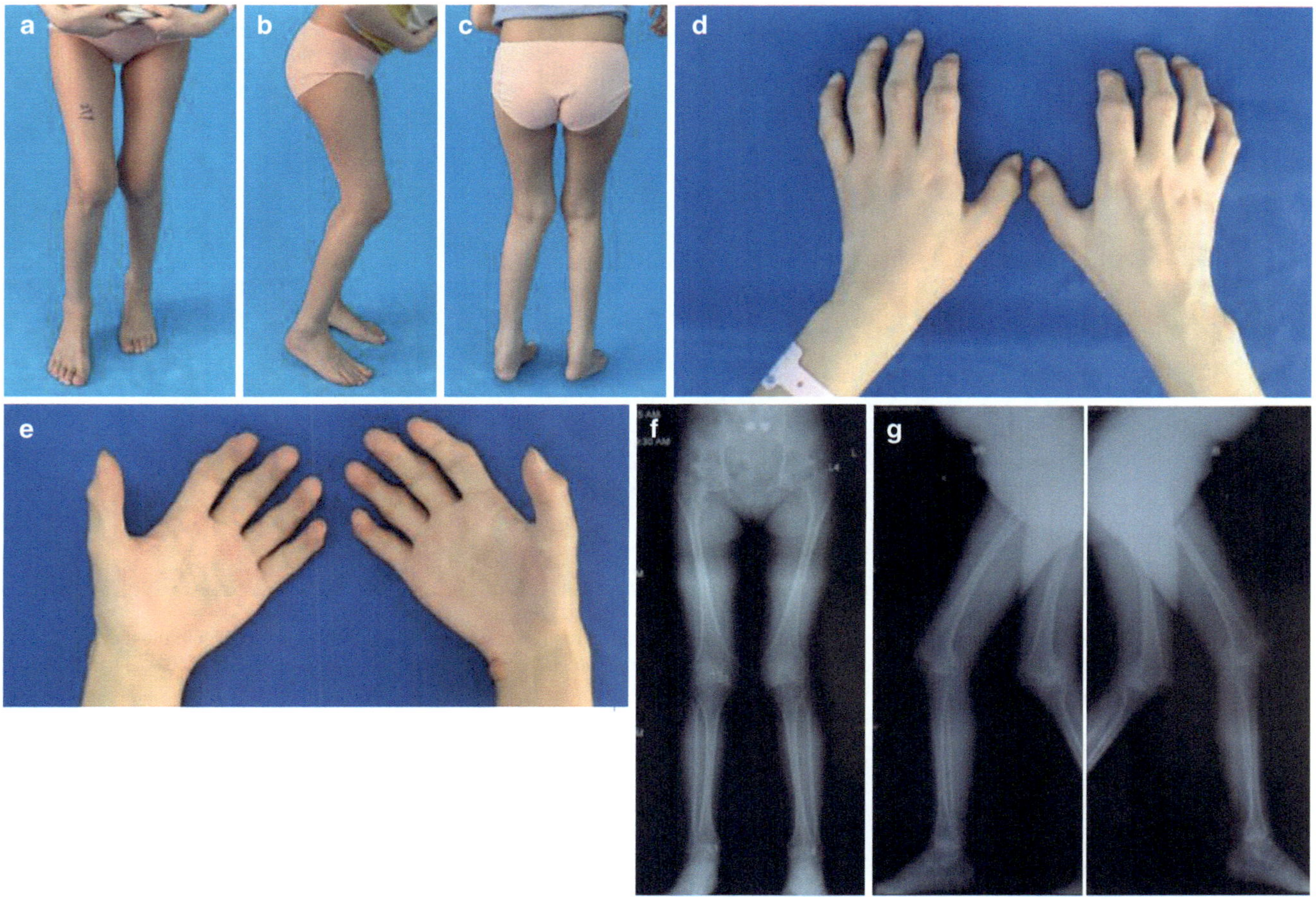

Fig. 5.2 Rheumatoid arthritis polyarticular deformity (**a**) View of both lower limbs standing in front; (**b**) View of both lower limbs standing in profile; (**c**) View from the back of both lower limbs standing; (**d**) View from the back of both hands; (**e**) View from the palms of both hands; (**f**, **g**). Full-length anteroposterior and lateral radiographs of both lower limbs in standing position

4. Oligoarticular type. This type is more common in female, and the onset is usually before the age of 5. Most of them are involved in large joints, such as knee, ankle, elbow or wrist, which are often asymmetric. Although arthritis is recurrent, it is rarely disabling. About 20% to 30% of children suffer from chronic iridocyclitis, resulting in visual impairment and even blindness.
5. The incidence of psoriatic arthritis was mostly female, and the ratio of female to male was 2.5:1. 40% of the patients had a family history of psoriasis.
6. Unclassified Juvenile idiopathic arthritis 。.

5.1.3.4 Treatment Principle

Reduce or eliminate joint pain and swelling, restore joint function, and ability to live and work to the greatest extent. Synovectomy and joint distraction can be performed to relieve joint contracture for the cases with ineffective conservative treatment, and Ilizarov technique can be used to correct the severe joint flexion contracture deformity and improve the limb shape and function.

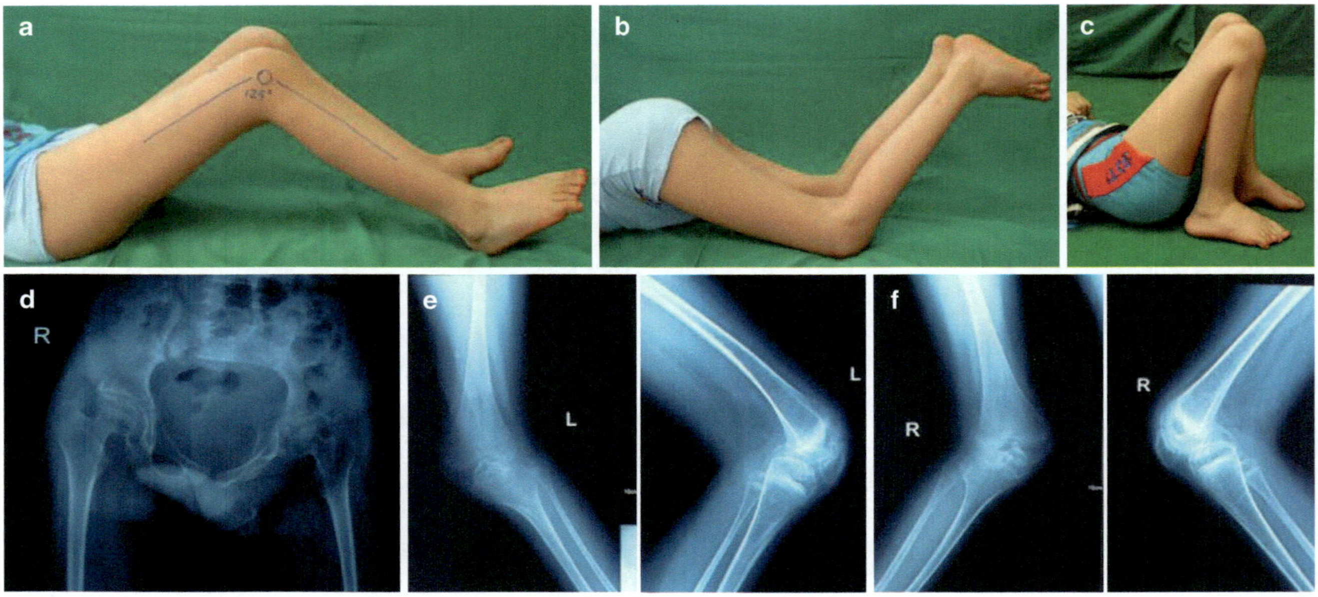

Fig. 5.3 Juvenile idiopathic arthritis. (**a**) Lateral view of the lower limb in the supine position; (**b**) View of the lower limb in prone position; (**c**) View of the flexion of both knees; (**d**) Pelvic anteroposterior radiography showed hip joint destruction. (**e**, **f**) On the anteroposterior and lateral X-ray films of both knees, the joint space was narrow

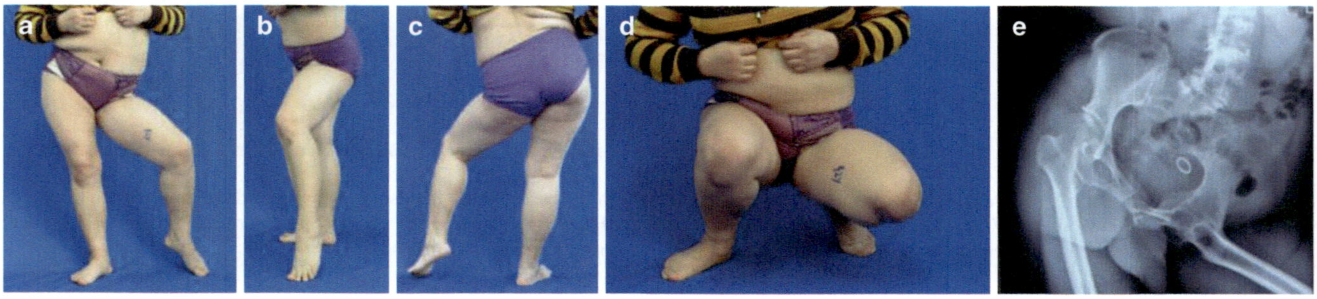

Fig. 5.4 Skeletal stiffness of flexion and abduction position of the left hip joint caused by synovitis. (**a**) Standing frontal view; (**b**) Standing lateral view; (**c**) Standing back view; (**d**) Squat front view; (**e**) Anteroposterior radiograph of pelvis

5.2 Immunity and Related Diseases

5.2.1 Stiffness Caused by Hip Synovitis

Hip synovitis is a multiple disease. If the synovitis is not treated correctly in the early stage, the articular cartilage will be destroyed, the hip joint fiber will be stiff and even the bone will be fused in the abnormal position.

5.2.1.1 Etiology

The cause of the disease is not yet clear but may be related to viral infection, trauma, bacterial infection, and allergy.

5.2.1.2 Clinical Manifestation

Unilateral hip or groin pain is the most common clinical symptom, and some patients may present with mid-thigh or knee pain. In very young children, it can be manifested as night crying. Children with synovitis of hip joint, if misdiagnosed, extensive destruction of articular cartilage, will inevitably be secondary to joint malformation, stiffness, and bony fusion (Fig. 5.4).

5.2.1.3 Treatment Principle

Surgical treatment should be performed as early as possible to improve the range of motion of the hip joint so that the hip joint can be restored to its functional position. In the late stage, the force line of the lower limb can be restored by osteotomy, and artificial joint replacement can be performed in accordance with the indications.

5.2.2 Scleroderma

Scleroderma is a disease characterized by localized or diffuse fibrosis or sclerosis of connective tissue of skin and internal organs, and finally atrophy. It is divided into localized scleroderma and systemic scleroderma.

5.2.2.1 Etiology

The etiology is unknown and is closely related to the following theories: (1) immune theory, (2) abnormal collagen synthesis theory, and (3) vascular theory. Dermal collagen fibers and arterioles were the main pathological changes.

5.2.2.2 Clinical Manifestation

Localized scleroderma lesions are mainly confined to the skin, early damage is often limited to the distal limbs such as ankle and finger skin, viscera are generally not involved, and the prognosis is better. Systemic scleroderma has widespread skin sclerosis, Raynaud's phenomenon and multisystem involvement, and the prognosis is uncertain and mostly good, but systemic scleroderma, especially diffuse, has a poor prognosis.

Another form of localized scleroderma, which causes limb deformities, is more common in girls from 1 to 14. Inflammation and sclerosis occur in the dermis, subcutaneous tissue, fascia, muscles, and bones of the limbs (Fig. 5.5), especially on the extension side, showing contractures of the hands, feet, elbows, and knees, rarely involving the viscera, without Raynaud's phenomenon. Patients may have sclerosing lichenoid lesions, and other parts of the body may have typical manifestations of morphea.

5.2.2.3 Treatment Principle

The goal of early treatment is to prevent new skin and organ involvement. The goal of late treatment is to improve existing symptoms. The methods include: (1) anti-inflammatory and immunomodulatory therapy, (2) treatment for vascular lesions, (3) anti-fibrosis therapy.

In the late stage of scleroderma, rigid joint contracture will inevitably lead to bone and joint deformities. Limited bone and soft tissue surgery combined with Ilizarov technique can partially correct deformities and improve limb morphology and function.

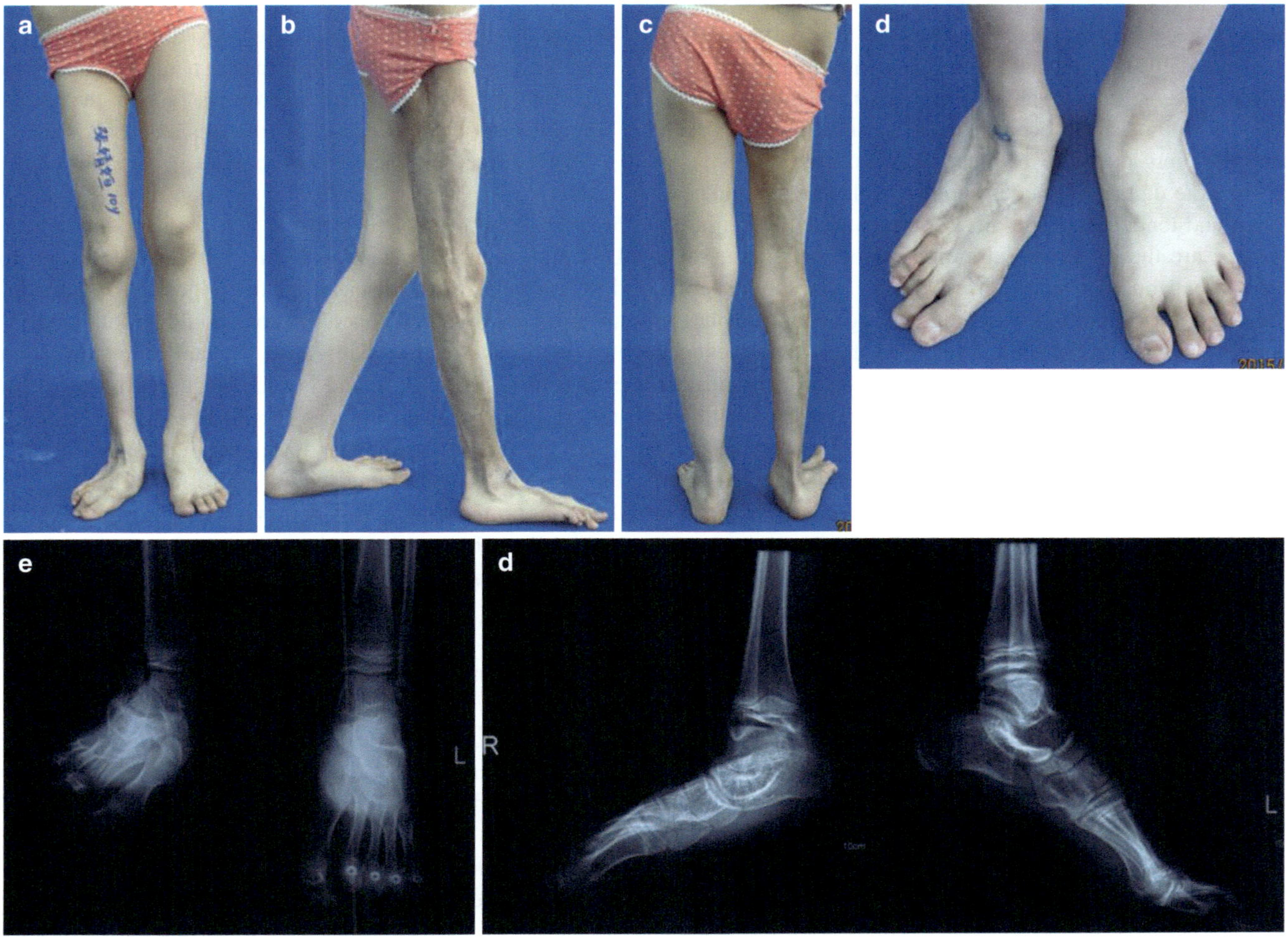

Fig. 5.5 Scleroderma. (**a**) Standing frontal view; (**b**) Standing lateral view; (**c**) Standing back view; (**d**) Bipedal frontal view; (**e**, **f**). Anteroposterior and lateral radiographs of both ankles

5.2.3 Dermatomyositis

Dermatomyositis (DM) is a non-suppurative inflammatory disease mainly involving striated muscle with lymphocyte infiltration, which may or may not be accompanied by a variety of skin lesions. Clinically, it is characterized by symmetrical weakness of limb girdle muscles, neck muscles, and pharyngeal muscles, often involving a variety of organs, and can also be accompanied by tumors and other connective tissue diseases.

5.2.3.1 Etiology

The exact cause of the disease is not yet clear, it is generally believed to be related to genetic and viral infection, and there is a genetic tendency.

5.2.3.2 Clinical Manifestation

The disease develops slowly, mainly involving skin and muscle, and the typical symptoms are skin lesions and muscle weakness. Skin lesions include purplish red spots on the eyelids, Gottron papules, and poikiloderma. Muscle weakness is symmetrical, causing weakness in lifting arms and legs, difficulty in chewing, etc. Muscle symptoms and skin lesions do not necessarily appear at the same time, about 2/3 of patients with skin lesions and muscle symptoms occur at the same time or first appear skin lesions, then muscle symptoms. Calcinosis may occur in the skin, subcutaneous tissue, around joints and diseased muscles in some children.

Muscle damage includes symmetrical muscle weakness, pain, and tenderness. The most commonly involved muscle groups are the proximal extremities, shoulder girdle, neck, and throat muscles, with corresponding symptoms such as raising hands, squatting, climbing, raising heads, dysphagia, and hoarseness. In the acute stage, the affected muscles may swell, and in severe cases, they may be bedridden and lose their voluntary movement completely. When the condition is serious, it can also involve the myocardium, resulting in arrhythmia and even heart failure. Muscle damage can also cause muscle contracture, resulting in secondary joint deformities, such as equinus (Fig. 5.6).

5.2.3.3 Treatment Principle

1. Treatment of dermatomyositis with drugs, including glucocorticoids, immunosuppressants, immunoglobulins, etc.
2. For secondary limb deformities, orthopedic surgery.

5.2.4 Multiple Sclerosis

Multiple sclerosis (MS) is a demyelinating disease of the central nervous system characterized by multiple lesions, remission, and recurrence in the course of the disease. It often occurs in young adults and is rare in children. There are racial differences in its incidence.

5.2.4.1 Etiology

The etiology is uncertain and may be related to the following factors: (1) Viral infection autoimmune diseases induced are generally accepted, (2) genetic factors, (3) environmental factors. The disease is characterized by multiple demyelinating plaques in the white matter of the central nervous system.

5.2.4.2 Clinical Manifestation

1. The onset of MS was mostly subacute. The course of the disease often has natural remission and recurrence.
2. Diversified clinical manifestations. Child patients often have central paralysis of limbs, encephalopathy, ataxia, visual, and language disorders as the first symptoms.
3. The main manifestations of brain stem involvement are: (1) internuclear muscle paralysis: when the child looks to one side, the contralateral eye cannot adduct, but the eyes are normal when they are cohesive; (2) nystagmus: horizontal, vertical, or rotatory; (3) facial paralysis; (4) medulla oblongae involvement: Dysphagia, slurred speech. (5) diplopia; (6) sensory disturbances (numbness, banding, burning, cold, and pain) may occur. In the late stage, spinal cord transverse sensory disturbances may occur; (7) motor dysfunction: spastic paralysis caused by corticospinal tract damage, cerebellar ataxia caused by cerebellar or spinocerebellar tract lesions, and sensory ataxia caused by sensory disturbances. (Fig. 5.7).

5.2.4.3 Treatment Principle

Different treatment measures should be taken according to different stages of the disease, and the principles of individualization, staging, and concretization should be followed.

For the dysfunction caused by skeletal deformity, joint contracture, dislocation, and instability caused by MS central paralysis, orthosis (brace) should be worn to stabilize joints and assist standing and walking in the early stage. Patients with obvious bone and joint deformities can achieve the goal of improving limb function by restoring the negative gravity line of lower limbs through orthopedic surgery and assisted by braces.

5.2.5 Acanthosis nigricans

Acanthosis nigricans (AN) is a skin marker that may indicate insulin resistance, diabetes, visceral malignancy, metabolic syndrome, and other syndromes.

5.2.5.1 Etiology

AN can be seen in short-limb skeletal dysplasia and craniosynostosis syndromes caused by fibroblast growth factor receptor mutations, including achondroplasia, chondrodysplasia, ectopic dysplasia, Apert syndrome, Crouzon syndrome, Pfeiffer syndrome, and Jackson-Weiss syndrome.

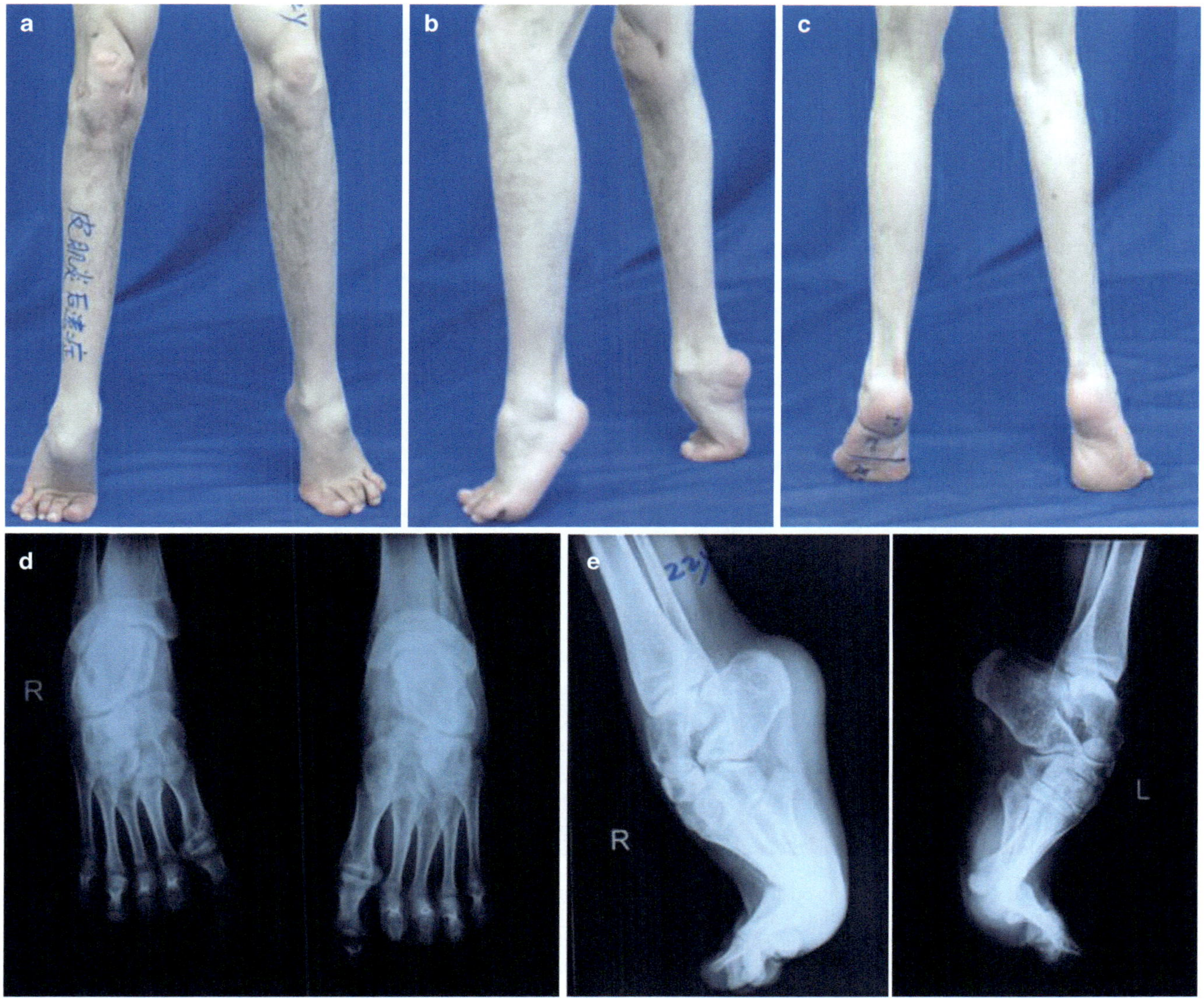

Fig. 5.6 Bilateral talipes equinus caused by dermatomyositis. (**A**) View of both lower limbs standing in front; (**b**) View of both lower limbs standing in profile; (**c**) View of both lower limbs from the back; (**d**–**f**) Anteroposterior and lateral X-ray films of both feet and ankles

5.2.5.2 Clinical Manifestation

AN is a skin keratosis characterized by skin pigmentation, hyperkeratosis, velvety hyperplasia, and verrucous vegetation, which often occurs in skin folds. When combined with Crouzon syndrome and Jackson-Weiss syndrome, it can also be manifested as skull deformity caused by craniosynostosis, wide eye distance, raised forehead, hand and foot abnormalities manifested as short and wide toes far away from other toes, fusion or dysplasia of phalanges, tarsus and phalanges. The dysplastic foot will gradually develop stress deformity during walking (Fig. 5.8).

5.2.5.3 Treatment Principle

There is no need to treat upper limb deformities that do not affect function. In view of the ankle deformity affecting walking, orthopedic surgery can be used to correct the deformity, restore the gravity line of the ankle, stabilize the joint, and improve the walking function.

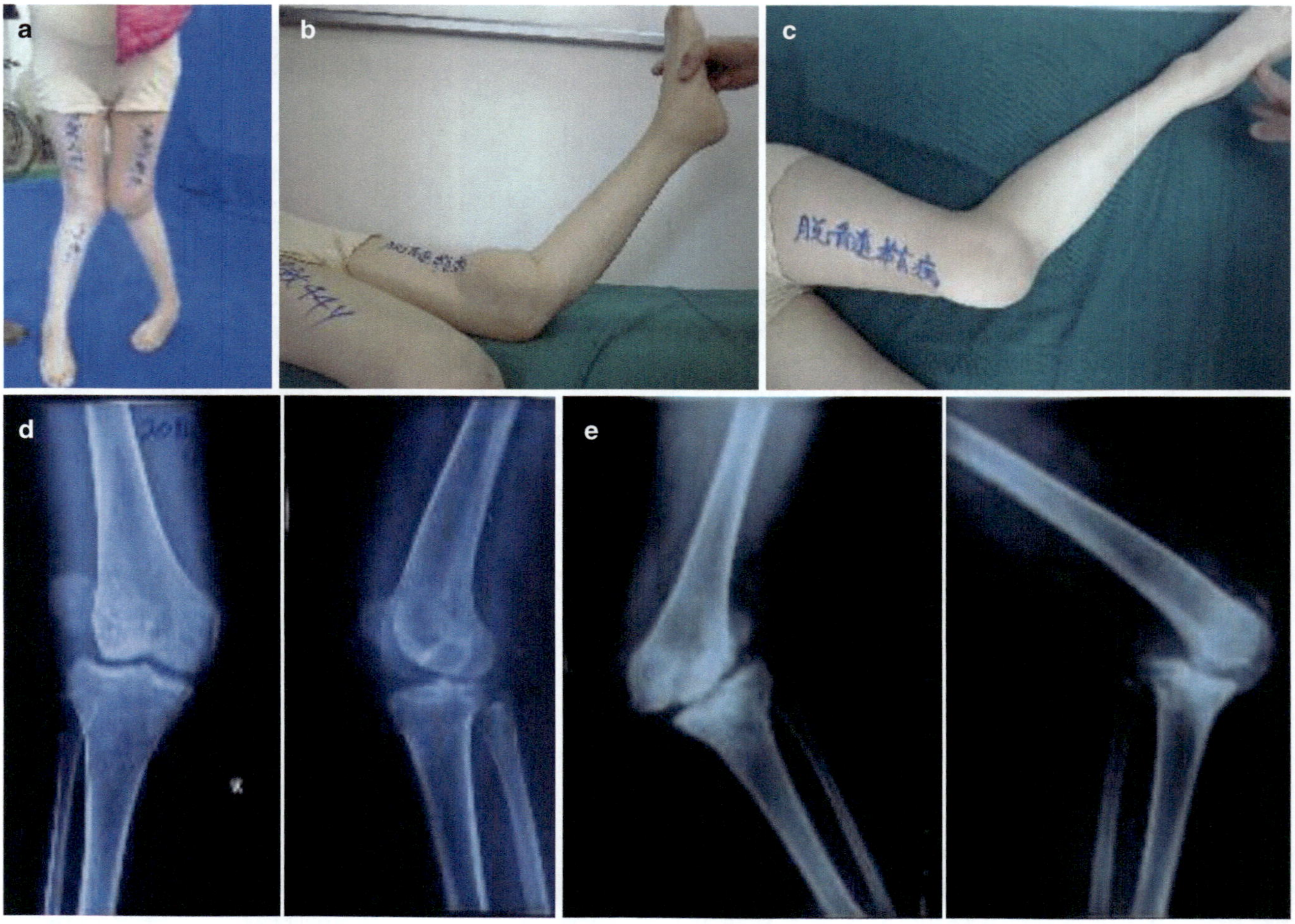

Fig. 5.7 a 44-year-old woman presented with bilateral knee laxity, retroflexion, and valgus deformity due to multiple sclerosis. (**a**) View of both lower limbs standing in front; (**b**) View of the left knee in passive maximum retroflexion (**c**) View of the left knee in the passive maximum valgus position; (**d**) Anteroposterior and lateral X-ray film of right knee joint; E. Anteroposterior and lateral X-ray film of left knee joint

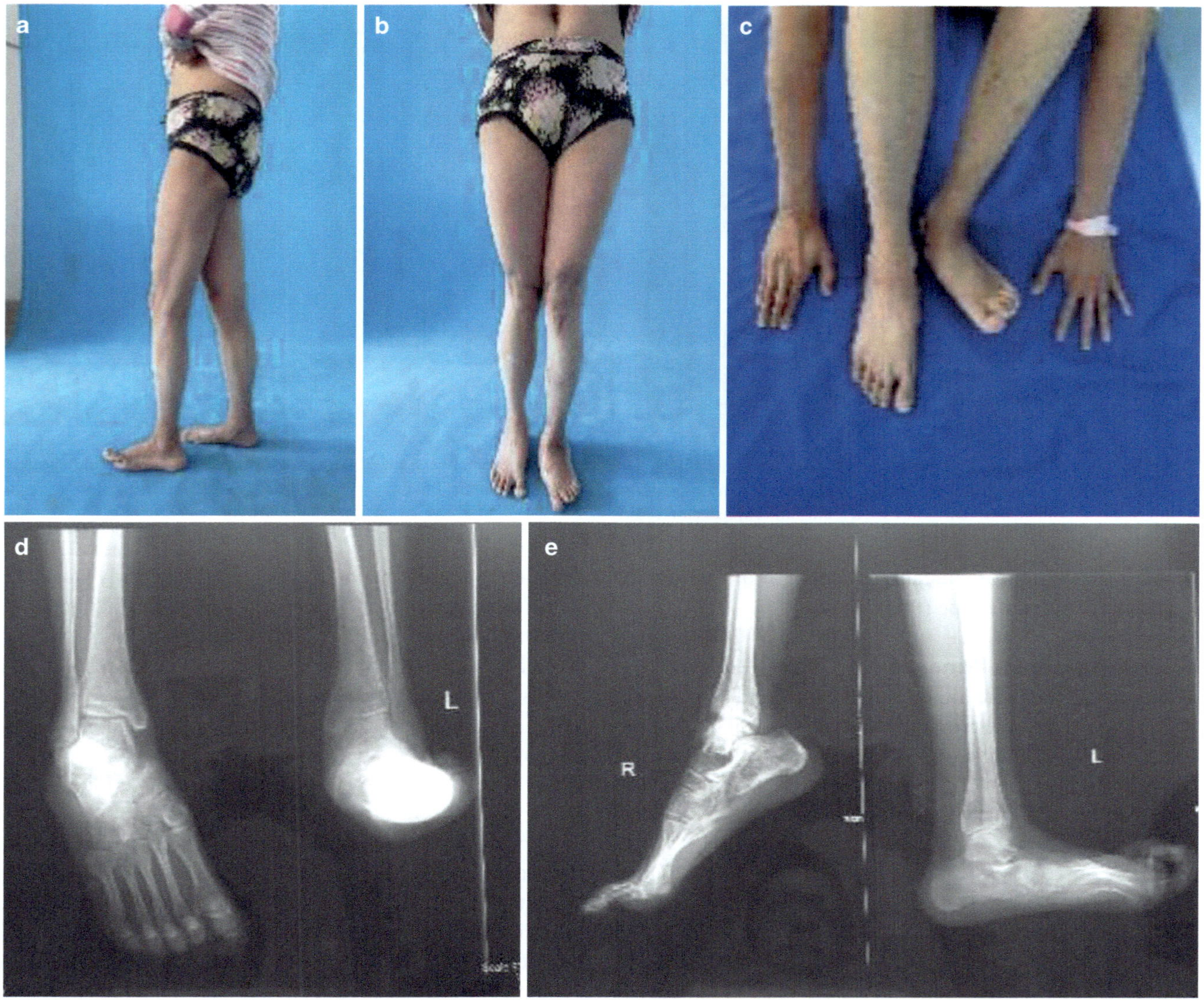

Figure 5.8 Female, 14 years old, deformity of both hands and left foot. (**a**) Lateral view of lower limbs; (**b**) frontal view of both lower limbs; (**c**) Bipedal frontal view photograph; (**d**) Anteroposterior X-ray film of both feet; (**e**) Lateral radiograph of both feet

5.3 Degenerative Changes

5.3.1 Coxa Plana

Coxa plana, also known as Legg-Cavle-Perthes disease (LCPD), is a self-healing, self-limiting, non-systemic disease of the femoral head in children.

5.3.1.1 Etiology

The cause of the disease is not yet fully understood. Local factors include trauma, synovitis, arthritis, increased intraosseous pressure, and intraarticular pressure. Systemic factors include: (1) coagulation and fibrinolysis system abnormalities, (2) endocrine and immune factors, (3) genetic, environmental, smoking, and so on. Because of the mismatch of joints, long-term weight-bearing walking results in joint wear and dislocation, which affects the function of standing and walking.

5.3.1.2 Clinical Manifestation

The peak age of LCPD is 8–14 years old, 10% of the cases are bilateral, male is more than female, the sex ratio is about 3:1. The pathological process is self-limited. In the recovery period, the abnormal shaping of the femoral head and the involvement of the metaphysis affect the normal development of the proximal femur, resulting in head enlargement, short neck or flat hip, and other deformities. The main clinical manifestation is claudication. In the late stage, the function of hip joint is seriously affected by joint degeneration due to long-term weight-bearing walking, pain, and limited movement of the affected hip joint. The X-ray features are

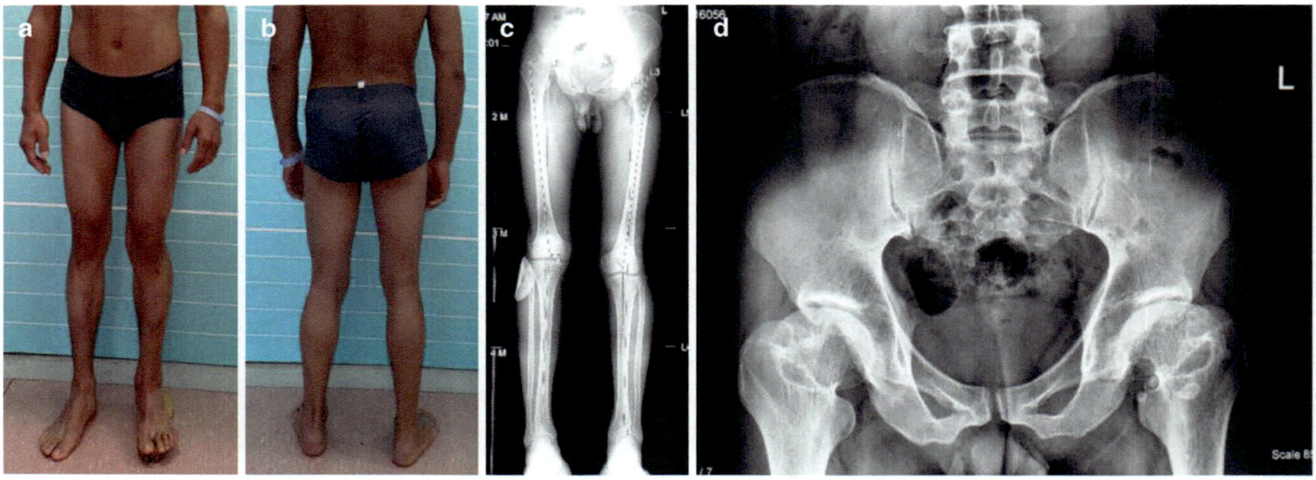

Fig. 5.9 Coxa plana. (**a**) The front view of both lower limb; (**b**) The rear view of both lower limb; (**c**) Full-length standing anteroposterior radiograph of both lower extremities; (**d**) The anteroposterior radiograph of the pelvis showed flattening of the femoral head and shortening of the femoral neck

cystic degeneration, fragmentation, collapse of the femoral head, and finally flat shape (Fig. 5.9).

5.3.1.3 Treatment Principle

Treatment methods are aimed at preventing and delaying the occurrence of adverse prognosis such as femoral head deformity and degenerative osteoarthritis. To reconstruct the structure and function of the hip joint, artificial joint replacement can be performed in adult patients with obvious pain symptoms.

5.3.2 Slipped Capital Femoral Epiphysis

Slipped capital femoral epiphysis (SCFE) is a hip disease in which the femoral neck is displaced relative to the femoral head epiphysis in children during adolescence.

5.3.2.1 Etiology

SCFE occurs in adolescent children. Because the proximal femoral epiphyseal plate is weak and unable to withstand shear force, the femoral neck is displaced and rotated relative to the femoral head epiphysis, which is mostly induced by obesity and trauma. The onset within 10 years old was related to endocrine, metabolic diseases, renal insufficiency, and other factors. Obese children have a higher incidence. SCFE can also be caused by sepsis, rickets, achondroplasia, and multiple epiphyseal dysplasia. Because of the mismatch of the hip joint on the affected side, long-term weight-bearing walking results in joint wear and dislocation, which affects the function of standing and walking.

5.3.2.2 Clinical Manifestation

Unilateral or bilateral epiphyseal spondylolisthesis occurs gradually, often manifested as hip pain, thigh pain, lameness, limited hip movement, and some knee pain as the first manifestation (obturator nerve stimulation). In the early stage, the X-ray film showed that the femoral neck was bent, the Kline line was destroyed, and the femoral head epiphysis was displaced posteriorly. In the late stage, hip dislocation and osteoarthritis were seen (Fig. 5.10). MRI showed that the synovial membrane of the hip joint was inflamed, the femoral medullary cavity was edematous, the epiphyseal plate was widened, the epiphysis slipped, and the anterior acetabular cartilage was destroyed.

Femoral head epiphyseal slippage in adults progresses to the sequelae stage, characterized by hip pain and short-limb claudication. X-ray showed osteoarthritis of the hip, posterior-inferior or medial-inferior slippage of the femoral head epiphysis, shortening of the femoral neck, and high position of the greater trochanter. According to the degree of epiphyseal displacement, it can be divided into early, mild, moderate, and severe slippage, which can lead to hip dislocation and stiffness in the late stage.

5.3.2.3 Treatment Principle

The goal of treatment is to restore the acetabulum relationship, relieve pain, and improve joint function. The methods vary according to different clinical stages and types, including non-surgical treatment, in situ fixation, femoral head osteotomy, femoral neck base and intertrochanteric osteotomy, pelvic osteotomy, and so on. Artificial joint replacement is feasible for patients with severe osteoarthritis pain in adulthood.

5.3.3 Hip Osteoarthritis

5.3.3.1 Etiology

Hip osteoarthritis (HOA) is a long-term bone and joint inflammation caused by repeated compression of hip joint, violent impact or cartilage degeneration in the elderly, result-

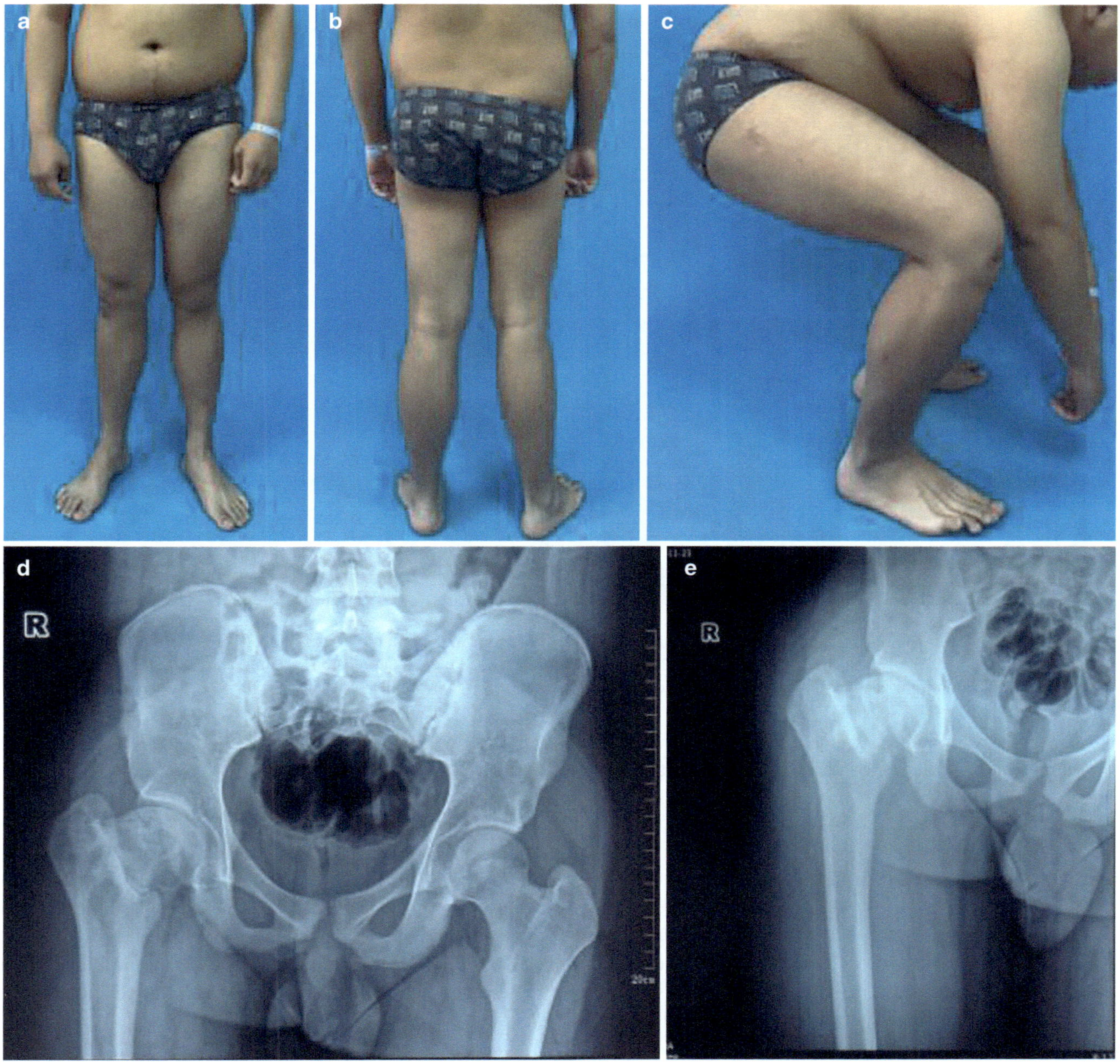

Figure 5.10 Slipped epiphysis of the right femoral head. (**a**) Both lower limbs stand and observe the photo from the front; (**b**) Both lower limbs stand and observe the photo from the back; (**c**) Squat side view photo; (**d**) Anteroposterior X-ray of pelvis; (**e**) Lateral radiograph of right hip

ing in cartilage destruction. It is characterized by degeneration of acetabular labrum and articular cartilage of femoral head, wear of acetabular cartilage, and formation of new bone under cartilage and around joint, which eventually leads to pain, deformity, and joint dysfunction. It is generally believed that it is related to aging, trauma, inflammation, obesity, metabolism, and heredity.

5.3.3.2 Clinical Manifestation

Osteoarthritis of the hip is characterized by abnormal gait and hip pain during activity or weight-bearing. Hip pain may radiate through the obturator nerve to the groin, thigh, and knee.

According to the severity of the disease, it can be divided into early stage, advanced stage, and late stage. If the hip joint space is narrowed and the bone around the joint and the femoral head are cystic, it is proved to be in the middle and late stages. In severe cases, the bone around the joint is hyperosteogeny and sclerosis, and the femoral head collapses and deforms (Fig. 5.11).

5.3.3.3 Treatment Principle

Treatment of osteoarthritis aims to relieve pain, delay disease progression, correct deformity, and improve or restore joint function. The principle of treatment is gradient and individualized treatment according to the patient's condition:

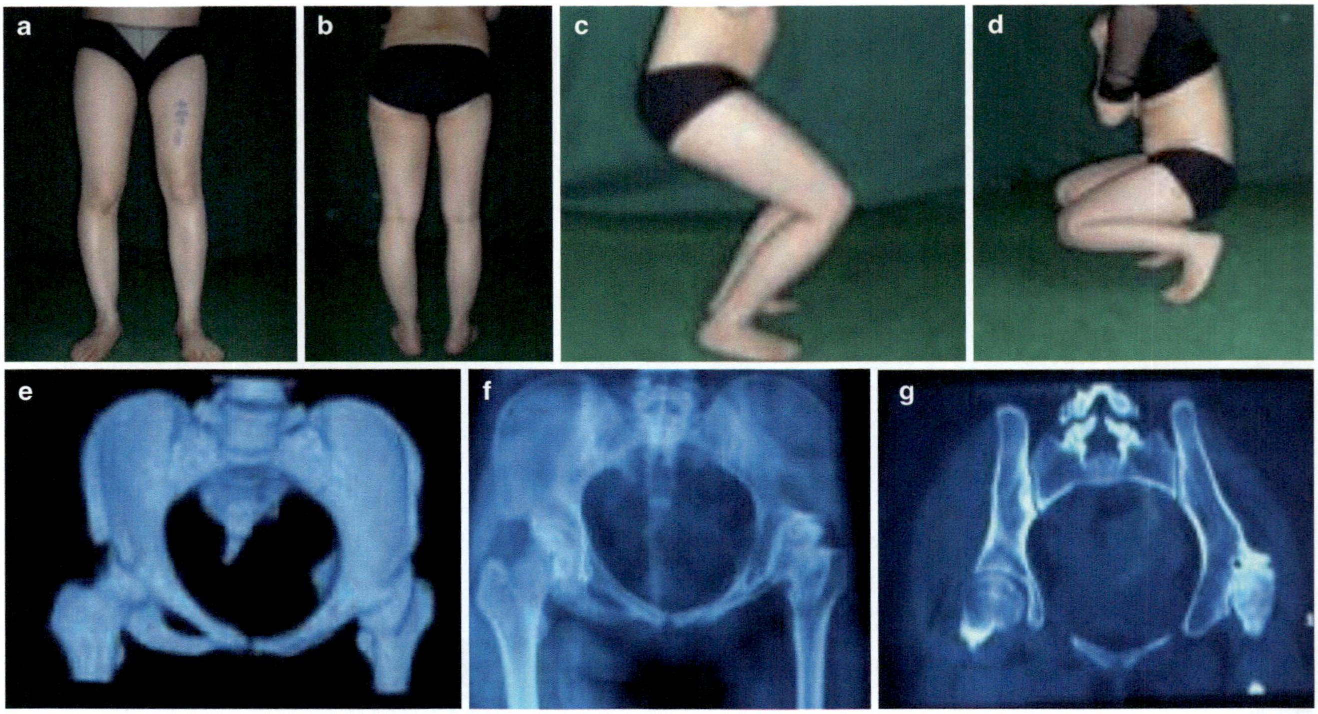

Fig. 5.11 Osteoarthritis of bilateral hip joints is severe in the right hip. (**a**) Front view of both lower limbs; (**b**) Back view of both lower limbs; (**c**) Lateral view of hip joint at maximum flexion; (**d**) Lateral view of knee joint at maximum flexion; (**e**) Keywords CT reconstruction of pelvis; (**f**) X; Pelvic anteroposterior radiograph; Coronal reconstruction of the (**g**) CT showed the destruction of the articular surface

(1) Hip preservation surgery, such as osteophyte resection, proximal femoral osteotomy, etc. (2) Femoral head or total hip arthroplasty.

5.3.4 Knee Osteoarthritis

5.3.4.1 Etiology

Knee osteoarthritis (KOA) is a chronic joint disease characterized by degeneration of knee cartilage and secondary hyperosteogeny, which is more common in middle-aged and elderly women than in men. At present, the etiology and pathogenesis of knee osteoarthritis are considered to be related to abnormal mechanical axis of lower limbs, cold and obesity of knee joint, living environment, overwork, long-term high-heeled shoes for women, and other factors. Genu varus deformity aggravates the process of degeneration of articular cartilage of femoral medial condyle.

5.3.4.2 Clinical Manifestations

Knee osteoarthritis is mostly accompanied by mild genu varum or leg torsion deformity, with early symptoms such as knee soreness and knee swelling. With the aggravation of genu varus deformity in the middle and late stages, the symptoms of knee pain, stiffness, and walking dysfunction became more obvious. X-ray examination showed that the joint space was narrow, the joint was destroyed, and the lower limb force line was abnormal (Fig. 5.12).

5.3.4.3 Treatment Principle

The primary goal of treatment of genu varum with osteoarthritis is surgical correction of genu varum deformity, restoration of normal mechanical axis of the lower limb, natural relief of pathological changes and clinical symptoms of osteoarthritis of the medial condyle, and artificial joint replacement if the joint has been significantly damaged.

5.3.5 Stress Knee Ligament Relaxation

The medial and lateral collateral ligaments of the knee play an important role in stabilizing and braking the movement of the knee joint. Once injured, it is easy to cause joint relaxation.

5.3.5.1 Etiology

Factors such as abnormal force line of lower limbs, trauma, and weak muscle strength around the joint lead to the vulnerability of the collateral ligament to injury when the knee joint is subjected to varus and valgus, rotation, and compound violence. Ligament relaxation is mostly caused by clinical misdiagnosis or inappropriate treatment after injury. Biomechanical changes of the knee joint after collateral ligament injury are often caused by clinical misdiagnosis or inappropriate treat-

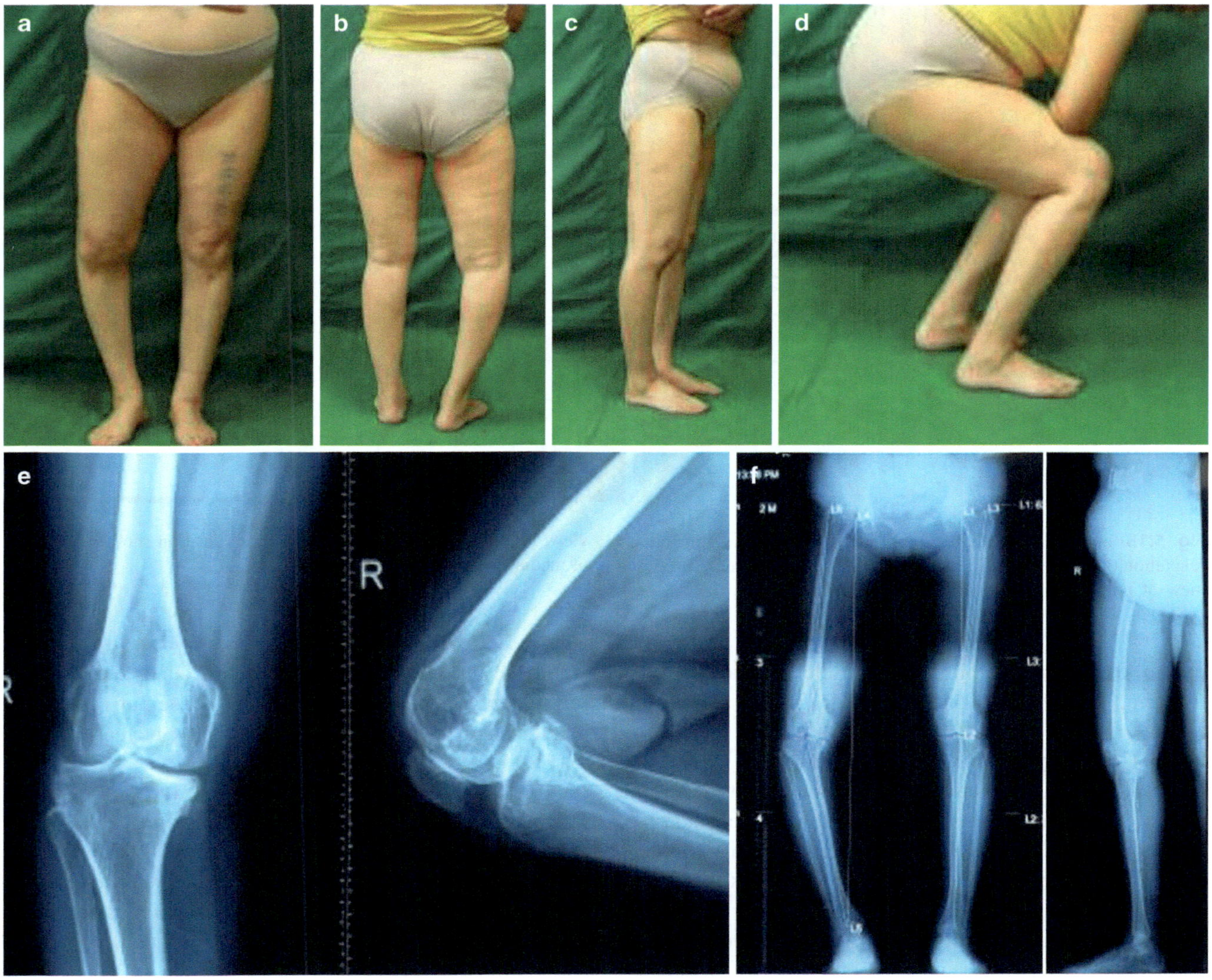

Fig. 5.12 Osteoarthritis of right knee with genu varum deformity. (**a**) Frontal view of both lower limbs; (**b**) Posterior view of both lower limbs; (**c**) Lateral view of lower limbs; (**d**) Maximum knee flexion lateral view photo; (**e**) Anteroposterior radiograph of the knee showed medial collapse of the tibial plateau; (**f**) Both lower limbs were standing in full-length normal position, and the mechanical axis of the lower limbs deviated to the medial side. (**g**) Standing full-length lateral radiograph of the right lower extremity

ment. Cartilage destruction of the medial femoral condyle and medial tibial plateau of the knee joint during long-term weight-bearing walking leads to secondary degenerative changes of the knee joint and eventually osteoarthritis.

5.3.5.2 Clinical Manifestation

The main manifestations are instability of the knee joint, instability of external rotation, and eversion of the knee joint in patients with severe relaxation of the medial collateral ligament after injury, instability of internal rotation and eversion in patients with severe relaxation of the lateral collateral ligament after injury, long-term lack of protection for weight-bearing walking, subluxation or dislocation of the knee under stress, joint swelling and pain, which seriously affect walking function. The X-ray film showed that the joint space was widened and mismatched, the articular cartilage was worn, and the bone was hyperosteogeny (Fig. 5.13).

5.3.5.3 Treatment Principles

Correct the gravity line of lower limbs, maintain the stability of joints, repair the natural contracture of loose collateral ligaments, restore the stability of knee joints, and improve the function of standing and walking.

5.3.6 Stress Knee Recurvatum Deformity

Knee joint hyperextension more than 10 degrees is knee flexion. Stress knee flexion refers to knee flexion formed and gradually aggravated by long-term weight-bearing walking

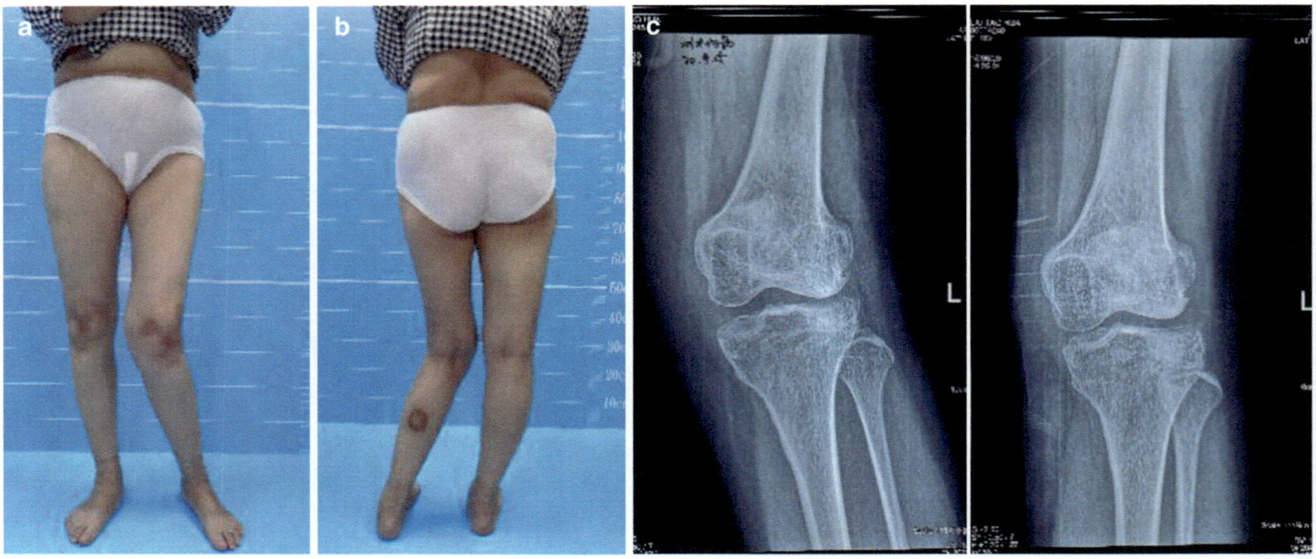

Fig. 5.13 a 48-year-old female presented with genu valgum due to relaxation of the medial collateral ligament of the left knee. (**a**) Frontal view of both lower limbs, left genu valgum deformity; (**b**) Posterior view; (**c**) X-ray film of knee joint in stress position showed relaxation of medial collateral ligament

due to knee joint instability and muscle imbalance around the joint.

5.3.6.1 Etiology

Congenital knee recurvatum, found at birth, is a type of joint contracture. Stress knee flexion is mostly secondary to neuromuscular diseases such as infantile paralysis. The muscles of lower limbs are widely paralyzed, the knee joint is relaxed, and even in a flail state. When bearing weight, the body's center of gravity moves forward, and the posture is maintained entirely by the interlocking ligaments in the knee joint and the tension of the posterior joint capsule. Or the hamstring muscle behind the knee joint is paralyzed, the quadriceps femoris loses antagonism and the knee recurves; it can also be secondary to the compensatory retroflexion of the knee joint during the walking process of the horseshoe foot. It is also seen in obese people, long-term weight-bearing walking without protection, and knee flexion occurs and gradually aggravates under stress.

5.3.6.2 Clinical Manifestation

The knee joint is in a relaxed state, the retroflexion is greater than 10 degrees, and in severe cases, it can exceed 70 degrees. The lateral movement is increased, the joint is unstable, and the tibial plateau can slide anterolaterally, the knee joint can be everted, and the subluxation can occur. Knee retroflexion from childhood to adolescence not only causes soft tissue relaxation but also bone and joint deformity. If knee retroflexion is used for lower limb weight-bearing for a long time, the X-ray film shows that the anterior part of the tibial plateau collapses, the articular surface tilts forward and downward, the anterior part of the femoral condyle is flat, the physiological anterior arch of the distal femur disappears, and the angle of the distal femoral condyle increases (≥ 100 °) (Fig. 5.14).

5.3.6.3 Treatment Principle

Individualized treatment should be adopted according to the patient's age, weight, type, and degree of retroflexion, and the bone line should be restored by distraction osteotomy of distal femur and proximal tibia. In childhood, epiphyseal stimulation can be adopted, stable fixation of knee flexion can be adopted, soft tissue contracture behind the knee joint can be promoted, and long-term treatment of external fixator, plaster, and brace can be used to restore the knee joint. Patients with severe genu recurvatum need to wear braces for a long time.

5.3.7 Middle-Aged and Elderly People with Flatfoot

Congenital or postural factors can lead to low arch or disappearance, foot valgus, arch collapse when standing and walking, fatigue or pain symptoms.

5.3.7.1 Etiology

The cause of flatfoot in middle and old age is acquired secondary factor. (1) Long-term weight-bearing standing, weight gain, excessive fatigue caused by long-distance travel, gradual weakening of soft tissues such as muscles, ligaments, joint capsules, and aponeuroses that maintain the

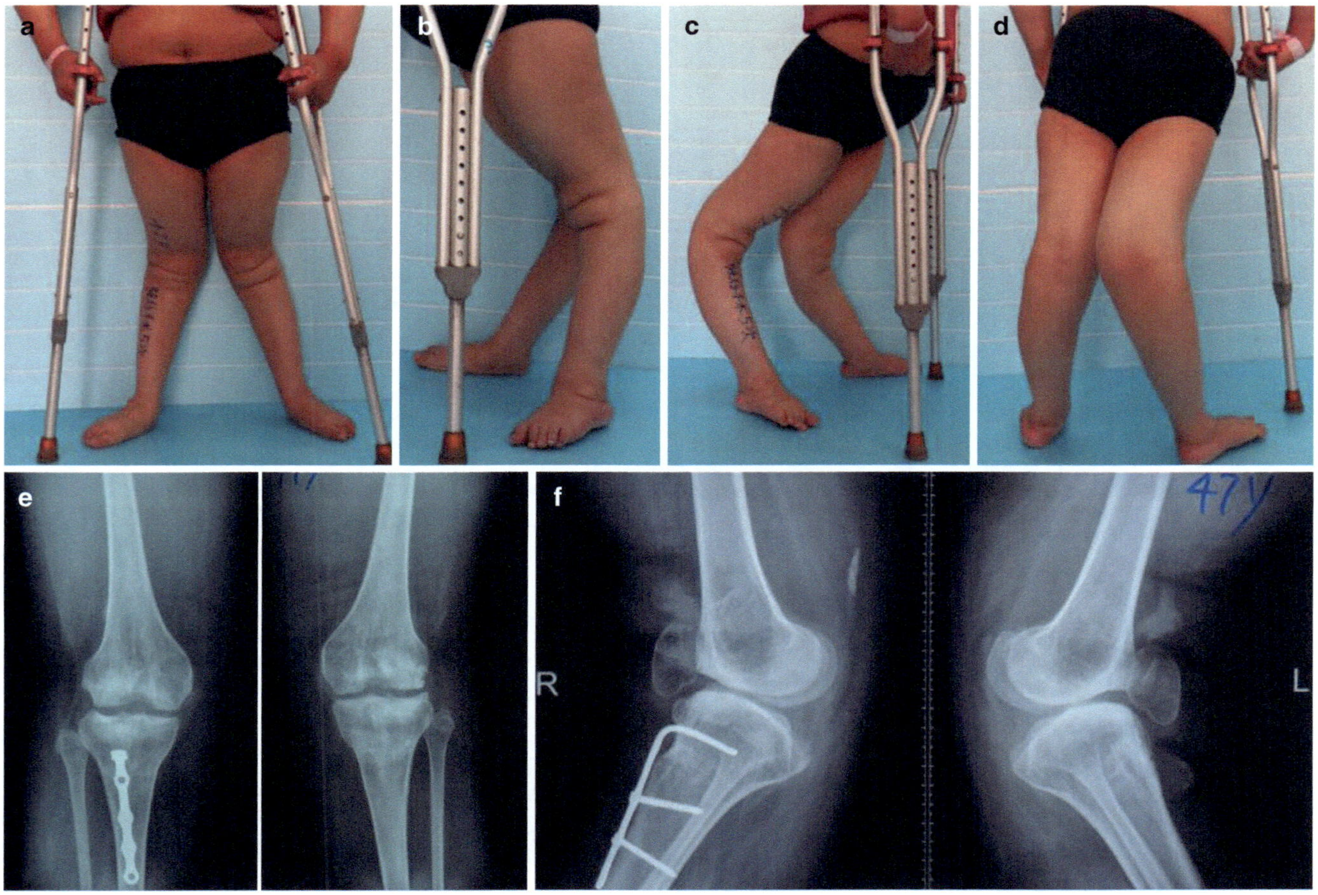

Fig. 5.14 Female, 47 years old, with progressive stress retroflexion of both knees due to poliomyelitis. (**a**) Frontal view of both lower limbs; (**b**, **c**) Lateral view of both lower limbs; (**d**) Photos from the back of both lower limbs; **e**, **f**. Anteroposterior and lateral radiographs of both knees

arch of the foot, and gradual flattening of the arch of the foot; (2) Lying in bed for a long time, lack of exercise, muscle atrophy, decreased tension, and foot arch subsidence during weight-bearing; (3) Improper wearing of shoes, too high heel, long-term forward weight movement, forward and downward inclination of calcaneus, and destruction of the longitudinal arch of the foot; (4) Foot osteopathy, such as rheumatoid arthritis bone and joint tuberculosis, etc. (5) Poliomyelitis Spina bifida, cerebral palsy and other foot internal and external muscle strength imbalance due to flat foot disease.

5.3.7.2 Clinical Manifestation

The early symptoms of flatfoot are anteromedial pain of ankle joint, aggravation of standing or walking for a long time, alleviation of rest and limitation of foot movement. Physical examination showed that the longitudinal arch of the medial foot collapsed, the heel was everted, the forefoot was abducted relative to the dorsum of the foot, and the standing load line moved inward beyond the ankle joint and the medial edge of the foot. Anteroposterior X-ray of ankle joint showed talocalcaneal tilt, lateral X-ray showed talar plantar flexion, and anteroposterior and lateral X-ray of weight-bearing foot showed adduction of the first metatarsal bone and hallux valgus. The metatarsus and calcaneus were overlapped, the transverse arch was destroyed, and the longitudinal arch collapsed. Inversion of the talus and eversion of the calcaneus, subluxation of the intertarsal joint and osteoarthritis can be seen in the late stage.

According to the clinical manifestations, it can be divided into: (1) Flexible flat foot: although the soft tissue is loose, it still maintains a certain degree of elasticity, the foot is flat when bearing weight, the foot can immediately return to normal after removing the gravity, and the long-term treatment effect is satisfactory. (2) Rigid flat foot: It is mostly caused by the syndesmosis of the tarsal bone of the foot, and the manipulation is not easy to correct. The plantar surface between the tarsal joints of the foot protrudes, the arch of the foot disappears, the calcaneus is everted, the bilateral Achilles tendons are splayed, the talus head moves inward, subluxation occurs, the medial talus protrudes, sometimes combined with spasm of the peroneus longus and brevis and the third peroneus muscle. Some patients may have secondary low back pain and hip and knee pain (Fig. 5.15).

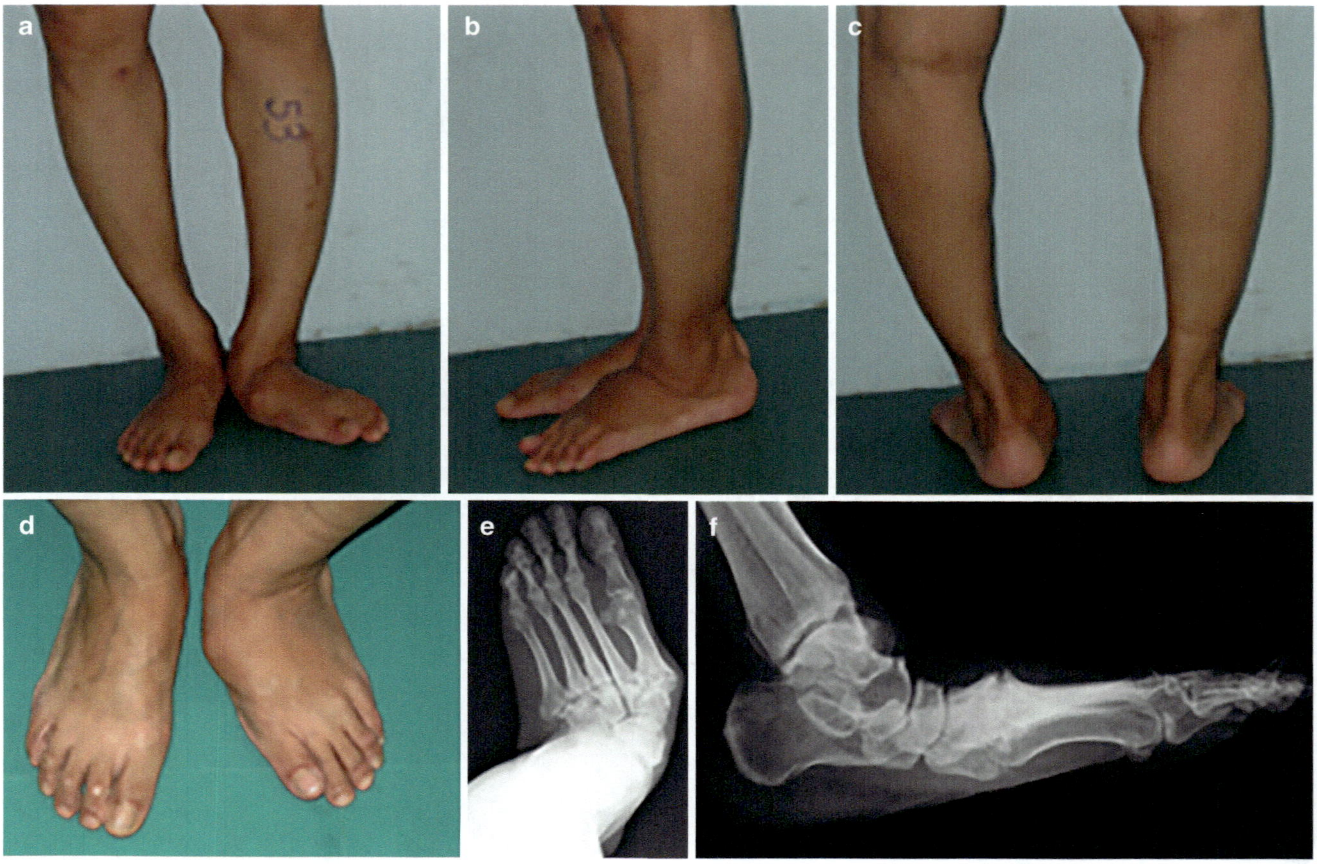

Fig. 5.15 Middle-aged and elderly people with flatfoot. (**a**) Foot-front view photo; (**b**) Anteroposterior contrast photograph of both feet; (**c**) Photos from the back of both feet; (**d**) Lateral X-ray film of ankle joint of both feet; (**e**) Foot weight-bearing anteroposterior radiograph. (**f**). Lateral X-ray of left foot in weight-bearing phase

5.3.7.3 Treatment Principle

Individualized treatment should be used, and non-surgical treatment can be used for flexible flat foot, such as physiotherapy, massage, functional exercise, wearing orthopedic shoes or orthopedic insoles. For rigid flatfoot, rehabilitation therapy and orthopedic shoes are ineffective, manual reduction and plaster fixation under anesthesia, soft tissue release, calcaneal osteotomy, subtalar joint fusion, and triple joint fusion can be used. For severe rigid foot valgus deformity, soft tissue release and limited osteotomy can be combined with Ilizarov technique.

5.3.8 Hallux Valgus

Hallux valgus is a common forefoot deformity in which the great toe is tilted laterally to the foot and the first phalanx is adducted.

5.3.8.1 Etiology

It is mostly related to heredity and shoe discomfort, more than 80% of them have family history, and women are more common. There is a strong ligament connection between the cuneiform bone and the metatarsal bone of the foot, but the connection between the medial cuneiform bone and the first metatarsal bone is weak. If standing too long or walking too much, especially often wear high-heeled or pointed shoes, the pressure on the medial cuneate bone and metatarsals will exceed 25%, which will cause the inward displacement of the first metatarsals and the collapse of the longitudinal and transverse arches of the foot. The great toe moves outward due to the traction of the adductor pollicis muscle and the extensor pollicis longus muscle, and the angle between the first and second phalanges increases. The bone of the first toe forms an osteophyte on the medial side of the foot, the eversion is gradually aggravated, the second toe is pushed dorsally by the first toe, and the interphalangeal joint is flexed to form a hammer-shaped toe.

5.3.8.2 Clinical Manifestations

Hallux valgus is often symmetrical and is more common in women. The metatarsophalangeal joint of the great toe may be dislocated, and osteophyte may be formed at the attachment of the medial joint capsule due to long-term traction. Because wear shoe to rub for a long time in metatarsal head inside out-

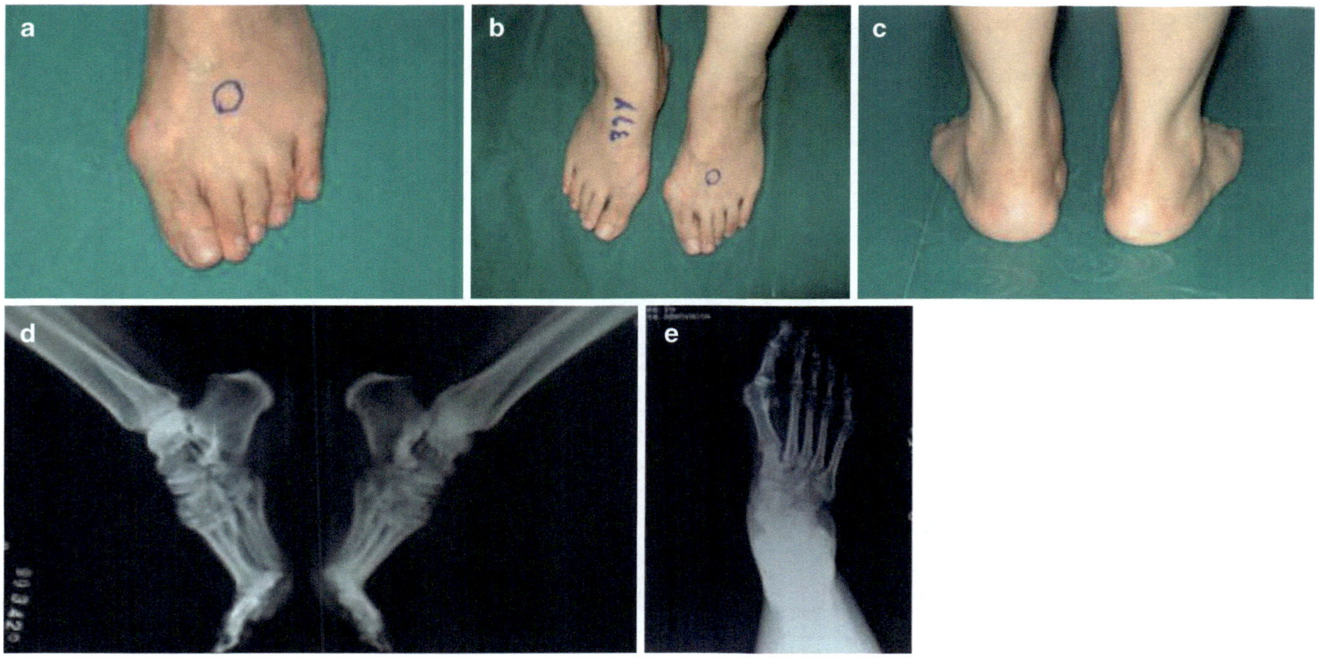

Fig. 5.16 Hallux valgus deformity. (**a**) Foot frontal view photo; (**b**) foot frontal view photo; (**c**) Photos from the back of both feet; (**d**) Lateral X-ray film of ankle joint of both feet; E. Foot weight-bearing anteroposterior radiograph

standing part, the skin is added thick, hypodermic produce bursa, red inflammation, form bursitis. In severe cases, the metatarsophalangeal joint of the hallux can produce osteoarthritis, causing pain. The skin on the metatarsal surface of the second and third metatarsal heads can form callus due to increased weight bearing. The skin on the dorsal side of the proximal interphalangeal joint of the second toe can form callus or corns due to friction with the vamp. It is often associated with flatfoot, severe hallux valgus with rotation deformity, local pain, and difficulty walking. Foot weight-bearing anteroposterior X-ray film showed increased intermetatarsal angle, increased hallux valgus angle, dislocation of the first metatarsophalangeal joint, severe dislocation of the second, third, and fourth metatarsophalangeal joints, varus deformity of the fifth toe, and lateral dislocation of the sesamoid bone under the first metatarsal head, which was osteoarthritis. Lateral radiographs showed flatfoot with collapsed arch. Axial radiographs of the calcaneus showed calcaneus valgus.

Clinical classification: (1) Mild: valgus angle <30 °, intermetatarsal angle <13 °, the joints are often matched, and the deformity may be caused by interphalangeal hallux valgus; (2) Moderate: valgus angle was 30 °–40 °, intermetatarsal angle was 13 °–20 °, metatarsophalangeal joint was often subluxated, and the second toe was compressed by hallux pronation; (3) Severe: valgus angle >40 °, intermetatarsal angle ≥20 °, hallux pronation, overlapping above or below the second toe, metatarsophalangeal joint dislocation, metastatic pain under the second metatarsal head, and arthritic changes (Fig. 5.16).

5.3.8.3 Treatment Principle

Individualized treatment should be carried out according to clinical stages: (1) early stage (early stage of subluxation): bunion is mild, pain is not serious, hammer-toe is not combined, non-surgical treatment is the main method, manipulative correction, auxiliary brace, insole, and so on can be used; (2) Middle stage (subluxation stage): If hallux valgus deformity is obvious, the pain of bunion is severe, and non-operative treatment is ineffective, it is suitable for the combination of osteotomy of the distal end of the first metatarsal bone and the base of the first phalanx or soft tissue surgery alone; (3) Late stage (osteoarthritis stage): In addition to the pain of bunion, the metatarsophalangeal joint was swollen and painful. In this stage, metatarsophalangeal osteotomy or metatarsal cuneiform joint fusion combined with soft tissue surgery was chosen for surgical treatment. The first metatarsal-phalangeal arthroplasty or fusion was rarely used, and the lateral toe surgery with deformity and symptoms was performed at the same time.

5.3.9 Fan-Shaped Foot

Congenital or postural factors can cause the transverse arch of the foot to be low and flat or disappear. When the affected foot stands and walks, if the anterior arch collapses obviously, it will stretch like a fan, and fatigue or pain symptoms will occur when standing and walking for a long time.

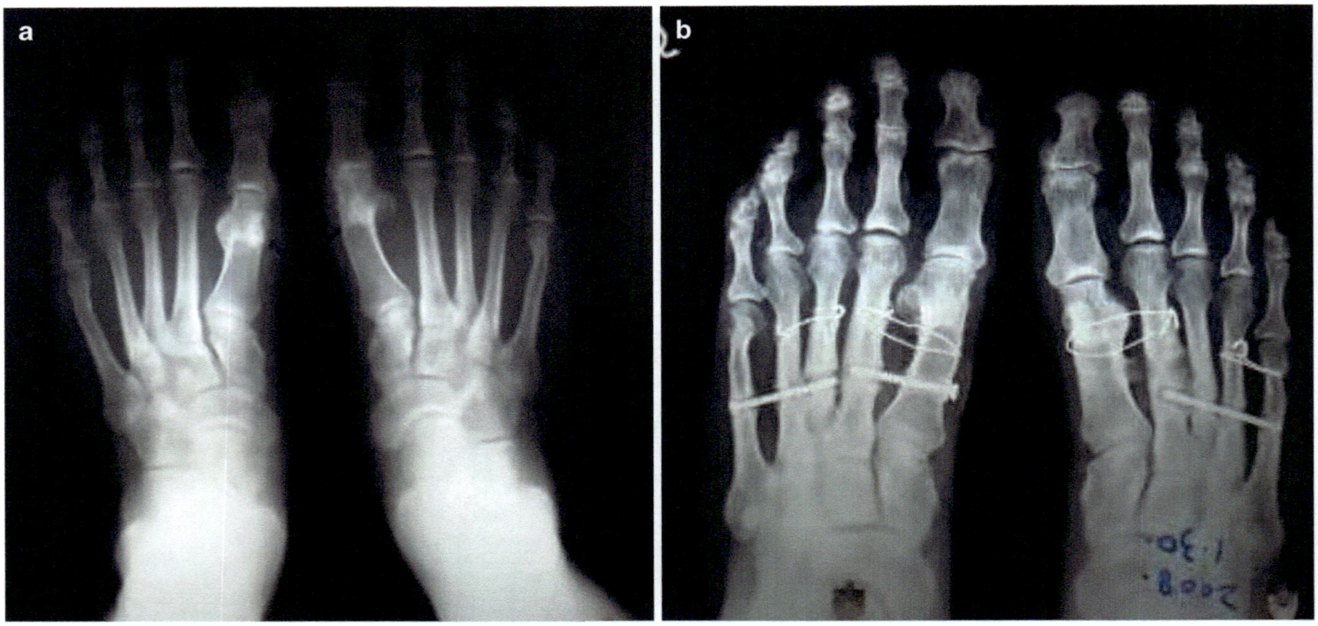

Fig. 5.17 Fan-shaped foot, male, 55 years old: (**a**) Preoperative anteroposterior X-ray of both feet, widening between the metatarsals of both forefeet; (**b**) X-ray examination after metatarsal binding showed narrowing of the forefoot

5.3.9.1 Etiology

The causes of arch collapse may be congenital dysplasia, mainly acquired secondary factors: (1) Long-term weight-bearing standing, weight gain, excessive fatigue caused by long-distance travel, gradual weakening of soft tissues such as muscles, ligaments, joint capsules, and aponeuroses to maintain the arch, and gradual flattening of the arch; (2) Lying in bed for a long time, lack of exercise, muscle atrophy, decreased tension, and foot arch subsidence during weight-bearing; (3) Improper wearing of shoes, too high heel, long-term forward weight movement, forward and downward inclination of calcaneus, and destruction of the longitudinal arch of the foot; (4) Foot osteopathy, such as rheumatoid arthritis bone and joint tuberculosis, etc. (5) Poliomyelitis sequelae, spina bifida, cerebral palsy, and other foot internal and external muscle strength imbalance left flat foot disease.

5.3.9.2 Clinical Manifestation

The main manifestations are the relaxation of the joints of the foot, the collapse of the transverse arch of the foot is the most typical, the gap between the metatarsal heads and the metatarsal bones is widened, showing a fan-shaped change, and the toes are also widened accordingly. Radiographs of the weight-bearing foot showed disappearance of the transverse arch of the foot, separation of the metatarsals, and eversion of the hindfoot (Fig. 5.17). It is often associated with hallux valgus.

5.3.9.3 Treatment Principle

1. Asymptomatic patients may not be treated or the forefoot may be bandaged with elastic bandage.
2. If it causes weakness in walking and foot pain during weight-bearing, metatarsal binding can be performed.

5.3.10 Ankle Osteoarthritis

Ankle osteoarthritis is an inflammatory disease caused by bone hyperplasia or wear around the joint due to joint degeneration, with typical symptoms of joint swelling and pain.

5.3.10.1 Etiology

Ankle osteoarthritis can be caused by degeneration caused by age or weight, deformity of lower limbs, rheumatic or rheumatoid diseases, gout, hemochromatosis, hemophilia, neurological diseases and infections. Other factors include: (1) chronic strain, (2) repeated twisting of the ankle, (3) joint trauma, (4) overweight, (5) poor or delayed reduction secondary to fracture and dislocation of the ankle.

5.3.10.2 Clinical Manifestation

The clinical manifestations are pain, stiffness, reduced range of motion, swelling, weakness, and ankle deformity. Pain is the most prominent clinical symptom of ankle osteoarthritis, which can cause post-exercise pain, exercise pain, and rest pain. When the joint movement is limited, there may be lameness, which is characterized by flat foot approach, small stride, and haste. X-ray film shows hyperplastic osteophyte. Osteochondritis dissecans was seen on MRI (Fig. 5.18).

Ankle osteoarthritis can be divided into primary and secondary. Primary osteoarthritis has no obvious cause and is often related to genetic and physical factors. It is common in the elderly and can be manifested as narrowing of joint space, osteophyte formation, cartilage wear and loss. Secondary osteoarthritis is common in young adults, mostly secondary to joint fracture, leading to early degeneration of the joint, resulting in ankle osteoarthritis.

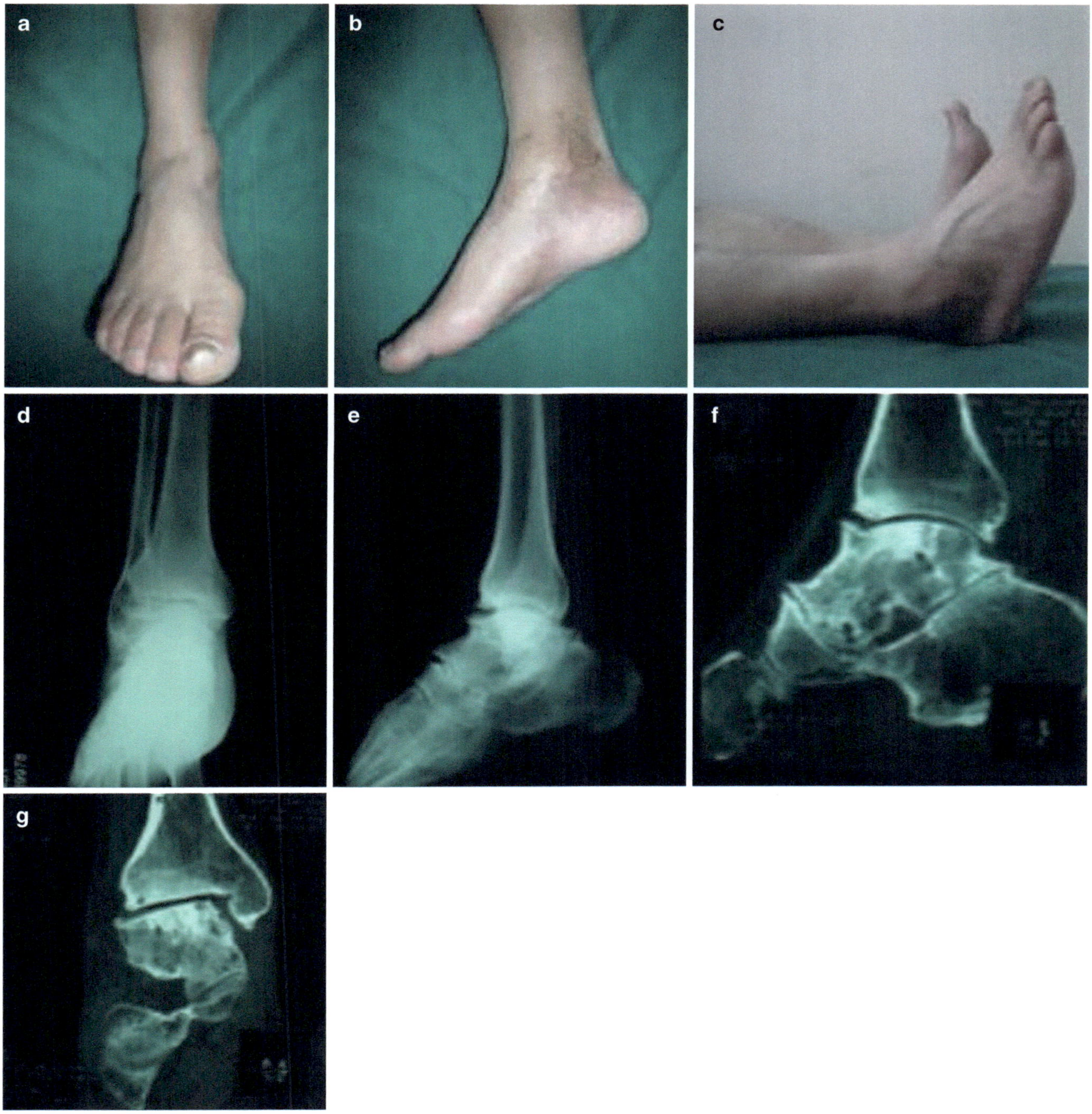

Fig. 5.18 Ankle osteoarthritis. (**a**) Ankle frontal view photograph; (**b**) Ankle lateral view photograph; (**c**) Ankle joint maximum dorsiflexion lateral view photo; (**d**) Ankle anteroposterior radiograph; (**e**) Lateral radiographs of the ankle; (**f**) Sagittal plane of CT reconstruction showed tibiotalar articular surface destruction; (**g**) Coronal view of CT reconstruction showing tibiotalar articular surface destruction

5.3.10.3 Treatment Principle

The treatment of osteoarthritis aims to relieve pain, correct deformity, slow down the development of deformity and lesions, improve joint function, and improve the quality of life of patients. The principle of treatment is gradient and individualized treatment according to the patient's condition. Non-operative treatment: (1) Rest and restriction of activities;(2) Physical therapy, hot and humid compress, massage, etc. (3) Drug therapy, symptomatic treatment with non-steroidal anti-inflammatory drugs; (4) Local block therapy; (5) Cartilage protective agent; (6) Brace. Surgical treatment: (1) Arthroscopic exploration and debridement of the ankle; (2) Ilizarov Ankle retractor; (3) Artificial ankle joint replacement; (4) Ankle arthrodesis.

6 Neoplastic Disease Leads to Deformity

Zhiwei Fang, Sihe Qin, and Shu Li

6.1 Craniocerebral and Spinal Cord Tumors

6.1.1 Intracranial Germ Cell Tumor

Intracranial germ cell tumors (ICGCTs) are a group of tumors with special pathological properties, clinical manifestations, and treatment options, which are derived from embryonic germ cells. The symptoms and signs are determined according to the location, nature, and size of the tumor.

6.1.1.1 Etiology

The etiology and pathogenesis of germ cell tumors remain unclear. According to the theory of Teilum (1965), germinoma originates from embryonic germ cells, and germ cells can evolve into full-potential cells and embryonic cancer stem cells, and further form embryonal carcinoma, choriocarcinoma, yolk sac tumor, and teratoma. Except for mature teratoma, all other germ cell tumors are malignant. Tumor cells can fall off in cerebrospinal fluid (CSF), implant and disseminate in the ventricles and subarachnoid space, and very few can metastasize to the outside of the central nervous system along the blood, such as lung, lymph nodes, bone, and so on.

6.1.1.2 Clinical Manifestation

The symptoms and signs are determined according to the location, nature, and size of the tumor. In addition to tumor mass effect and compression of adjacent brain tissue, it can also obstruct the circulation of cerebrospinal fluid, causing increased intracranial pressure and ventricular dilatation; tumors in the pineal region often cause increased intracranial pressure and eye movement disorder; there are often polydipsia, polyuria, and developmental retardation in the sellar region. Larger tumors can obstruct the foramen of Monro, resulting in increased intracranial pressure and bilateral ventricular enlargement, manifested as headache vomiting. Tumor growth compresses or invades the motor center, causing motor central nervous system injury, resulting in corresponding motor dysfunction, and gradually secondary limb deformities, with talipes equinovarus in the lower limbs (Fig. 6.1).

6.1.1.3 Treatment Principle

First, treat the primary tumor, relieve the central nervous system compression, recover the secondary limb deformity that has not improved for more than 2 years, and perform surgical correction to improve the limb motor function.

6.1.2 Craniopharyngioma

Craniopharyngioma is a common embryonic residual tissue tumor developed from the epithelial cells of the residual craniopharynx formed by ectoderm. It is the most common congenital intracranial tumor, which often occurs in children and is rare in adults.

6.1.2.1 Etiology

Craniopharyngiomas are derived from remnants of epithelial cells or Rathke's bursa of the craniopharynx (ameloblastic type) or from remnants of squamous epithelial cells of the primitive fovea (papillary type). Craniopharyngioma can occur from any point of the pituitary-hypothalamic axis and develop along this axis. Tumors can be located from the sella turcica to the third ventricle of the brain. About 50% of tumors originate from the infundibulum and (or) tuberculum cinereum area at the level of the third ventricle floor, mainly developing toward the third ventricle.

Z. Fang · S. Li
Department of Bone and Soft Tissue Tumor, Peking University Cancer Hospital, Key laboratory of Carcinogenesis and Translational Research (Ministry of Education/Beijing), Beijing, China

S. Qin (✉)
Department of Orthopaedics, Rehabilitation Hospital of the National Research Center for Rehabilitation Technical Aids, Beijing, China

S. Qin et al. (eds.), *Atlas of Limb Deformity*, https://doi.org/10.1007/978-981-97-0999-1_6

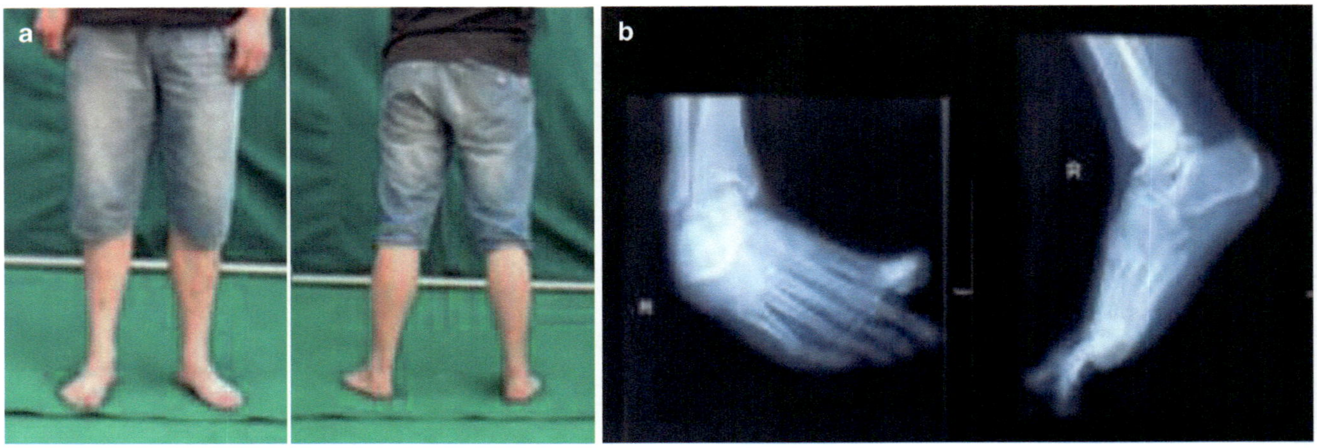

Fig. 6.1 Right foot varus caused by intracranial germ cell tumor

6.1.2.2 Clinical Manifestation

Craniopharyngiomas are usually slow-growing, insidious in onset, and are often diagnosed 1–2 years after the onset of symptoms. Common symptoms include endocrine dysfunction, visual impairment, and intracranial hypertension. Craniopharyngioma often leads to endocrine dysfunction, such as hypothyroidism, orthostatic hypotension, short stature, diabetes insipidus, impotence, amenorrhea, etc., but in a few cases, some endocrine hyperfunction may also occur, such as precocious puberty in children, obesity in adults, and so on. Classical bitemporal hemianopsia is caused by tumor compression of the optic chiasm. Secondary hydrocephalus can be caused when the tumor increases to a certain extent and the occupying effect blocks the foramen of Monro, the third ventricle or the aqueduct, and patients may have symptoms of intracranial hypertension such as headache, nausea, and vomiting. Lower limb deformities caused by craniopharyngioma are mainly spastic paralysis and increased muscle tension. Fixed deformities, such as talipes equinovarus deformity and knee flexion contracture, occur in patients with a longer course of disease (Fig. 6.2).

6.1.2.3 Treatment Principle

The primary tumor was resected and the nerve compression was relieved. Lower limb deformities secondary to nerve injury can be corrected by orthopedic surgery to balance muscle strength, correct bone and joint deformities, and improve lower limb walking function.

6.1.3 Spinal Cord Glioma

Spinal cord glioma (spinal cord glioma, SPG) is one of the central nervous system tumors with low incidence, accounting for 10% of the total intraspinal tumors, while the proportion in foreign countries is slightly higher than 15%. It originates from the ectoderm of the spinal cord, such as glial cells and ependymal cells, so it is an intramedullary tumor. Astrocytoma and ependymoma are common, accounting for about 40% each.

6.1.3.1 Etiology

Spinal cord gliomas can occur at all ages, and the exact cause of the disease is not yet clear. Spinal cord injury caused by spinal cord glioma leads to incomplete paralysis below the level of injury, weakening or loss of the muscles of the lower limbs innervated by the affected nerves, and imbalance of muscle strength, which gradually results in bone and joint deformities of the lower limbs.

6.1.3.2 Clinical Manifestation

Gliomas of the spinal cord were distributed segmentally, mainly in the cervical, thoracic, and lumbar segments, among which ependymoma and astrocytoma were the most common pathological types. Ependymomas are more common in adults, with men slightly more than women, accounting for about 56.9%. Spinal cord ependymoma grows slowly, the course of disease is generally longer, accompanied by cystic degeneration or hemorrhage, the condition can be suddenly aggravated. When some patients were admitted to the hospital, the symptoms were only limb movement disorder, numbness, weakness or banding sensation of one side of the limb, some involved the contralateral limb, and some patients were accompanied by sensory disorders, which mostly developed from top to bottom, and the sensory plane was not obvious. There may be vesico-rectal disorders. Some patients had deformity of lower limbs, which was common in talipes equinovarus (Fig. 6.3).

6.1.3.3 Treatment Principle

Surgical resection is the most effective treatment strategy for most spinal cord gliomas. Orthopedic surgery can achieve satisfactory results for secondary lower limb deformities.

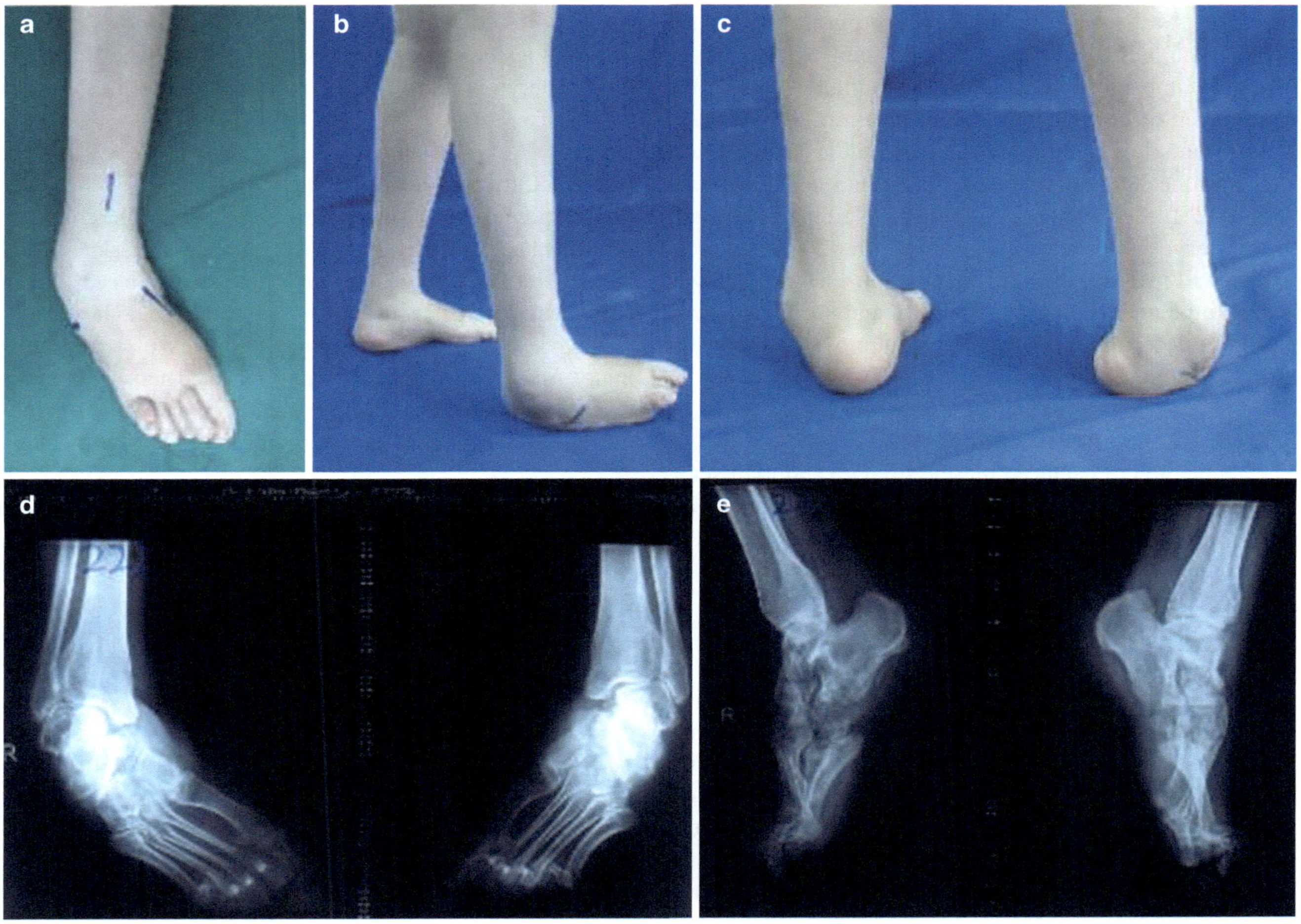

Fig. 6.2 Patient, female, 22 years old, craniopharyngioma, endocrine disorder, right talipes equinovarus deformity

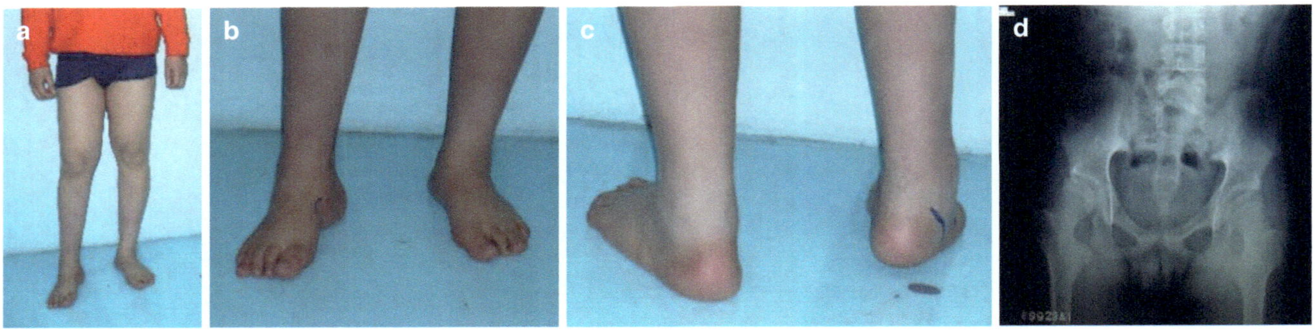

Fig. 6.3 Right talipes equinovarus following spinal glioma. (**a**) frontal view of standing position; (**b**) partial frontal view of both feet; (**c**) dorsal view of both feet; (**d**) Anteroposterior radiograph of pelvis

6.1.4 Spinal Neurofibroma

Spinal neurofibroma (SN), also known as spinal neurofibroma, originates from dorsal spinal nerve roots and can also produce subpial infiltration when it grows centripetally, which is more common in cases of rhomboid neurofibroma. Neurofibromas of the brachial or lumbar plexus may invade the central dura along multiple nerve roots.

6.1.4.1 Etiology

The etiology of this disease is unknown or related to genetic factors.

6.1.4.2 Clinical Manifestation

Symptoms of nerve root compression and stimulation may occur in the early stage, such as needling or knife-like pain, which can be aggravated by coughing and sneezing. As the tumor continues to progress, the spinal cord is compressed, which is manifested by the disturbance of limb movement below the tumor level and the disturbance of contralateral limb sensation. Severe cases lead to paraplegia, complete loss of motor, sensory, urinary and fecal functions below the spinal cord compression level. If the spinal cord is not completely compressed or the nerve is permanently injured after fibroma resection, it will lead to paralysis of some muscles of the lower limbs, imbalance of muscle strength, and secondary bone and joint deformities, with talipes equinovarus being the most common (Fig. 6.4).

6.1.4.3 Treatment Principles

The application of balanced muscle strength and joint stabilization to correct foot and ankle deformities can improve the weight-bearing walking function of lower limbs.

6.1.5 Hemangioblastoma

Spinal cord hemangioma, also known as hemangioblastoma (HB), is about 1/3 combined with cerebral retinal hemangiomatosis, about 1/2 occurs in the thoracic spinal cord, 40% in the cervical spinal cord, 80% in single lesions, 75% in intramedullary lesions, or in both intramedullary and extramedullary dura mater, attached to the pia mater on the dorsal side of the spinal cord. Epidural hemangioblastoma is rare, accounting for about 10–15% of all cases.

6.1.5.1 Etiology

The etiology is unknown, and some scholars believe that the early embryo is related to the mechanical injury of embryonic tissue.

6.1.5.2 Clinical Manifestation

The main symptom of spinal cord hemangioma is the compression of spinal cord nerves, such as numbness, weakness, and paralysis of limbs. If hemangioma ruptures and bleeds, it can cause acute subarachnoid hemorrhage or intramedullary hematoma, resulting in corresponding symptoms of acute nerve injury. Acute nerve injury or chronic repeated nerve injury may result in limb deformity and dysfunction, and talipes equinovarus is more common in lower limb deformity (Fig. 6.5).

6.1.5.3 Treatment Principle

1. To treat the primary disease, the spinal cord hemangioma was removed by the neurosurgeon.
2. Secondary limb deformities were corrected by soft tissue release and muscle strength balance. If the course of disease is long and bony deformity occurs, arthrodesis or osteotomy should be performed at the same time to correct limb deformity and improve walking function of lower limbs.

6.1.6 Spinal Meningioma

The incidence of spinal meningioma (SM) is similar to that of spinal schwannoma. SM can occur in any age group, but it is more common in 50–70 years old, and 75–85% of SM

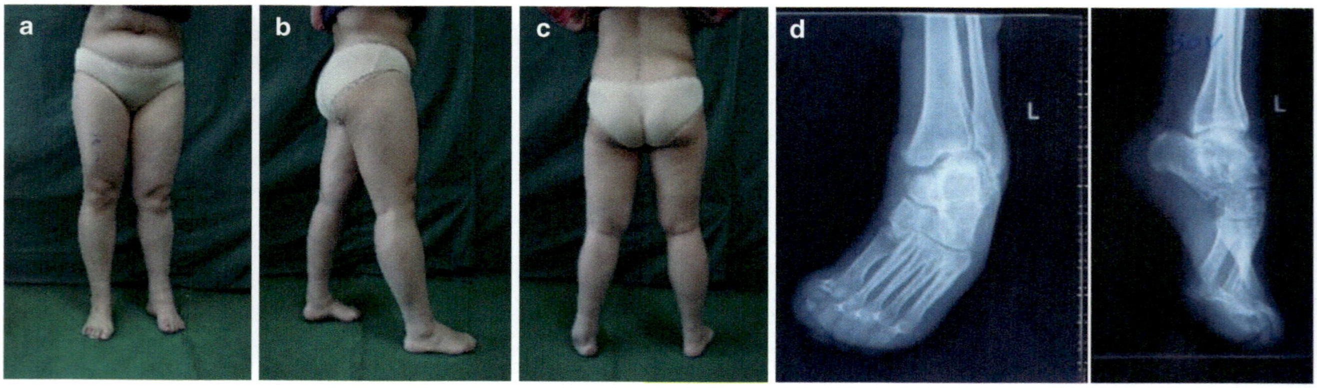

Fig. 6.4 Female, 30 years old, left foot varus caused by spinal neurofibroma. (**a**) frontal view in standing position; (**b**) right lateral view; (**c**) dorsal view, surgical incision scar in the middle of the waist, left foot varus; (**d**) Anteroposterior and lateral radiographs of the left foot

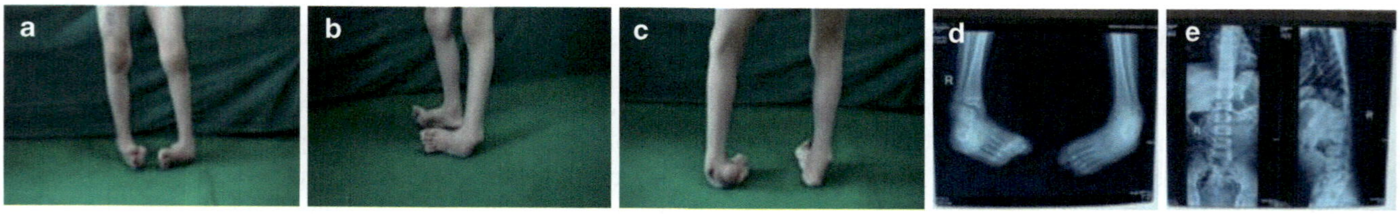

Fig. 6.5 Patient, male, 7 years old, bilateral talipes equinovarus secondary to hemangioma of spinal cord

occur in women. 80% of them were located in the thoracic spinal canal, and the upper cervical vertebra and the foramen magnum were also the predilection sites. The vast majority of meningiomas grow within the dura mater of the spinal cord, and about 10% grow across the dura mater or completely outside the dura mater of the spinal cord. Meningiomas usually occur in the arachnoid cap cells around the nerve roots near the dura mater of the spinal cord, which may explain why meningiomas often occur laterally in the spinal canal. Meningiomas may also originate from fibroblasts of the pia mater or dura mater of the spinal cord, suggesting that they may originate from mesodermal tissue.

6.1.6.1 Etiology

The cause is not clear.

6.1.6.2 Clinical Manifestation

Meningioma growth is slower, inchoate symptom is more not apparent, reason medical history is longer. The common first symptom was the numbness of the limbs corresponding to the location of the tumor, followed by fatigue, and radicular pain ranked third. Tumor growth compresses the spinal cord or nerve root, or tumor resection injures the spinal nerve, which can cause different degrees of muscle paralysis, muscle imbalance, and gradually secondary limb deformity (Fig. 6.6).

6.1.6.3 Treatment Principle

(1) The primary tumor is resected by a neurosurgeon; (2) Lower limb deformity secondary to nerve injury caused by tumor compression or resection. After the condition is stable, surgery should be performed to correct the deformity, restore the shape of lower limb, and improve walking function.

6.1.7 Spinal Cord Teratoma

Teratoma is a common type of ovarian germ cell tumor, which is divided into mature teratoma (benign teratoma) and immature teratoma (malignant teratoma). Benign teratomas contain many

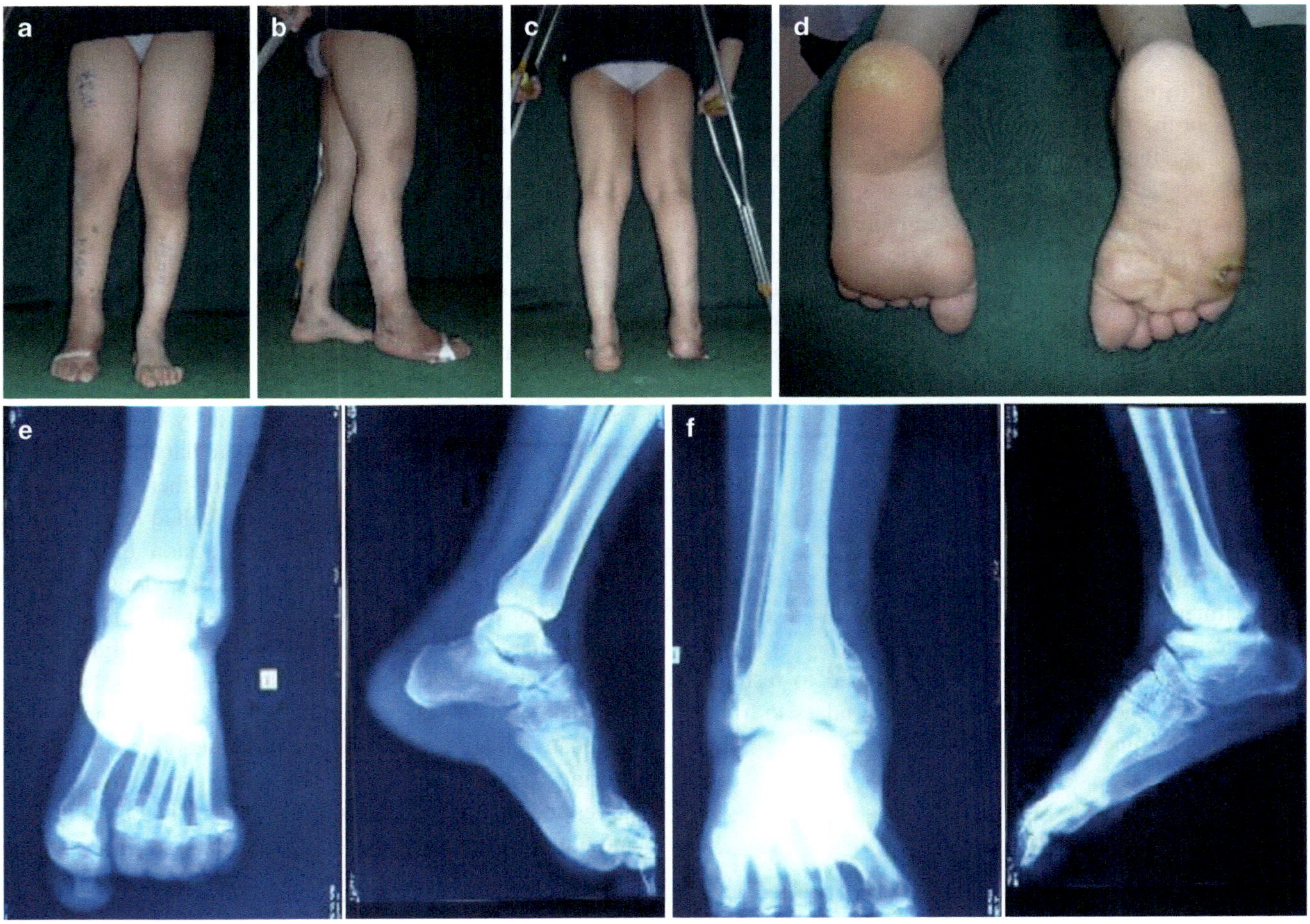

Fig. 6.6 Male, 14 years old, with spinal meningioma, resulting in deformity of both lower limbs, who had been operated for eight times. (**a**) frontal view in standing position; B. lateral view in standing position; (**c**) dorsal view in standing position; (**d**) plantar view, dysesthesia ulcer at the head of the fifth metatarsal bone; E. anteroposterior and lateral X-ray film of the left ankle; (**f**) Anteroposterior and lateral radiographs of the right ankle

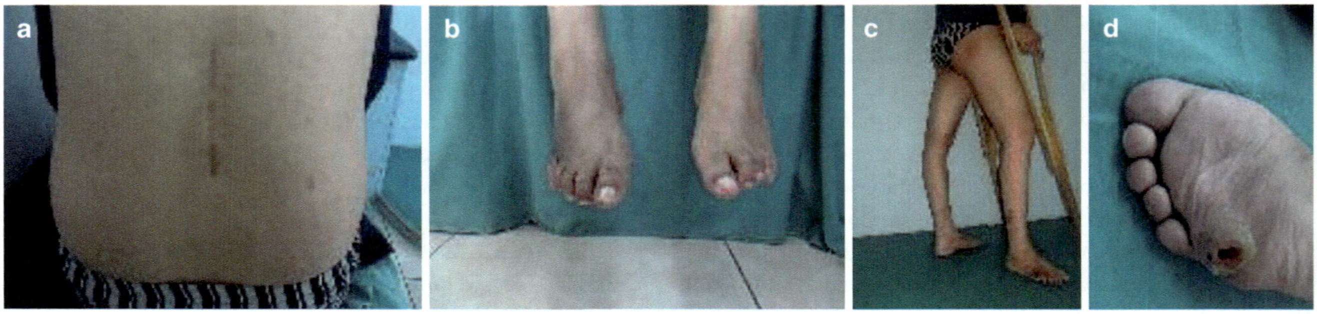

Fig. 6.7 Male, 36 years old, suffered from spinal teratoma after operation, with right foot varus and incomplete paralysis of both lower limbs. (**a**) incision scar after surgical resection of teratoma of thoracolumbar spinal cord; (**b**) anteroposterior view of both feet; (**c**) lateral view of both feet in standing position, right foot varus; (**d**) Ulcer at the base of the fifth metatarsal head of the right foot

components, including skin, hair, teeth, bone, oil, nerve tissue, and so on. Malignant teratomas are poorly differentiated, have little or no formed tissue, and are poorly structured. Most of the early teratomas have no obvious clinical symptoms, and most of them are found accidentally during physical examination.

6.1.7.1 Etiology

The etiology is unknown, which may be related to abnormal differentiation of germ cells in embryonic stage.

6.1.7.2 Clinical Manifestation

It occurs in the spinal cord teratoma, compresses the spinal cord to cause the nerve symptom, appears the corresponding area skin sensation to drop, the numbness, the limb myodynamia to weaken, and so on the symptom; if not treated in time, the symptoms will gradually worsen, resulting in spastic paralysis of lower limbs and secondary limb deformities. During the surgical treatment of spinal teratoma, spinal cord nerve injury is prone to occur, causing paralysis of different muscles of the lower limbs, and the deformity of the lower limbs gradually occurs. The deformity of talipes equinovarus is more common. If sensory nerve damage occurs at the same time, neurotrophic ulcer in the weight-bearing area of the foot will occur (Fig. 6.7).

6.1.7.3 Treatment Principle

1. Treatment of primary disease, surgical resection of teratoma.
2. Orthopedic surgery should be performed to restore the shape and function of lower limbs secondary to irreversible nerve injury.

6.2 Soft Tissue Tumor

6.2.1 Lymphangioma

Lymphangioma (LA) is a congenital benign tumor composed of dilated and endothelial cell proliferated lymphatic vessels and connective tissue, containing lymph, lymphocytes or mixed with blood.

6.2.1.1 Etiology

The etiology of this disease is unknown, and it is caused by many factors, such as genetic susceptibility, geographical environmental factors, and endocrine factors. Moreover, viral infection and autoimmune deficiency are also related to this disease. Lower extremity lymphangioma invades muscles, causing muscle contracture and traction of bone and joint, which can cause deformity of bone and joint.

6.2.1.2 Classification

Clinically and pathologically, it can be divided into three types: simple lymphangioma, cavernous lymphangioma, and cystic lymphangioma.

6.2.1.3 Clinical Manifestation

The clinical manifestations of lymphangioma in different parts may be different. It is a multilocular cyst with thin wall, large cavity, lymph, soft, unclear boundary, and no firm adhesion with mucosa and skin. Most of them occur in the posterior triangle of the neck, which is called tension mass. When breathing and coughing, the tension of the mass increases. It occurs in the armpit, chest or abdominal cavity and can cause respiratory disorders. When there is no infectious damage, the transparent test can transmit light. When there is a huge mass in the left axilla and left chest, the tumor boundary is not clear, cystic, and the chest is deformed. Limb lymphangioma invades fascia, muscle, and other soft tissues, causing contracture of fascia and muscle, resulting in deformities and dysfunction of knee joint and ankle joint (Figs. 6.8 and 6.9).

6.2.1.4 Treatment Principle

Release the contracted fascia and tendon, correct the deformity of bone and joint, restore the force line of lower limbs, and improve the function of lower limbs.

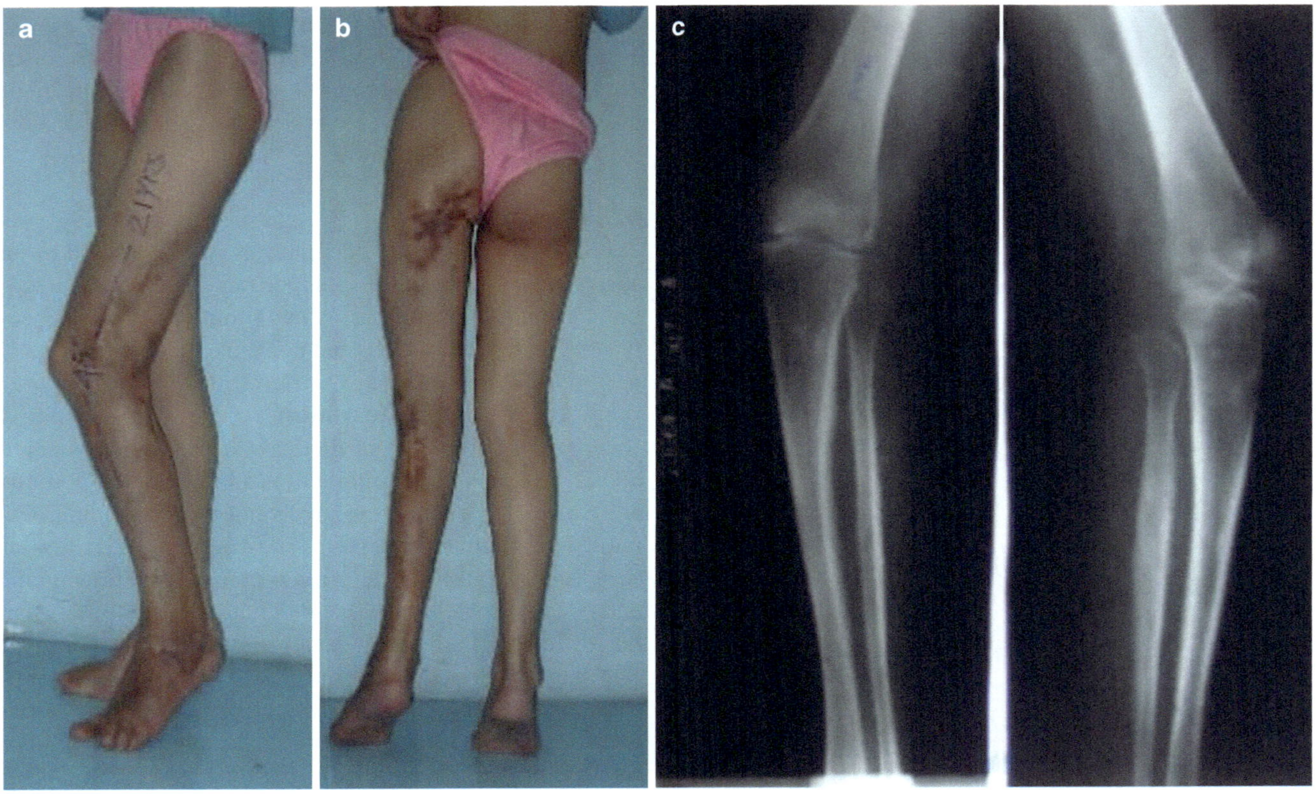

Fig. 6.8 Left flexion equinus caused by lymphangioma: (**a**) left lateral view in standing position; (**b**) dorsal view; (**c**) Anteroposterior and lateral X-ray film of left knee joint

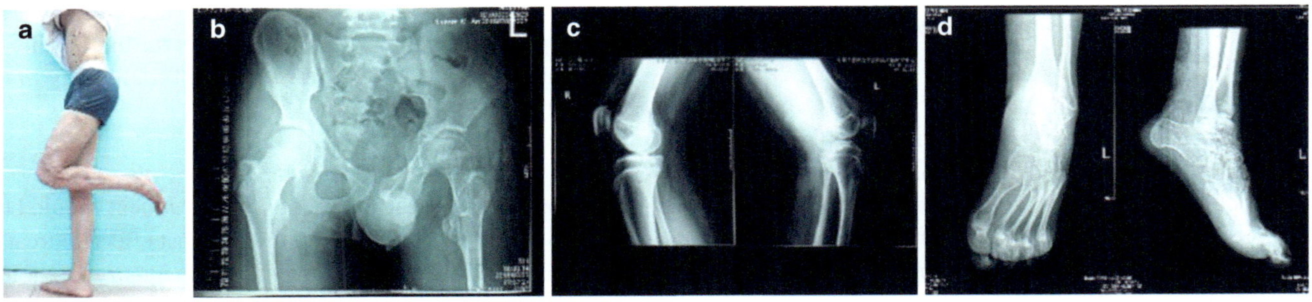

Fig. 6.9 Left flexion equinus caused by lymphangioma. (**a**) left side view in standing position; (**b**) anteroposterior X-ray film of pelvis; (**c**) lateral X-ray film of knee joint; (**d**) Anteroposterior and lateral X-ray film of left ankle and foot

6.2.2 Cutaneous Neurofibroma

6.2.2.1 Etiology

Cutaneous neurofibroma is a peripheral neurocutaneous manifestation of neurofibromatosis. It is an autosomal dominant genetic disease, often accompanied by cafe au lait spots. Plexiform nodules of the skin are distributed according to the course of nerve fibers and can occur anywhere on the body surface, mostly on the chest and back (Fig. 6.10).

6.2.2.2 Treatment Principle

Dermatofibroma generally does not require surgical excision, if accompanied by skeletal problems can be considered surgery.

6.2.3 Intermuscular Lipoma

The intramuscular lipoma is a benign tumor tissue composed of mature fat cells, which grows between the striated muscles. It often occurs in the large muscles of the limbs. It has no capsule and grows infiltratively.

6.2.3.1 Etiology

At present, the etiology of this disease is not completely clear, which may be related to inflammatory stimulation of connective tissue degeneration, abnormal metabolism and disorders of adipose tissue, abnormal secretion of gonadal hormones in anterior pituitary, congenital dysplasia, intestinal malnutrition, and other factors.

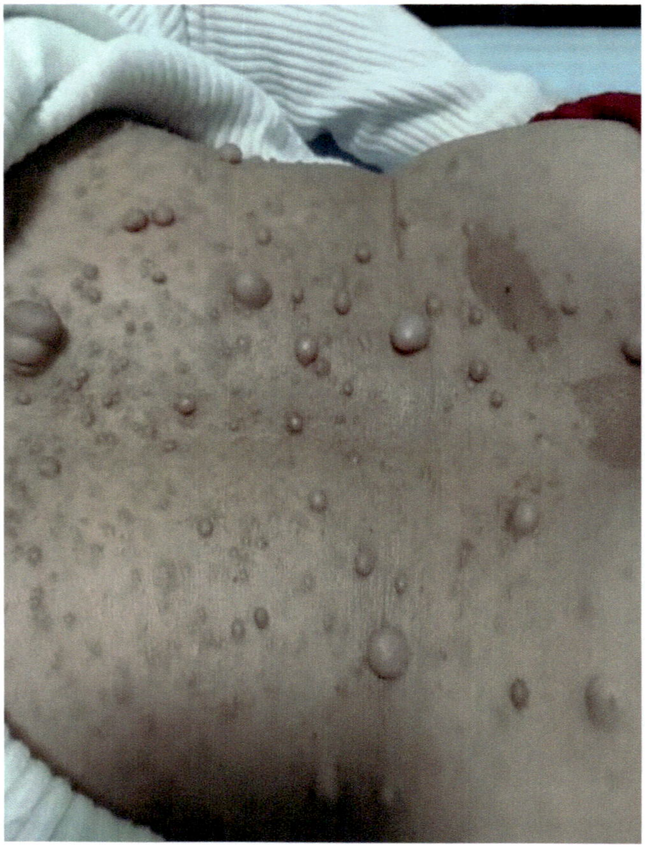

Fig. 6.10 Plexiform nodules of the skin are distributed according to the course of nerve fibers and can occur anywhere on the body surface

6.2.3.2 Clinical Manifestation

Smaller intermuscular lipomas are usually asymptomatic or mildly painful, except for local masses, and do not cause dysfunction. If the tumor enlarges obviously, it will cause compression symptoms, limb deformities and dysfunction, mostly manifested as knee flexion and horseshoe deformity (Fig. 6.11).

6.2.3.3 Treatment Principle

Smaller lipomas may be left untreated if clinically asymptomatic; For larger lipomas, if they cause pain and discomfort, or even limb deformities, they should be actively resected, while correcting deformities and improving limb function.

6.2.4 Malignant Peripheral Nerve Sheath Tumor

Malignant peripheral nerve sheath tumor (MPNST) is a rare tumor of the peripheral nervous system. It originates from Schwann cells, so it is also called malignant Schwann cell tumor. This kind of tumor often occurs in young and middle-aged men, and often occurs in limbs or scalp and neck. Tumors grow slowly, usually more than 5 years, often accompanied by neurofibroma or schwannoma. About 2/3 of the cases are based on the recurrence and malignant transformation of these two diseases.

6.2.4.1 Etiology

This disease is a neuroectodermal abnormality caused by an aberrant dominant gene, resulting in multiple tumor-like proliferation of peripheral nerves and proliferation of connective tissue in nerve sheaths and nerve fibers.

6.2.4.2 Clinical Manifestation

It can occur in any part of the body, and its symptoms are diverse and lack of specificity. It is more common in limbs and trunk, and sciatic nerve involvement is common. Local mass is a common symptom, mostly painless, a few of which are painful mass, or mass compression symptoms and distant limb numbness and radiating pain. Tumors can invade locally, and distant lymph nodes and blood circulation metastasis can also occur. Mass is a common symptom, mostly painless, and difficult to differentiate from other sarcomas. Some performance is painful sex bump, or bump is oppressive appear far limb is coma reach radiate painful. Deep tumors show corresponding symptoms due to local invasion, such as chest pain, suffocation (posterior mediastinum), low back and leg pain (lumbar nerve root invasion), diplopia (retrobulbar invasion), etc. Others may be asymptomatic and lumps may be found during physical examination. Nerve injury can cause limb deformity and dysfunction (Fig. 6.12).

6.2.4.3 Treatment Principle

For primary tumors, early detection and treatment should be carried out, and surgical resection is the most effective treatment. For the limb deformities secondary to tumor resection, surgical correction was performed after the condition was stable.

6.2.5 Non-ossifying Fibroma

Non-ossifying fibroma (NOF) is a kind of metaphyseal hamartoma composed of tissue fibroblasts, also known as metaphyseal fibrous defect, non-osteogenic fibroma, histiocytic fibroma, metaphyseal hamartoma, and fibrous cortical defect. At present, small lesions, no clinical symptoms, lesions confined to the periosteum or cortex are called metaphyseal fibrous defects or fibrous cortical defects, while larger lesions, lesions that can expand into the medullary cavity and often combine with pathological fractures are called non-ossifying fibroma or non-ossifying fibroma. Therefore, non-ossifying fibroma and fibrous cortical defect

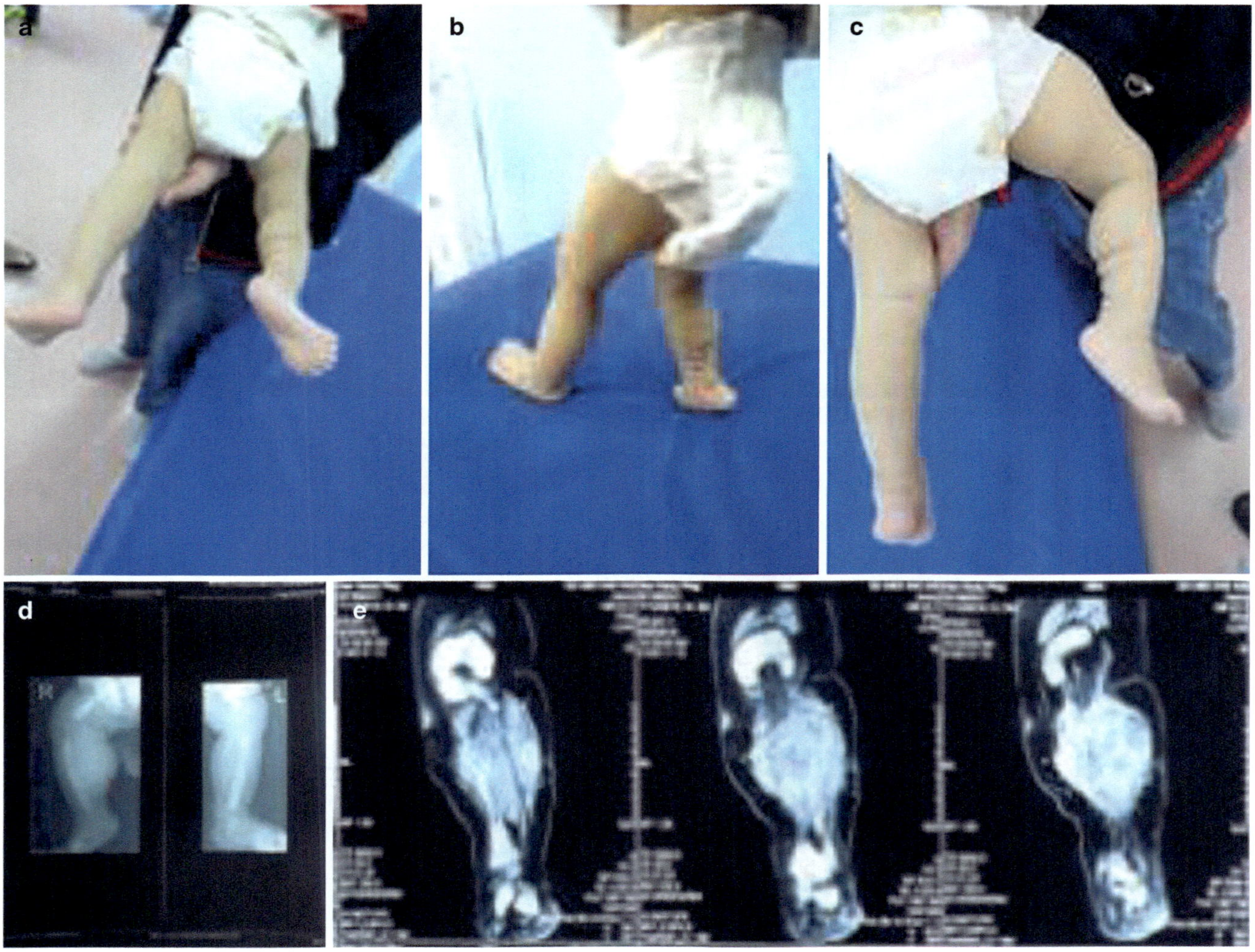

Fig. 6.11 Shortening deformity of leg caused by intermuscular lipoma

are two diseases of non-ossifying fibroma or two different manifestations of the same disease.

6.2.5.1 Etiology

The cause of the disease is unknown.

6.2.5.2 Clinical Manifestation

Non-ossifying fibroma is most common in children and adolescents, and is most common between the ages of 5 and 20. The most common site of the disease was the long bone of the lower limb, mainly around the knee joint. The distal femoral metaphysis was the most common, followed by the proximal tibia and distal metaphysis, and the proximal fibula metaphysis was also common. Multiple lesions are most commonly found in one or both lower extremities or may involve the pelvis.

Non-ossifying fibroma can cause limb deformities, even severe limb deformities and bone resorption in children (Fig. 6.13).

6.2.5.3 Treatment Principle

Bone fibrous cortical defect is the early manifestation of non-ossifying fibroma, which has a tendency of self-healing, can invade the medullary cavity and develop into non-ossifying fibroma, and surgical treatment should be chosen when progressive enlargement occurs. In patients with secondary bone and joint deformities, the lesions were thoroughly removed and soft tissue release and osteotomy were performed to restore the shape and function of the limbs.

6.2.6 Desmoid Fibromatosis

Desmoid fibromatosis, also known as desmoid fibroma, aggressive fibroma, and fibromatosis, is a fibroblastic clonal proliferative lesion located in deep soft tissue, characterized by infiltrative growth and local recurrence, but not metastasis. The disease can occur in all parts of the body, more common in the abdominal wall, can also occur in the abdomen and skeletal muscle.

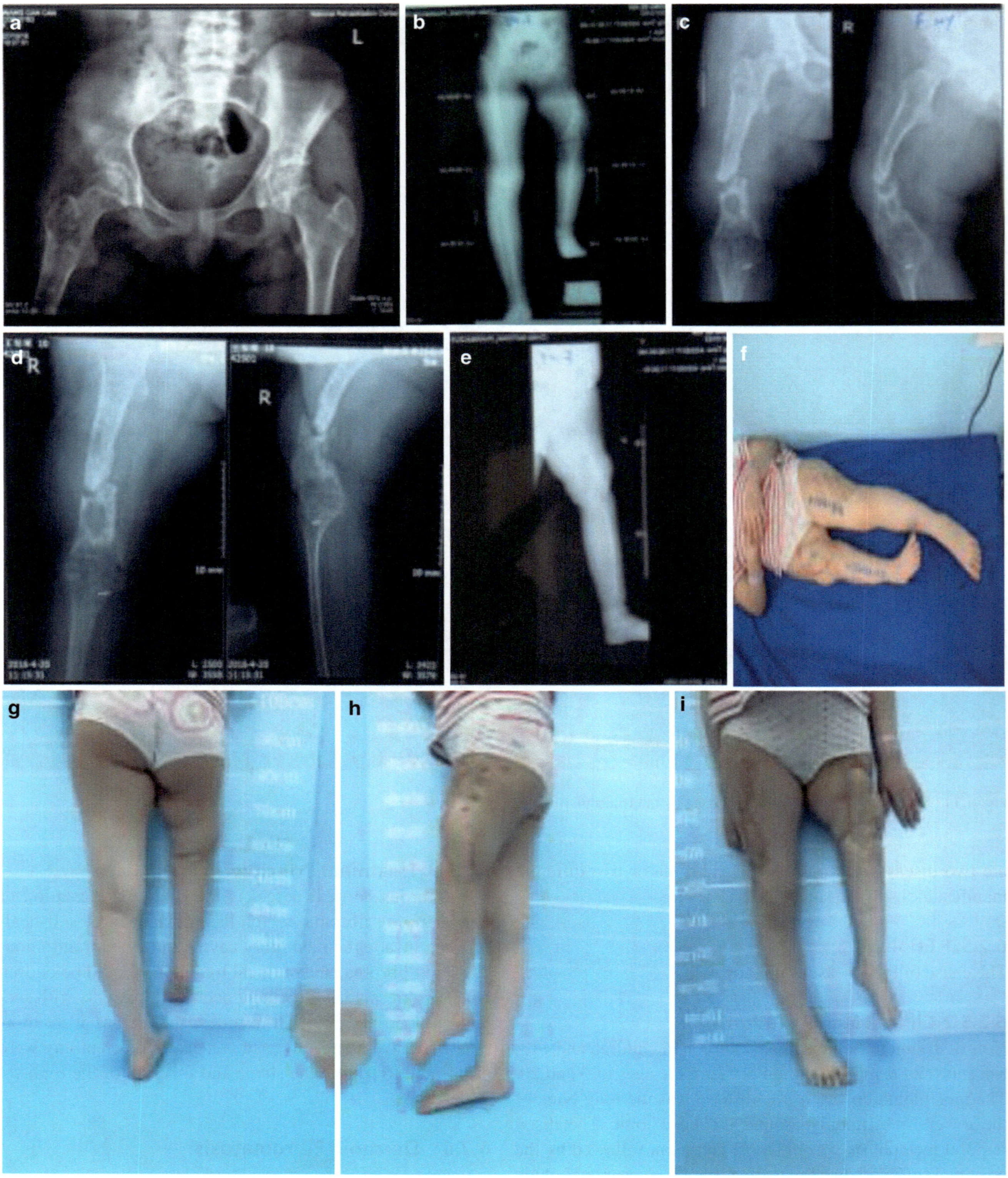

Fig. 6.12 Shortening and nonunion of left femur caused by malignant peripheral nerve sheath tumor

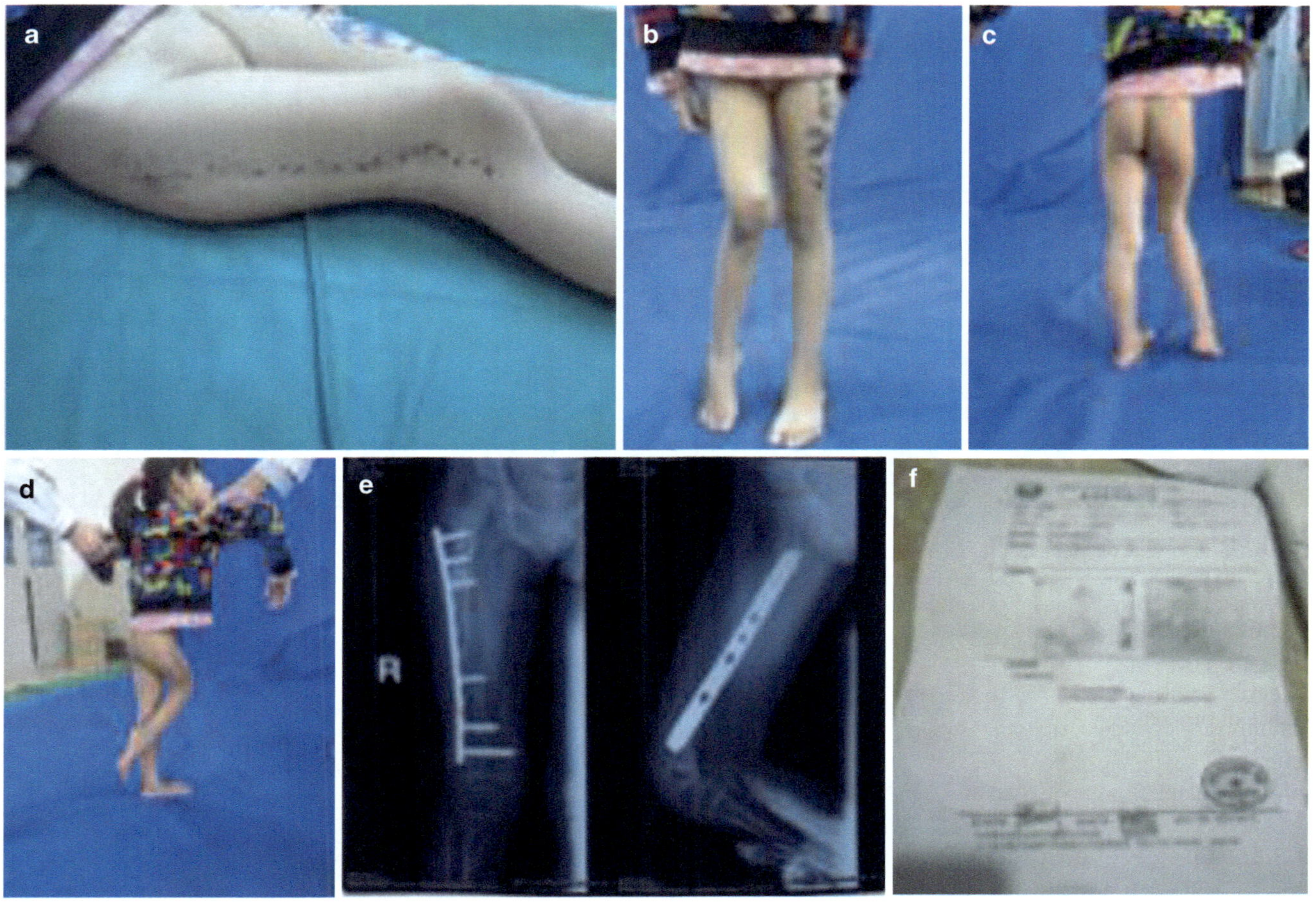

Fig. 6.13 Bone resorption after non-ossifying fibroma surgery

6.2.6.1 Etiology

Causes include genetic, endocrine, and physical factors. Patients with familial adenomatous polyposis are prone to desmoid tumors, known as Gardner syndrome. High estrogen and progesterone levels may also be associated with morbidity. Trauma is also an important factor.

6.2.6.2 Clinical Manifestation

The typical manifestation of desmoid fibromatosis is a deep, ill-defined, hard mass that is difficult to detect and is slightly painful or painless. Some lesions are multifocal. Ligamentous fibromatosis of the lower extremities invades muscles, joint capsules, and other tissues, causing joint contracture and deformity, such as hip stiffness in the deformed position, knee flexion deformity, etc. (Fig. 6.14). Desmoid tumors in children often occur in the buttocks, which can easily cause pelvic tilt, unequal length of lower limbs, and scoliosis.

6.2.6.3 Treatment Principle

(1) At present, it is believed that the initial diagnosis of desmoid fibroma should be observed conservatively, and if the tumor does not grow, it will not be treated. If the tumor continues to progress, only the abdominal wall desmoid fibroma is the first choice for surgery, and the rest of the site is the first choice for drug treatment. Medications include low-dose chemotherapy with methotrexate plus vinorelbine (Fig. 6.15), doxorubicin liposome-based chemotherapy, and targeted therapies such as imatinib, sorafenib, and pezopanib. Radiotherapy is not recommended for young patients, especially for minors. (2) The deformity of hip, knee, and ankle caused by tumor was corrected by Ilizarov slow traction technique. (3) Deformities caused by tumors should be treated with orthopedic surgery after tumor control, otherwise tumor recurrence will cause the recurrence of deformities.

6.2.7 Rhabdomyosarcoma

Rhabdomyosarcoma is one of the most common soft tissue malignant tumors in children. It originates from striated muscle cells or striated muscle differentiated mesenchymal cells. It is more common in children under 10 years old. Embryonal rhabdomyosarcoma occurs before 8 years old and is common in limbs, head, and neck. After surgery, chemotherapy and radiotherapy, rhabdomyosarcoma of the lower extremities was basically cured, but resulting in muscle necrosis on the flexor side of the joint, fibrosis contracture of tendons and fascia, and different types and degrees of deformities in the growth and development of children (Fig. 6.16).

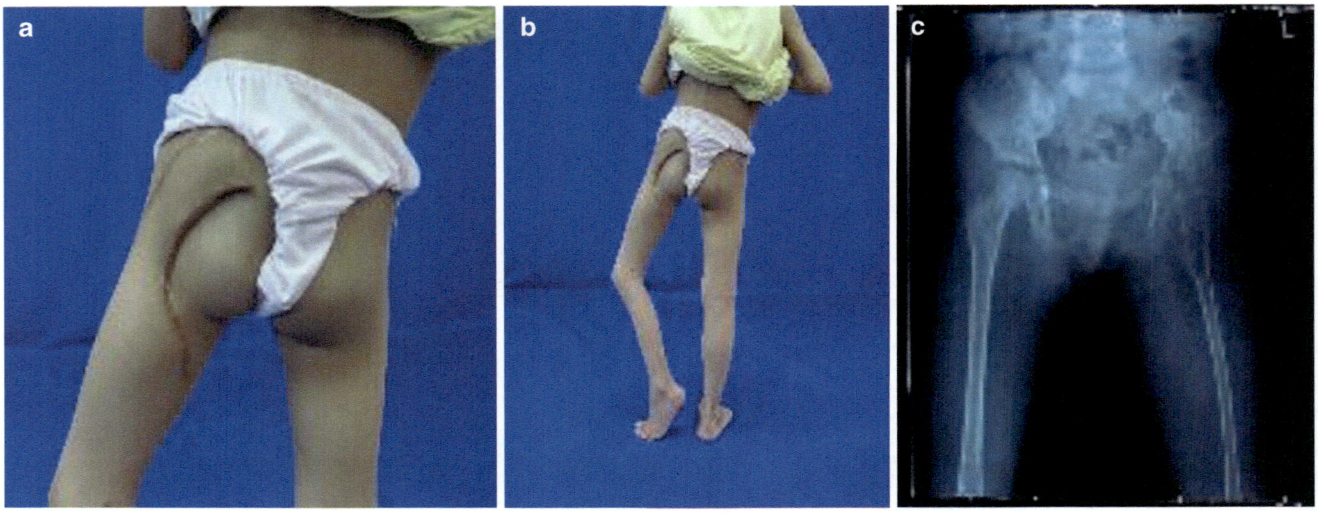

Fig. 6.14 A 6-year-old female presented with ankylosis of the hip caused by ligamentous fibromatosis of the left buttock. Surgery was performed to remove the tumor. (**a**) left buttock incision, (**b**) left hip joint stiffness, standing pelvis right upward, postural knee flexion horseshoe foot performance; (**c**) Pelvic radiograph showed narrowing of the left hip joint space

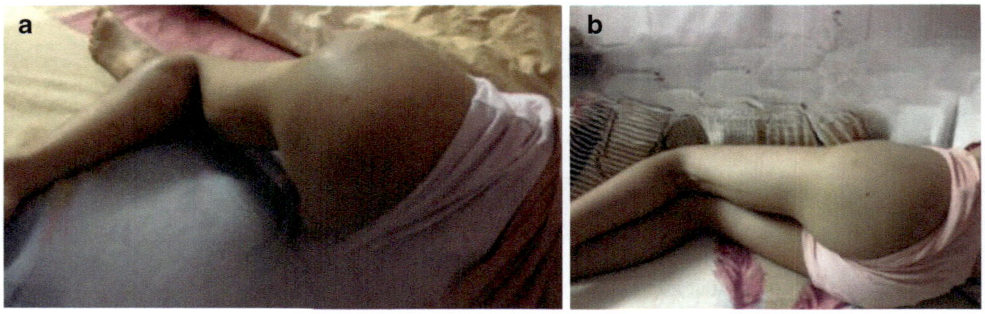

Fig. 6.15 Desmoid fibromatosis of left buttock. (**a**) before chemotherapy; (**b**) After chemotherapy (photo provided by Zhiwei Fang)

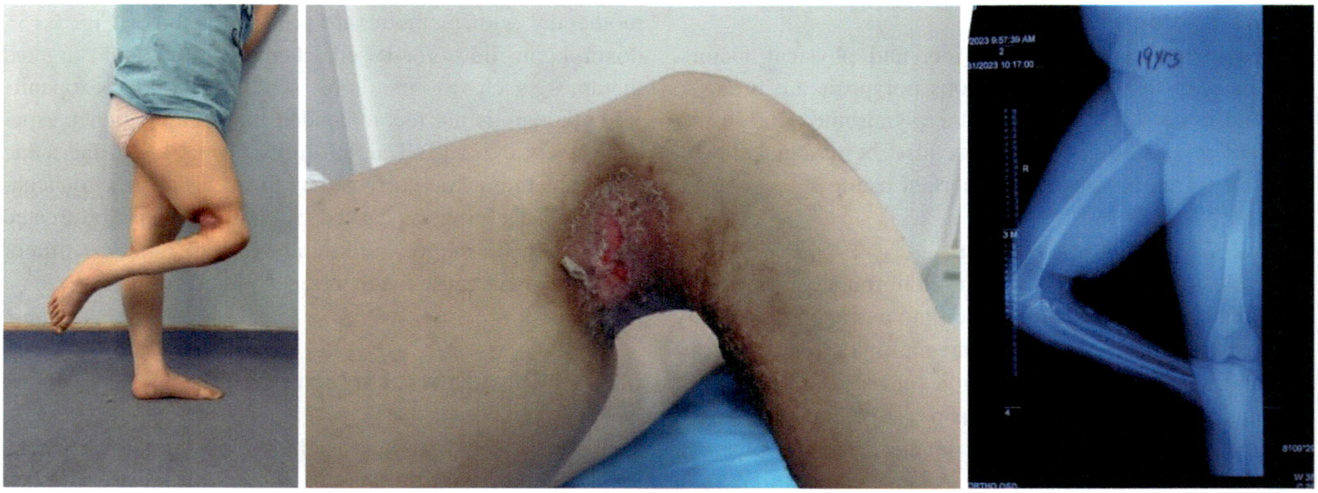

Fig. 6.16 Rhabdomyosarcoma was found behind the knee joint of the right lower limb in a 19-year-old female at the age of 3. After surgery and radiotherapy, sclerosing scar appeared behind the knee. During the development of the patient, severe knee flexion contracture deformity was gradually developed, the scar skin of the popliteal fossa was often ulcerated, and the X-ray showed that the angle of the anterior arch of the lower end of the femur increased

6.3 Skeletal Tumor

6.3.1 Endophytic Chondroma

If enchondroma occurs in bone, it is called central type, and if it occurs on the surface of bone, it is called marginal type (periosteal chondroma). The disease may be a single lesion or multiple lesions (enchondromatosis). Endophytic chondroma is a tumor caused by embryonal ectopic tissue. Solitary endophytic chondroma is slow growing, small in size, and may be asymptomatic for a long time. Multiple enchondroma has symptoms and signs in early childhood, leading to limb shortening and bending deformity, causing limb dysfunction. Multiple osteochondromas with malformations are called Ollier's disease, and multiple osteochondromas with soft tissue hemangiomas of the extremities are called Maffucci's syndrome.

6.3.1.1 Etiology

A tumor caused by embryonal ectopic tissue.

6.3.1.2 Clinical Manifestation

Solitary endogenous Chondroma It grows slowly, is small in size, and can be asymptomatic for a long time. The enchondroma in the tubular of the hands and feet often causes swelling and pain due to bone expansion and stimulation or pain due to pathological fractures, often leading to deformity of the fingers or toes. In the long bones of the limbs, most of them are asymptomatic and are discovered during X-ray examinations for other diseases or pathological fractures. Multiple enchondromas often lead to limb shortening and bending deformities. Symptoms and signs are manifested in early childhood and are discovered early. In the hand, the lesion is spherical or nodular swelling, when the lesion is severe, the fingers are shortened, deviated from the axis, and generally painless; At the metaphysis of the limb, there may be slight swelling, and with the development of the skeleton, there may be shortening deformity (Fig. 6.17). Some enchondromas may become chondrosarcomas.

6.3.1.3 Treatment Principle

(1) Asymptomatic small enchondroma cannot be treated, and surgical treatment is mainly curettage and bone grafting. (2) For limb deformity and shortening caused by tumors, surgery should be performed to completely remove the lesions and correct the deformity, restore the length of the limbs and improve the function of the limbs.

6.3.2 Fibrous Dysplasi

Fibrous dysplasia (FD) refers to the proliferation and degeneration of fibrous tissue of bone, and the bone formed by metaplasia is immature interwoven bone. It is also called fibrous dysplasia of bone. This disease is the first in tumor-like lesions (38.42%). It is more common in young people

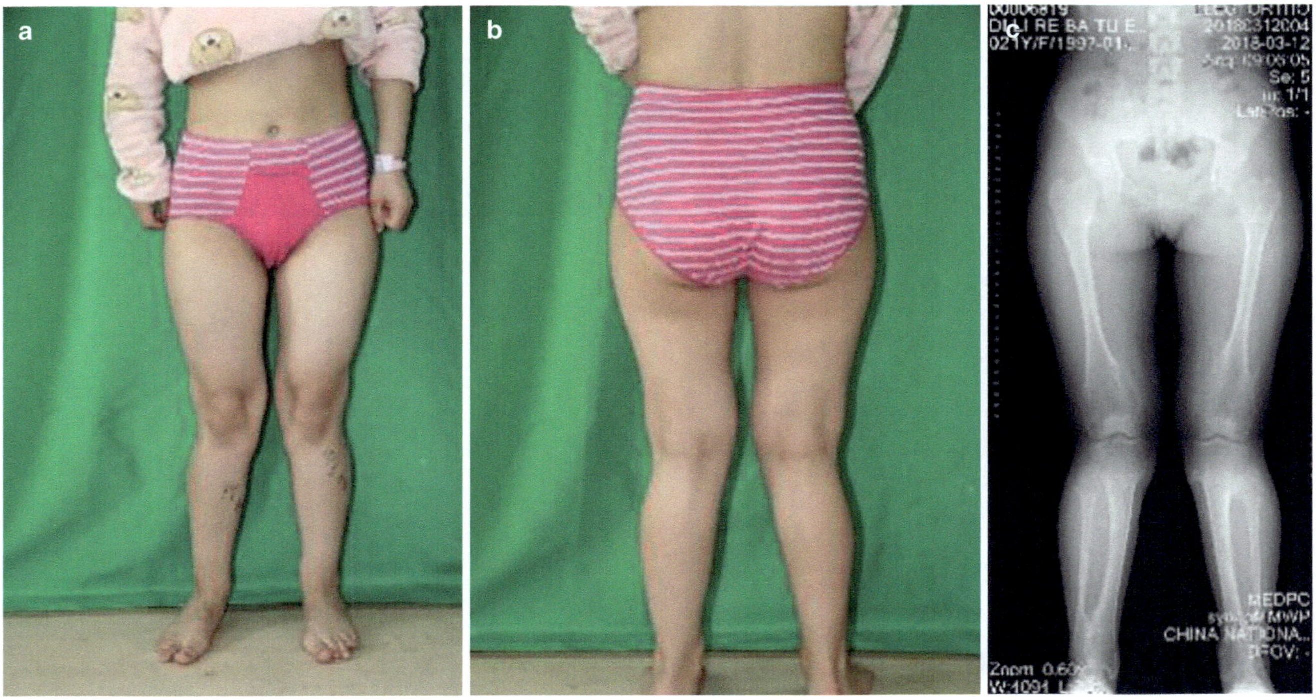

Fig. 6.17 Female, 21 years old, multiple enchondroma with complex deformity of lower limbs. (**a**) view from the front in standing position; (**b**) view from the back in standing position; (**c**) Full-length X-ray film of both lower extremities in standing position

aged 11–30 years old, and the ratio of male to female is 1.1: 1. The predilection sites were mainly in the femur and tibia, followed by the jaw and ribs.

6.3.2.1 Etiology

The etiology of fibrous dysplasia of bone is unknown, which may be related to gene mutation, congenital dysplasia of bone, bone formation disorders, and endocrine abnormalities.

6.3.2.2 Clinical Manifestation

Fibrous dysplasia of bone often occurs around the age of 10, often in adolescence, accompanied by endocrine disorders can occur at the age of 3–4, and even have symptoms after birth. The disease can occur in any bone, limb solitary lesions are often located in the proximal end of the bone, can be localized or spread to the diaphysis, mostly in the femur, tibia, fibula and pelvis, often on one side of the limb; Bilateral involvement is not symmetrical. Upper limb lesions can be seen in the skull at the same time. Trunk lesions may involve several ribs and vertebral bodies and their appendages. The disease is mainly on one side of the upper and lower limbs. The severity of clinical symptoms is related to age, course of disease and damaged parts, and the younger the age, the more severe the symptoms. The lesion may remain asymptomatic for many years in its early stages, followed by pain, dysfunction, arcuate deformity, or pathological fracture (Fig. 6.18). Fractures can be caused by mild trauma, pain, swelling, dysfunction, rarely displacement, and most of them can heal after immobilization.

X-ray examination showed solitary fibrous dysplasia of bone, which was described as "frosted glass" with a blurred radiolucent (low density) area in the medullary cavity. Irregular bone markings can be seen, the bone cortex is thinned, the boundary between the lesion area and the normal bone is clear, reactive sclerosis can be seen, there is no periosteal reaction, and the lesion rarely invades the epiphyseal cartilage. Sickle-shaped deformity may occur at the femoral neck or upper end of the femur, which is called "shepherd's stick" deformity (Fig. 6.19). The lesions of the spine are well defined, with low density areas on X-ray, and may collapse due to pathological fractures.

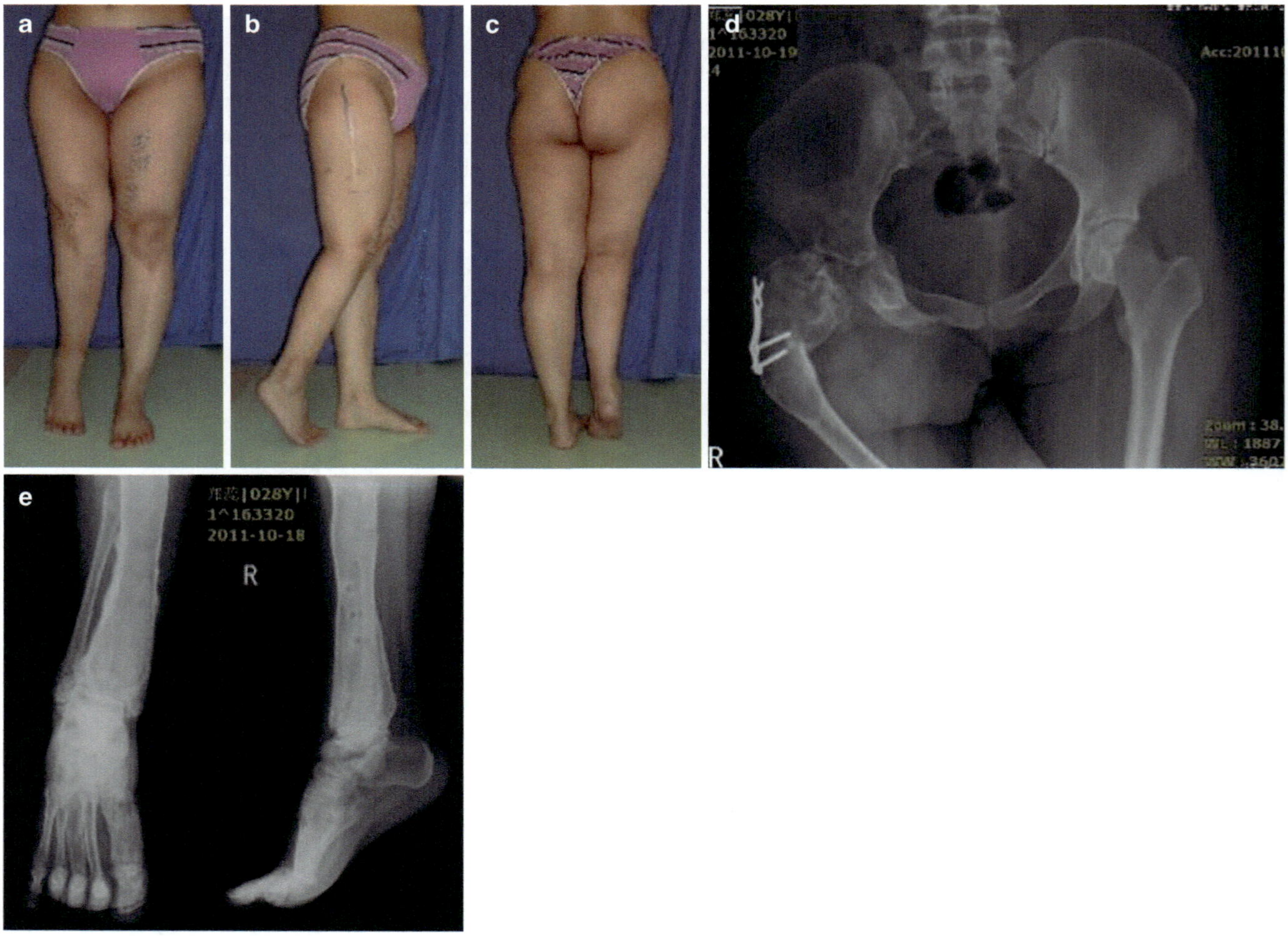

Fig. 6.18 Deformity of right lower limb in fibrous dysplasia of bone. (**a**) standing frontal view; (**b**) right lateral view; (**c**) dorsal view; (**d**) pelvic anteroposterior radiograph; (**e**) X-ray film of right ankle

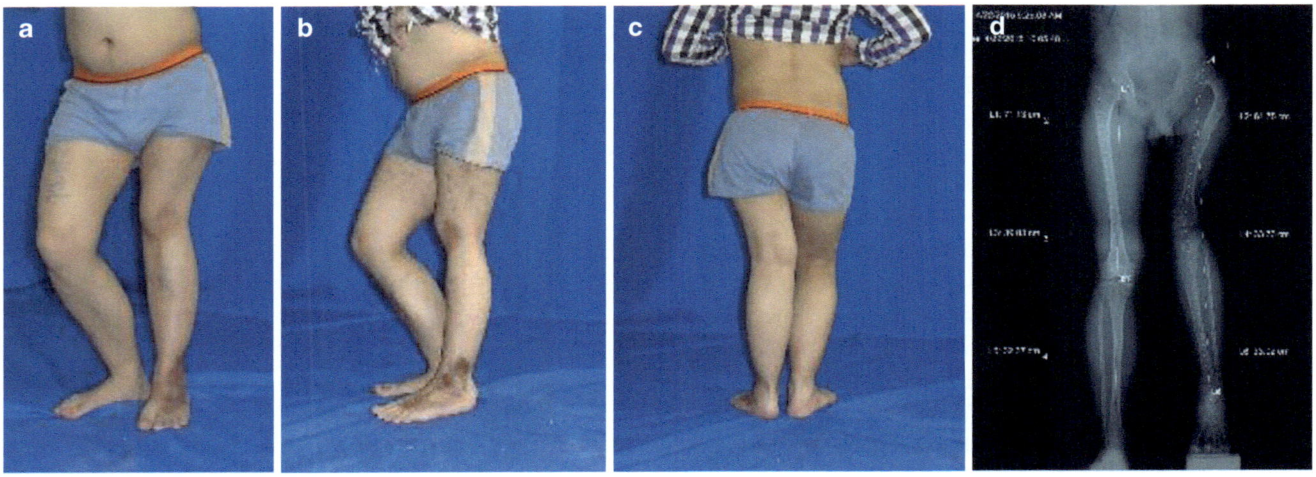

Fig. 6.19 Male, 28, fibrous dysplasia of bone, "shepherd's stick" deformity of right femur. (**a**) preoperative appearance, left lower limb shortening, hip adduction deformity; (**b**) standing lateral view, left lower limb shortening; (**c**) standing dorsal view; (**d**) Full-length anteroposterior radiograph of both lower extremities in standing position

6.3.2.3 Treatment Principle

(1) For asymptomatic lesions, no treatment is required in principle. (2) When the skeletal deformity caused by pathological changes affects the function of limbs, it is feasible to remove the focus and osteotomy at the same time to restore the normal shape and function of limbs.

6.3.3 Ossifying Fibroma of Three Long Bones

Ossifying fibroma was first reported by Menzel in 1872 and occurs primarily in the jaw. In 1966, Kempson introduced ossifying fibroma of the long bones of the extremities, and the name of the disease has been used up to now.

6.3.3.1 Etiology

The cause of the disease is not yet clear, but it may be congenital dysplasia of skeletal structure.

6.3.3.2 Clinical Manifestation

The disease often occurs before the age of 10, and most of them occur within the age of 5. The incidence is higher in men than women. The tibia was the most common, followed by the fibula. Most of the lesions were unilateral, and occasionally bilateral. Located in 1/3 of the diaphysis or distal and proximal parts, the subjective symptoms are not obvious, mostly painless swelling or mass, or tibial bending and deformation. Pathological fracture and pseudarthrosis were occasionally seen. X-ray showed that the lesions were unilocular or multilocular cystic clear areas with calcified plack-like shadows.

6.3.3.3 Treatment Principle

The treatment plan is determined based on the course of disease, nature, growth rate, X-ray morphology and histological examination. There is occasional possibility of self-healing before the age of 5, and conservative treatment is the main treatment. When the patient is 5–10 years old, the operation should be postponed as far as possible. Surgery is necessary when there is extensive disease, severe swelling and bone weakness, or pseudarthrosis. Surgical treatment is needed at the age of 10–12 years, and the commonly used method is complete curettage or resection, with osteotomy to correct the deformity.

6.3.4 Osteosarcoma

Osteosarcoma, also known as osteosarcoma, is a common malignant bone tumor occurring in adolescents or children under the age of 20. It is the most common malignant bone tumor in children, accounting for about 5% of children's tumors. The 5-year survival rate of osteosarcoma is about 70%.

6.3.4.1 Etiology

Osteosarcoma is one of the most common bone malignant tumors, which develops from mesenchymal cell lines. The rapid growth of tumors is due to the direct or indirect formation of tumor osteoid tissue and bone tissue by cartilage stage. Under the action of external factors (such as trauma), the weight-bearing bones of lower limbs cause cell mutation, which may be related to the formation of osteosarcoma.

6.3.4.2 Clinical Manifestation

The prominent symptom of osteosarcoma is pain at the tumor site, which is intermittent in the early stage and gradually develops into persistent pain. A fixed mass appeared at the site of pain, local skin temperature increased, and superficial veins filled. Osteosarcoma of the lower extremities may present with painful claudication. Osteosarcoma mostly occurs in the metaphysis of long bones. X-ray films mainly show bone trabecular destruction, periosteal reaction, and irregular new bone formation (Figs. 6.20 and 6.21).

6.3.4.3 Treatment Principle

Osteosarcoma is sensitive to chemotherapy, and chemotherapy can significantly prolong the survival time of patients, so the treatment principle of osteosarcoma is preoperative adjuvant chemotherapy, surgery, postoperative adjuvant chemotherapy. Limb salvage methods for osteosarcoma include tumor-type artificial joint replacement, devitalized tumor bone replantation, and allogeneic bone transplantation. For minor patients, the bone defect formed after tumor resection (Fig. 6.22) can be repaired by Ilizarov bone transfer technique to preserve the shape and function of the patient as much as possible. Replacement with an extendable prosthesis may also be considered.

6.3.5 Multiple Enchondromatosis

Multiple enchondromatosis is a rare nonhereditary benign neoplasm caused by a predominantly asymmetrical distribution of cartilaginous lesions within the bone and subperiosteal deposits. In the long and short tubular bones of the body, the disease can occur in unilateral or bilateral bones. It is also called Ollier's disease because it was first described by Ollier in 1899. Clinically, a palpable painless mass often invades the hand or foot, resulting in disability. The disease has the possibility of malignant transformation.

6.3.5.1 Etiology

Multiple enchondromatosis is the development of ectopic epiphyseal plate during skeletal development.

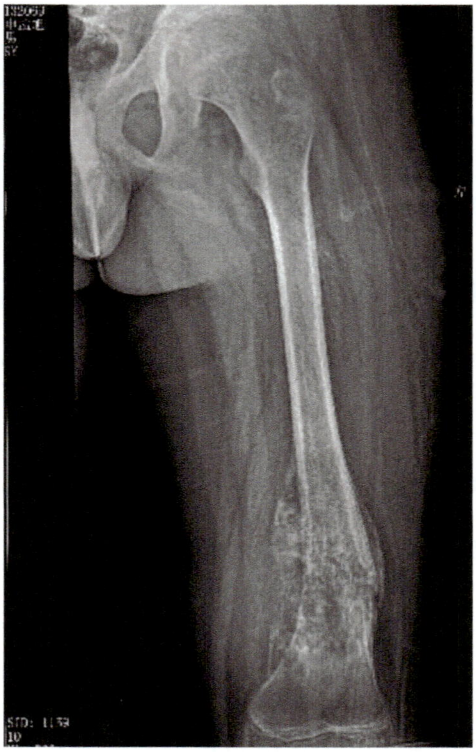

Fig. 6.21 A 9-year-old male presented with osteosarcoma of the left distal femur

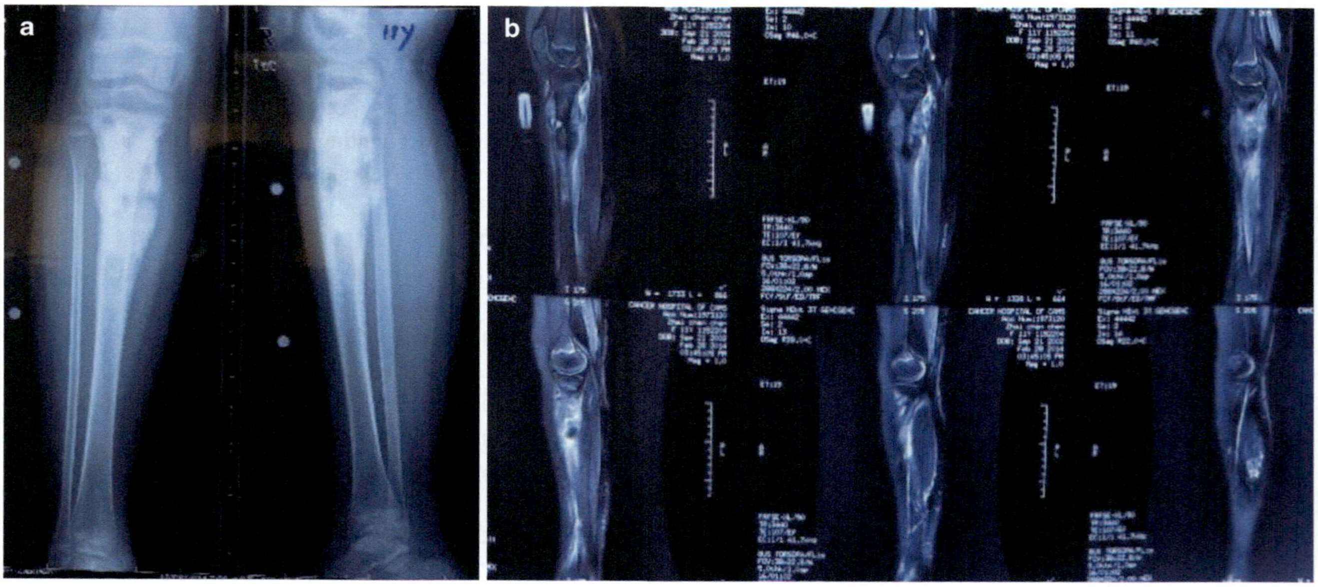

Fig. 6.20 Osteosarcoma, male, 11 years old. Osteosarcoma of the upper segment of the right tibia: (**a**) X-ray of the right tibia and fibula; (**b**) MRI of right lower leg

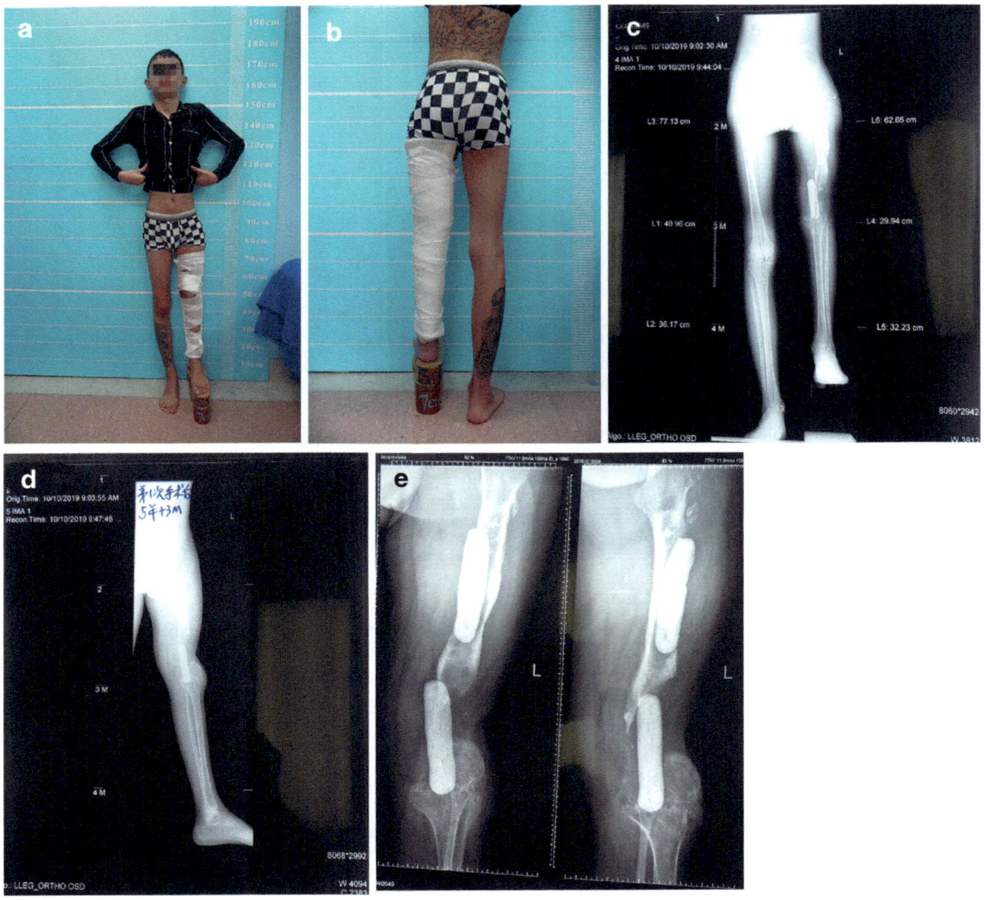

Fig. 6.22 Nonunion of left femur after osteosarcoma

6.3.5.2 Clinical Manifestation

The onset age of multiple enchondromas is less than 10 years old, and males are more than females. Symptoms appear in childhood, obvious deformities appear in adolescence, and then gradually stabilize. The clinical manifestation is a palpable painless mass, which can invade the hands or feet, resulting in disability. The lesions invaded the long tubular bone, so that the endogenic cartilage could not ossify normally, the epiphyseal plate could not grow normally, and the limbs were shortened and bent. Such as the deformity of the genu valgum of the lower limbs (Fig. 6.23). Tumors can stop growing in adult patients. Malignant transformation can occur in adults, and the malignant transformation rate is 5–25%.

6.3.5.3 Treatment Principle

Symptomatic treatment is fine. Asymptomatic patients may not be treated; those who cause limb deformities are corrected by osteotomy.

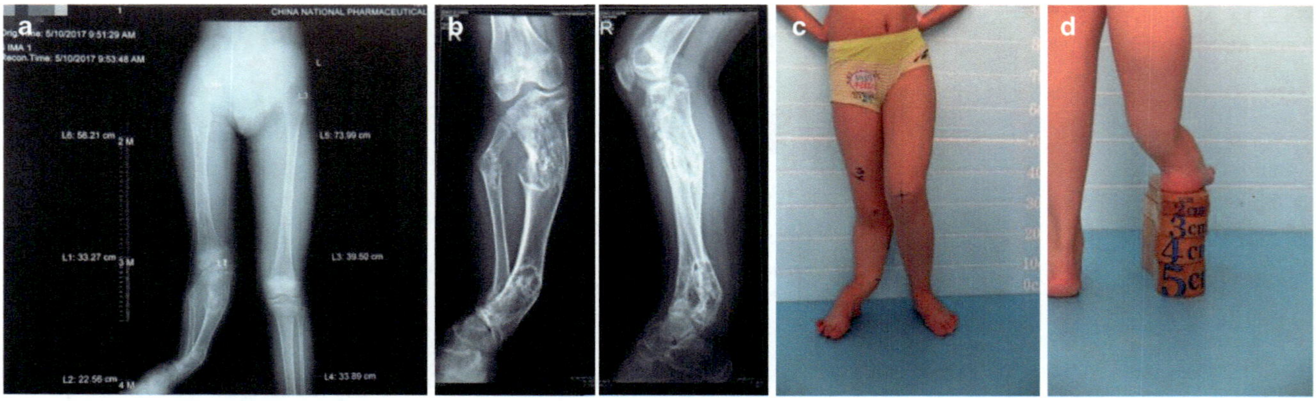

Fig. 6.23 A 13-year-old female with multiple enchondromatosis resulting in deformity of the right lower limb. (**a**) Full-length standing radiograph of the lower extremity; (**b**) Most of the right tibia and fibula are tumor-like lesions; (**c**) Standing anterior view; (**d**) Lower limb shortening 15 cm

Suggested Reading

1. Chen J, Chen X. Diagnosis and treatment of intracranial germ cell tumors (with clinical analysis of 38 cases). Chin J Clin Neurosurg. 2002;7(1):28–9.
2. Zhang B, Xu W, Sun W, et al. Comprehensive treatment of intracranial germ cell tumors. 1996;12(4):219–21.
3. Gao X, Wang Y, Bai M. Research progress on intracranial germ cell tumors. Clin Med Progress. 2020;10(3):270–8.
4. Huang G, Qi S. Characteristics and origin of craniopharyngioma research. Int J Neurol Neurosurg. 2005;32(6):4.
5. Lu Y, Peng L. Surgical treatment of spinal gliomas and discussion of related clinical issues. Chin Med Inf Bull. 2018;33(8):1.
6. Li J, Yang X, Zhang J, et al. Current research on the diagnosis and treatment of cerebral and spinal cavernous hemangiomas. Chin J Neurosurg. 2012;28(4):429–32.
7. Yi C, Ding H, Tu Q, et al. Clinical diagnosis and surgical treatment of intraspinal meningiomas. J Neck Back Pain. 2011;32(2):4.
8. Xue Y, Luo N, Dong Y. Imaging features and clinical analysis of malignant peripheral nerve sheath tumors. Chin J Clin Radiol. 2020;39(2):377–81.
9. Yu C, Jia X. Advances in the diagnosis and treatment of malignant peripheral nerve sheath tumors. Chin J Hand Surg. 2021;37(3):223–6.
10. Li S, Fan Z, Fang Z, Liu J, Bai C, Xue R, Zhang L, Gao T. Efficacy of vinorelbine combined with low-dose methotrexate for treatment of inoperable desmoid tumor and prognostic factor analysis. Chin J Cancer Res. 2017;29(5):455–62. (IF 3.0)
11. Li S, Fan Z, Liu J. Analysis of the efficacy of imatinib in the treatment of inoperable desmoid tumors with ligament-like characteristics. Chin J Cancer Prevention Treatment. 2018;25(8):591–4.
12. Li S, Fang Z, Liu J. Preliminary exploration of the efficacy of liposomal pirarubicin combined with dacarbazine in the treatment of inoperable hard fibromas. Chin J Clin Oncol. 2021;48(14):716–20.

Vascular, Blood, and Lymphatic Diseases Lead to Deformity

7

Sihe Qin, Shaofeng Jiao, Dingwei Zhang, and Qikai Hua

7.1 Cerebral and Spinal Vascular Diseases

7.1.1 Sequelae of Cerebrovascular Embolism

7.1.1.1 Etiology

Cerebrovascular embolism refers to various emboli in the blood (such as mural thrombus in the heart, atherosclerotic plaque, fat, tumor cells or air, etc.) enter the cerebral artery with the blood flow and block the blood vessel. When the collateral circulation cannot compensate, it causes ischemic necrosis of the brain tissue in the arterial blood supply area. Focal neurologic deficits were present. If it affects the language center, it will lead to language disorders or even aphasia and other corresponding symptoms. If it affects the motor center, it will appear. Hemiplegia Ataxia and other movement disorders, long-term poor posture after paralysis will lead to limb deformities.

7.1.1.2 Clinical Manifestation

According to the dysfunction of brain tissue innervated by different vascular innervated areas, it was divided into ischemic stroke symptoms of internal carotid artery system and vertebrobasilar artery system. In the acute stage, it is characterized by unilateral facial or limb weakness or paresthesia, various aphasia, blurred vision, cognitive dysfunction, limb weakness or paresthesia, and crossed limb dyskinesia. Sequelae include coxa adduction, circling gait, knee flexion contracture or retroflexion deformity, and talipes equinovarus (Fig. 7.1).

7.1.1.3 Treatment Principle

Active treatment of primary diseases in acute stage, such as maintenance of basic vital signs, thrombolysis, anticoagulation, thrombectomy, etc., and recovery of motor system usually occur 3–4 months after onset, which can greatly improve gait. Orthopedic surgery can be used to balance muscle strength, reduce muscle tension, stabilize ankle joint, and improve walking function.

7.1.2 Sequela of Cerebral Vasculitis

7.1.2.1 Etiology

Cerebral vasculitis is a kind of disease, which is caused by inflammation and necrosis of blood vessel wall due to invasion of intracranial artery by cerebral artery or other diseases, resulting in pathological changes such as cerebral ischemia, infarction, and intracranial hemorrhage. According to the etiology, it can be divided into primary vasculitis and secondary vasculitis.

7.1.2.2 Clinical Manifestation

Limb deformities caused by cerebral vasculitis are rare, which can be manifested as focal neurological signs, headache, and cognitive impairment, such as hemiplegia, quadriplegia, ataxia, etc. When the nervous system is damaged, the specific nerve parts involved can be manifested as spastic paralysis of limbs to varying degrees, followed by limb deformities, such as hip and knee flexion contracture, talipes equinovarus, valgus, and so on (Fig. 7.2).

7.1.2.3 Classification

According to the etiology, it can be divided into primary vasculitis and secondary vasculitis: (1) Primary vasculitis: its etiology is not yet clear, but the autoimmune mechanism has

S. Qin (✉) · S. Jiao
Department of Orthopaedics, Rehabilitation Hospital of the National Research Center for Rehabilitation Technical Aids, Beijing, China

D. Zhang
Department of Orthopedic Surgery, Central Hospital of Mianyang, Mianyang, Sichuan, China

Q. Hua
Department of Bone and Joint Surgery, the First Affiliated Hospital of Guangxi Medical University, Nanning, Guangxi, China

S. Qin et al. (eds.), *Atlas of Limb Deformity*, https://doi.org/10.1007/978-981-97-0999-1_7

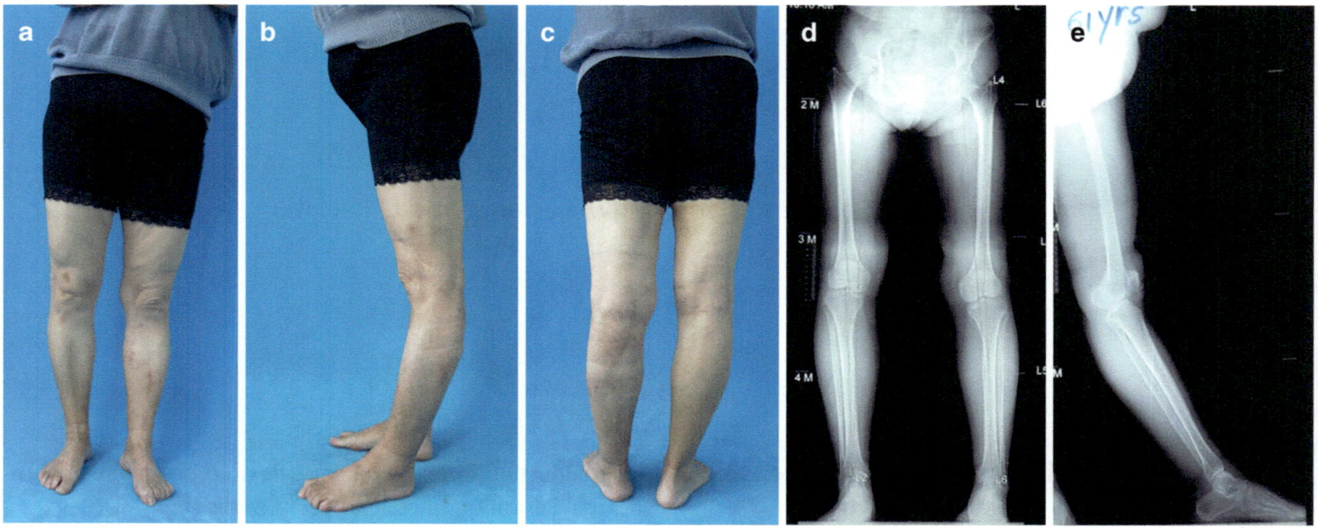

Fig. 7.1 Male, 61 years old, sequela of cerebrovascular embolism. (**a**) frontal view in standing position; (**b**) lateral view; (**c**) dorsal view; (**d**) full-length anteroposterior X-ray film of both lower limbs in standing position; (**e**) Full-length lateral X-ray of both lower limbs in standing position, with recurved deformity of the left knee

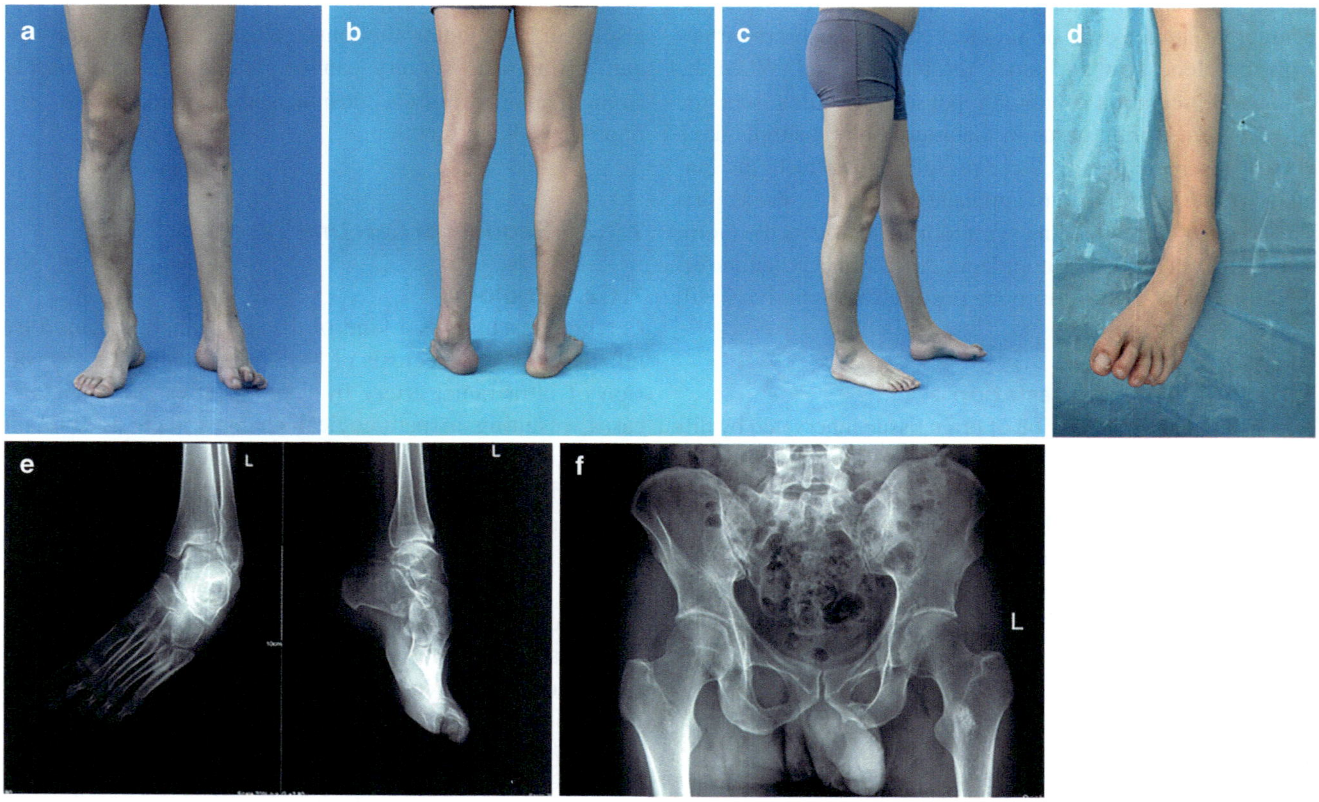

Fig. 7.2 Varus deformity of left foot after cerebral vasculitis. (**a**) frontal view; (**b**) dorsal view; (**c**) lateral view; (**d**) Front view of the left foot; (**e**) Anteroposterior and lateral radiographs of the left foot; (**f**) X-ray of the pelvis in the anteroposterior position

been widely recognized. (2) Secondary vasculitis: common primary causes include connective tissue disease, viral and fungal infections, parasitic infections, and drug-induced infections.

7.1.2.4 Treatment Principle

In the acute stage, anti-inflammatory, control of inflammatory reaction, and immunosuppressant were the main methods. When the condition is prolonged and deteriorated, it can cause irreversible central nervous system injury, leading to limb deformity, orthopedic surgery can be used to balance ankle muscle strength, stabilize joints, and cooperate with braces to facilitate patients to exercise and walk.

7.1.3 Cerebrovascular Malformation

7.1.3.1 Etiology

Cerebrovascular malformation (CVM) is a congenital, non-neoplastic developmental abnormality of cerebral vessels, including the number and structure of local cerebral vessels, which affects the normal cerebral blood flow. When combined with hypertension, malformed blood vessels can spontaneously rupture and bleed, causing intracerebral hemorrhage or hematoma, compressing brain tissue, and causing brain ischemia, causing brain damage. It is more common in young people, with an average age of 20–40 years.

7.1.3.2 Clinical Manifestation

The general condition is insidious, without obvious clinical manifestations, mostly found during physical examination or symptoms of cerebral hemorrhage, and the diagnosis mainly depends on imaging examination. The clinical manifestations were epilepsy and cerebral hemorrhage, manifested as nausea, headache, vomiting, acute intracranial hypertension, and seizures. If the amount of bleeding was small, it could be manifested as refractory headache and other symptoms. If hemorrhage or epileptic nerve damage involves the motor center, the acute stage shows delayed paralysis, and the later stage shows spastic paralysis. Muscle tension increases, tendon reflexes become hyperactive, muscle strength generally decreases, and motor dysfunction occurs. In the long run, secondary bone and joint deformation will lead to changes in the gravity line of lower limbs and limb deformities. The main manifestations of the lower limbs were adduction and internal rotation of the affected limbs and talipes equinovarus deformity of the foot (Fig. 7.3).

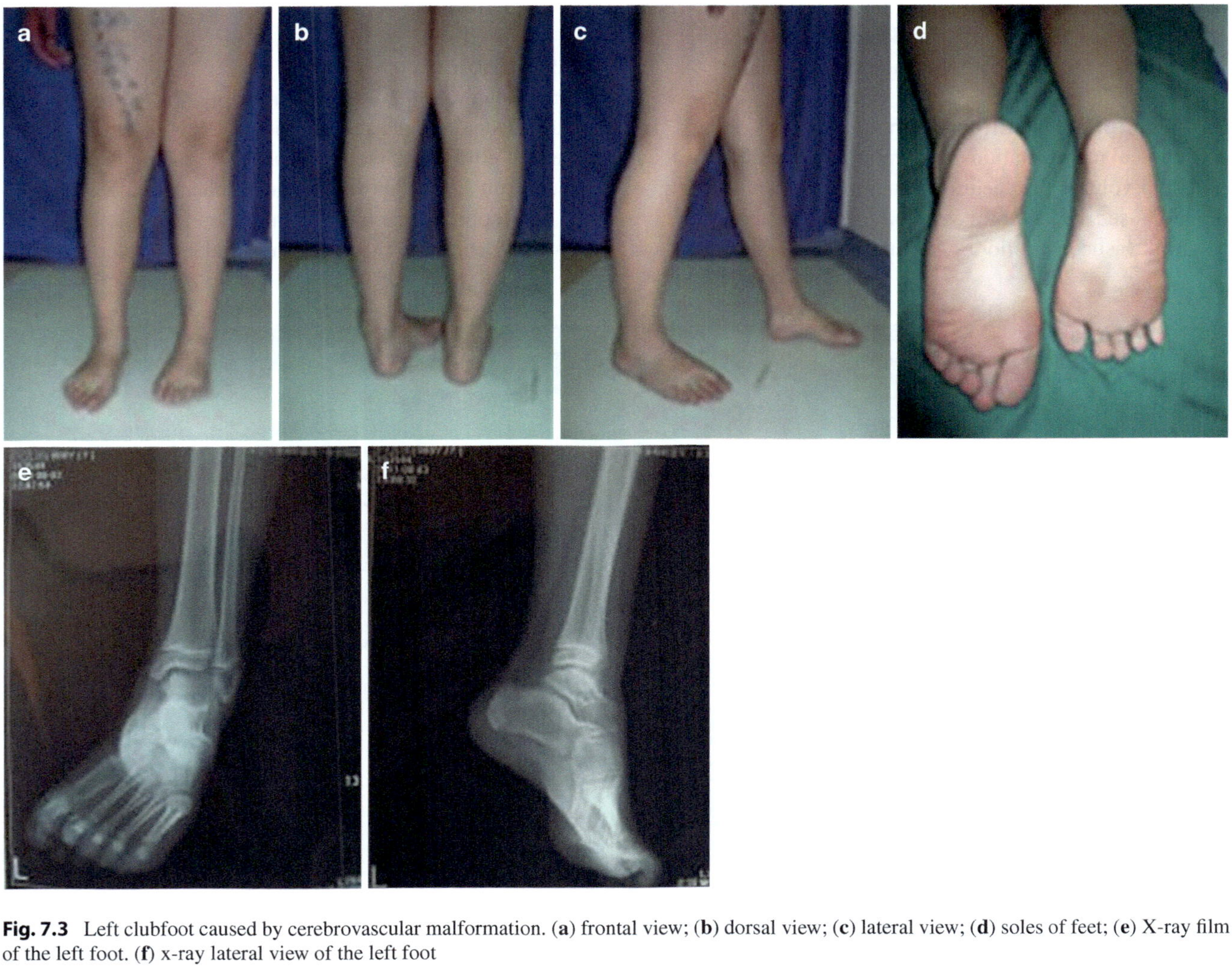

Fig. 7.3 Left clubfoot caused by cerebrovascular malformation. (**a**) frontal view; (**b**) dorsal view; (**c**) lateral view; (**d**) soles of feet; (**e**) X-ray film of the left foot. (**f**) x-ray lateral view of the left foot

7.1.3.3 Treatment Principle

1. Early detection, early treatment, according to the clinical manifestations of patients, hematoma and lesion resection, reduce the occurrence of sequelae;
2. Long-term spastic paralysis leads to deformity of lower limbs, such as talipes equinovarus, which can be treated by orthopedic surgery.

7.1.4 Cerebral Hemorrhage

7.1.4.1 Etiology

Cerebral hemorrhage refers to the hemorrhage caused by the rupture of blood vessels in the non-traumatic brain parenchyma. The cause is related to cerebrovascular disease. Most patients with cerebral hemorrhage are accompanied by hypertension, and the common cause is hypertension combined with arteriolar sclerosis. Emotional excitement and sudden exertion are the causes of the disease. In the early stage of the disease, the mortality rate is very high due to intracranial hypertension and other reasons, and most of the survivors have different degrees of hemiplegic dyskinesia, cognitive impairment, speech impairment, and other sequelae.

7.1.4.2 Clinical Manifestation

The clinical manifestations were related to the etiology, location, and volume of bleeding. Patients with cerebral hemorrhage caused by cerebral venous embolism and reversible cerebral vasoconstriction syndrome showed headache and discomfort several days or weeks before onset. Cerebral arteriovenous malformations (AVMs) are often associated with migraine with aura. Cerebral cavernous hemangiomas often present with rebleeding at the same site. Hemorrhagic stroke has a high rate of disability and mortality, and its sequelae can lead to spastic paralysis on one side of the body and secondary limb deformities (Fig. 7.4).

7.1.4.3 Treatment Principle

After the control of acute cerebral hemorrhage, the patient's vital signs are stable and the condition is no longer progressing, and rehabilitation should be carried out. Early and staged comprehensive rehabilitation therapy is beneficial to the recovery of neurological function and the improvement of quality of life. It is generally believed that 6 months is the golden period of rehabilitation, and orthopedic surgery is feasible for patients with secondary limb deformities affecting function in the later period.

7.1.5 Fanconi Syndrome

7.1.5.1 Etiology

Fanconi syndrome (FS) is a clinical syndrome of multiple proximal renal tubular reabsorption dysfunction caused by a variety of etiologies. The proximal renal tubule reabsorption defect results in the loss of a large number of glucose, amino acids, phosphate, bicarbonate, and so on in urine, leading to acidosis. Electrolyte disorders (hypokalemia, hyponatremia,

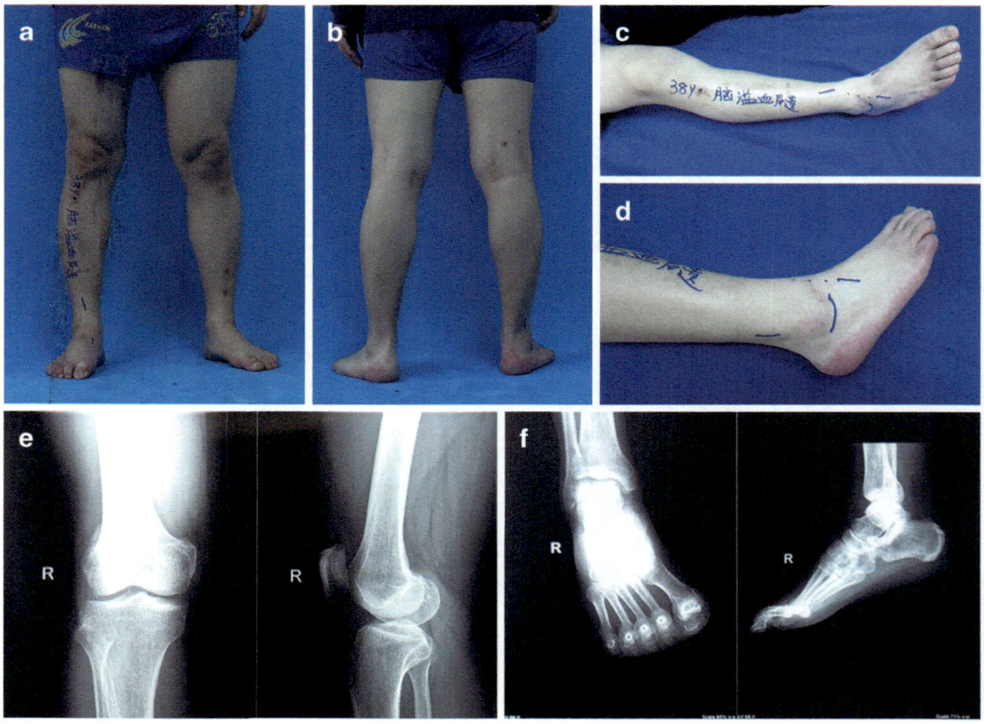

Fig. 7.4 Deformity of right lower limb after cerebral hemorrhage. (**a**) frontal view; (**b**) dorsal view; (**c**) Right lower limb; (**d**) Right ankle; (**e**) anteroposterior and lateral radiographs of right knee joint; (**f**) X-ray anteroposterior and lateral film of right ankle

and hypophosphatemia), renal function and bone metabolism disorders, growth retardation, etc. The causes are primary and secondary: ① The primary disease is mostly related to heredity, which is chromosomal dominant or recessive inheritance, and symptoms occur in infants or within 1 year after birth; ② In secondary cases, all diseases with extensive involvement of proximal renal tubular reabsorption function may be secondary to this disease. Long-term renal dysfunction leads to vitamin D deficiency and osteomalacia in adults, which can be secondary to bone and joint deformities.

7.1.5.2 Clinical Manifestations

1. The disease is rare, and infantile Fanconi syndrome occurs more often than 6–12 months after birth, with vitamin D-resistant rickets and severe malnutrition. The adult type starts after 10–20 years old and has a variety of renal tubular dysfunction. The prominent symptom is adult osteomalacia, which leads to bone deformation of the whole body. When the lower limbs are affected, femoral or tibial varus, joint contracture, and other deformities occur (Fig. 7.5).

7.1.5.3 Treatment Principles

1. Treatment of primary diseases and correction of metabolic abnormalities.
2. For secondary bone and joint deformities, orthopedic surgery was used to correct limb deformities, restore the mechanical axis and joint line of lower limbs, and improve walking and motor function.

7.1.6 Hemophilic Arthropathy

7.1.6.1 Etiology

Hemophilic arthropathy is a joint disease complicated by hemophilia and characterized by joint hematoma and ankylosis. It often occurs in joints with more activities and gravity, such as knee, ankle, elbow and hip joint, of which knee joint is the most common. The pathological changes of hemophilic arthropathy are mainly caused by repeated intra-articular hemorrhage: (1) Intra-articular hemorrhage: It causes joint space widening, hemosiderin deposition, synovial fibrosis, and hyaline cartilage decomposition, resulting in chronic synovitis, cartilage degeneration, and joint surface erosion. (2) Intraosseous hemorrhage (subchondral hemorrhage): It causes osteolysis or cystic degeneration and cystic lesions near the joint. (3) Subperiosteal hemorrhage rarely occurs, causing periosteal reaction, cortical thickening, and pressure erosion. (4) Hemophilic pseudotumor: Osteolytic destruction, combined with soft tissue mass and periosteal reaction, is prone to pathological fracture.

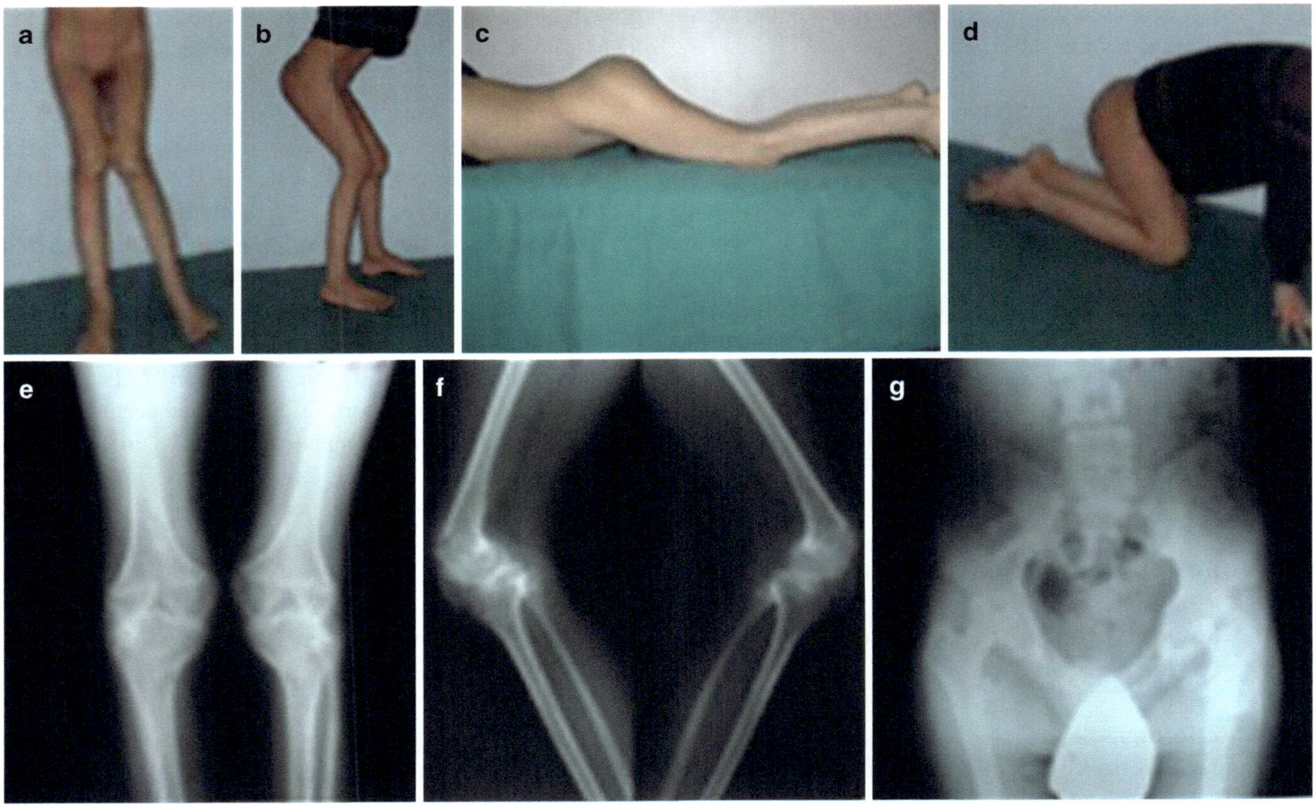

Fig. 7.5 Bilateral flexion of hip and knee caused by Fanconi syndrome. (**a**) frontal view; (**b**, **c**) lateral view; (**d**) General view: flexion of knee and flexion of hip; (**e**) X-ray: bilateral knee joint anteroposterior film; (**f**) X-ray: bilateral knee joint lateral film; (**g**) X-ray pelvic anteroposterior film

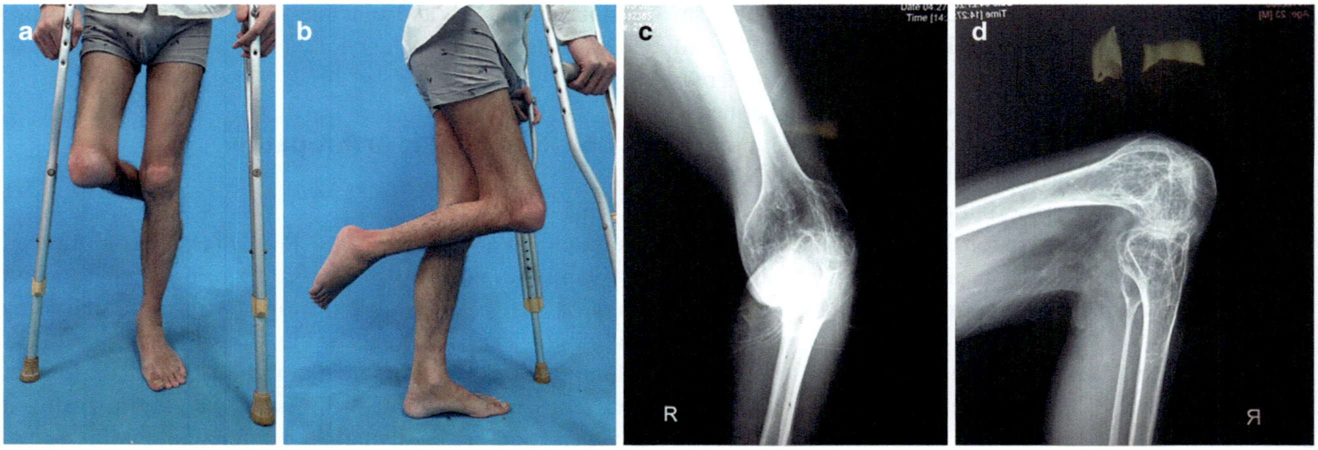

Fig. 7.6 Severe knee flexion deformity of right lower limb caused by hemophilic arthropathy, walking with left lower limb with double crutches. (**a**) Gross view from the front of both lower extremities; (**b**) Gross view of both lower extremities; (**c**) X-ray anteroposterior film of right knee joint; (**d**) Lateral X-ray film of right knee joint

7.1.6.2 Clinical Manifestations

Repeated bleeding leads to iron deposition in joints, synovial hyperplasia and neovascularization, as well as cartilage and subchondral bone injury, resulting in severe bone and joint destruction. Clinically, the upper limbs often occur in the elbow joint, which is characterized by swelling of the elbow joint and joint flexion contracture deformity. The lower limb occurs in the knee joint, showing knee joint swelling, knee flexion contracture deformity, and loss of walking function (Fig. 7.6). It occurs in the ankle joint, showing ankle swelling, foot drop, and varus deformity.

7.1.6.3 Treatment Principles

1. Correction of coagulation abnormalities: supplement of factor VIII to prevent intra-articular bleeding injury;
2. Patients with flexion and talipes equinovarus deformity were not corrected by large skin incision surgery, but by subcutaneous surgery with a sharp knife to release the contracture tendon, and then Ilizarov circular external bindings was installed with a needle, and the flexion and ankle deformity were corrected by slow traction after operation. After correction of knee flexion deformity, artificial joint replacement was performed in patients with severe knee joint destruction.

7.2 Peripheral Vascular Disease

7.2.1 Lower Limb Deformity Secondary to Hemangioma

7.2.1.1 Etiology

Hemangioma is a vascular malformation caused by the proliferation of hemangioblasts during the embryonic period. It is found at birth or shortly after birth, and its etiology is unknown. Hemangioma can occur in all parts of the body, cavernous or racemose hemangioma invasion of muscle, fascia tissue can cause muscle, fascia contracture, resulting in secondary deformity near the bone and joint.

7.2.1.2 Clinical Manifestations

It can be manifested as skin venous dilatation or local cavernous mass, involving multiple tissues and organs in severe cases. Its growth rate is basically synchronized with the growth of the body, and it will not degenerate by itself, and there is no gender difference in the incidence. The local mass is soft, compressive, and non-pulsatile, and its size can change with the change of body position or the speed of venous return. If the lesion is located in the extremities, the lesion shrinks when the extremities are elevated, and the lesion fills and enlarges when the extremities are lowered or the tourniquet is applied. Venous thrombosis is characterized by repeated local pain and tenderness. When the tumor grows and enlarges gradually, it can cause heavy feeling and dull pain. Lesions invading the joint cavity can cause local soreness and abnormal flexion and extension. Subcutaneous venous malformations can affect the adjacent skeletal changes, which are mostly manifested as decalcification and atrophy of the limbs, causing joint deformities of the limbs, such as knee flexion deformity and talipes equinovarus deformity (Fig. 7.7).

7.2.1.3 Treatment Principles

To correct the deformity, the contracture tendon and fascia were properly released by limited surgery, and the hemangioma was protected from injury. After the operation, the Ilizarov circular external bindings were slowly stretched to correct the deformity. After the removal of the external bindings, the brace should be worn for a long time to prevent the recurrence of the deformity.

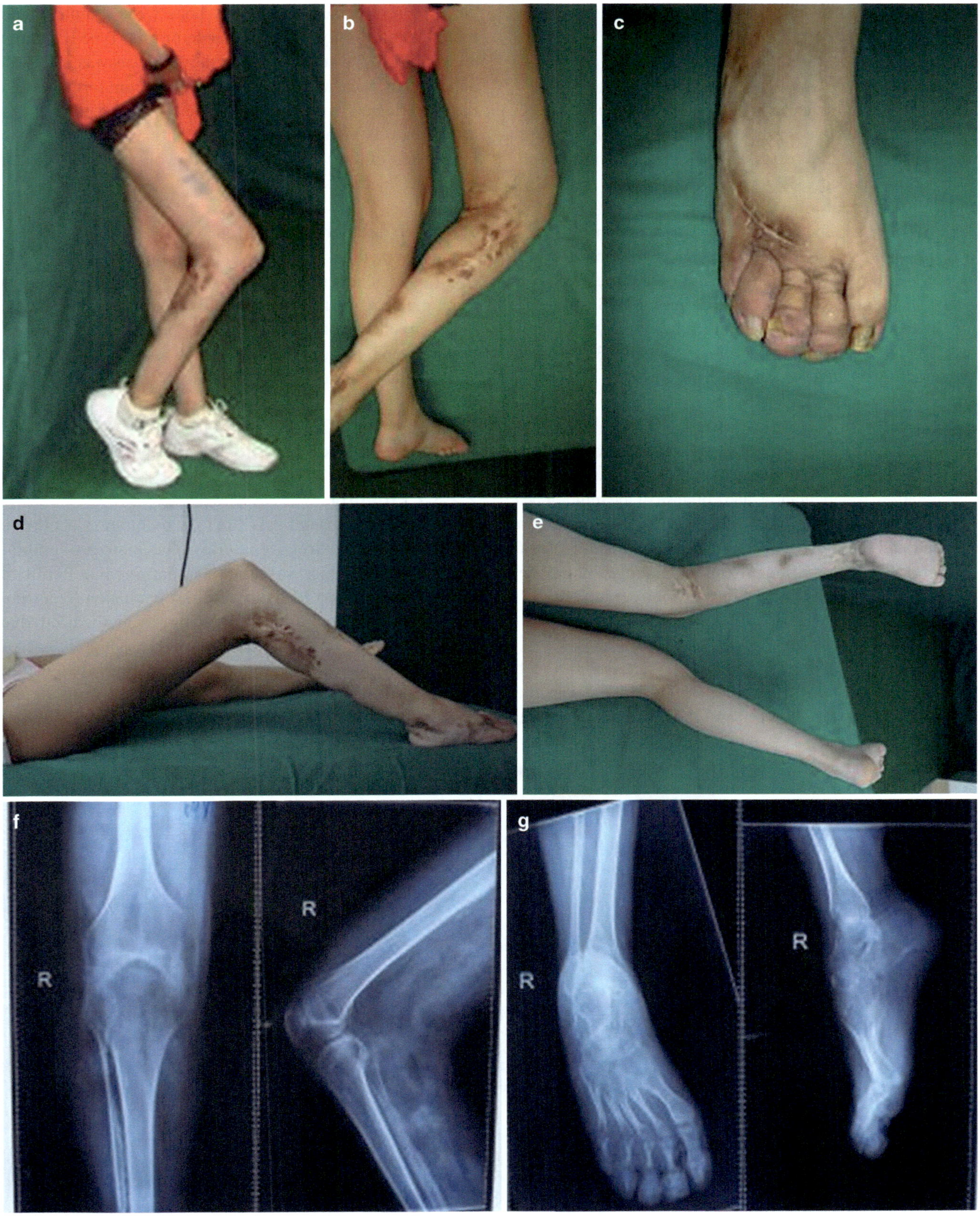

Fig. 7.7 Secondary deformity of knee flexion and foot drop caused by hemangioma of right lower limb. (**a**) Lateral view; (**b**) dorsal view; (**c**) Frontal view; (**d**) Lateral view of knee flexion deformity; (**e**) Knee flexion dorsal view; (**f**) Anteroposterior and lateral X-ray film of right knee joint; (**g**) Anteroposterior and lateral film of right ankle joint

7.2.2 Avascular Necrosis of Femoral Head in Children

7.2.2.1 Etiology

Osteonecrosis of the femoral head epiphysis in children, also known as Legg-Calve-Perthes disease, is a self-limited, self-healing, non-systemic disease of the femoral head in children. Children aged 2–12 years can suffer from this disease, and children aged 4–8 years are more common. The incidence of male and female is 4:1, and most of them are unilateral. Its pathogenesis is not yet clear, local factors include trauma, birth position, anatomical abnormalities, synovitis, arthritis and increased intra-articular pressure. Systemic factors include: (1) coagulation and fibrinolysis system abnormalities; (2) endocrine and immune factors; (3) cytokines; (4) heredity and adverse living environment.

7.2.2.2 Clinical Manifestations

Clinically, the main manifestations were claudication, hip pain, and limitation of movement. The X-ray signs were cystic degeneration, fragmentation, and collapse of the femoral head. During the recovery period, the abnormal shaping of the femoral head and the involvement of the metaphysis affected the normal development of the proximal femur, resulting in head enlargement, short neck or flat hip deformity (Fig. 7.8).

7.2.2.3 Classification

Catterall classification: Type I: only the anterior part of the epiphysis (< 1/2) was involved, the femoral head was intact without collapse, the absorption of the necrotic area, and the creeping replacement of the new bone were complete, and there was no or only mild residual deformity. Type II: a large area (>1/2) of the anterior side of the epiphysis was involved, and the femoral head collapsed and sequestrum formed when the necrotic part was absorbed. In the X-ray film, the sequestrum area was V-shaped. In type III, only a small part of the lateral side of the epiphysis was not involved. Type IV: total epiphyseal necrosis.

7.2.2.4 Treatment Principles

Treatment methods are aimed at preventing and delaying the occurrence of adverse prognosis such as femoral head deformity and degenerative osteoarthritis, hoping to improve the blood circulation of femoral head, restore the containment of femoral head, avoid or reduce the collapse of femoral head, and maintain the function of hip joint.

7.2.3 Sequelae of Popliteal Artery Embolism

7.2.3.1 Etiology

Popliteal artery thrombosis (PAT) is a common occlusive disease of lower extremity arteries. The sources of emboli include cardiogenic, vascular, and iatrogenic. Popliteal artery embolization leads to vascular occlusion, resulting in soft tissue ischemia of the leg. After recanalization, due to a long period of ischemia, irreversible ischemic necrosis, fibrosis, and gradual contracture of the calf muscles occur, resulting in secondary talipes equinovarus deformity.

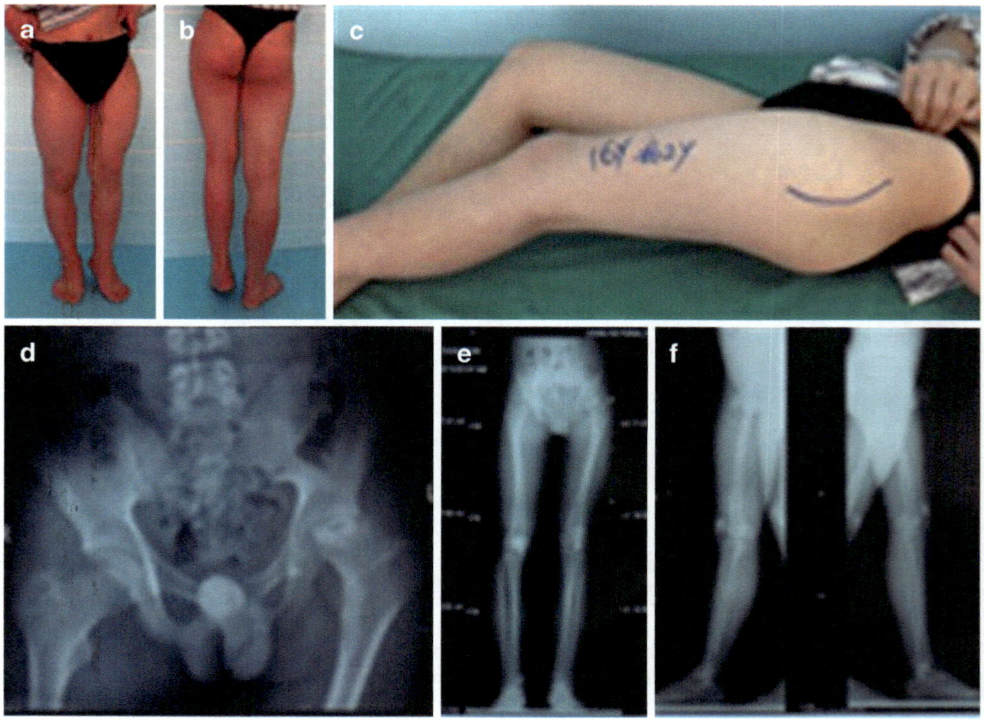

Fig. 7.8 Avascular necrosis of femoral head in children. (**a**) Frontal view; (**b**) dorsal view; (**c**) Lateral view; (**d**) pelvic anteroposterior radiograph; (**e**) anteroposterior radiograph of the whole length of both lower limbs; (**f**) Full-length lateral radiographs of both lower extremities

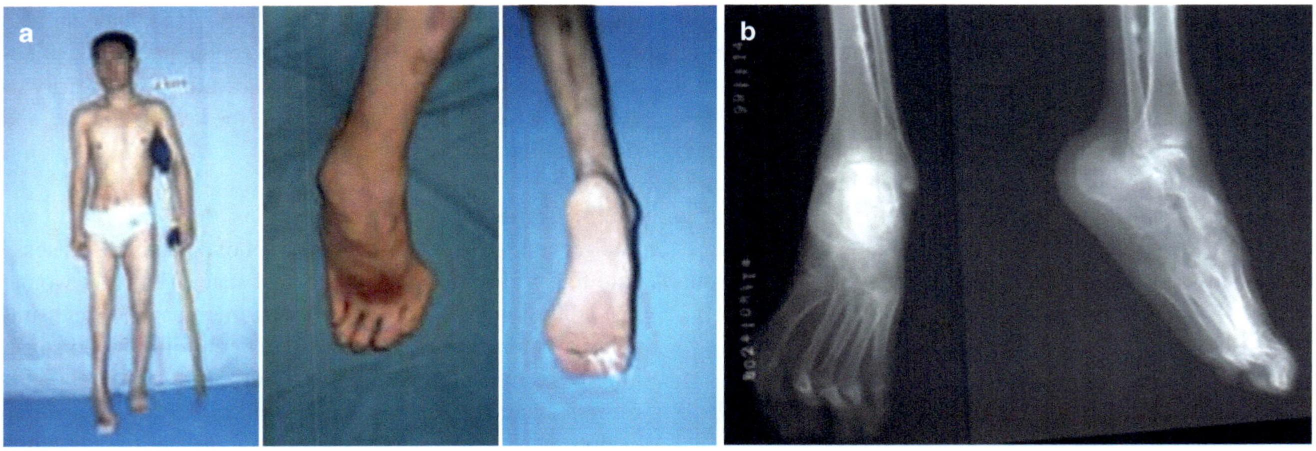

Fig. 7.9 Right rigid talipes equinovarus caused by sequelae of popliteal artery embolism. (**a**) Front view and front and back view of right foot; (**b**) Anteroposterior and lateral radiograph of right foot

7.2.3.2 Clinical Manifestations

Acute popliteal artery embolism can cause ischemia of the leg and foot, resulting in soreness, numbness, cold, and pain of the leg. In severe cases, it can cause extensive necrosis of the leg muscle, secondary deformity, amputation, and other adverse consequences. Embolization of the popliteal artery eventually leads to ischemic muscle contracture and rigid clubfoot deformity with poor blood circulation (Fig. 7.9).

7.2.3.3 Treatment Principles

Soft tissues such as contracture tendons and fascia were released by surgery, and Ilizarov technique was used to slowly pull them to correct foot and ankle deformities. Patients with long course of disease and bony deformity should be treated with osteotomy or arthrodesis.

7.2.4 Thromboangiitis Obliterans

7.2.4.1 Etiology

Thromboangiitis Obliterans (TAO) is also known as Buerger's disease, commonly known as "vasculitis," the etiology is not yet completely clear, may be related to genetic, androgen, immune dysfunction, cold, and smoking are closely related to the disease, the disease often occurs in young adults.

7.2.4.2 Clinical Manifestations

The lesions occur in the small and medium arteries and veins of the distal extremities, showing a segmental vasculitis, especially in the lower extremities, but rarely in the large arteries. In the early stage, the skin of the extremities is pale, the skin temperature is low, the limbs are cold, sore, and weak, and intermittent claudication may occur, which is the period of local ischemia. It is followed by dystrophy, characterized by dry skin, desquamation, thickening and deformation of fingernails and toenails, and rest pain. Finally, extreme ischemia can lead to necrosis of the extremities, mostly dry gangrene, such as "mummification," or even self-shedding. The patient suffered from unbearable severe and persistent pain, which could not be effectively relieved by analgesics, resulting in amputation.

7.2.4.3 Treatment Principles

To improve microcirculation, because the lesions occur in small arteries and veins, the effect of conventional vascular reconstruction surgery is not good.

In recent years, the technique of transverse tibial bone transfer has been used to stimulate the establishment of peripheral collateral circulation and alleviate the symptoms of distal limb ischemia to a certain extent (Figs. 7.10, 7.11 and 7.12).

7.2.5 Diabetic Foot

7.2.5.1 Etiology

Diabetic foot (DF) is a disease cause by diabetic peripheral neuropathy, including peripheral nerve sensory disturbance and autonomic nerve damage, peripheral arteriolar occlusion cause by lower extremity vascular disease-arteriosclerosis, or foot pain, foot ulcer and foot gangrene caused by skin microvascular disease and bacterial infection. Ischemia, neuropathy, and infection often act in concert. Minor trauma can lead to severe ulcers and infections, and eventually the destruction of foot bones, leading to foot deformities, mostly manifested as flat arch, disappearance, and even the formation of "rocking chair foot" deformity.

7.2.5.2 Clinical Manifestations

The main manifestations of patients are foot paresthesia, such as numbness and itching, or hypoesthesia, such as sock feeling, which can lead to Charcot foot deformity in severe cases (Fig. 7.13), pain and dry gangrene due to ischemia (Fig. 7.14), difficulty in walking or even inability to stand and walk. Because the skin damage of the foot can lead to infection that is difficult to contain (Fig. 7.15) and wet necrosis, the infection can spread rapidly from the local to the surrounding, leading to osteomyelitis (Fig. 7.16), and can also spread to the whole body, leading to septicopyemia, septicemia, and even septic shock, thus aggravating the severity of the disease. Even after amputation, the quality of life and survival time are not optimistic.

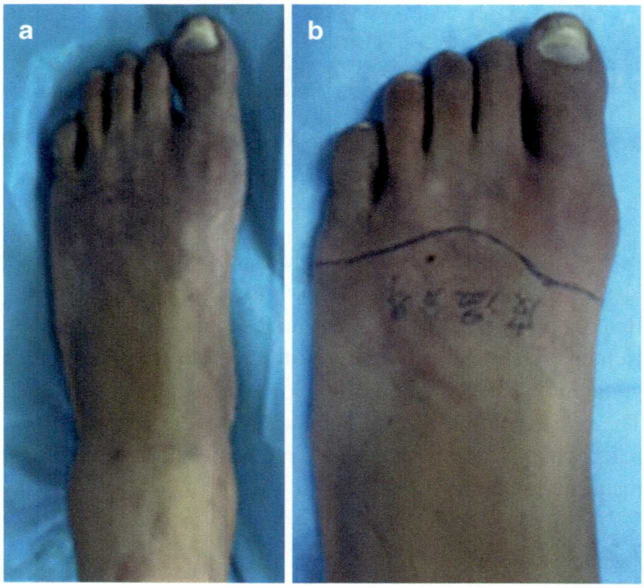

Fig. 7.10 Thromboangiitis obliterans with chronic ischemic "thin" toe deformity. (**a**) Left foot front view; (**b**) A partial photograph of the left forefoot

7.2.5.3 Treatment Principles

The general principle for the treatment of diabetic foot disease is to transform the local pathological state of the foot wound into a physiological state and create a microenvironment suitable for wound repair, including strict control of blood sugar, improvement of peripheral circulation, anti-infection, supportive treatment, and maintenance of the stability of the internal environment. In recent years, a large number of Ilizarov tibial transverse transfer operations have been carried out in China, and satisfactory results have been achieved.

7.2.6 Atherosclerotic Angiitis Obliterans

7.2.6.1 Etiology

Atherosclerotic angiitis obliterans (ASO) is a common teratogenic and disabling ischemic disease of the lower extremities. Pathological changes generally start from the intima of the artery, lipid deposits inside and outside the intima of the artery, forming yellow atheromatous lipid accumulation on the surface of the intima, which can lead to the decrease of arterial elasticity and gradual hardening. If combined with abnormal glucose metabolism (diabetes mellitus), uric acid metabolism disorders and other diseases, atherosclerosis will occur earlier and progress rapidly, eventually leading to vascular embolism.

Fig. 7.11 Typical manifestations of ischemic necrosis of thromboangiitis obliterans. (**a**) Right dorsum of foot; (**b**) Right foot sole

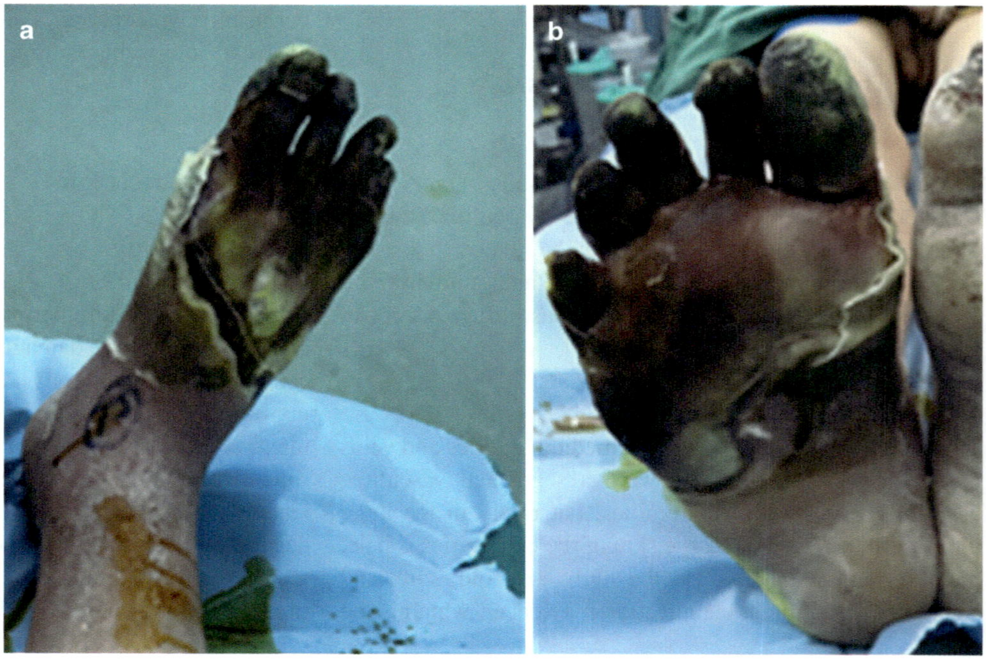

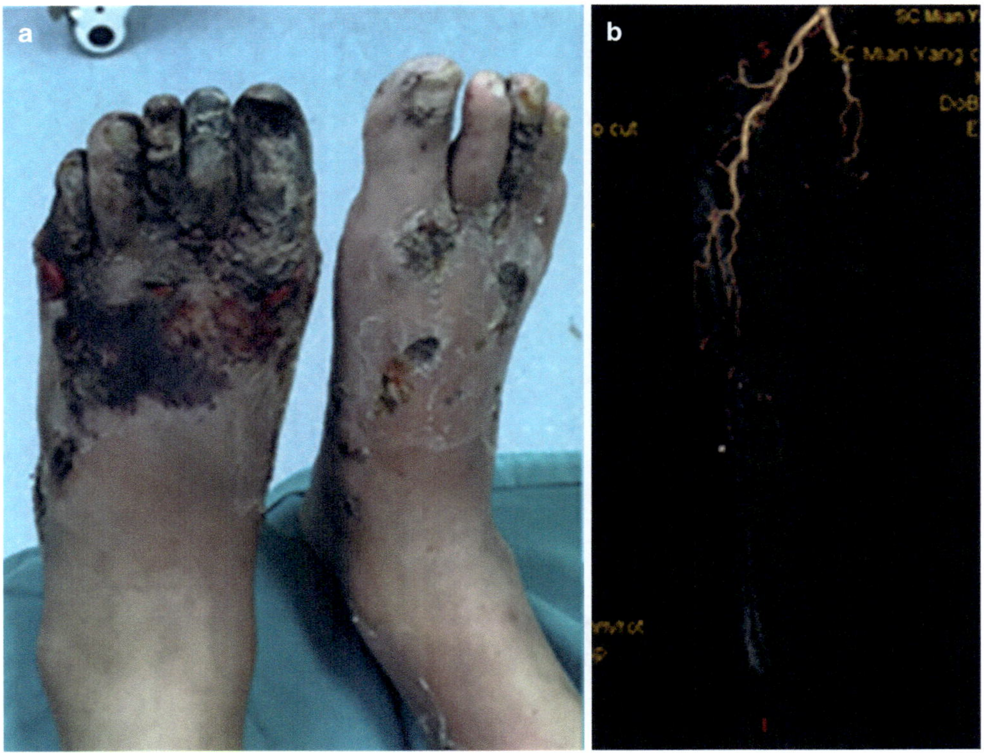

Fig. 7.12 Dry gangrene of both feet caused by thromboangiitis obliterans. (**a**) Generally according to the front view of both feet; (**b**) Angiography of both lower limbs

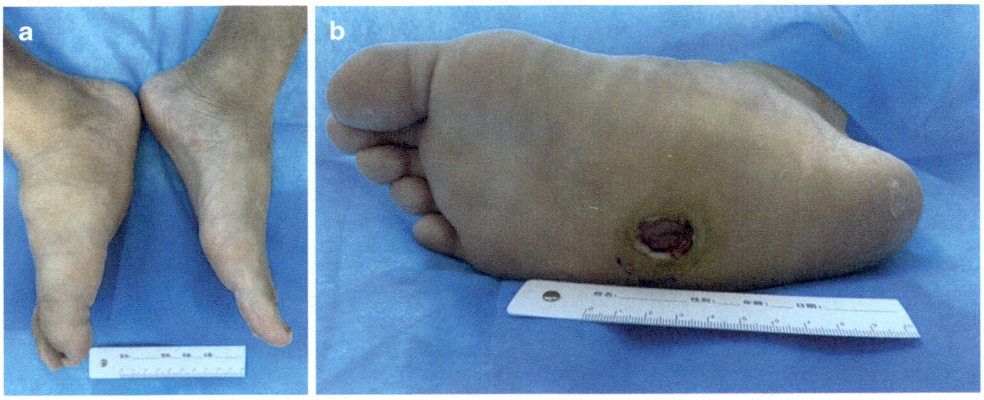

Fig. 7.13 Charcot deformity caused by diabetic foot. (**a**) Lateral view; (**b**) Right plantar ulcer

7.2.6.2 Clinical Manifestations

Sclerosis and vascular occlusion occurring in the blood supply arteries of the limbs are bound to be secondary to extremity necrosis (Fig. 7.17). A small number of patients will not have obvious ischemia in the limbs, and may only have mild coldness or soreness. However, patients with vascular collateral circulation cannot be compensated, manifested as expanding skin ulcers and severe pain, and eventually necrosis and exfoliation of acral tissue (Fig. 7.18).

7.2.6.3 Treatment Principles

Lumbar sympathectomy, great saphenous vein graft bypass or arterial thromboendarterectomy can be performed if non-operative treatment is ineffective. After the limitation of the necrotic border of the extremities, the wound was expanded and the necrotic tissue was removed under aseptic conditions. For patients with distal gangrene, amputation should be considered.

7.2.7 Venous Stasis Ulcer

7.2.7.1 Etiology

Venous stasis ulcer (VSU) is mostly caused by venous diseases, including primary venous valve insufficiency of lower extremities, deep venous thrombosis syndrome of lower extremities, and so on. The above causes lead to venous reflux or reflux disorder, long-term increase of venous pressure, blood stasis, local tissue hypoxia, capillary wall damage, increased vascular permeability, and fibrin exudation.

Fig. 7.14 Dry necrosis of diabetic foot. (**a**) Right sole; (**b**) Lateral view of right foot; (**c**) Ulcer on right dorsum of foot

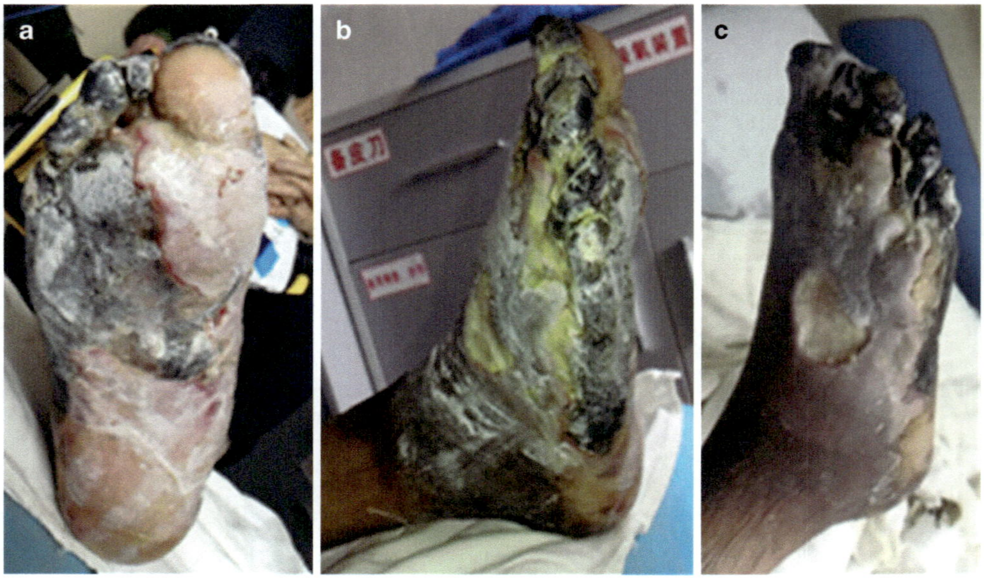

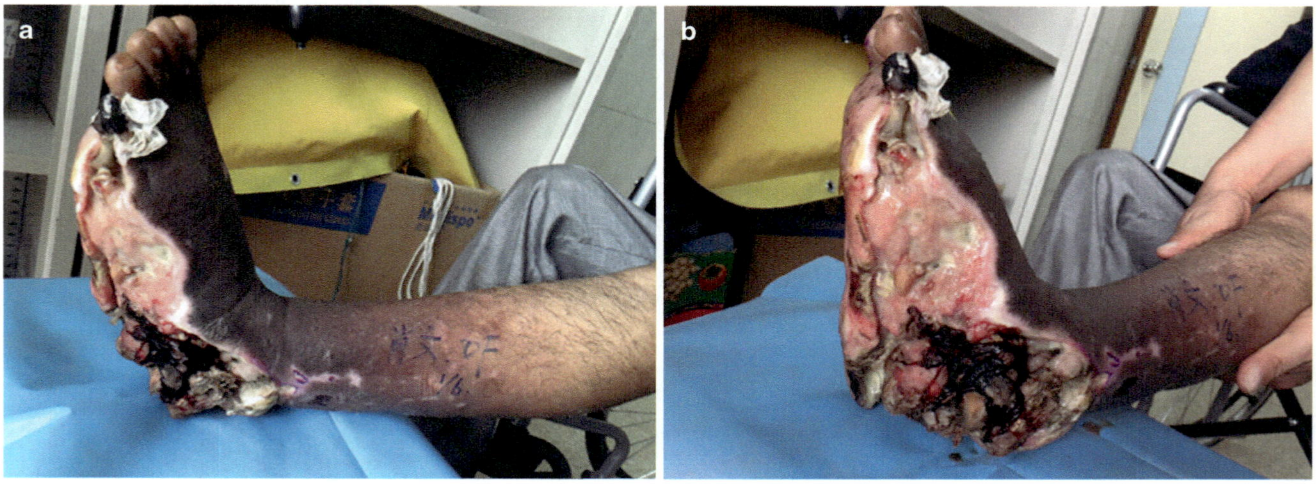

Fig. 7.15 Severe infection and necrosis of bone and soft tissue caused by diabetic foot. (**a**) Oblique view of left foot; (**b**) Lateral view of left foot

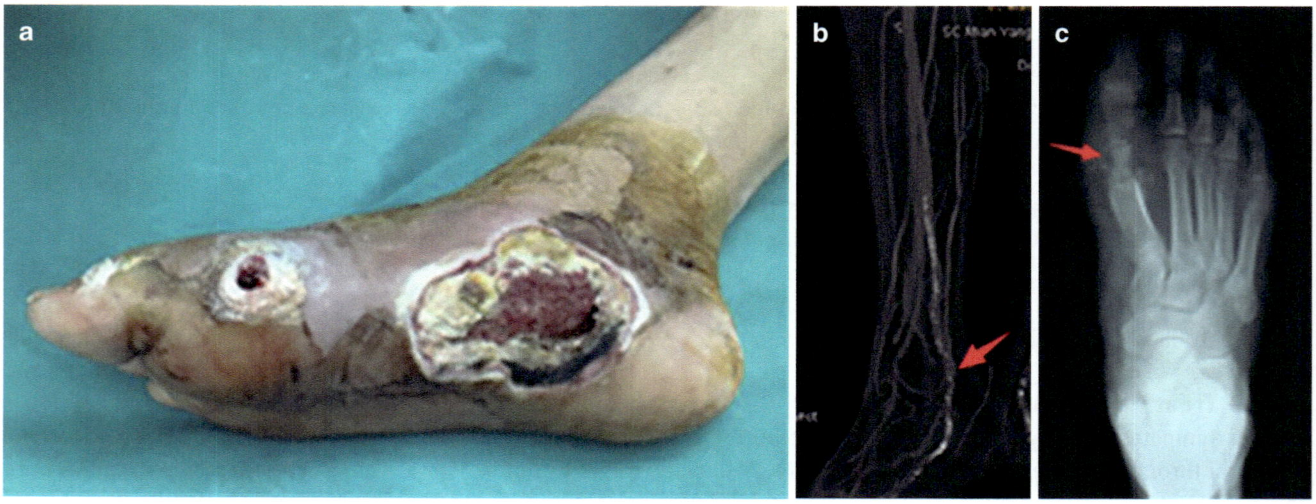

Fig. 7.16 Foot gangrene infection and osteomyelitis caused by diabetic foot. (**a**) The lateral view of the right foot shows multiple gangrene with sinus tracts; (**b**) Angiography of right leg; (**c**) X-ray of the right foot showed infection and destruction of the first metatarsal bone of the right foot

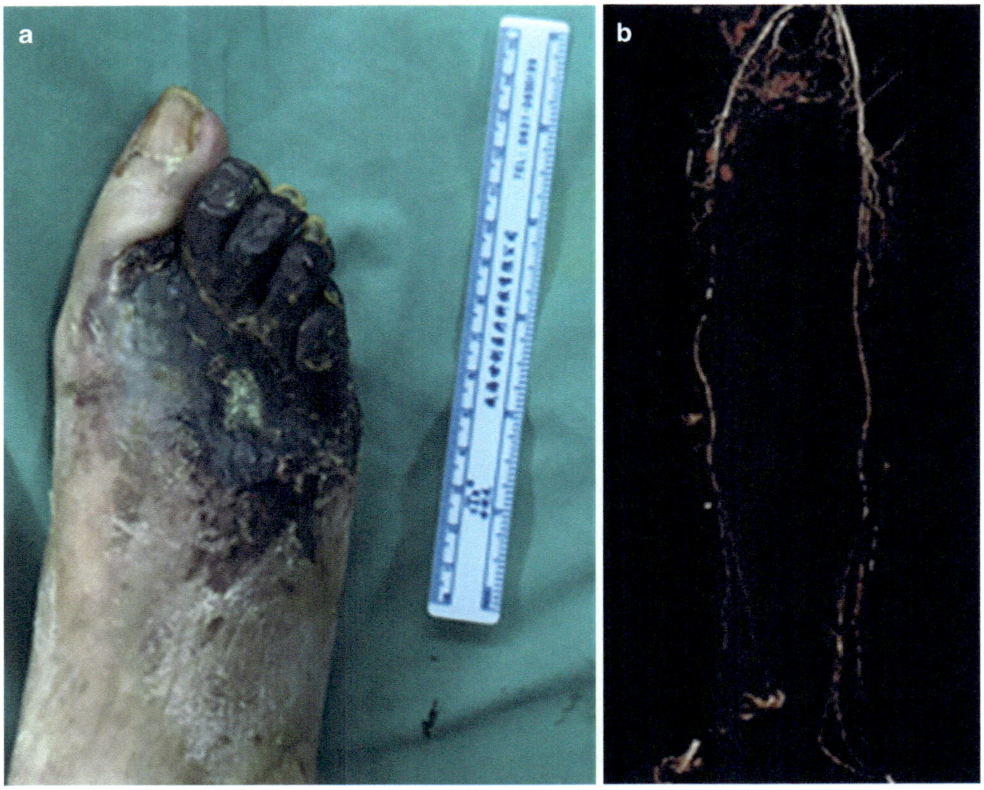

Fig. 7.17 Peripheral ischemic necrosis caused by atherosclerotic angiitis obliterans. (**a**) Frontal view of the right foot shows dry gangrene of the second to fourth toes of the right foot. (**b**) Angiography of both lower extremities

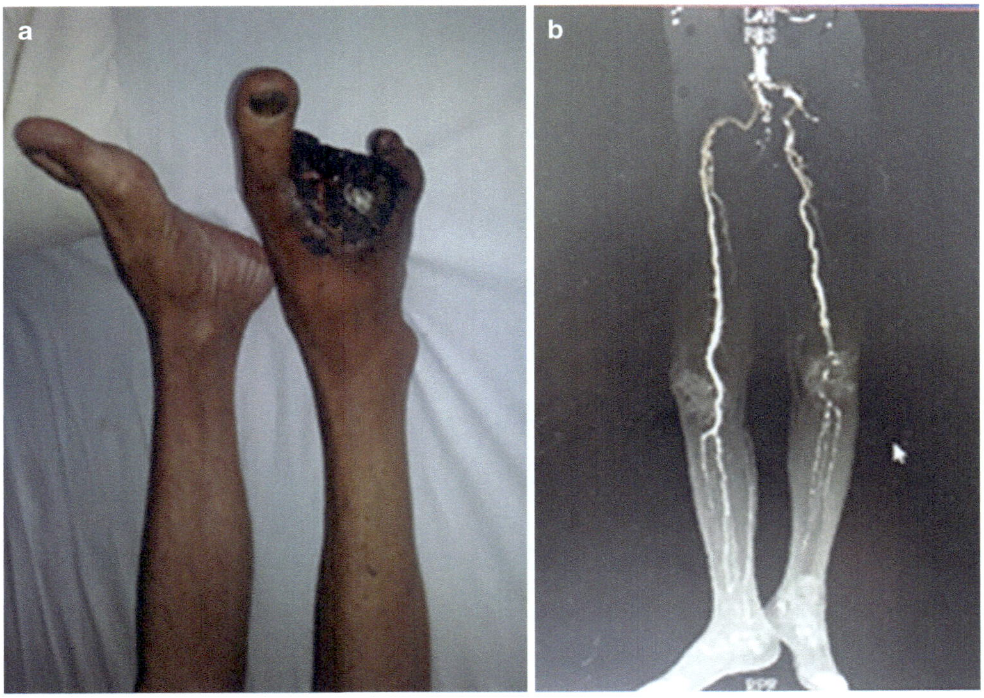

Fig. 7.18 Ischemic necrosis and desquamation of toes caused by atherosclerotic occlusive vasculitis. (**a**) The appearance of both feet showed necrosis and exfoliation of the right toe. (**b**) Angiography of both lower extremities

After trauma, ulcers can be formed because of the obstruction of wound healing due to circulatory disorders. This kind of ulcer happens in crus more below 1/3 inside or outside, and much companion has skin pigment ad cool-headed, ulcer lasts for a long time does not heal.

7.2.7.2 Clinical Manifestations

In the early stage of the disease, it may only be inflammatory exudation, followed by ulceration, gradually expanding, and eventually necrosis of the whole skin. The skin around the ulcer is affected, atrophied and blackened, causing eczema,

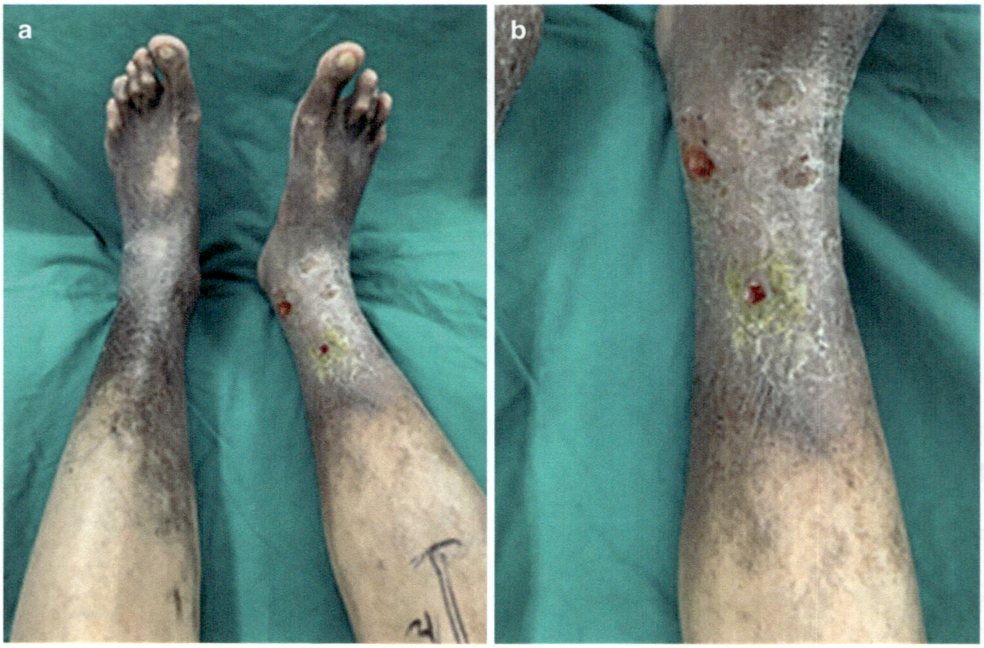

Fig. 7.19 Skin pigmentation, dry desquamation, and skin ulcer caused by venous stasis ulcer. (**a**) Appearance of both lower limbs; (**b**) Appearance of ulcer on right ankle

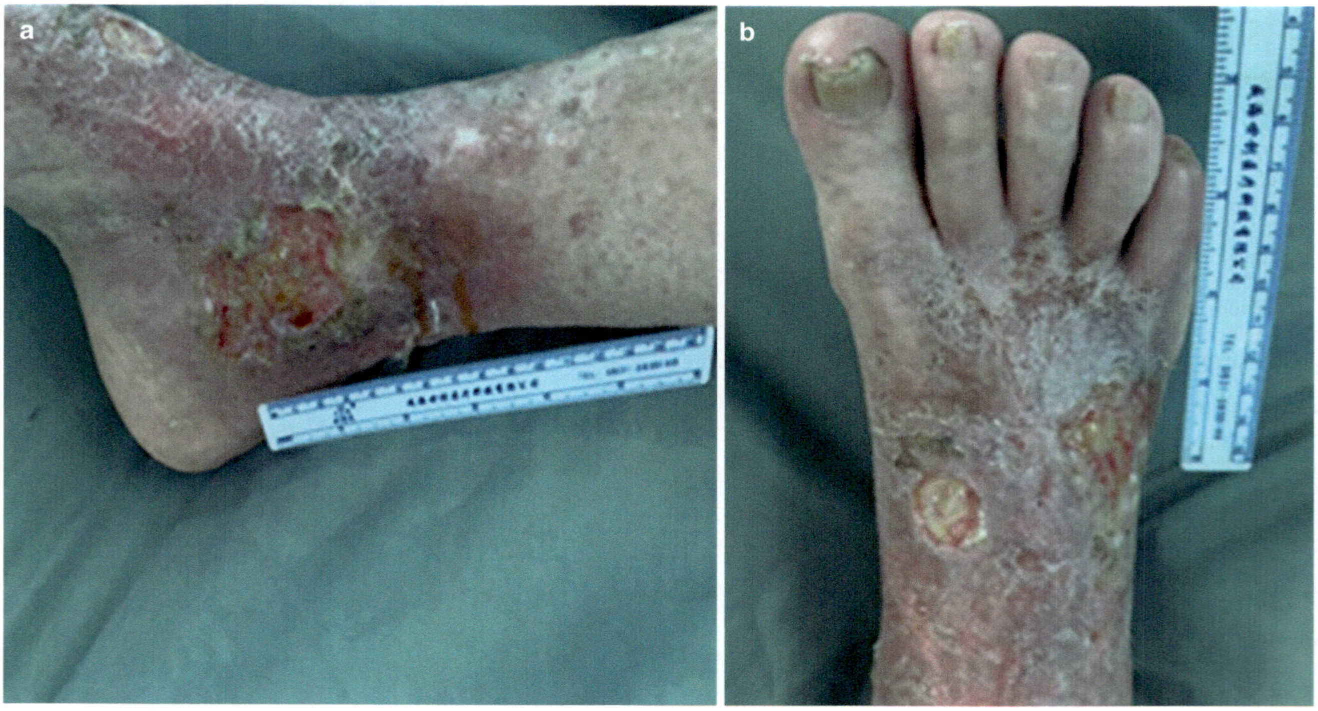

Fig. 7.20 Venous stasis ulcer causes skin ulceration at the dorsum of the foot and ankle joint. (**a**) Appearance of right ankle joint; (**b**) Appearance of right dorsum of foot

manifested as desquamation, itching, and other symptoms (Figs. 7.19 and 7.20).

7.2.7.3 Treatment Principles

Improve the blood circulation of lower limbs and promote blood reflux, including drug treatment, pressure treatment, surgical treatment, etc. Ilizarov's transverse tibial bone transfer can reconstruct microcirculation and promote wound healing.

Neurogenic Disease Leads to Deformity

8

Sihe Qin, Lei Shi, and Jiancheng Zang

8.1 Encephalic Disease

8.1.1 Cerebral Palsy

8.1.1.1 Definition of Cerebral Palsy

Cerebral palsy (CP) refers to organic lesions that cause motor and postural disorders due to various factors damaging the immature brain tissue of the fetus or infant during the gestational and perinatal periods, and is often accompanied by impairments in intelligence, behavior, and sensation.

8.1.1.2 Etiology

Brain damage that causes cerebral palsy can occur during the prenatal, intrapartum, and postpartum periods. The mechanism of limb deformity in cerebral palsy is due to the dysfunction of upper motor neurons, which leads to the disorder of the regulation mechanism of lower motor neurons.

8.1.1.3 Clinical Manifestation

The clinical manifestations of cerebral palsy include: (1) hypertonia, hyperreflexia, and positive ankle clonus; (2) existence of primitive reflex; (3) different degrees of motor disorders; (4) abnormal posture and walking: such as scissors gait; pointed gait; knee-bending semi-squat gait, etc.; (5) spastic or fixed deformities such as hip flexion, knee flexion, foot drop, foot varus, foot valgus, etc. Torsional spasms can lead to the coexistence of multiple deformities of the whole body.

S. Qin (✉)
Department of Orthopaedics, Rehabilitation Hospital of the National Research Center for Rehabilitation Technical Aids, Beijing, China

L. Shi
Department of Orthopaedics, Rehabilitation Hospital, National Research Center for Rehabilitation, Beijing, China

J. Zang
Department of Hand and Foot Surgery, Beijing University of Chinese Medicine Third Affiliated Hospital, Beijing, China

8.1.1.4 Classification and Typing of Cerebral Palsy

The classification and typing of cerebral palsy are complex, including etiology, pathophysiology, clinical signs, and so on. According to the clinical manifestations, it is divided into the following types (American Cerebral Palsy Association):

1. Spastic hypertonia, tendon hyperreflexia, positive ankle clonus, elbow and wrist flexion, and thumb adduction deformity. Adduction of bilateral lower limb at the hip, and knee flexion, both lower limbs are crossed legs, the most common ankle is talipes equinovarus or flatfoot valgus deformity (Fig. 8.1).
2. Athetosis is difficult to control by will. Involuntary movement (Fig. 8.2).
3. Ataxia is characterized by non-sustainability. Sexual position control, coordinate movement disturbance, manifested as imbalance, muscular proprioception articulated position sense loss, muscle tension descending, fatiguing, may be accompanied by distance-measuring disorders, eyeball and limb tremor (Fig. 8.3).
4. Rigid and rigid cerebral palsy is characterized by resistance to passive movement. Because ankylosing cerebral palsy belongs to extrapyramidal injury, the biggest difference between ankylosing cerebral palsy and spastic cerebral palsy is that ankylosing cerebral palsy has no hyperreflexia, ankle clonus, and involuntary movement (Fig. 8.4).
5. Mixed symptoms of several types of cerebral palsy are mixed together and concentrated in one patient, in which spasticity is the main cause of secondary lower limb deformities (Fig. 8.5).

8.1.1.5 Cerebral Palsy Is Classified According to the Affected Parts

1. Quadriplegia. The lower limbs are stiff, straight, and crossed in a scissors shape. Hip and knee flexion, internal rotation of lower limbs, scissors gait, severe spasm of both upper limbs, often abnormal postures such as

S. Qin et al. (eds.), *Atlas of Limb Deformity*, https://doi.org/10.1007/978-981-97-0999-1_8

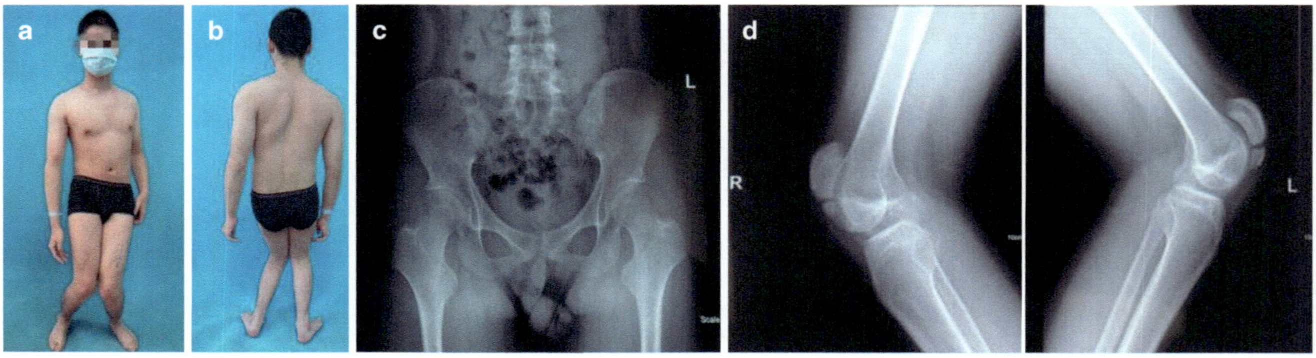

Fig. 8.1 Spastic cerebral palsy. (**a**) Front view, bilateral knee flexion; (**b**) Rear view; (**c**) Pelvic plain film; (**d**) Bilateral knee joint lateral film, bilateral patella high, patella lower pole due to muscle spasm rupture

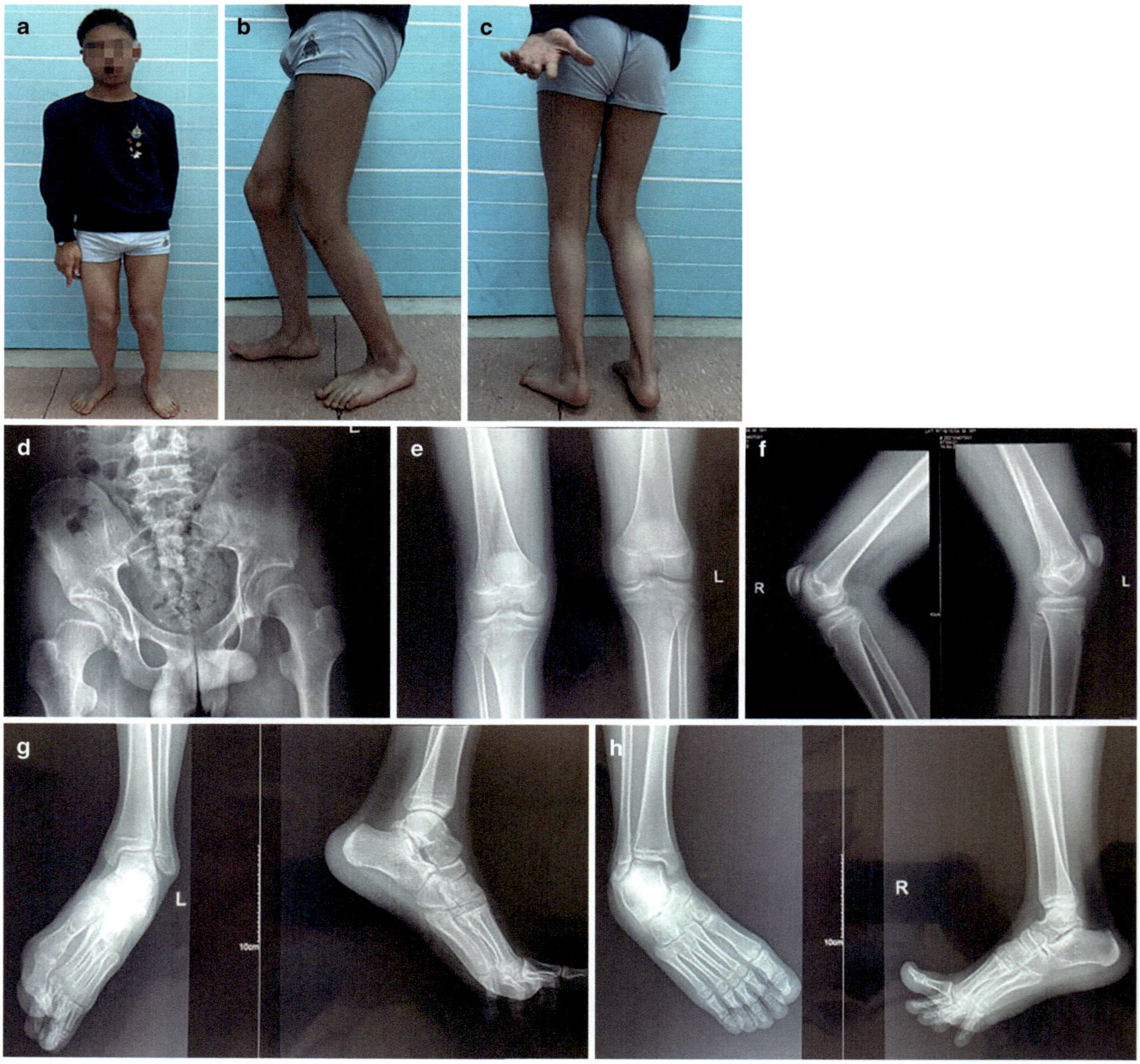

Fig. 8.2 Athetoid cerebral palsy. (**a**) Positive view; (**b**) Lateral view of both lower limbs, flexion deformity; (**c**) Posterior view of both lower extremities, flexion of the knees, mild equinus deformity; (**d**) Pelvic obliquity; E-F. Bilateral anteroposterior and lateral radiographs of knee joint; (**g**, **h**). Anteroposterior and lateral radiographs of the ankle joints of both feet, and eversion of both feet

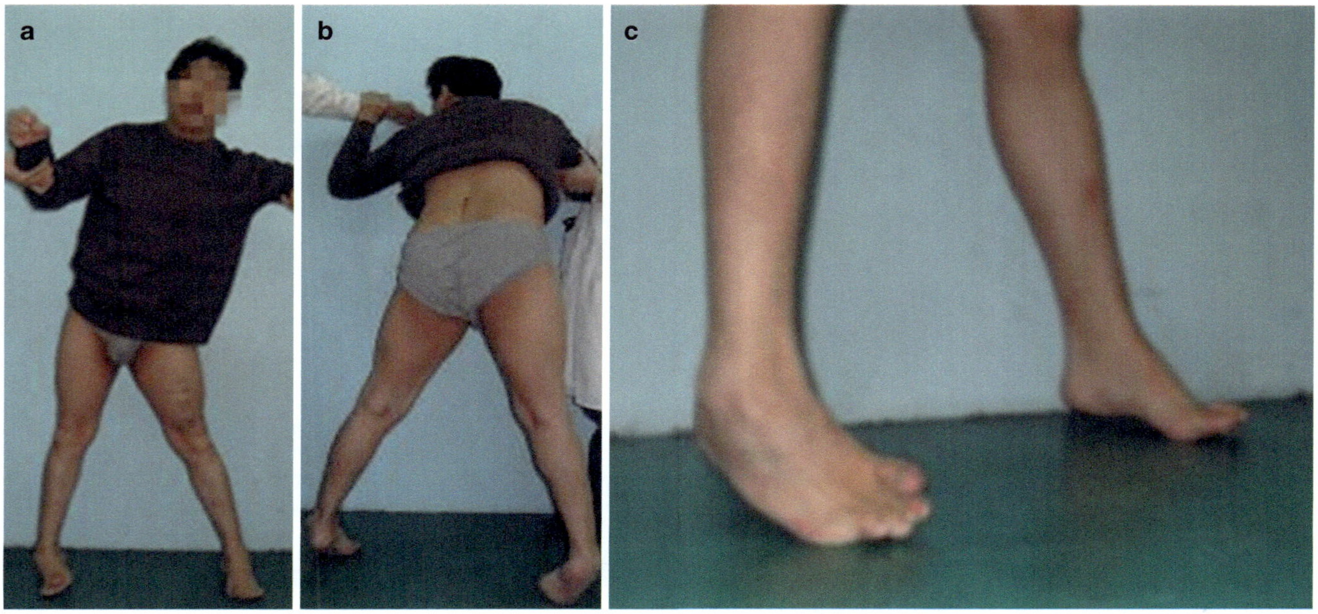

Fig. 8.3 Ataxic cerebral palsy, not persistent sexual position control, coordinate movement disturbance, imbalance, left foot with talipes equinovarus deformity

forearm pronation, thumb adduction, shoulder girdle adduction, and internal rotation (Fig. 8.6).

2. The prominent manifestation of diplegia is the increase of muscle tension of both lower limbs. The lower extremities are stiff, straight, and crossed in a scissor shape. Upper limb involvement is mild, often manifested as abnormal upper limb posture when walking, but hand function involvement is not obvious (Fig. 8.7).
3. Adduction and internal rotation of paraplegic lower limbs, increased muscle tension, hyperactive tendon reflexes, and positive pathological reflexes (Fig. 8.8).
4. Triplegia of both lower limbs with spastic paralysis of the right upper limb (Fig. 8.9).
5. Hemiplegia is characterized by spastic paralysis of one limb (Fig. 8.10).
6. Paralysis of one of the monoplegic limbs (Fig. 8.11).
7. Double hemiplegic limbs are involved, both upper limbs are heavier than both lower limbs, and one side is heavier than the other. Classification by degree:
   (a) Mild: completely self-care, able to stand and walk (Fig. 8.12).
   (b) Moderate: The patient takes care of himself partially and needs help (Fig. 8.13).
   (c) Severe: completely unable to take care of oneself, take a wheelchair for activities, and need complete help (Fig. 8.14).

8.1.1.6 Principles of Surgical Treatment of Limb Deformities in Cerebral Palsy

(1) Partially relieve spasm; (2) correction of deformity; (3) Cooperate with rehabilitation training.

8.1.2 Patella Fatigue Fracture Separation Caused by Severe Knee Flexion Deformity in Cerebral Palsy

8.1.2.1 Etiology

Spastic cerebral palsy (spastic cerebral palsy) leads to knee flexion contracture, while the quadriceps femoris muscle strength is relatively weakened, patellar ligament is stretched for a long time, severe cases occur patellar pole avulsion fracture or patellar ligament heterotopic ossification.

8.1.2.2 Clinical Manifestation

Spasmodic knee flexion contracture, quadriceps femoris muscle strength is relatively weakened, patella is high or knee pain, patella separation can be seen in lateral knee radiograph (Fig. 8.15), which further weakens the knee extension strength of quadriceps femoris and aggravates knee flexion deformity.

8.1.2.3 Treatment Principle

After correction of knee flexion deformity, the separated patella was repositioned and fixed.

8.1.3 Sequelae of Encephalitis

8.1.3.1 Etiology

Encephalitis refers to the central nervous system lesions caused by pathogens invading meninges and brain parenchyma (such as encephalitis B). If the injured part involves the motor center, secondary motor dysfunction will occur after cure, and gradually secondary limb deformities will occur.

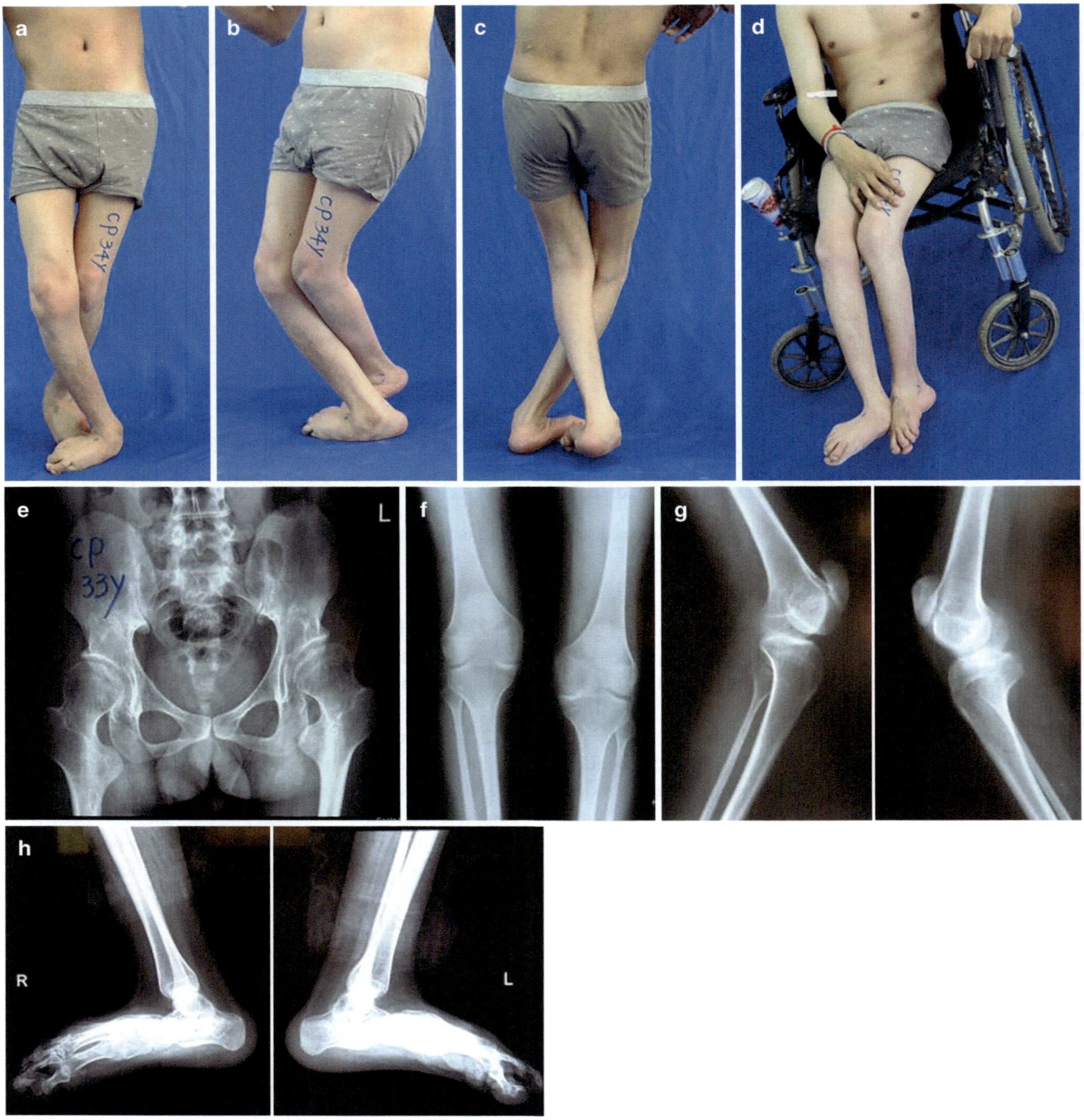

Fig. 8.4 Rigid cerebral palsy. (**a**) Front view of both lower limbs, adduction, and internal rotation of both lower limbs; (**b**) Side view of both lower limbs, hip, and knee flexion of both lower limbs; (**c**) In the posterior view of both lower limbs, both feet were severely deformed, especially on the right side; (**d**) The patient is unable to walk upright and requires a wheelchair; (**e**) Plain radiograph of pelvis; (**f–h**) Bilateral anteroposterior and lateral radiographs of knee joint; (**i**) Stiff Feet

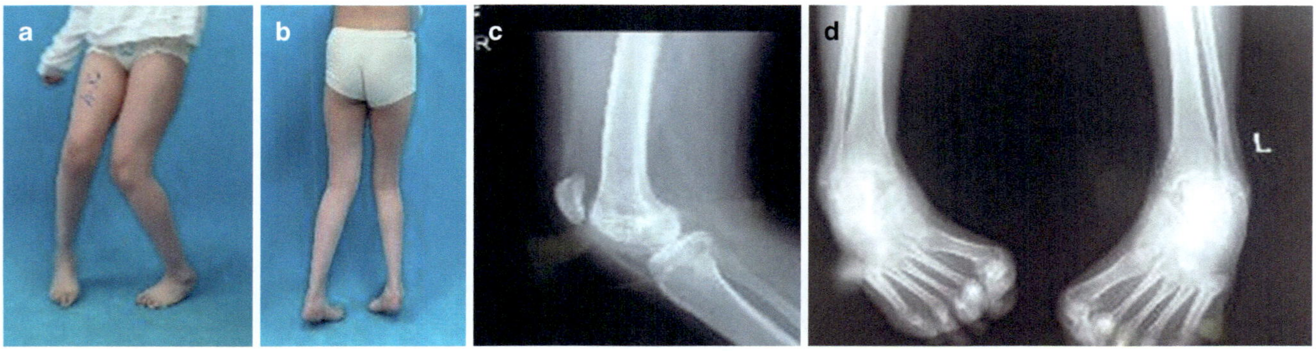

Fig. 8.5 Bilateral knee flexion and horseshoe deformity in mixed cerebral palsy. (**a**) Front view of both lower limbs; (**b**) Posterior view of both lower extremities; (**c**) Knee X-ray: knee flexion, patella alta; (**d**) Bipedal varus

Fig. 8.6 Quadriplegia. (**a**) Positive view in standing position; (**b**) In the standing lateral view, the extremities are involved, with bilateral hip and knee flexion

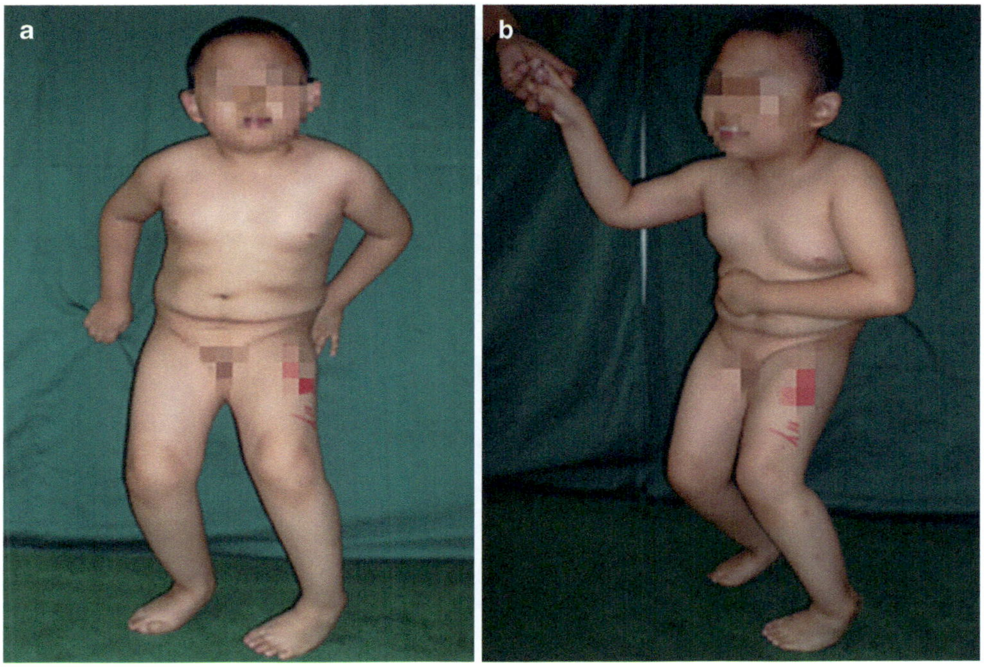

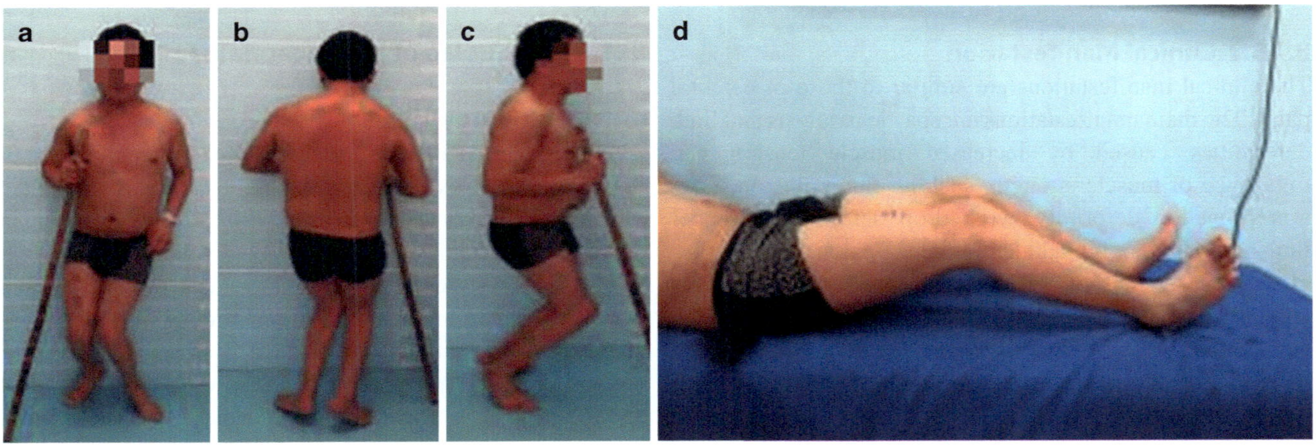

Fig. 8.7 Diplegia, limbs involved, lower limbs heavier than upper limbs, bilateral knee flexion. (**a**) Positive view; (**b**) Rear view; (**c**) Side view; (**d**) Supine position, lateral view of lower extremity

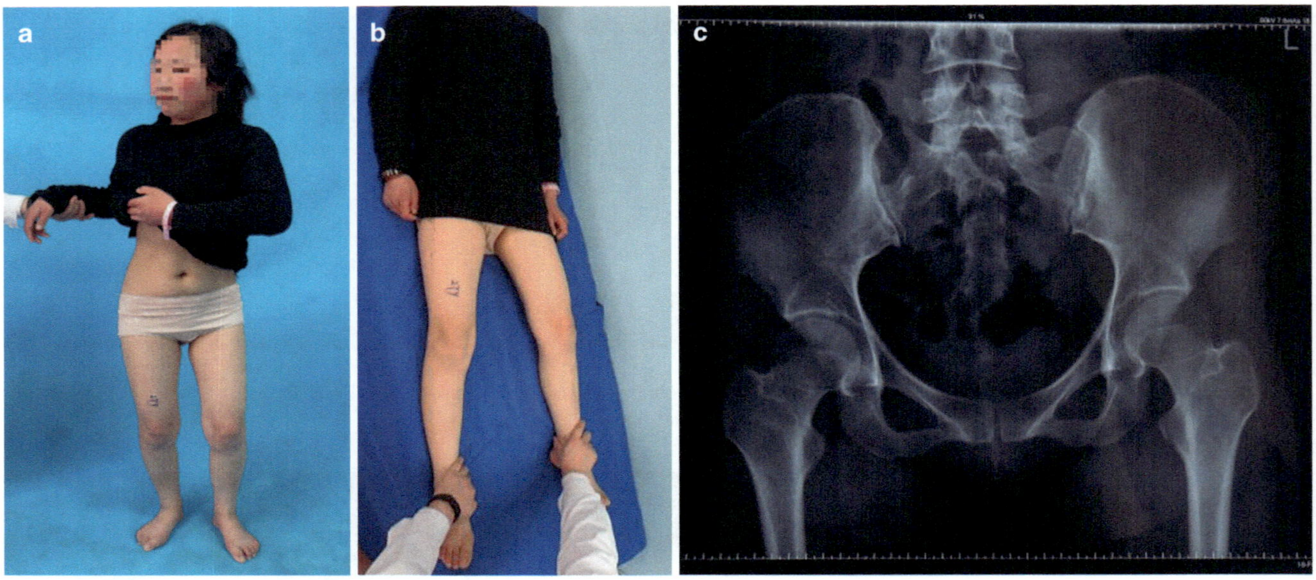

Fig. 8.8 Paraplegia, simple spastic paralysis of both lower limbs. (**a**) Front view, simple spastic paralysis of both lower extremities; (**b**) In the supine position, the full length of both lower limbs is viewed from the front, and both lower limbs are adducted. (**c**) X-ray plain film of pelvis

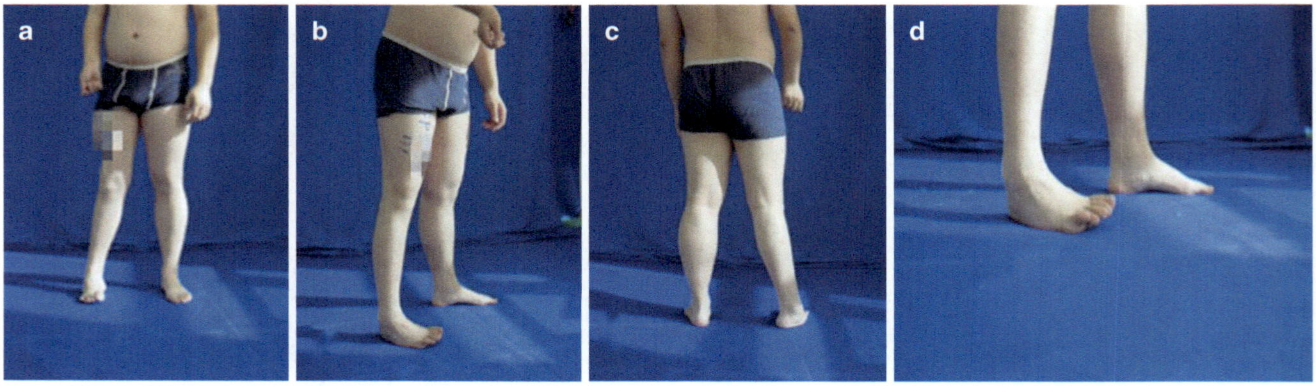

Fig. 8.9 Triplegia. (**a**) Full length frontal view of lower limbs, paralysis of both lower limbs and left upper limb, right foot varus deformity; (**b**) Full-length lateral view of the lower limb; (**c**) Posterior view of the whole length of lower limbs; (**d**) Lateral view of both feet, right foot varus

8.1.3.2 Clinical Manifestation

The clinical manifestations are similar to those of cerebral palsy. The main manifestations are spastic paralysis and limb deformities caused by increased muscle tension and imbalance of muscle strength, such as elbow flexion, forearm pronation deformity, wrist drop deformity of upper limbs, hip flexion, hip adduction, knee flexion, talipes equinus varus or flatfoot valgus deformity of lower limbs (Fig. 8.16).

8.1.3.3 Treatment Principle

(1) Correction of fixed deformity of limbs. (2) Moderate reduction of muscle tension. (3) Balance muscle strength and improve gait.

8.1.4 Sequelae of Hydrocephalus

8.1.4.1 Etiology

Hydrocephalus is a kind of disease caused by brain disease or trauma, which leads to excessive secretion of cerebrospinal fluid or (and) circulatory obstruction and malabsorption, resulting in increased intracranial cerebrospinal fluid volume, enlargement of ventricular system or (and) enlargement of subarachnoid space, secondary to compression and atrophy of brain parenchyma. The severity of neurological dysfunction caused by hydrocephalus is positively correlated with the severity of hydrocephalus. Severe cranial nerve damage affects the motor center, causing spastic paralysis of limbs, increased muscle tension, unbalanced muscle strength, and gradually secondary limb deformities.

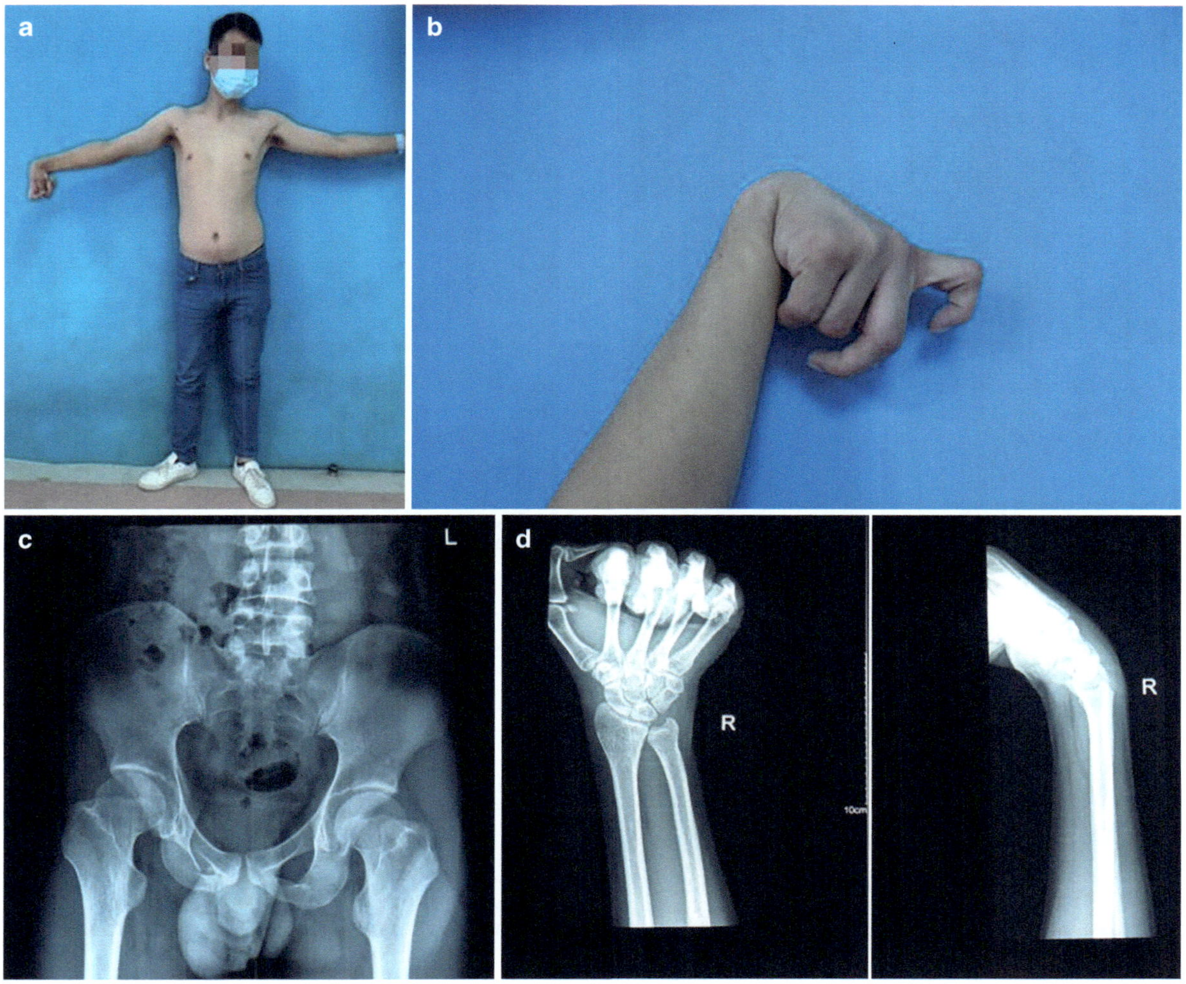

Fig. 8.10 Hemiplegia, right limb spastic paralysis. (**a**) Front view of the whole body, right limb spastic paralysis, right upper limb is the most serious; (**b**) Local view of the right hand, flexion of the wrist and fingers; (**c**) X-ray plain film of pelvis; (**d**) Anteroposterior and lateral film of right wrist joint, flexion deformity of wrist

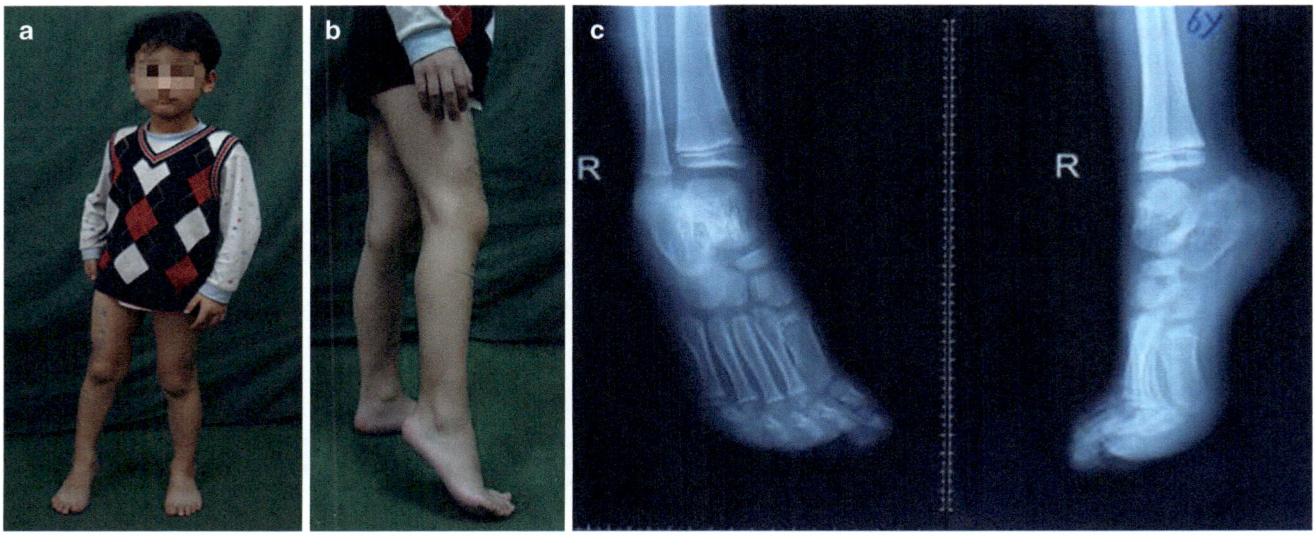

Fig. 8.11 Monoplegia. (**a**) Front view of both lower extremities, right lower extremity involved; (**b**) From the side view of both lower limbs, the right foot showed horseshoe change. (**c**) Anteroposterior and lateral X-ray film of right ankle joint, change of right talipes equinus

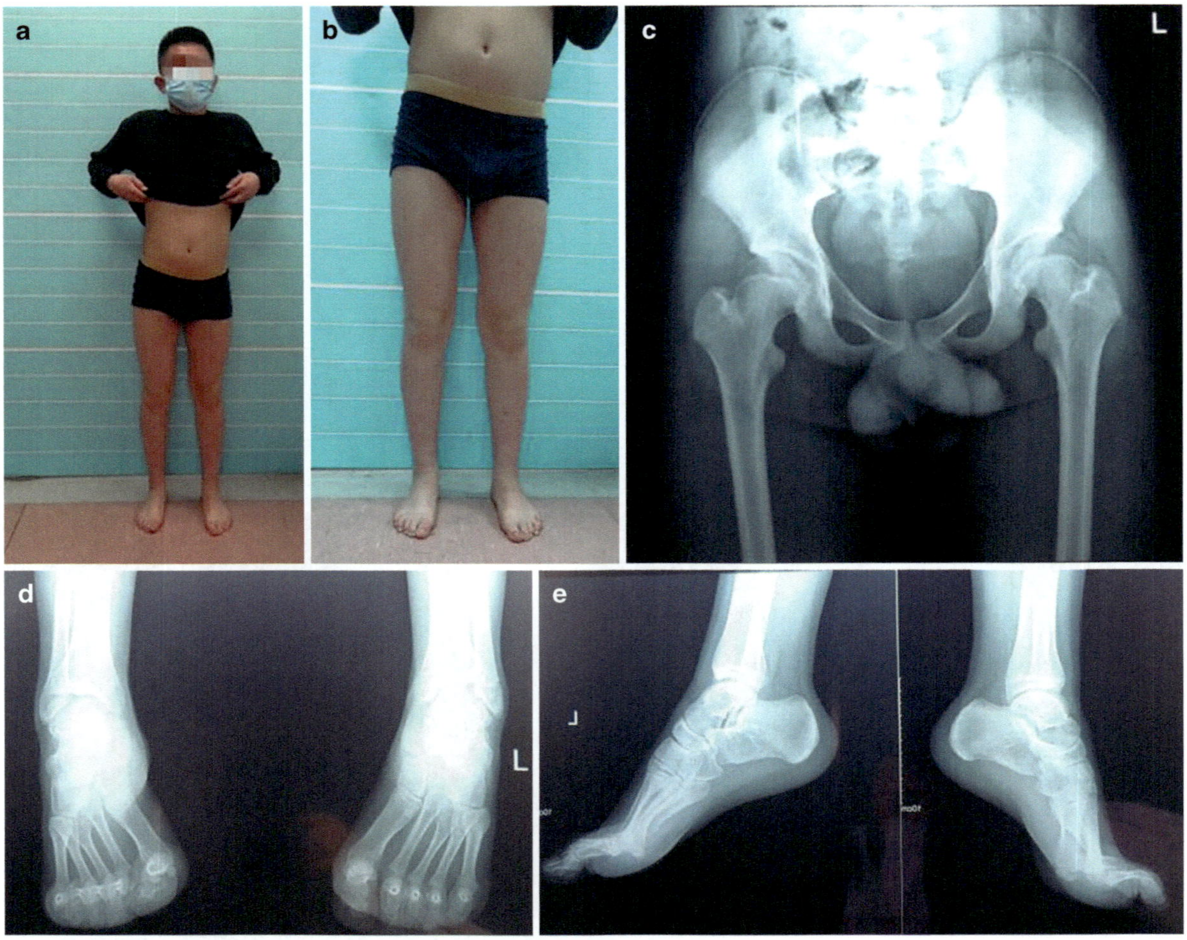

Fig. 8.12 Double hemiplegia (mild). (**a**) Full-body frontal view; (**b**) Full length frontal view of both lower extremities, no obvious deformity; (**c**) X-ray of pelvis; (**d**, **e**), anteroposterior and lateral X-ray of ankle joints of both feet, mild varus deformation

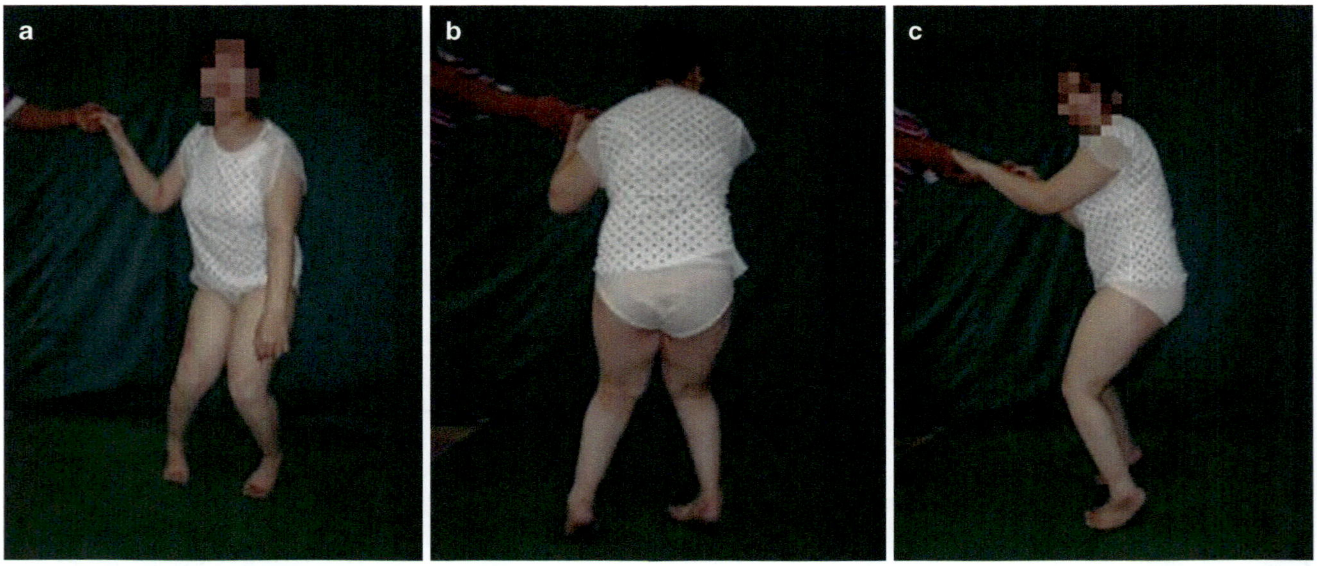

Fig. 8.13 Double hemiplegia (moderate). (**a**) Whole body frontal view, bilateral hip and knee flexion deformity; (**b**) Back view of the whole body, bilateral knee flexion, horseshoe foot deformation; (**c**) Whole body profile view

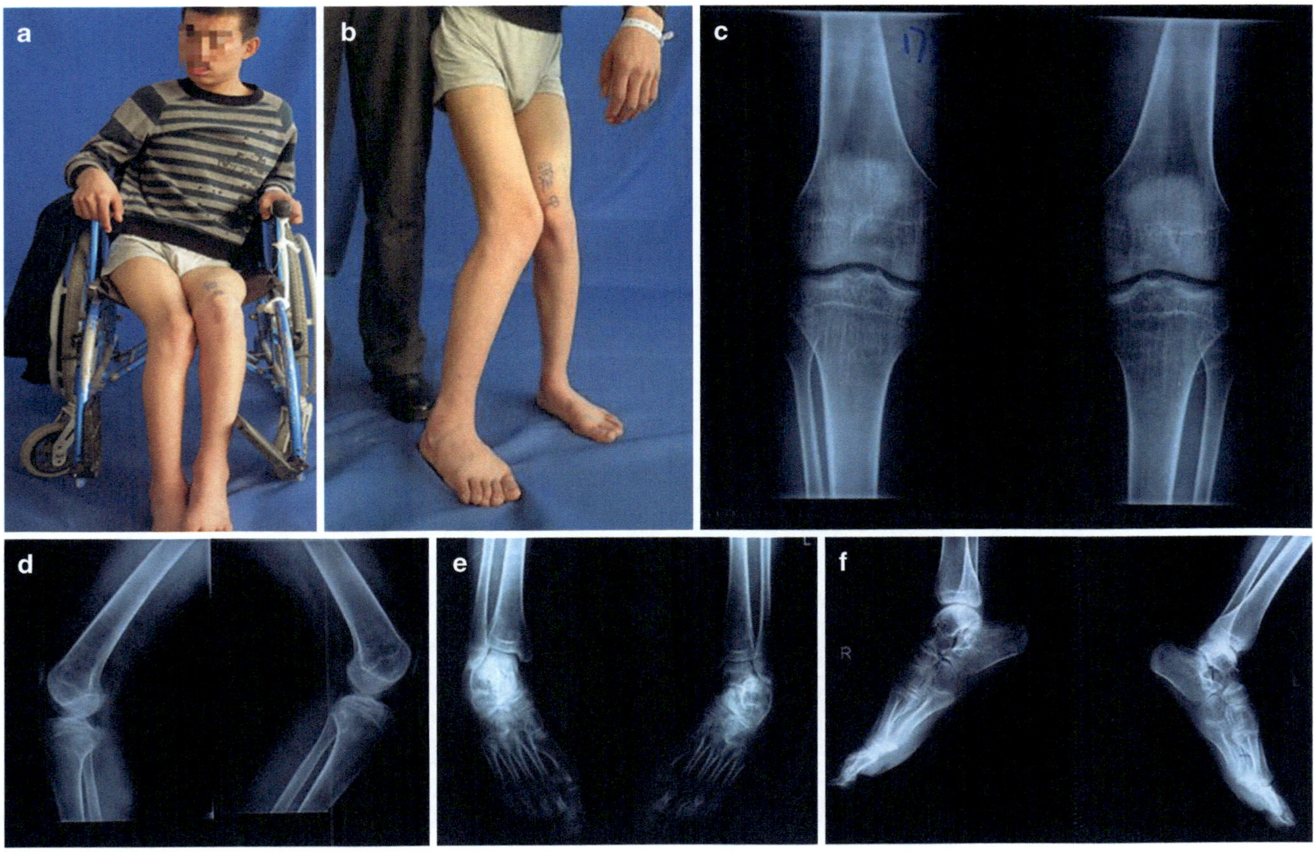

Fig. 8.14 Double hemiplegia (severe). (**a**) Limb deformity, wheelchair mobility; (**b**) Need a chaperone to help you stand; (**c**, **d**). Bilateral antero-posterior and lateral radiographs of knee joints; (**e**, **f**). Anteroposterior and lateral radiographs of bilateral ankle joint

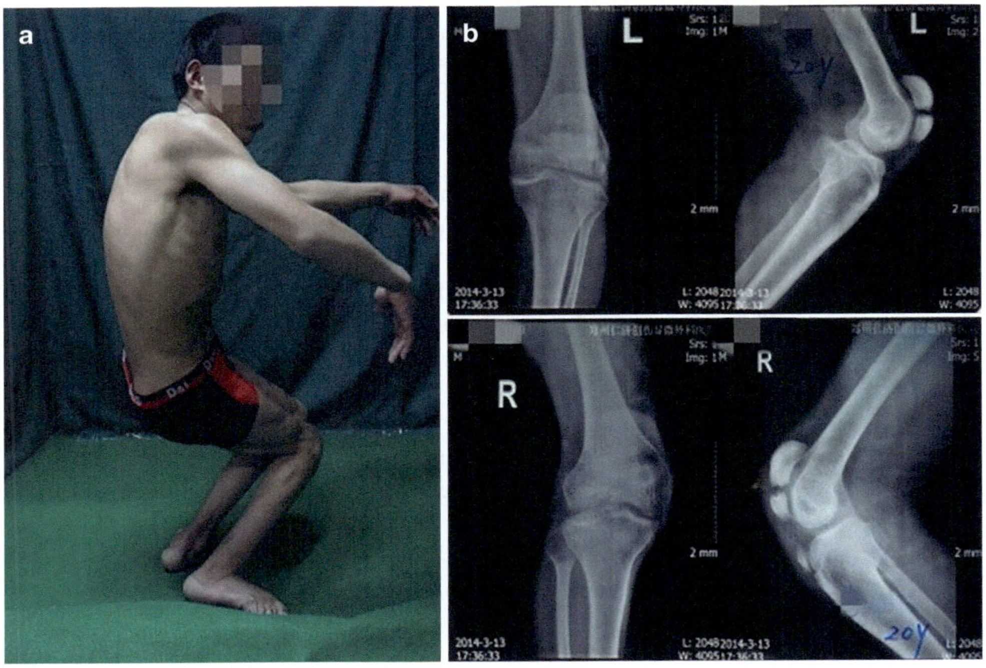

Fig. 8.15 Male, 20 years old, with spastic severe knee flexion deformity, sitting and walking. X-ray examination showed bilateral patellar high position with fatigue fracture separation, and right tibial tubercle showed bone fragment separation. Heterotopic ossification of patellar ligament was found in the left knee joint

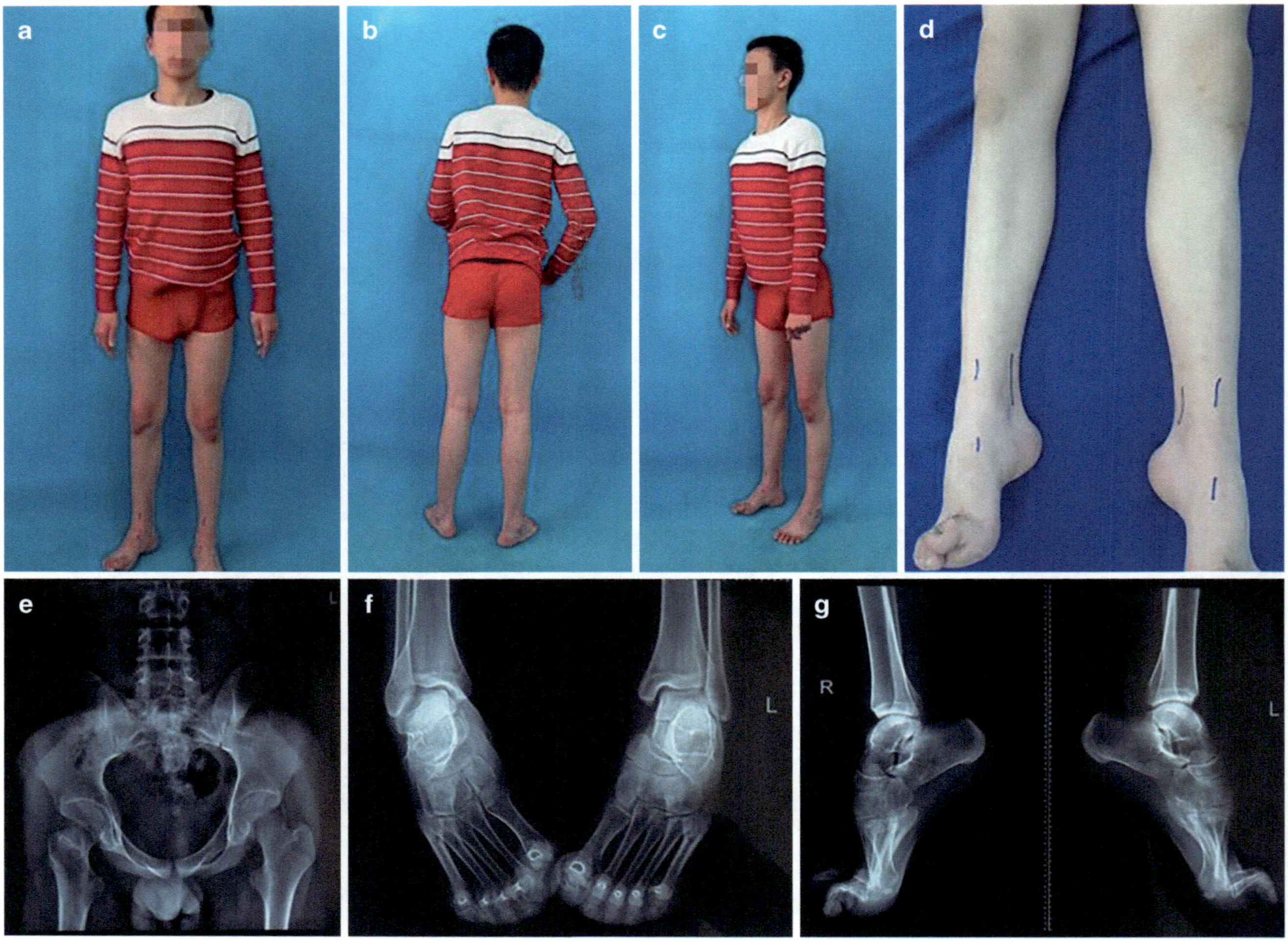

Fig. 8.16 Sequelae of encephalitis. (**a**) The clinical manifestations were similar to those of cerebral palsy, mainly spastic paralysis; (**b**) Full-length posterior view of lower limbs; (**c**) Lateral view of the whole length of the lower limb; (**d**) Bilateral talipes equinovarus, preoperative plan; (**e**) X-ray of pelvis; (**f**, **g**). Anteroposterior and lateral radiographs of bilateral ankle joint

8.1.4.2 Clinical Manifestation

In patients with hydrocephalus, the circumference of the head is increased, the reaction is often slow, the muscle tension of the lower limbs is increased, the abduction of the hip joint is limited, the deformity of the foot is horseshoe inversion or eversion, and tendon hyperreflexia and spastic paralysis may occur (Fig. 8.17).

8.1.4.3 Treatment Principle

(1) Cerebrospinal fluid shunt should be performed as early as possible. (2) Secondary fixed limb deformities were treated with orthopedic surgery.

8.1.5 Sequelae of Stroke

8.1.5.1 Etiology

Stroke (cerebral apoplexy) is a group of cerebral ischemia and hemorrhagic injury symptoms as the main clinical manifestations of the disease, also known as "stroke" or "cerebrovascular accident," with a very high. When brain injury affects the motor center, hemiplegia will occur, the muscle tension of the affected limbs will increase, the muscle strength will be unbalanced, and the secondary deformity will gradually occur, which is more common in talipes equinovarus.

8.1.5.2 Clinical Manifestation

The main manifestations are increased Muscle tension, tendon hyperreflexia, present Pathological reflex, Spastic paralysis. The main manifestations of the lower limbs were adduction and internal rotation of the affected limbs and talipes equinovarus deformity of the foot (Fig. 8.18). If the patient bears weight with abnormal stress in the condition of foot deformity, the progression of deformity will be accelerated.

8.1.5.3 Treatment Principle

(1) In the acute stage, brain injury was mainly treated to protect brain cells and reduce the degree of brain damage as much as possible. (2) Early rehabilitation intervention to reduce the degree of limb dysfunction. (3) When deformity

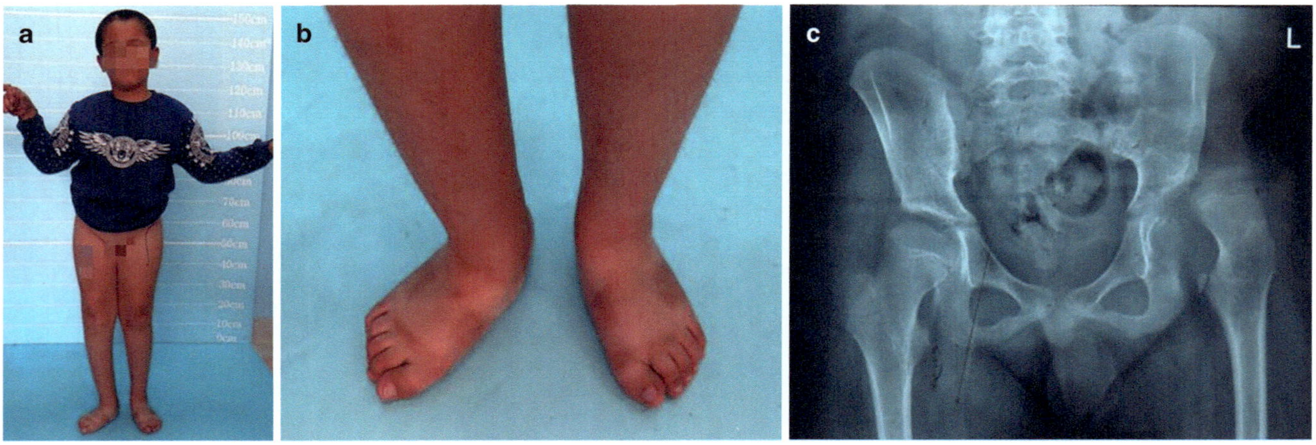

Fig. 8.17 Sequelae of hydrocephalus. (**a**) Full length frontal view of both lower extremities, the patient has undergone craniocerebral surgery; (**b**) Partial frontal view of both feet, bilateral flatfoot valgus; (**c**) X radiograph showing pelvic obliquity and dislocation of left hip

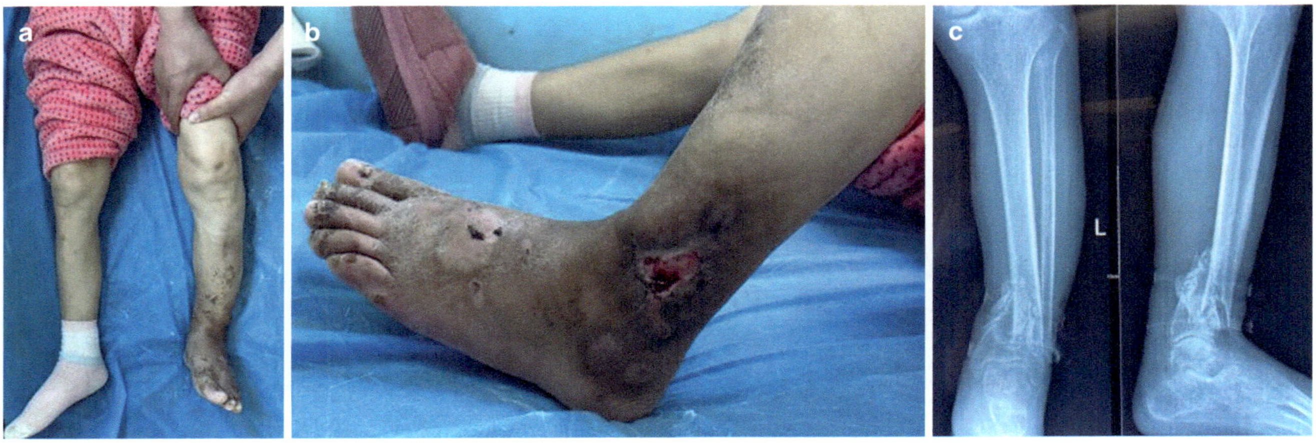

Fig. 8.18 Lower limb deformity after stroke and chronic osteomyelitis of tibia after trauma. (**a**) The left limbs were paralyzed after stroke, and the fracture of the distal end of the left tibia was not healed after falling. (**b**) Left leg distal sinus with bone exposure; (**c**) Ancient nonunion of left distal tibia with osteoporosis

of lower limbs, such as talipes equinovarus, occurs in the later stage, which affects walking and rehabilitation training, orthopedic surgery is feasible.

8.1.6 Sequelae of Hepatolenticular Degeneration

8.1.6.1 Etiology

Hepatolenticular degeneration (HLD) is an autosomal recessive inherited disorder of copper metabolism, which is characterized by liver cirrhosis and basal ganglia damage. When the basal ganglia of the brain is damaged, the extrapyramidal system will be damaged, and the muscle tension of the limbs will gradually increase, and the muscle strength will be out of balance. If not controlled in time, the bone and joint deformities of the limbs will gradually occur, and the multi-joint deformities of the lower limbs will gradually lose their walking function.

8.1.6.2 Clinical Manifestation

The Neurological symptoms are prominently manifested as extrapyramidal system damage, mainly choreiform movements, athetosis and dystonia, as well as facial oddity, dysphagia, dysarthria, bradykinesia and myotonia. Nervous system damage can be secondary to lower limb muscle spasm, contracture, and secondary deformity, affecting the motor function of patients. The main phenotypes affecting the lower limbs are the decrease and imbalance of muscle strength, the increase of muscle tension, knee flexion deformity, foot talipes equinovarus deformity, claw toe, and other manifestations (Fig. 8.19).

8.1.6.3 Treatment Principle

Control copper intake and promote copper excretion, correction of secondary limb deformities, reduce muscle tension, imbalance of muscle strength, if secondary bone and joint deformities, the implementation of orthopedic surgery to correct.

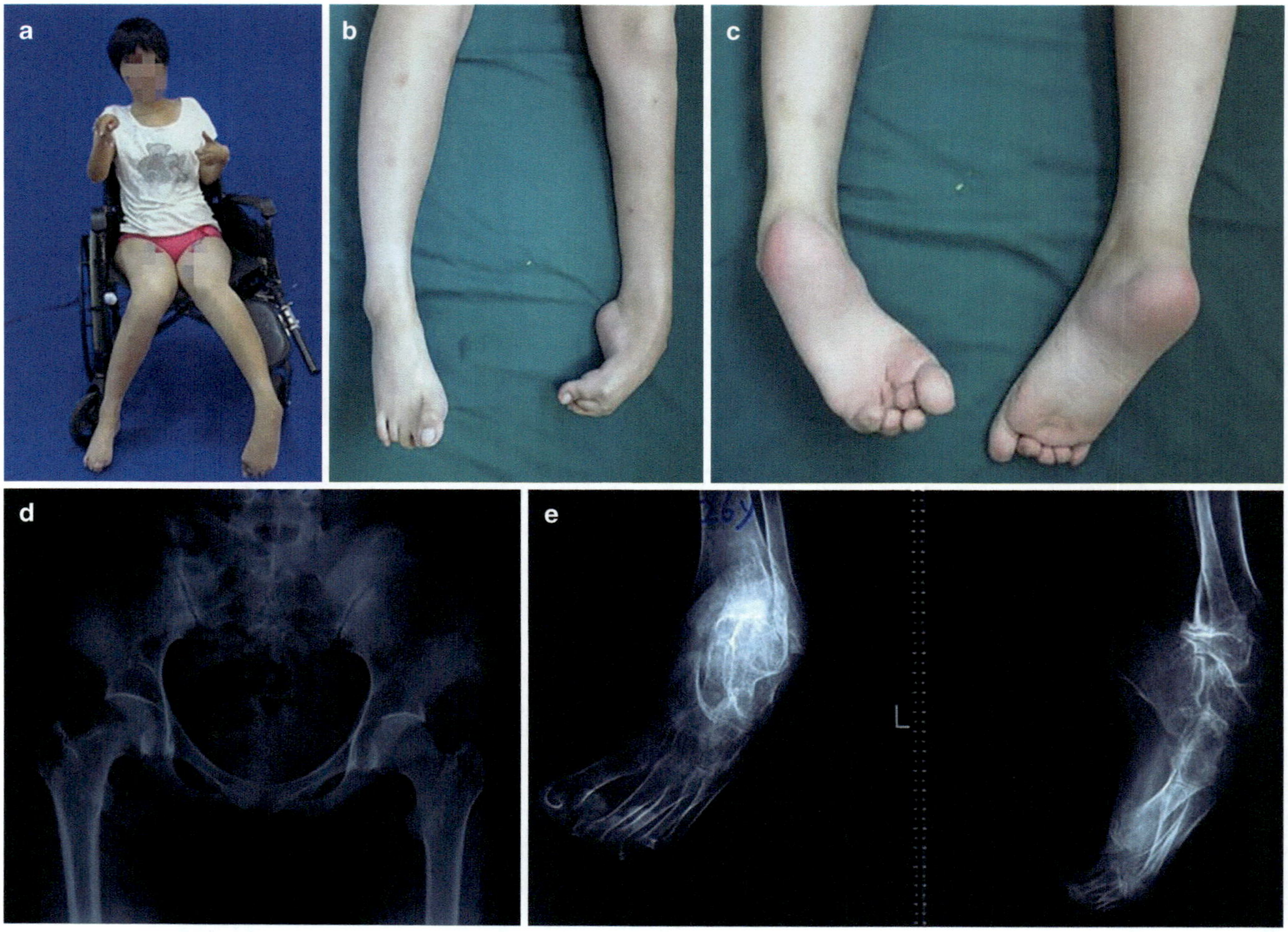

Fig. 8.19 Sequelae of hepatolenticular degeneration. (**a**) Patients with increased muscle tension of limbs, muscle spasm, wheelchair activities; (**b**, **c**) Bilateral clubfoot deformity; The toes are claw-shaped; (**d**) X-ray of pelvis; E. Anteroposterior and lateral radiographs of left ankle joint

8.1.7 Sequelae of Parkinson's Disease

8.1.7.1 Etiology

Parkinson's disease (Parkinson's disease, PD) is a common neurodegenerative disease. Its main pathological change is the degeneration and death of dopaminergic neurons in the substantia nigra of the midbrain, which leads to the significant decrease of dopamine in the striatum. Parkinson's disease generally progresses slowly, and very few patients may have secondary deformity of lower limbs in the later stage, which is common in talipes equinovarus.

8.1.7.2 Clinical Manifestation

Clinical manifestations mainly include resting tremor, bradykinesia, myotonia, and postural gait disorders, while patients may be accompanied by non-motor symptoms such as depression, constipation, and sleep disorders. Due to persistent muscle tremor and myotonia, some patients may suffer from ankle deformity and unstable standing and walking due to dynamic imbalance. Abnormal stress loading in the deformity state aggravates the deformity progress (Fig. 8.20).

8.1.7.3 Treatment Principle

(1) Control tremor symptoms with drugs; (2) Secondary talipes equinovarus deformity was treated with orthopedic surgery. (3) Orthopedic surgery is based on the principle of balancing muscle strength, correcting deformity, stabilizing foot and ankle joints, and improving walking function of patients.

8.1.8 Sequelae of Subarachnoid Hemorrhage

8.1.8.1 Etiology

Subarachnoid hemorrhage (SAH) is a clinical syndrome caused by the rupture of diseased blood vessels at the base or surface of the brain and the direct flow of blood into the subarachnoid space. The common causes were: (1) intracranial aneurysm; (2) Cerebral vascular malformation; (3) Abnormal vascular network disease at the base of brain; (4) Others: dissecting aneurysm, vasculitis, thrombosis of intracranial venous system, connective tissue disease, hematological disease, intracranial tumor, coagulation disorder, complications of anticoagulant therapy, etc.

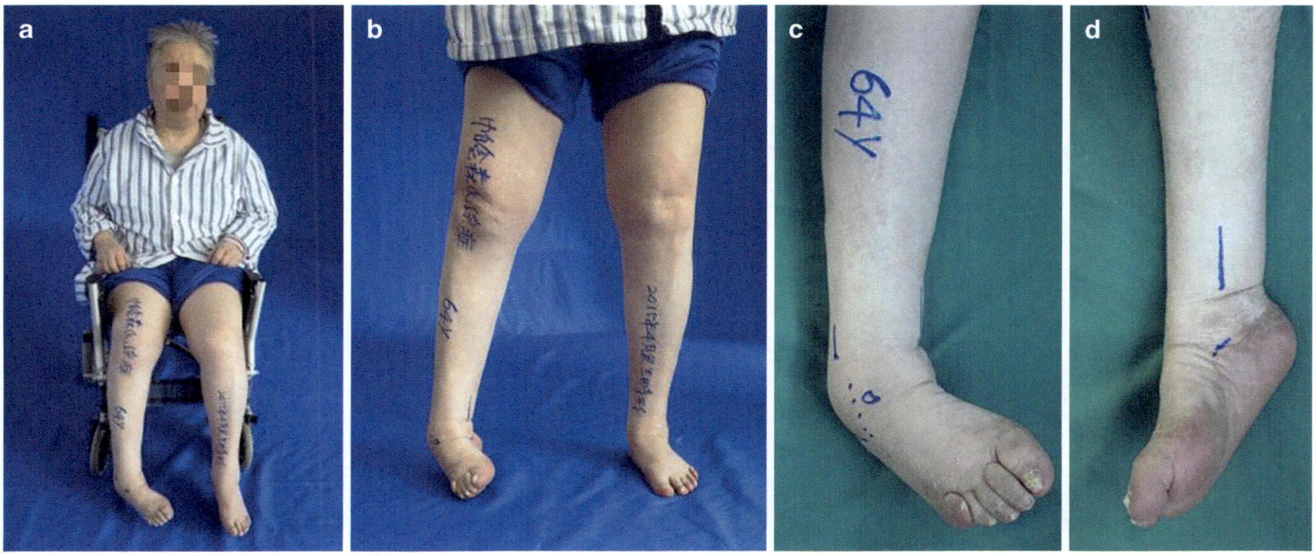

Fig. 8.20 Lower limb deformity after Parkinson's disease. (**a**) The right foot varus deformity was caused by continuous muscle tremor and myotonia in wheelchair; (**b**) Positive view in standing position; (**c**, **d**). Preoperative planning

8.1.8.2 Clinical Manifestation

The typical clinical manifestations in the acute phase are sudden onset of severe headache, nausea, vomiting, and meningeal irritation, with or without focal signs. If the treatment of subarachnoid hemorrhage is delayed or improper, it will cause central nervous system injury, which may lead to spastic paralysis of limbs, and gradually lead to bone and joint deformity of limbs (Fig. 8.21).

8.1.8.3 Treatment Principle

(1) Treatment of primary diseases in acute stage, protection of nerves and prevention of central nervous system nerve injury; (2) Secondary limb deformities can be corrected by soft tissue release, tendon transfer, and osteotomy to improve gait.

8.1.9 Limb Deformity Caused by Epilepsy

8.1.9.1 Etiology

Epilepsy, commonly known as "Epilepsy" or "Epilepsy," is a chronic disease of sudden abnormal discharge of neurons in the brain, leading to transient brain dysfunction.

8.1.9.2 Clinical Manifestation

Seizures are divided into partial/focal seizures, generalized seizures, and unclassifiable seizures. Long-term uncontrolled epilepsy can easily lead to limb deformities, mainly manifested as adduction and internal rotation deformity of lower limbs, valgus deformity of knee joint, talipes equinovarus deformity of foot, fixed deformity or bony changes in the long course of disease, foot valgus deformity in a few patients, and instability in standing and walking in severe cases (Fig. 8.22).

8.1.9.3 Treatment Principle

(1) At present, the main purpose of epilepsy treatment is to reduce seizures. (2) Secondary limb deformities were corrected by soft tissue release, tendon displacement, and osteotomy.

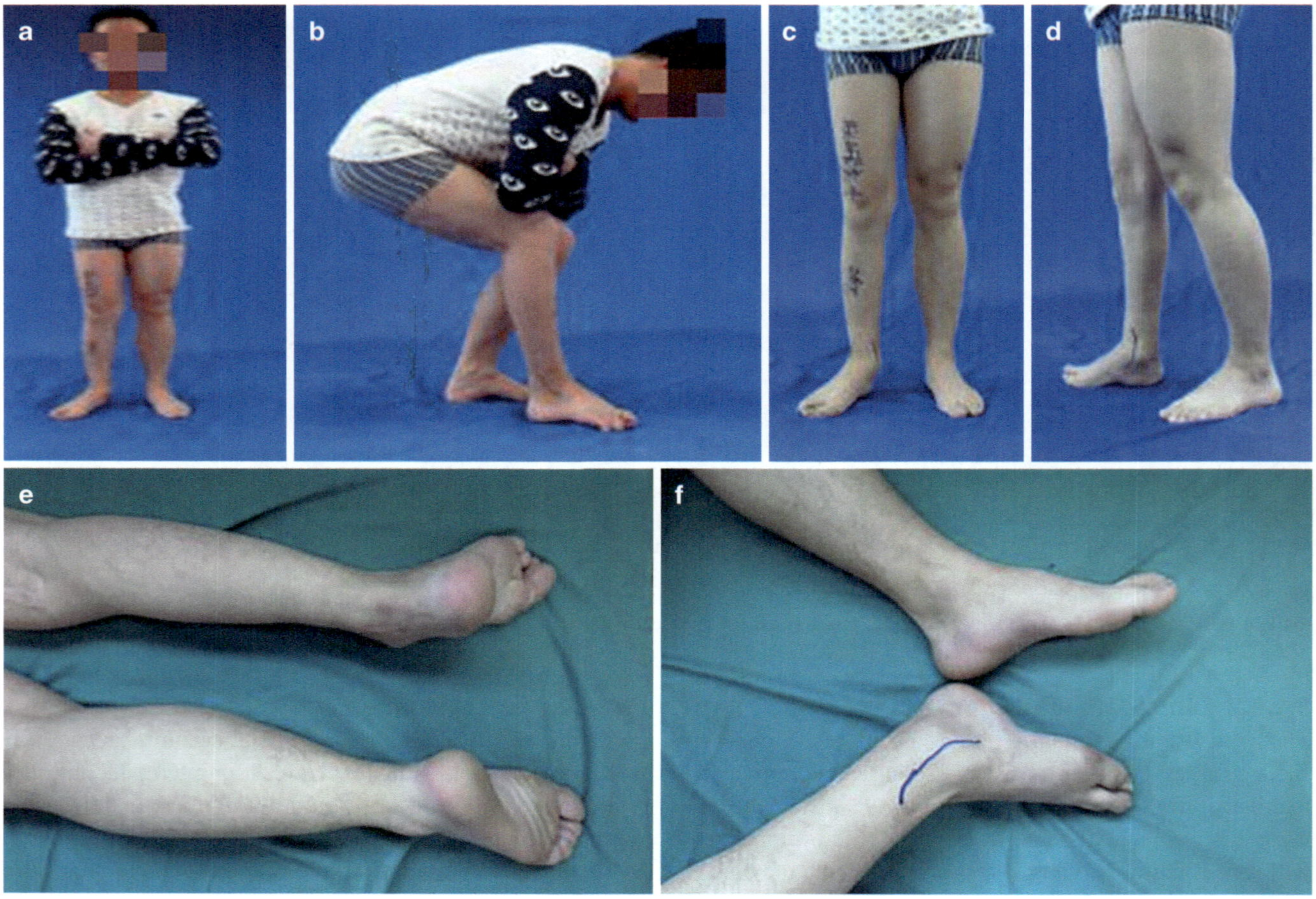

Fig. 8.21 Right lower limb deformity after subarachnoid hemorrhage. (**a**) Full length frontal view of both lower extremities; (**b**) Spasm of both lower limbs, unable to walk upright; (**c**) Full length partial frontal view of both lower extremities; (**d**) Local profile view of the whole length of both lower limbs; (**e**) In the prone position, the back view of the whole length of both lower limbs; (**f**) Partial profile view of both feet and preoperative plan of operation

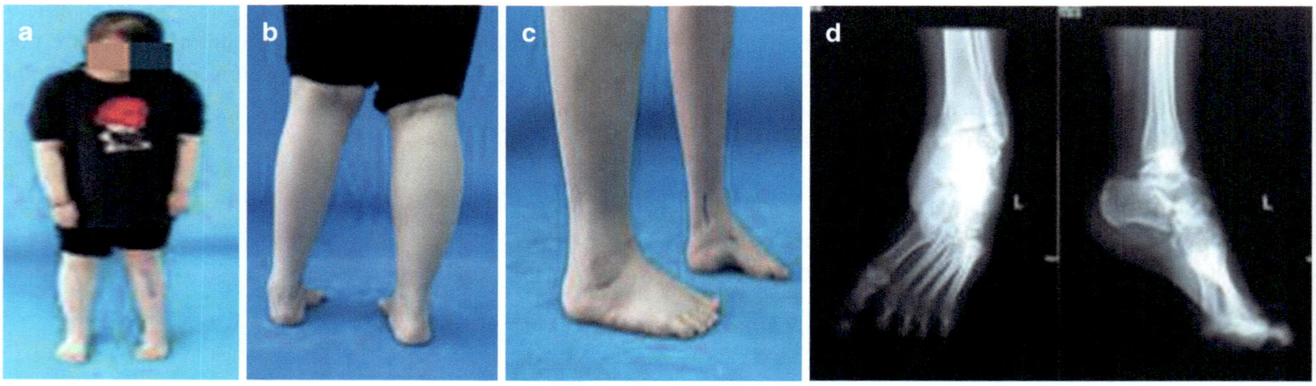

Fig. 8.22 Left foot deformity after long-term epilepsy, left lower limb adduction and internal rotation deformity, knee valgus, and high arch varus deformity. (**a**) Full length frontal view of both lower extremities; (**b**) Full-length posterior view of both lower extremities; (**c**) Partial profile view of both feet; X-ray film of (**d**). X: left foot varus

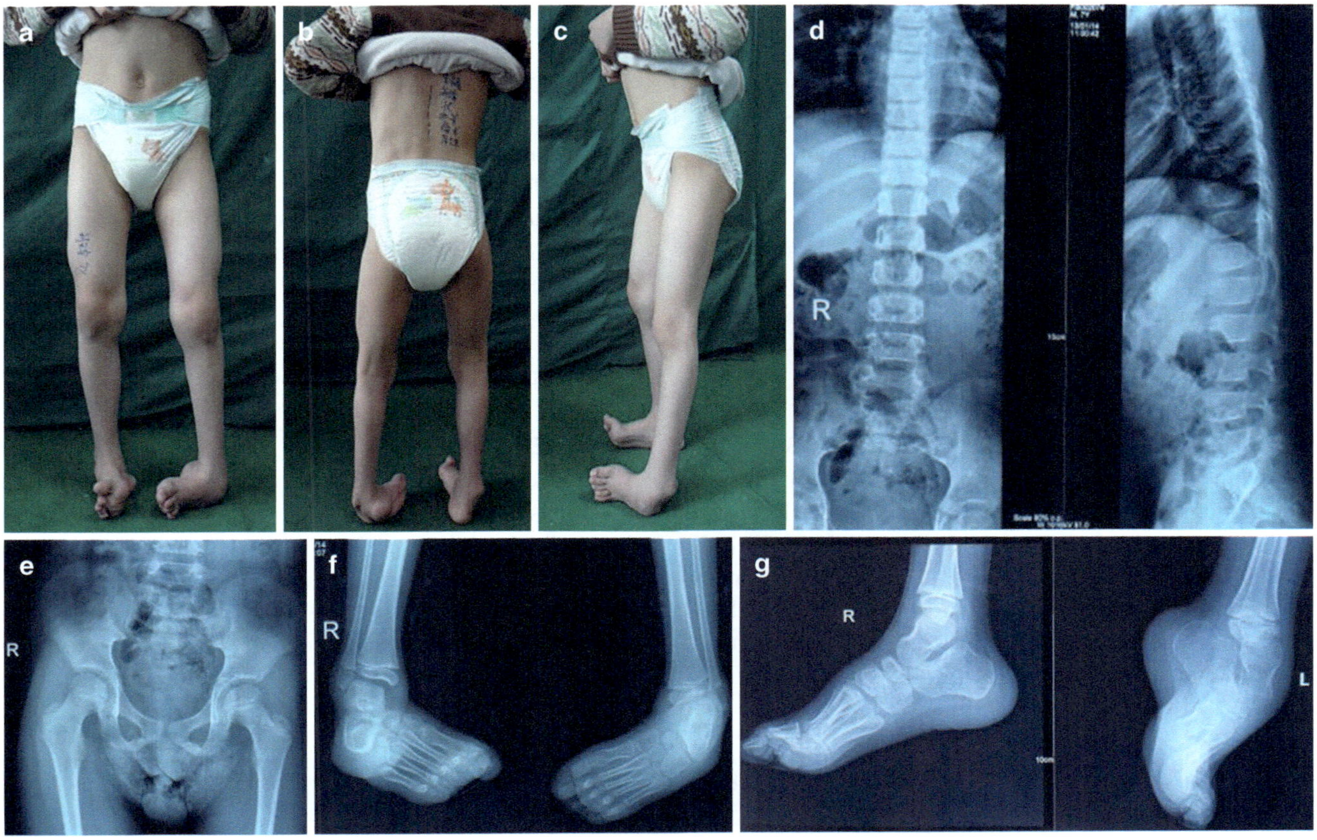

Fig. 8.23 Deformity of both lower limbs after thoracolumbar cavernous hemangioma. (**a**) Frontal view of the full length of both lower limbs, bilateral knee flexion, talipes equinovarus deformity. (**b**) Full-length posterior view of both lower extremities; (**c**) Left side view of the whole length of both lower limbs; (**d**) Full-length anteroposterior and lateral radiographs of the spine; (**e**) X-ray of pelvis; (**f, g**) Anteroposterior and lateral radiographs of bilateral ankle joint

8.2 Spinal Cord Disease

8.2.1 Spinal Cavernous Hemangioma Secondary to Lower Limb Deformity

8.2.1.1 Etiology

Spinal cavernous hemangioma (spinal cavernous hemangioma) is one of the occult vascular malformations of the spinal cord, accounting for 5–12% of vascular diseases of the spinal cord, which can occur in different parts of the spinal cord. Its origin and mechanism are congenital, non-angiomatous dysplasia of spinal cord blood vessels. According to its location, it can be divided into intramedullary type, intradural extramedullary type, extradural type, and vertebral type, among which intramedullary type is the most common and has the greatest impact on the nervous system. Secondary deformities of the lower extremities are often associated with subarachnoid hemorrhage. Neurological dysfunction causes muscle imbalance of lower limbs and secondary limb deformities.

8.2.1.2 Clinical Manifestation

The main symptoms are related to spinal cord nerve center injury, such as sensory and motor dysfunction of lower limbs, increased muscle tension, hyperreflexia of tendons, and unbalanced reduction of muscle strength, resulting in secondary foot and ankle deformities, which are gradually aggravated (Fig. 8.23).

8.2.1.3 Treatment Principle

1. Treatment of primary disease: Resection of spinal cord hemangioma and relief of spinal cord compression.
2. Correct the deformity of foot and ankle and improve the function of foot and ankle.

8.2.2 Sequelae of Spina Bifida

8.2.2.1 Etiology

Spina bifida (spina bifida) is the most common congenital defect of neural tube development. The core pathological change is tethered spinal cord, which leads to the spinal cord being pulled, compressed, and fixed, unable to rise and move with the growth of the spine, and then produces spinal cord nerve damage syndrome, mainly including urinary and fecal disorders and incomplete paralysis of lower limbs.

8.2.2.2 Clinical Manifestation

Local bulging or excessive hair growth can be seen on the back (Fig. 8.24). Spina bifida occurs above the conus medullaris and causes spinal cord injury, which is mainly manifested as spastic paralysis below the level of injury. If spina bifida occurs below the conus medullaris, the main manifestations below the level of injury are flaccid paralysis and urinary and urinary disorders (Fig. 8.25). Because the nerve injury caused by spina bifida includes both motor nerve and sensory nerve, in addition to muscle strength decline or even paralysis, bone and joint deformity, it is often combined with sensory disorders, and secondary to neurotrophic ulcers in weight-bearing areas that do not heal for a long time, severe cases lead to osteomyelitis and spontaneous toe amputation (Fig. 8.26).

8.2.2.3 Treatment Principle

1. Spinal cord nerve tethered operation was released to relieve the traction of nerve root.
2. Correct the deformity of lower limbs, especially the deformity of foot and ankle, and restore the gravity line of lower limbs.
3. Pay attention to the prevention of complications, such as skin ulcer, osteomyelitis, urinary retention, hydronephrosis, uremia, etc.

8.2.3 Sequelae of Acute Myelitis

8.2.3.1 Etiology

Acute myelitis refers to the acute transverse myelitis caused by various autoimmune reactions (mostly induced by infection, individually by vaccination or iatrogenic causes), also known as acute transverse myelitis. The main pathological changes were swelling and loss of myelin sheath, significant proliferation of peripheral lymphocytes, axonal degeneration, and infiltration of perivascular inflammatory cells. Tho-

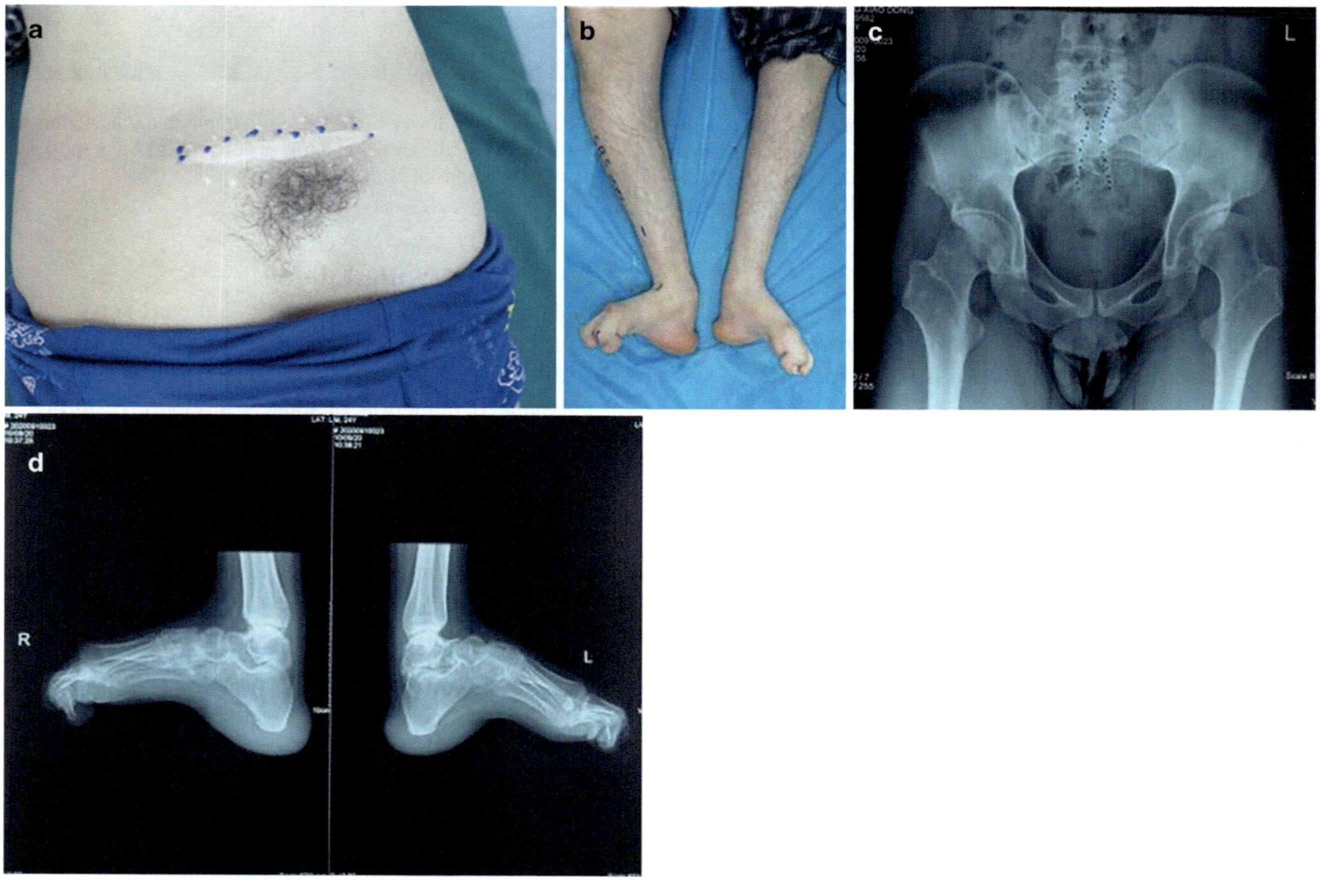

Fig. 8.24 Spina bifida sequelae. (**a**) Hair hyperplasia in the lumbosacral region, with previous lumbar tethered nerve release; (**b**) Bilateral severe calcaneus deformity; (**c**) Lumbosacral spina bifida was seen on pelvic X-ray. (**d**) Lateral radiographs of bilateral ankle joints, severe calcaneal deformity

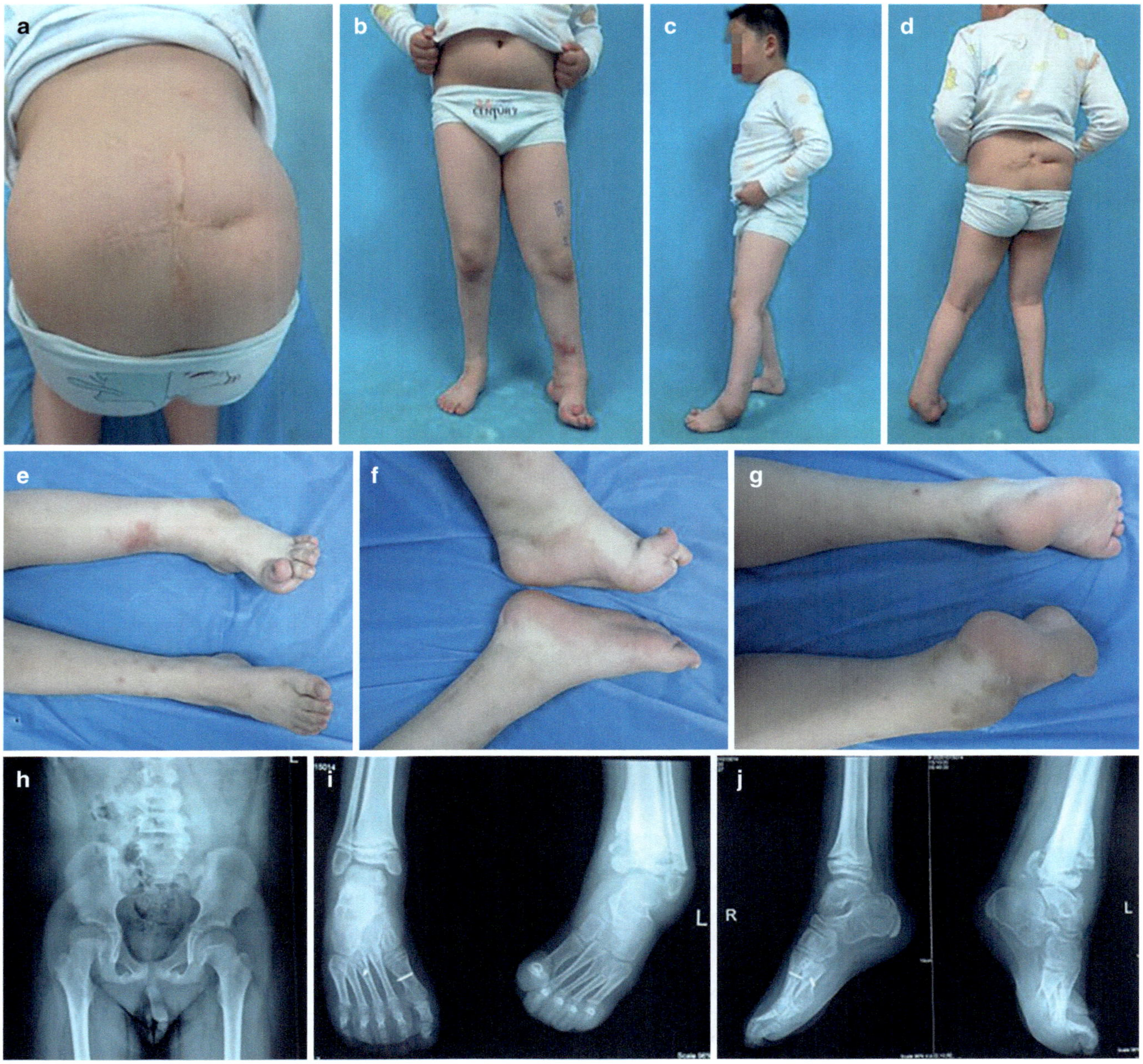

Fig. 8.25 Spina bifida with bilateral deformity. (**a**) Postoperative changes in the lumbodorsal region, local bulging; (**b**) Full-length frontal view of both lower extremities; (**c**) Full-length profile view of both lower extremities; (**d**) Full-length posterior view of both lower extremities; (**e–g**). Bipedal local view; (**h**) Lumbosacral spina bifida was seen on pelvic radiograph. (**i, j**) Right foot varus, left ankle Charcot joint

racic spinal cord was most frequently involved, and the clinical features were paralysis of the limbs below the lesion level, conduction bundle sensory disturbance, and defecation and urination disorders.

8.2.3.2 Clinical Manifestation

Acute myelitis is an acute onset, with low fever, nerve root pain at the lesion site, numbness and fatigue of the limbs, and band sensation at the lesion site. Dyskinesia below the level of involvement, loss of sensation, and dysfunction of bladder and rectal sphincter occur in most cases within a few hours or days. Dyskinesia is the manifestation of spinal cord shock in the early stage, which usually lasts for 2–4 weeks, with gradual increase of muscle tension and pathological reflex. In the later stage, because the degree of paralysis and recovery of the lower limb muscles are different, the muscle strength is unbalanced, and the lower limb deformity is gradually secondary, which is more common in knee flexion and talipes equinovarus, affecting the walking function (Fig. 8.27).

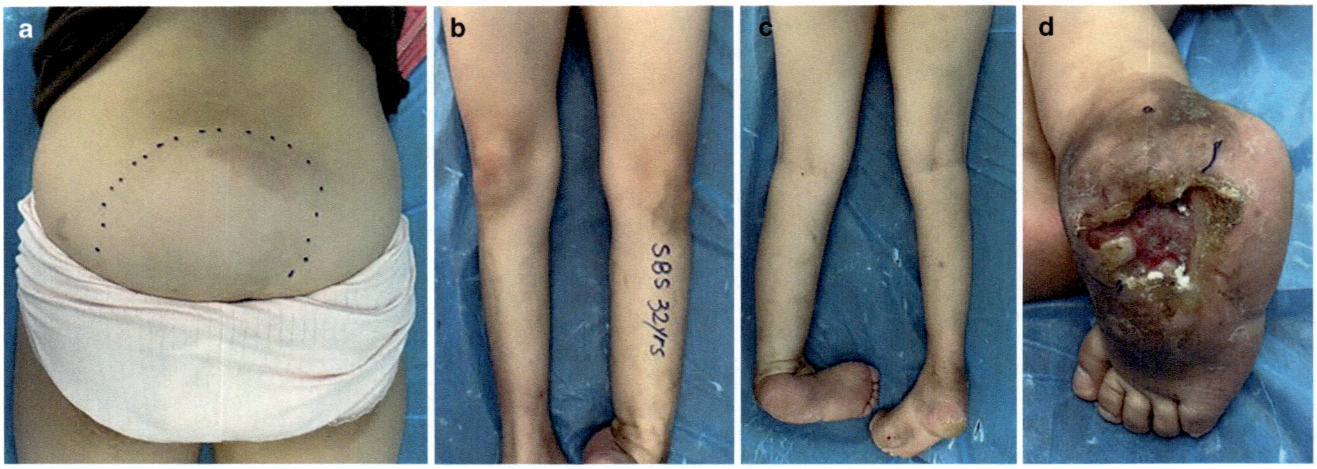

Fig. 8.26 Left foot deformity after spina bifida. (**a**) Local bulging of the lumbar and back; (**b**) Supine position, full-length frontal view of both lower limbs, left foot varus; (**c**) In the prone position, the full length of both lower limbs is viewed from the back, and the left foot is varus. (**d**) Local view of the left foot, the lateral malleolus ulcer has not healed for more than 20 years

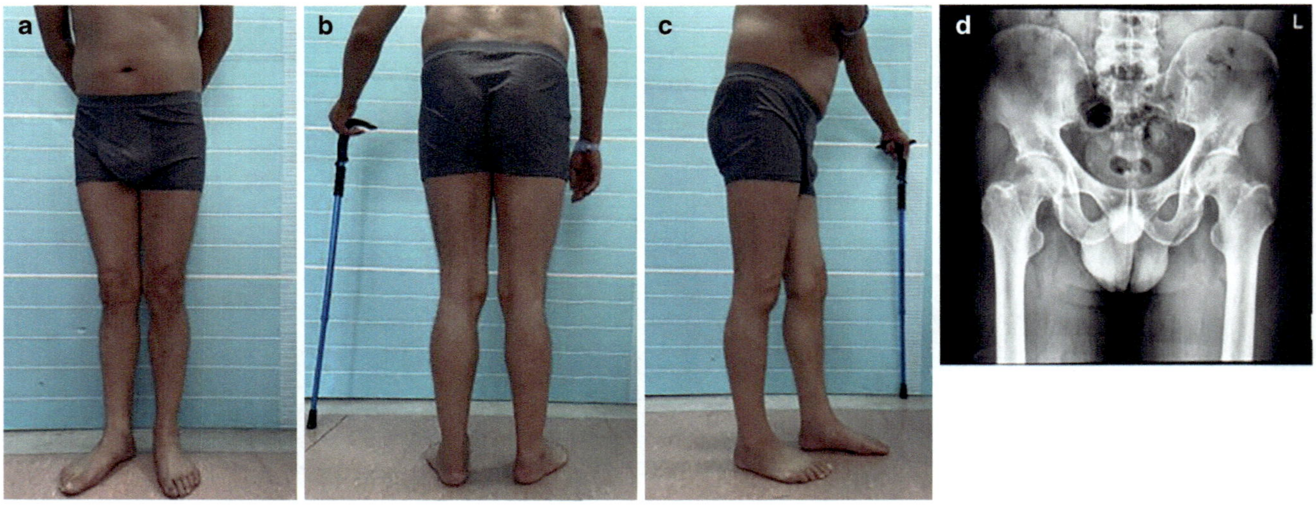

Fig. 8.27 Sequelae of acute myelitis: deformity of both lower limbs. (**a**) Full length frontal view of both lower limbs, spasticity of both lower limbs, need to walk with crutches; (**b**) Full-length posterior view of both lower extremities; (**c**) Full-length profile view of both lower limbs; (**d**) Pelvic plain film, bilateral hip adduction, internal rotation

8.2.3.3 Treatment Principle

In the sequelae stage, the treatment goal is to correct limb deformity, balance muscle strength, and improve walking function of patients.

8.2.4 Sequelae of Spinal Arachnoiditis

8.2.4.1 Etiology

There are many causes of spinal arachnoiditis, such as infection, spinal cord trauma, adjacent tissue lesions or foreign body stimulation, and non-specific infection, resulting in arachnoid thickening and spinal cord, spinal nerve root adhesion or cyst formation, resulting in spinal cord dysfunction caused by blocking the medullary cavity.

8.2.4.2 Clinical Manifestation

Most of them are chronic onset, slow progress, and acute or subacute onset. Because of the different parts involved, the clinical manifestations are diverse, there may be single or multiple nerve root pain, sensory disorders are mostly nerve root type, segmental type or patchy irregular distribution, bilateral asymmetry. Dyskinesia is asymmetric paraplegia, monoplegia or quadriplegia, with different degrees of limb muscle paralysis, imbalance of muscle strength, and gradual secondary deformity of lower limbs, affecting walking func-

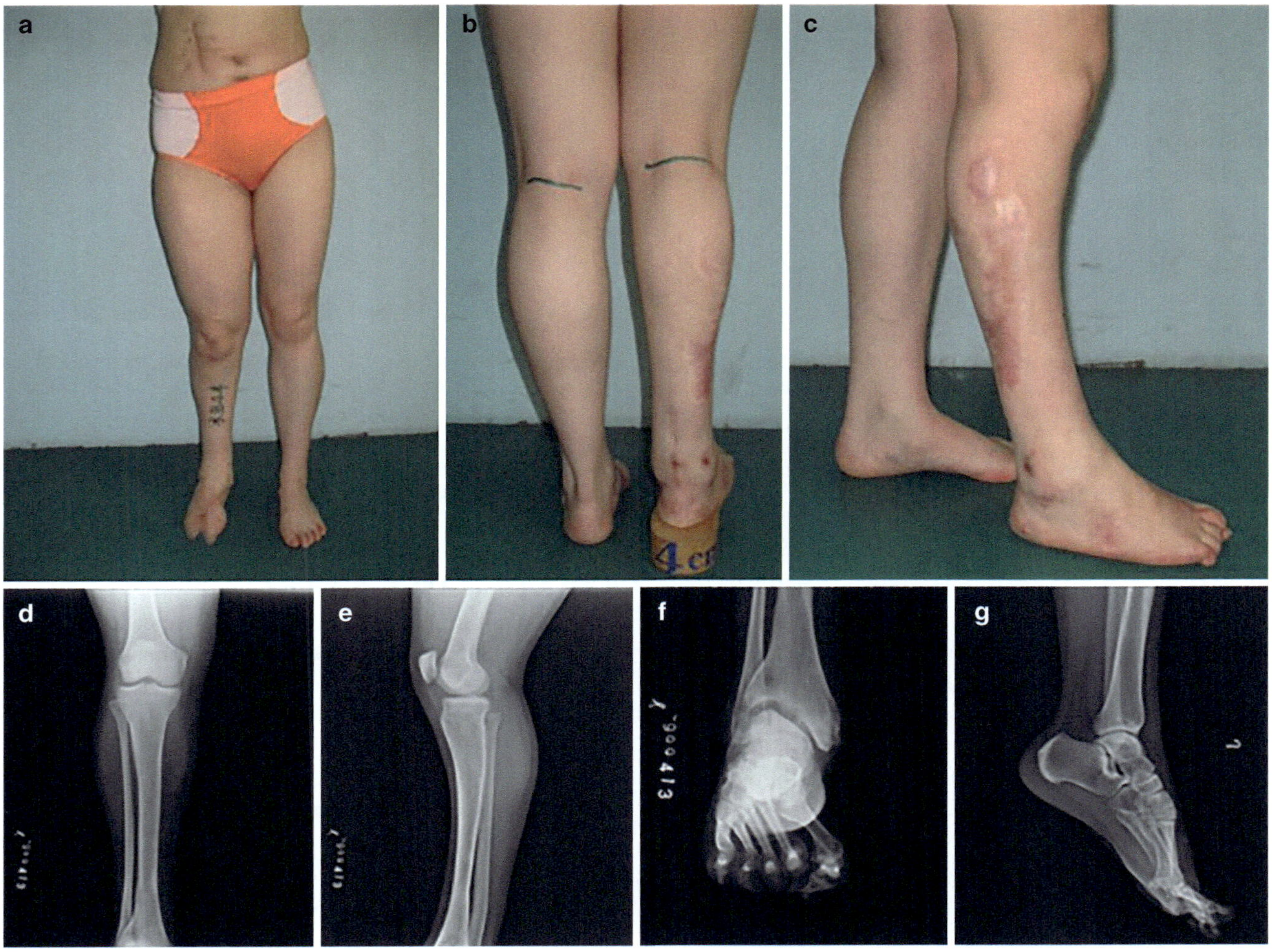

Fig. 8.28 Spinal arachnoiditis sequelae. Right lower limb deformity. (**a**) Full length frontal view of both lower extremities; (**b**) Back view of the whole length of both lower limbs, the right lower limb is shortened; (**c**) Full-length profile view of both lower extremities; (**d**, **e**) Anteroposterior and lateral radiographs of knee joint; (**f**, **g**) Ankle facet tilt

tion (Fig. 8.28); Sensory disturbances may be secondary to Charcot's arthropathy.

8.2.4.3 Treatment Principle

Patients with secondary limb paralysis and deformity were treated with orthopedic surgery to restore limb shape and improve walking function.

8.2.5 Sequelae of Spinal Cord Compression

8.2.5.1 Etiology

There are many causes of spinal cord compression, including: (1) Congenital diseases, such as spinal vascular malformation, syringomyelia, meningocele, etc. (2) Trauma: such as spinal fracture and dislocation, traumatic hematoma, etc. (3) Inflammation: such as spinal tuberculosis, epidural and subdural abscess, adhesive arachnoiditis, etc.; Tumors: including spinal cord, spine, adjacent tissues, and metastatic tumors. (4) Others: such as spinal cord parasitosis, spondyloarthropathy, and intervertebral disc herniation compress the thoracic spinal cord or thoracic nerve, resulting in neuromuscular dysfunction and limb deformity.

8.2.5.2 Clinical Manifestation

After the cause of spinal cord compression is relieved, the symptoms of nerve injury are left behind, such as sensory disturbance in the corresponding innervated area; after partial loss of muscle strength of the lower limbs, the deformity of the lower limbs is gradually secondary. The common deformity includes knee flexion and valgus deformity, foot horseshoe, varus and valgus deformity, and claw toe deformity (Fig. 8.29).

8.2.5.3 Treatment Principle

Correct the deformity of the lower limbs, restore the weight-bearing line of the lower limbs, correct the deformity of the ankle, balance the muscle strength, and increase the weight-bearing stability of the ankle.

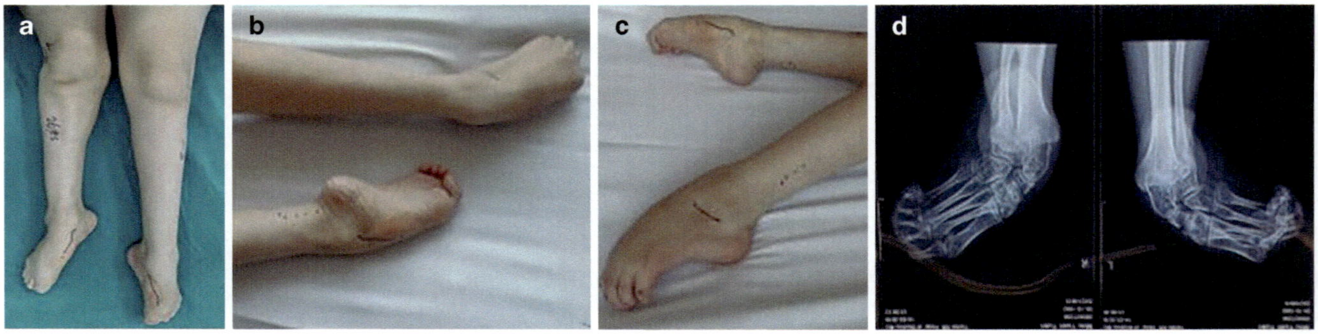

Fig. 8.29 Spastic paralysis of both lower limbs and talipes equinovarus caused by sequelae of thoracolumbar spinal cord tumor. (**a**) Supine position, frontal view of both lower extremities; (**b**) Supine position, local view of right foot; (**c**) Supine position, local view of left foot; X-ray film of (**d**). X showed talipes equinovarus on both sides

8.3 Peripheral Nerve Disease

8.3.1 Lumbar Disc Herniation

8.3.1.1 Etiology

Lumbar disc herniation is one of the most common spinal diseases in clinic. It is mainly because the nucleus pulposus and annulus fibrosus that make up the intervertebral disc, under the action of external factors, the annulus fibrosus ruptures and the nucleus pulposus protrudes, stimulating the nerve roots, resulting in decreased sensation in the innervated area of the nerve, decreased muscle strength, and even paralysis.

8.3.1.2 Clinical Manifestation

The corresponding segment of the corresponding innervated area is hypoesthesia, and the muscle strength of the innervated muscle is reduced, or even completely paralyzed. If not treated in time, the compression will be relieved, resulting in permanent injury, which will result in secondary joint deformity changes, such as foot drop, due to the imbalance of muscle strength.

8.3.1.3 Treatment Principle

(1) Early detection, early treatment, treatment of primary diseases, relief of nerve root compression; (2) For limb deformities caused by permanent nerve root injury, muscle strength balance is performed to correct deformities and improve functions.

8.3.2 Peripheral Nerve Injury Caused by Drug Poisoning

8.3.2.1 Etiology

There are many drugs causing peripheral nerve injury, especially antineoplastic drugs and antibacterial drugs. Some drug poisoning is caused by improper dosage and type of drugs used by medical staff, resulting in nerve damage, secondary muscle spasm, paralysis and deformity of lower limbs.

8.3.2.2 Clinical Manifestation

Drug poisoning can be found soon after medication. Besides systemic symptoms, the secondary nerve damage of limbs is mainly sensory and motor disorders. In severe cases, there may be muscle atrophy, paralysis, hand and foot contracture deformity (Fig. 8.30).

8.3.2.3 Treatment Principle

1. Prevention first, early detection and early treatment.
2. For limb deformities caused by peripheral nerve injury, muscle strength balance is performed to correct deformities and improve functions.

8.3.3 Limb Deformity after Sensory Disturbance Peripheral Neuropathy

8.3.3.1 Etiology

Various physical and chemical factors, chronic poisoning, and endocrine abnormalities can lead to nerve root, nerve plexus, nerve trunk or nerve endings damage, which has different clinical manifestations according to the location, degree, and scope of injury.

8.3.3.2 Clinical Manifestation

In addition to paresthesia and muscle dysfunction in the innervated area, when most peripheral nerve endings are damaged, various sensory disorders at the ends of symmetrical limbs occur, which are distributed like gloves and socks, accompanied by motor and autonomic nerve dysfunction. Due to sensory disorders, extremity ulcers or Charcot arthropathy are often caused (Fig. 8.31). Spontaneous amputation (fingers and toes) in severe cases (Fig. 8.32).

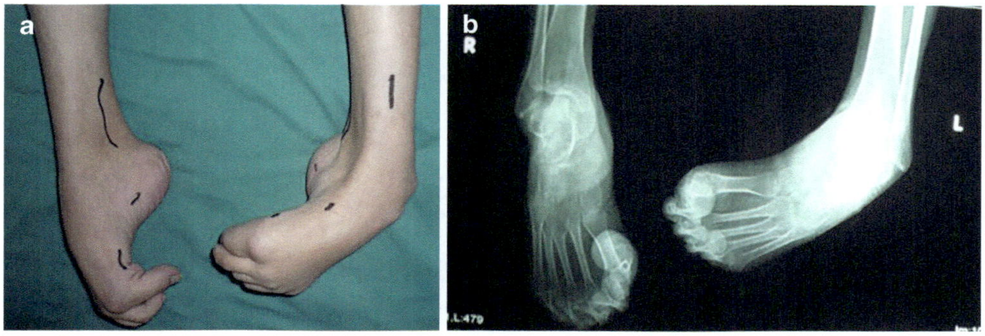

Fig. 8.30 A 21-year-old female presented with spastic deformity of both feet after intravenous injection at the age of 12. (**a**) Partial photograph of both feet, right horseshoe foot, toe flexion deformity. Left talipes equinovarus with flexion deformity; (**b**) Anteroposterior radiographs of both feet

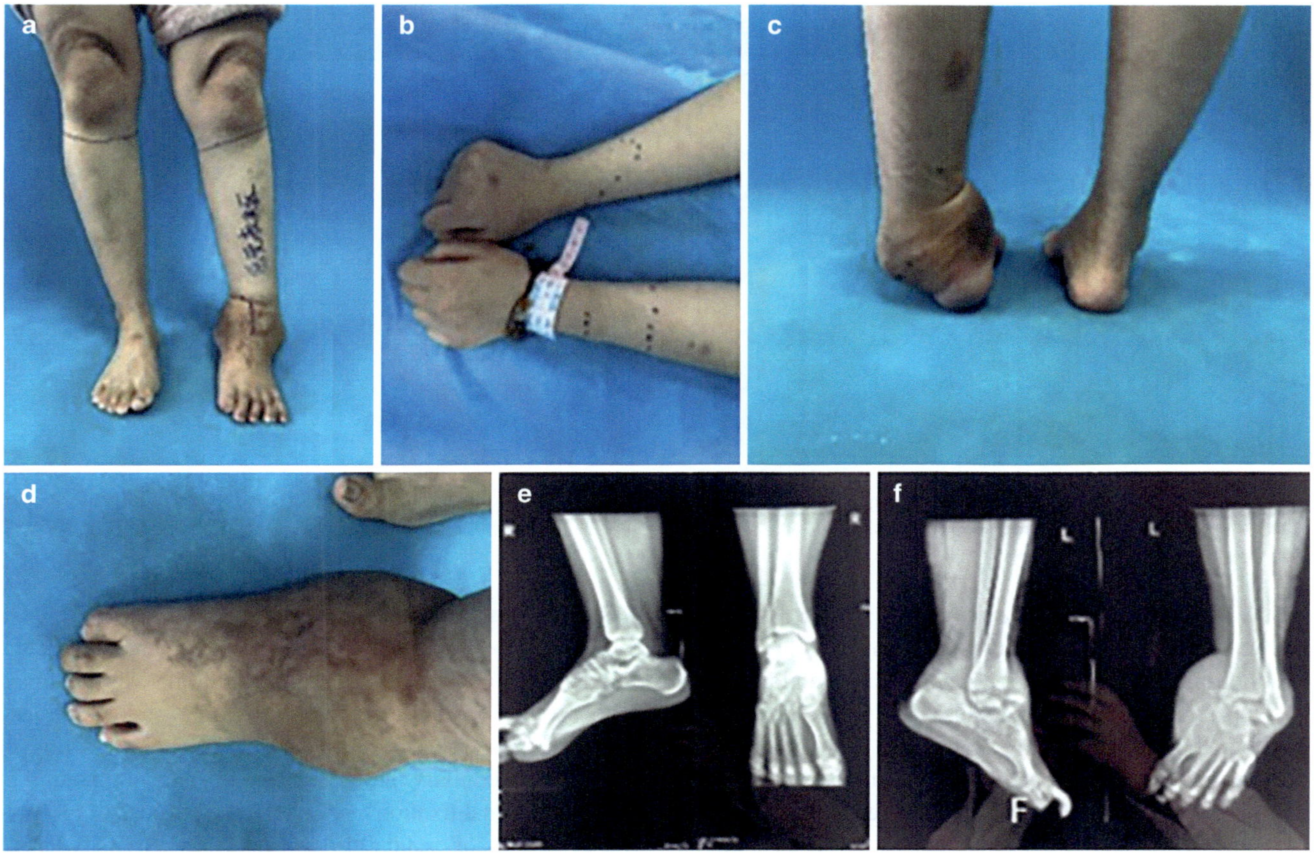

Fig. 8.31 Female, 18 years old, sensory disturbance peripheral neuropathy, distal sensory disturbance of limbs, partial amputation of fingers and toes, swelling of left ankle joint. (**a**) Full-length frontal view of both lower limbs; (**b**) Gloved paresthesia of both hands; (**c**) Left foot varus; (**d**) Swelling of left ankle joint; (**e**) Charcot's arthropathy of the left ankle. (**f**) X-rays showed severe damage to the left ankle

8.3.3.3 Treatment Principle

(1) Active treatment according to the cause of disease; (2) Early detection and treatment of mild limb deformities.

8.3.4 Lower Limb Deformity Caused by Neurofibromatosis

8.3.4.1 Etiology

Neurofibromatosis (NF) is a benign peripheral nerve sheath tumor originating from Schwann cell, which is an autosomal dominant genetic disease with incomplete penetrance. Neurofibromatosis was classified into neurofibromatosis type 1 (NF1) and neurofibromatosis type 2 (NF2) by the National Institutes of Health (NIH) in 1988 according to its clinical manifestations and gene localization. NF1 is characterized by skin café au lait spots and multiple neurofibromas of peripheral nerves, with high penetrance, and its gene is located on chromosome 17q 11.2. NF2, also known as central neurofibromatosis or bilateral acoustic neuromatosis, is located on chromosome 22q.

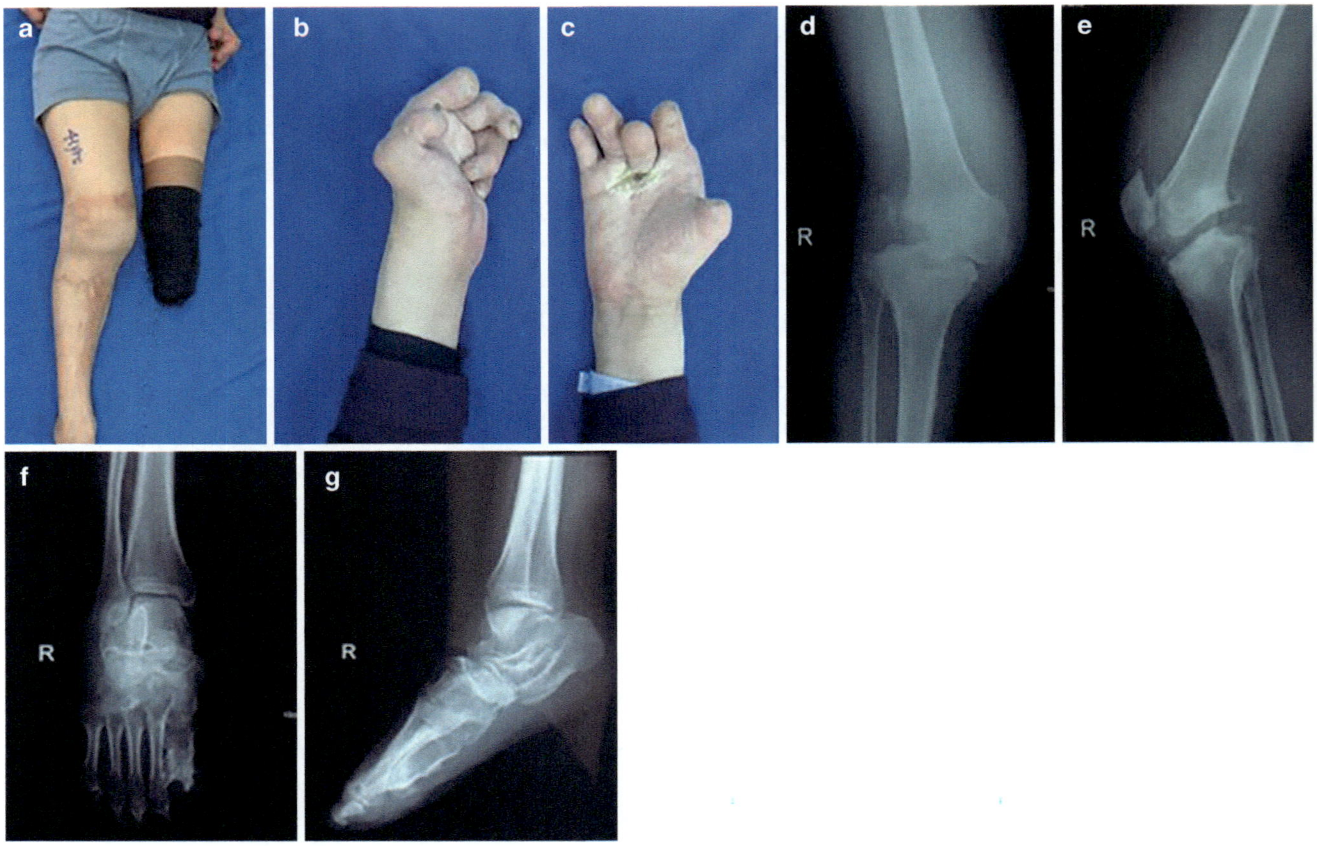

Fig. 8.32 A 40-year-old man with sensory peripheral neuropathy suffered from spontaneous amputation. (**a**) Amputation of left lower limb; (**b**) Partial amputation of fingers of both hands; (**c**) X-ray film showed destruction of bone of right knee joint. The UNK1X radiograph showed the change of right talipes equinus

8.3.4.2 Clinical Manifestation

The two most common features are skin café au lait spots and multiple neurofibromas. It can appear in childhood and develop significantly after adolescence. Most of them are distributed on the trunk, limbs, and face. Tumors are mostly nodular, pedunculated or pedunculated, smooth surface, generally without pain and tenderness. However, neurofibromas located in superficial nerves may have pain, occasional tenderness, and even pain and paresthesia along the nerve trunk. Tumors vary in size and number, and most of them increase with age. The main manifestations of bone damage are dystrophic scoliosis and tibial pseudarthrosis located in the middle and lower part of the leg, resulting in severe limb shortening and angular deformity (Fig. 8.33).

8.3.4.3 Treatment Principle

Orthopedic treatment mainly includes the treatment of deformity and dysfunction caused by neurofibromatosis combined with scoliosis and pseudarthrosis of tibia of lower limbs. Through the resection of pseudarthrosis, bone grafting of ilium, intramedullary fixation, correction and lengthening of Ilizarov external fixation technology, the purpose of promoting the healing of pseudarthrosis, restoring the gravity line of limbs, equaling the length of limbs, and improving the appearance and function is achieved.

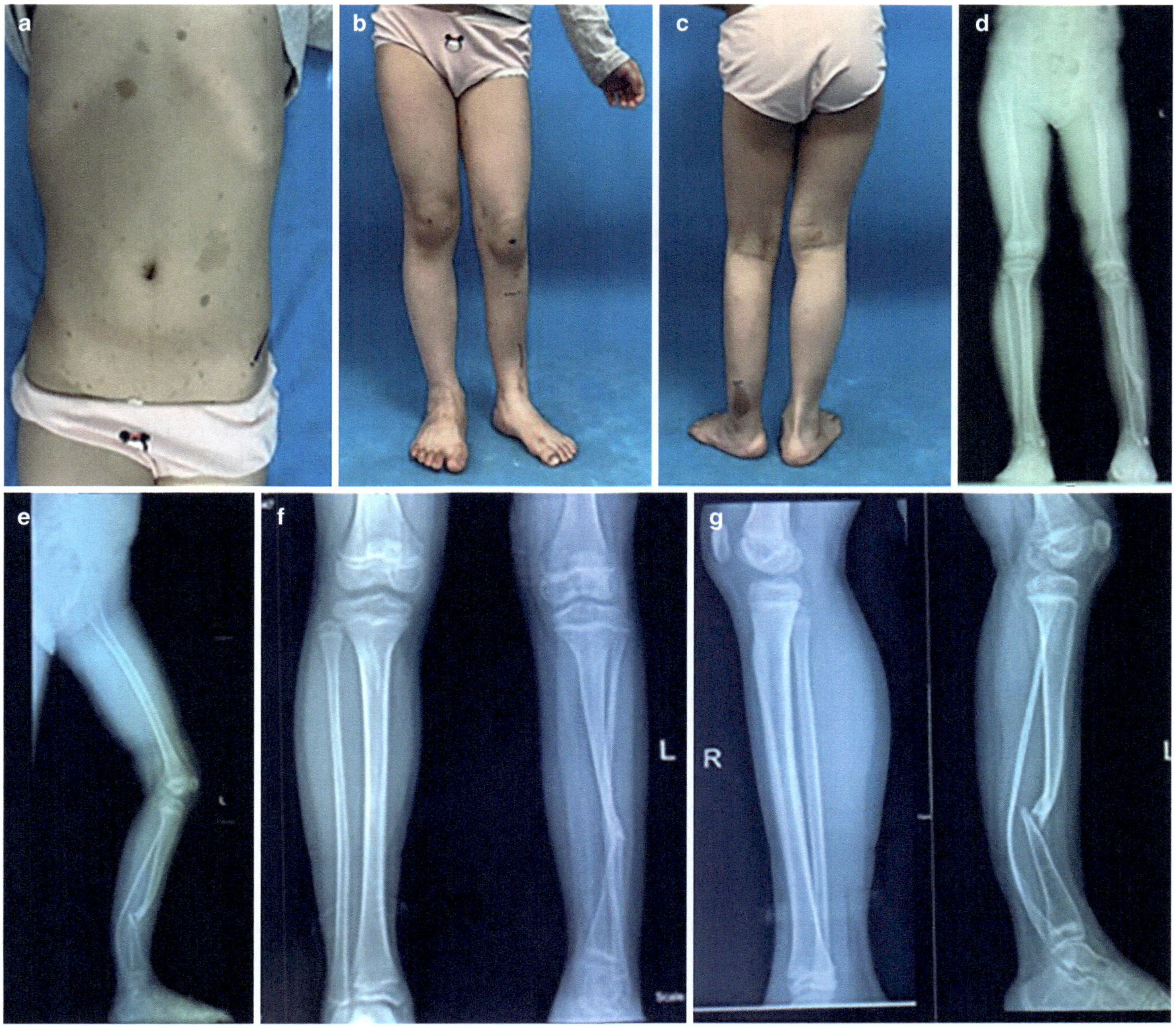

Fig. 8.33 Familial neurofibromatosis. (**a**) Cafe-au-lait spots on the abdomen; (**b**) Full-length frontal view of both lower extremities; (**c**) Full-length posterior view of both lower extremities; (**d**) Full-length anteroposterior radiographs of both lower extremities, shortening of the left lower extremity; (**e**) The whole length of both lower limbs was viewed from the side, and the knee joint was flexed. (**f**, **g**) X-ray film of bilateral tibia and fibula, pseudarthrosis of left tibia, small and curved left fibula

8.4 Motor Nerve Disease

8.4.1 Lower Limb Deformity Secondary to Amyotrophic Lateral Sclerosis

8.4.1.1 Etiology

Amyotrophic lateral sclerosis (amyotrophic lateral sclerosis, ALS), commonly known as "frozen human disease," is one of the five common motor neuron diseases, suffered by physicist Hawking. The disease mainly involves the upper Motor neurons (Brain, Brain stem, Spinal cord), which in turn affects the lower motor neurons (Cranial nerves Nuclear, Anterior horn of spinal cord Cell) and the trunk, limbs, and head and face that it controls Muscle A chronic progressive degeneration disease. Clinically, it is often manifested as a mixed paralysis with combined injury of upper and lower motor neurons.

8.4.1.2 Clinical Manifestation

Amyotrophic lateral sclerosis is usually caused by hand and foot. Usually, hand muscle weakness and atrophy are the first symptoms Generally, it starts from one side and then spreads to the opposite side. With the development of the disease, the symptoms of mixed damage of upper and

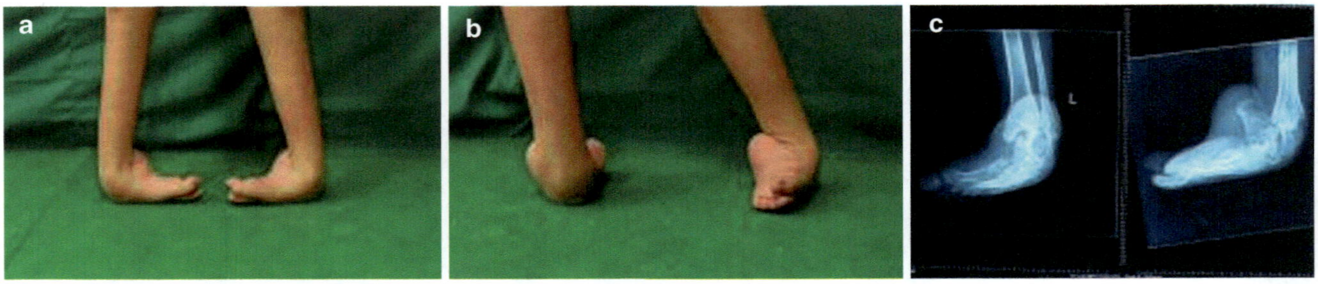

Fig. 8.34 Lateral sclerosis foot deformity, bilateral clubfoot deformity. (**a**) bipedal anterior view; (**b**) View from the back of both feet; (**c**) Anteroposterior and lateral radiograph of left foot

lower motor neurons appear. Most of the upper limbs are distal. Muscle atrophy mainly in the thenar and hypothenar Muscles and Interosseous muscle, at the same time accompanied by Muscle Bundle Vibrating, feeling normal. Bitateral lower limbs show Spastic paralysis, Increased muscle tension, tendon hyperreflexia, and positive pathological reflexes on both sides (Fig. 8.34). In addition, breathing muscle involvement occurs. It is hard to breathe.

8.4.1.3 Treatment Principle

(1) At present, there is no effective treatment for this disease, and the treatment adopted is symptomatic treatment. (2) Prevention Ankylosis Contracture, adhere to proper physical exercise and Physical therapy; (3) Patients with limb deformities can be treated with orthopedic surgery to improve limb function.

8.4.2 Limb Deformity Secondary to Spinal Muscular Atrophy

8.4.2.1 Etiology

Spinal muscular atrophy (SMA) is one of the most common autosomal recessive genetic diseases, also known as "progressive spinal muscular atrophy" and "spinal muscular atrophy." It is a typical neurogenic injury disease because of the damage of motor neurons caused by the defect of genetic material, which affects muscle contraction. Spinal muscular atrophy (SMA) is the most common neurogenic disease in infants and children, which leads to motor development disorders. Electromyography shows neurogenic damage, and muscle biopsy shows typical neurogenic damage.

8.4.2.2 Clinical Manifestation

The typical clinical manifestations are as follows: (1) Signs of lower motor neuron damage, such as decreased muscle tension and loss of tendon reflexes. (2) Decreased muscle strength is more severe in the lower extremities than in the upper extremities, more severe in the proximal extremities than in the distal extremities, and severe deformities of multiple parts of the extremities may occur in severe cases (Fig. 8.35). (3) Patients with paralysis of the scapular girdle muscles have a pronounced winged scapular deformity (Fig. 8.36).

8.4.2.3 Treatment Principle

At present, there is no effective treatment for this disease, and the treatment adopted is symptomatic treatment. Patients with limb deformities can be treated with orthopedic surgery to improve limb function.

8.4.3 Charcot-Marie-Tooth Disease

8.4.3.1 Etiology

Charcot-Marie-Tooth (CMT), also known as hereditary motor-sensory neuron disease (HMSN), has significant genetic characteristics. The main clinical feature is the progressive muscle weakness and atrophy of the distal extremities with sensory disturbance. According to the clinical and electrophysiological characteristics, CMT can be divided into two types: demyelinating type (CMT1 type), nerve conduction velocity slow down. Axonal type (CMT2 type), nerve conduction velocity is normal or slightly slow. Because of muscle atrophy of lower limbs and legs, accompanied by muscle imbalance, it is often followed by high arch of horseshoe and claw toe deformity.

8.4.3.2 Clinical Manifestation

Both lower limbs are in the shape of an inverted wine bottle or crane legs, and at the same time, there are high arches, claw toes, talipes equinovarus deformity, etc. (Fig. 8.37); When walking, it shows special striding gait, such as muscle weakness, muscle atrophy, tendon hyporeflexia, glove-sock-like deep and shallow sensory disorders and a series of autonomic nervous and nutritional metabolic disorders at the extremities in a few cases, local skin bluish purple, low skin temperature, ulcer formation, etc.

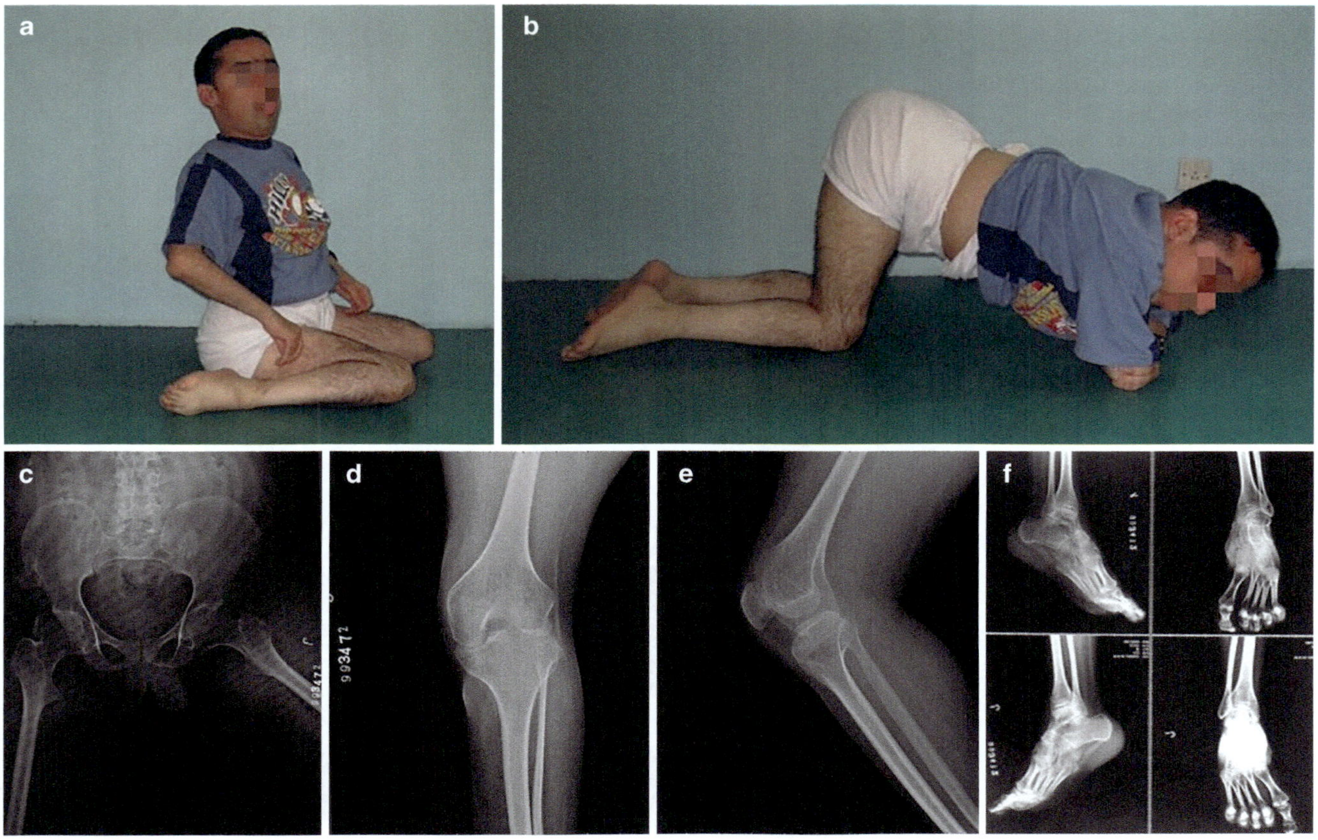

Fig. 8.35 Male, 25 years old, progressive (spinal) muscular atrophy, spinal muscular atrophy, hip flexion, knee flexion, horseshoe foot deformity of both lower limbs, three times of spinal cord stem cell transplantation. (**a**) Severe hip flexion deformity, unable to stand; (**b**) Limitation of hip and knee joint movement; (**c**) Prone position, inability to extend limbs; (**d**) Bilateral hip anteroposterior radiographs; (**e**) Lateral radiographs of bilateral knee joints; (**f**) Anteroposterior and lateral radiographs of bilateral ankle joint

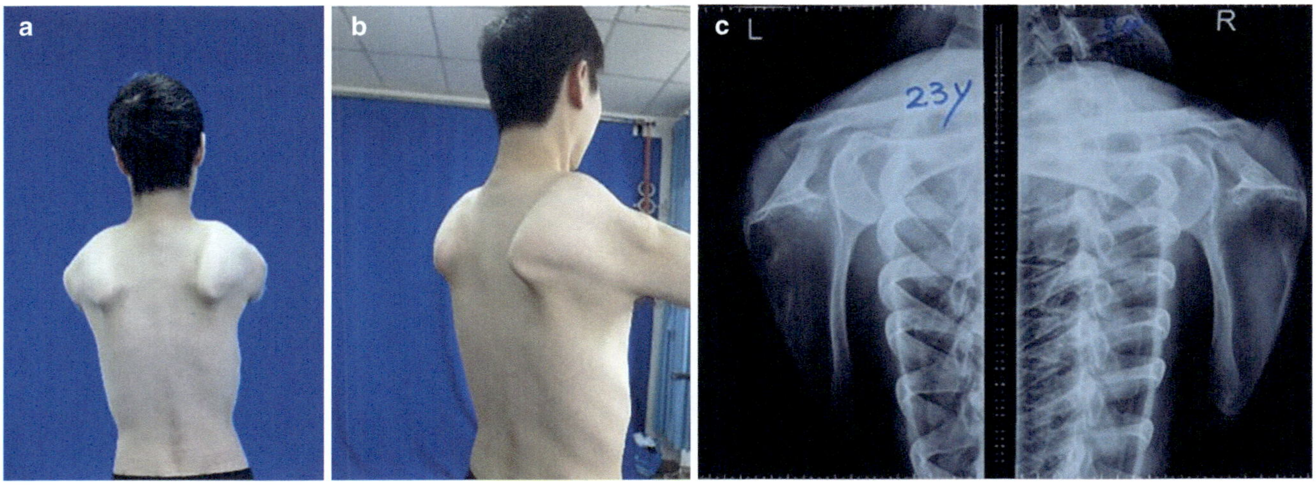

Fig. 8.36 A 23-year-old man with spinal muscular atrophy and bilateral alar scapular deformity. (**a**) dorsal appearance, bilateral scapular wing-like protuberance; (**b**) lateral view, bilateral scapular protuberance; (**c**) Bilateral shoulder radiograph

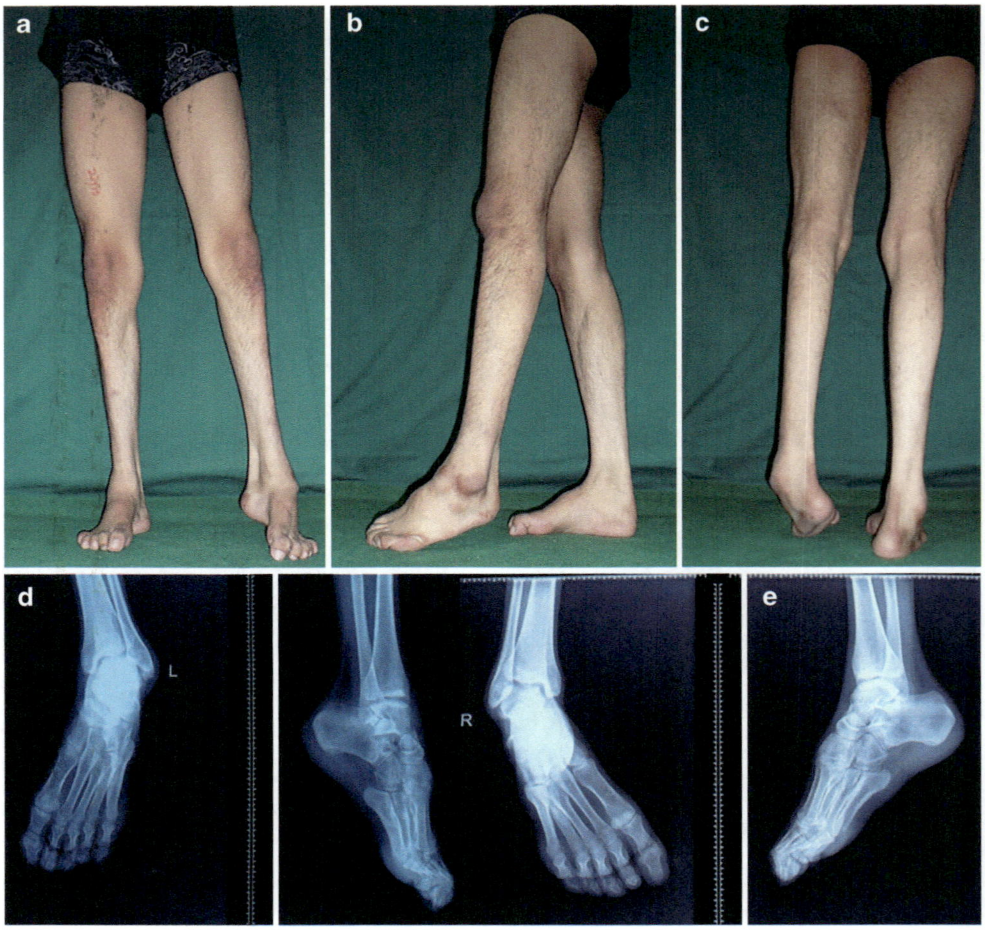

Fig. 8.37 Charcot-Marie-Tooth disease. (**a**, **b**, **c**) Male, 22 years old, Charcot-Marie-Tooth disease, slender legs, high arched claw toes; (**d**, **e**) X examination of varus cavus deformity of left foot

8.4.3.3 Treatment Principle

1. At present, there is no effective treatment for CMT in clinic, and some symptomatic and supportive therapies are mainly adopted for patients.
2. Orthopedic treatment mainly aims at the correction of limb deformities and the improvement of function. The focus of deformity correction is talipes cavus and claw toe deformity, which can significantly improve the weight-bearing walking ability of the affected limb.

9 Infectious Diseases Lead to Deformity

Sihe Qin

9.1 Bacterial Infection

9.1.1 Chronic Osteomyelitis

9.1.1.1 Etiology

Chronic osteomyelitis refers to the infection of bone 6 weeks after the initial infection, usually caused by bacteria, fungi, etc. According to the pathogenic mechanism, the disease can be divided into exogenous or hematogenous. After chronic osteomyelitis is cured, problems such as unequal length of lower limbs and angular deformity are often left behind. Repeated healing of soft tissue sinus tract causes skin scar contracture, which has a great impact on limb function and may be accompanied by muscle atrophy. If the site of the disease is close to the joint, the function of the joint will be destroyed, resulting in joint contracture or stiffness.

9.1.1.2 Clinical Manifestation

During the period of chronic inflammation, there are local swelling, bone thickening, rough surface, and tenderness. If there is a sinus, the wound will not heal for a long time, and occasionally a small piece of sequestrum will be discharged. Sometimes the wound heals temporarily, but because the infection focus persists, when the general health is poor and the immunity is reduced, the inflammation spreads, which can lead to acute attack, which is characterized by elevated body temperature and local redness and swelling. After incision and drainage, or self-perforation, or drug control, systemic symptoms disappeared, local inflammation gradually subsided, wound healing, and so on. When the infection is completely controlled, it will enter the sequelae of osteomyelitis, which can be manifested as limb shortening, limb deformity, bone nonunion, bone defect, etc. (Fig. 9.1).

S. Qin (✉)
Department of Orthopaedics, Rehabilitation Hospital of the National Research Center for Rehabilitation Technical Aids, Beijing, China

9.1.1.3 Treatment Principle

Osteotomy can be used to correct the joint deformity left by chronic osteomyelitis. Limb lengthening is feasible for patients with limb shortening; Nonunion and bone defects can be treated by the Ilizarov technique.

9.1.2 Sequelae of Suppurative Arthritis

9.1.2.1 Etiology

Invasion of joints by pyogenic bacteria causes joint destruction and loss of function, which can be caused by hematogenous dissemination, direct inoculation of wounds or surgical incisions, and spread of adjacent osteomyelitis or cellulitis. It can occur at any age, but severe sequelae of infection often occur in children. Suppurative arthritis was most common in weight-bearing joints of the lower extremities (61–79%). Hematogenous involvement is mostly a single large joint of the limbs, such as hip, knee, and elbow joints. More than 50% of the pathogenic bacteria were Staphylococcus aureus, followed by Streptococcus, Diplococcus pneumoniae, Escherichia coli, Haemophilus influenzae, and so on. Because suppurative arthritis leads to different degrees of joint synovium destruction, even articular cartilage destruction, after inflammation is cured, joint function is often limited, fibrous stiffness, and even bone stiffness in non-functional position, affecting limb function.

9.1.2.2 Clinical Manifestation

The acute stage is characterized by local swelling, pain, and obvious tenderness. The joint fluid increased and fluctuated, which was more obvious in superficial joints such as knee joint, and the floating patella sign was positive. Patients often place the knee joint in a semi-bending position to relax the joint capsule to reduce tension. The above symptoms are sometimes not obvious in newborns, and symptoms such as erythema, swelling, fever, and pain may be mild or absent, so diagnosis is sometimes difficult. After infection control, the

S. Qin et al. (eds.), *Atlas of Limb Deformity*, https://doi.org/10.1007/978-981-97-0999-1_9

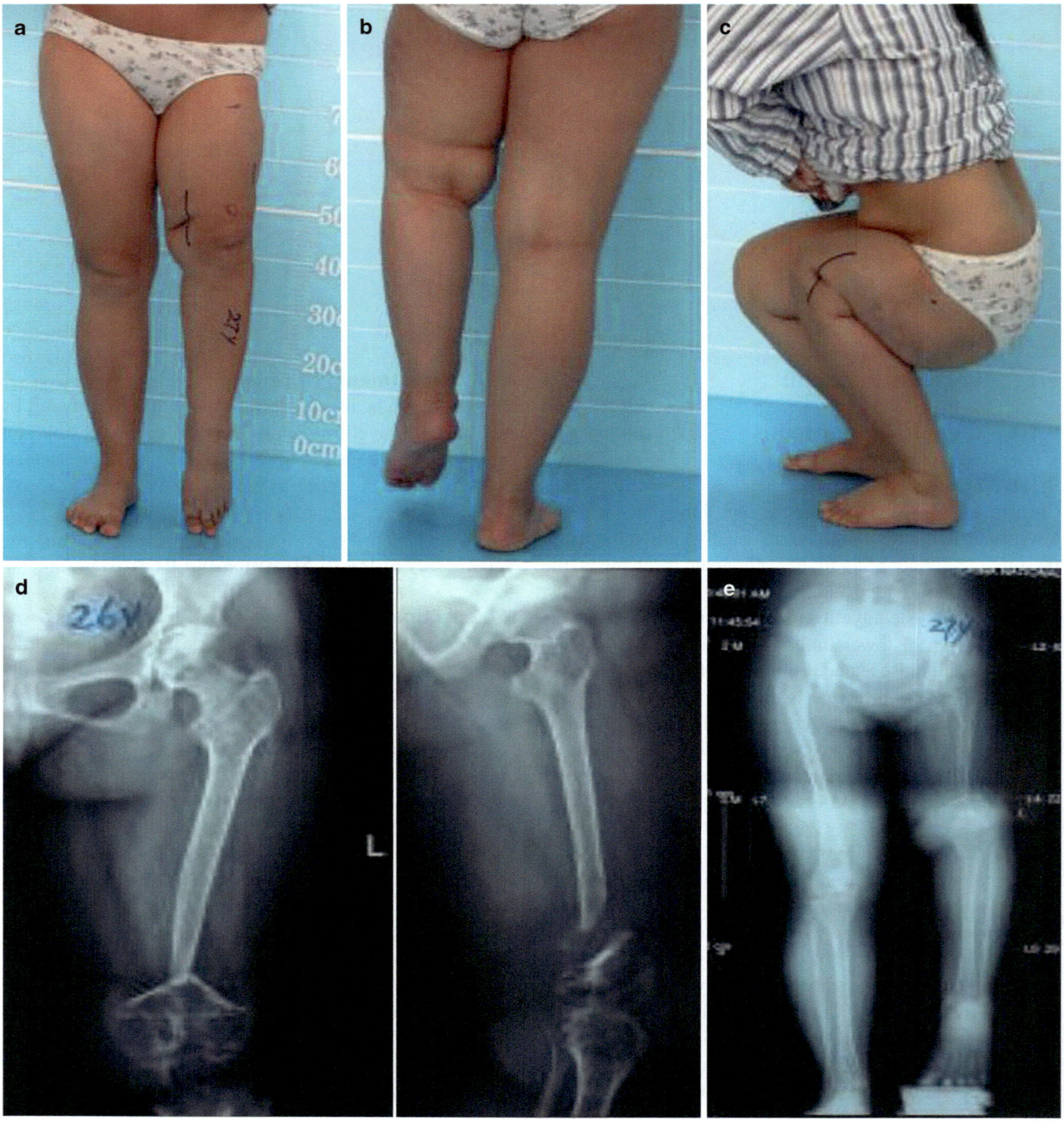

Fig. 9.1 Deformity after chronic osteomyelitis of left femur. (**a**) In the frontal view of the standing position, the left lower limb is shortened; (**b**) Dorsal view in standing position; (**c**) View from the left side of the squat position, with the left thigh shortened; (**d**) Anteroposterior and lateral radiographs of left femur; (**e**) Full-length anteroposterior radiographs of both lower extremities in standing position

joints were damaged to varying degrees and entered the sequelae period. If the lesion occurs in the hip joint, it may occurs joint dislocation, femoral head necrosis, even complete destruction and absorption, non-functional joint fiber stiffness, joint bony fusion, etc. (Fig. 9.2); Occurs in the knee joint, may appear the knee joint fiber stiffness, or the osseous fusion, if the joint destruction is serious, the stiffness or the osseous fusion in the non-function may simultaneously appear the knee joint flexion or the varus and valgus deformity; Suppurative arthritis of the ankle is rare and may result in ankle stiffness in plantar flexion with secondary talipes equinus.

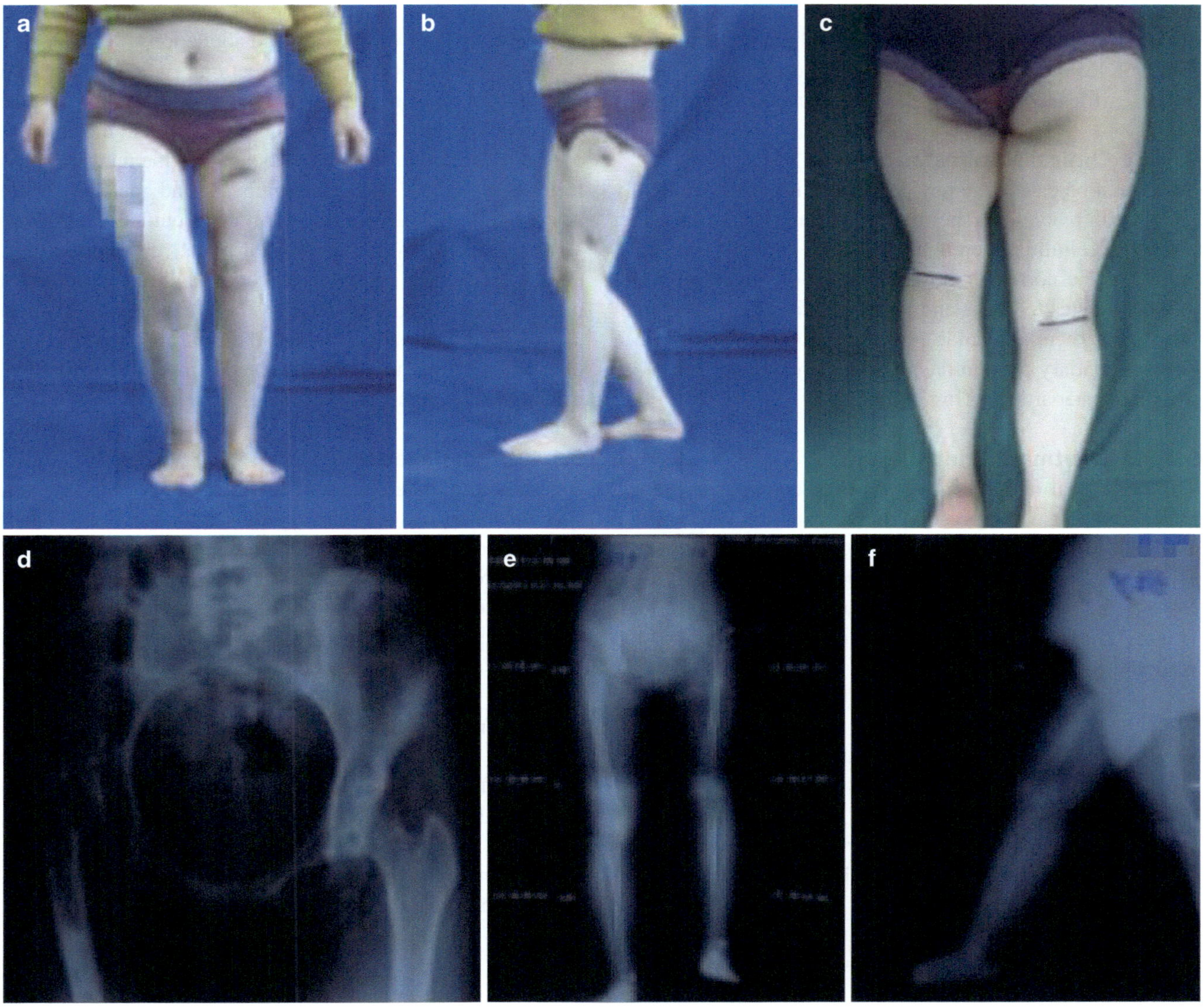

Fig. 9.2 Sequelae of suppurative arthritis of right hip joint. (**a**) General view of the front of both lower limbs; (**b**) Gross view of both lower extremities; (**c**) General view of the back of both lower limbs; Pelvic anteroposterior film of (**d**). X line; Anteroposterior film of the whole length of both lower limbs of (**e**). X line; (**f**) Full-length lateral X-ray film of the right lower limb

9.1.2.3 Treatment Principle

The principle of treatment for acute infection is to control infection and reduce joint destruction, including joint irrigation, arthroscopy, antibiotic application, and other methods. For the treatment of sequelae of suppurative arthritis, the principle of orthopedic surgery is to restore joint function or fuse joint in functional position to the greatest extent, correct contracture deformity of joint, restore the gravity line of lower limbs, equal-length limbs, improve the function of standing and walking, and provide conditions for long-term joint replacement.

9.1.3 Sequelae of Sepsis (Juvenile Osteomyelitis)

9.1.3.1 Etiology

Sepsis refers to the systemic inflammatory response syndrome caused by infection, which is clinically confirmed to have the presence of bacteria or highly suspicious foci of infection. Although sepsis is caused by infection, it causes systemic inflammatory response syndrome, leading to further destruction of the body's physiological function. Pathogenic microorganisms include bacteria, fungi, viruses, and parasites. Bacteria in blood migrate to joints, bones, and other places with blood flow, and multiply in large numbers, infecting local tissues, resulting in the destruction of joints, bones, cartilage, and soft tissues, and causing deformities.

9.1.3.2 Clinical Manifestation

Sepsis can be caused by any part of the infection, clinically common in pneumonia, peritonitis, cholangitis, urinary tract infection, cellulitis, meningitis, abscess, and other manifestations of the corresponding symptoms of infection. When sepsis migrates to bones and joints (it can occur in any joint of the hip, knee, and ankle), bone and joint deformities can occur secondary to joint damage, with symptoms similar to pyogenic osteoarthritis (Fig. 9.3).

9.1.3.3 Treatment Principle

The main goal of acute infection is to control the inflammatory response and preserve organ function. When bone and joint destruction leads to limb dysfunction, orthopedic surgery is needed to correct bone and joint deformity, restore the weight-bearing line of lower limbs, equal-length limbs, and improve the function of standing and walking.

9.1.4 Osteoarticular Tuberculosis

9.1.4.1 Etiology

Osteoarticular tuberculosis is a destructive disease caused by the invasion of Mycobacterium tuberculosis into bone or joint. Tuberculosis occurs mostly in the lungs, but it can also occur in any organ of the body. About 50% of patients with bone tuberculosis are complicated with pulmonary tuberculosis. Tuberculosis lesions first occur in the lungs. After pulmonary infection, they can spread to all parts of the body through the circulatory system, leading to tuberculosis of the skeletal system, urinary system, digestive system, and so on. Bone and joint tuberculosis is characterized by destruction of bone, synovium, and articular cartilage, resulting in stiffness and deformity of bone and joint.

9.1.4.2 Clinical Manifestation

The local symptoms of bone and joint tuberculosis include dysfunction, swelling, sinus tract, pain, and deformity, especially in early cases. The symptoms and signs are not specific and can also be seen in inflammatory joint diseases of other causes. About 94% of cases of joint tuberculosis are single lesions, so single joint lesions can be regarded as a feature of joint tuberculosis. In the early stage of the disease, in order to relieve pain, the affected joints are forced to be in special positions, such as knee and elbow tuberculosis in semi-flexion position (Fig. 9.4); ankle tuberculosis was maintained in plantar flexion. In the early stage of hip tuberculosis, the position was abduction and external rotation, and in the late stage, the position was flexion and adduction.

X-ray findings: (1) Bone destruction: The bone trabecula was blurred, like frosted glass, showing bone defect. Bone destruction is easy to occur in the epiphysis and metaphysis, can be in the central part of the bone or in the marginal part, forming a defect, often the epiphysis and metaphysis are destroyed at the same time, forming a unified destruction area not limited by the epiphyseal plate; (2) Joint destruction: It starts from the bilateral edges, and the central joint plate surface is lighter, which is the characteristic of bone and joint tuberculosis. However, the central part of the knee joint and shoulder joint can also be destroyed, because there is less closely connected cartilage.

9.1.4.3 Classification

Bone and joint tuberculosis is divided into bone tuberculosis, synovial tuberculosis, and total joint tuberculosis. Bone tuberculosis is divided into cancellous bone tuberculosis, cortical bone tuberculosis, and metaphyseal bone tuberculosis. If simple bone tuberculosis and synovial tuberculosis are not treated in time, they can develop into total joint tuberculosis, and even if they are cured, fibrous or bony ankylosis will occur.

9.1.4.4 Treatment Principle

The basis of orthopedic treatment is that tuberculosis has been effectively controlled or cured. For the sequelae of bone and joint deformity, the treatment principle is to correct the deformity, restore the joint line and lower limb weight-bearing line, fuse the damaged joint to the functional position, and improve the function of standing and walking.

9.1.5 Sequelae of Meningitis

9.1.5.1 Etiology

Meningitis is caused by the invasion of pia mater by various biological pathogenic factors such as bacteria, viruses, fungi, spirochetes, protozoa, rickettsiae, tumors, and leukemia. Inflammatory reaction can invade the brain parenchyma, so the disease is also known as meningoencephalitis. If it affects the motor center of the cerebral cortex and causes damage to the motor center, it will lead to secondary motor dysfunction and gradually secondary limb deformity.

9.1.5.2 Clinical Manifestation

Neurological symptoms caused by meningitis are characterized by motor neuron damage, extensive nervous system damage, increased muscle tension, pathological signs, tendon hyperreflexia, seizures, and signs of cerebral cortex and hypothalamus damage. Nervous system damage can be secondary to muscle spasm and contracture of lower limbs, leading to bone and joint deformities (Fig. 9.5), affecting the motor function of patients.

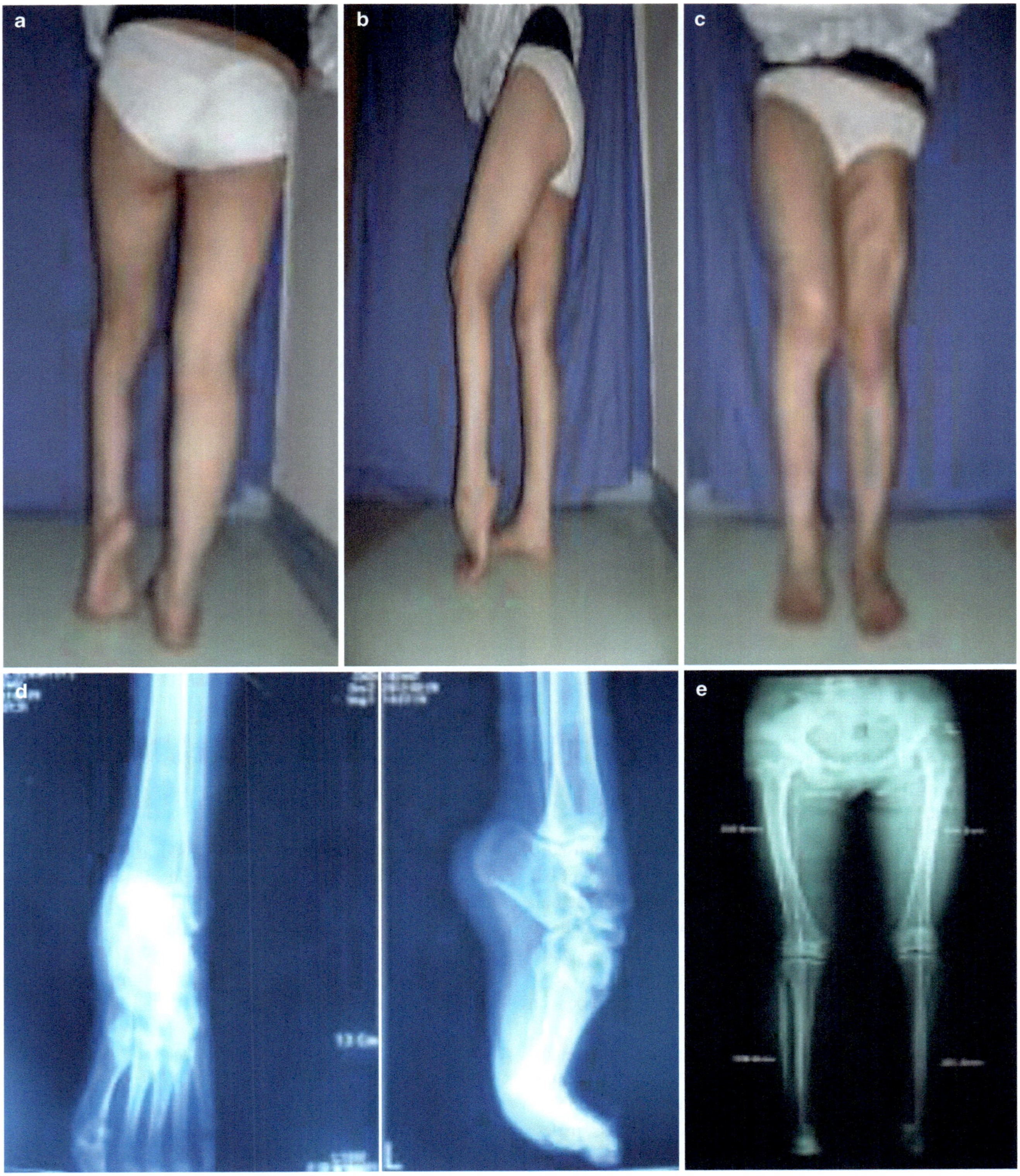

Fig. 9.3 Left lower limb deformity caused by sepsis. (**a**) Gross view from the back of both lower limbs; (**b**) Gross view of both lower extremities; (**c**) General view: frontal view of both lower limbs; (**d**) X line: anteroposterior and lateral radiographs of left ankle; (**e**) Full-length X-ray films of both lower extremities

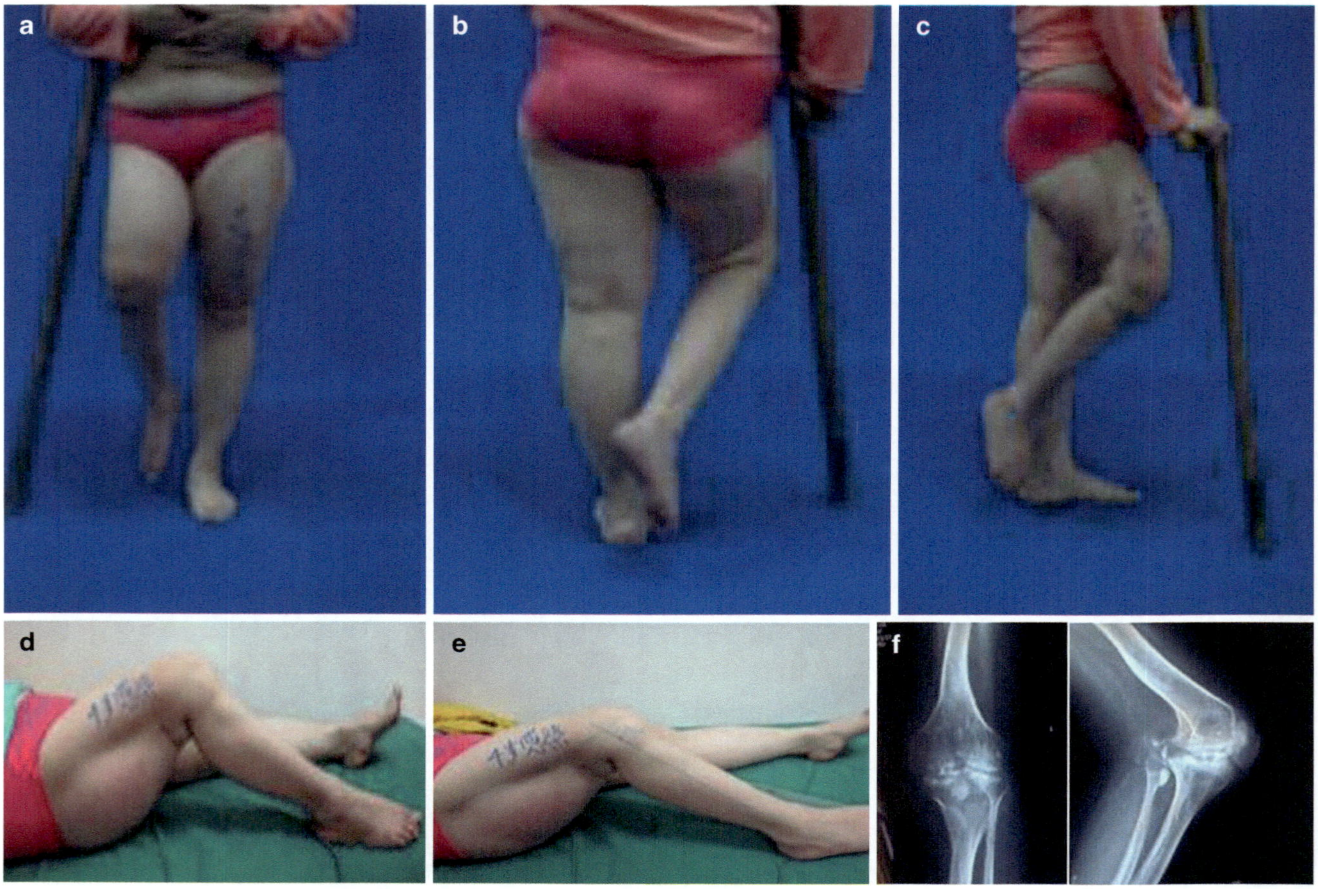

Fig. 9.4 Bending deformity of right knee joint after bone tuberculosis. (**a**) Gross view from the front of both lower extremities; (**b**) Gross view from the back of both lower limbs; (**c**) Gross view of both lower extremities; (**d**) The maximum flexion position of the right knee joint was generally observed; (**e**) The maximum extension position of the right knee joint was generally observed. (**f**) X-ray anteroposterior and lateral film of right knee joint

9.1.5.3 Classification

Purulent meningitis is a meningeal inflammation caused by various pyogenic bacteria, which is a major category of bacterial meningitis. It is one of the serious intracranial infections, often accompanied by suppurative encephalitis and brain abscess. There are three common types of pathogenic bacteria, namely Haemophilus influenzae type B, Neisseria meningitidis (diplococcus), and Streptococcus pneumoniae (diplococcus pneumoniae).

Tuberculous meningitis is a non-suppurative inflammation of the meninges caused by tubercle Bacillus. There may be symptoms of tuberculosis poisoning such as low fever, night sweat, loss of appetite, general fatigue and weakness, listlessness, meningeal irritation, and increased intracranial pressure.

Viral meningitis is an infection of the central nervous system caused by many viruses.

Meningitis can also be caused by fungi. The most common one is Cryptococcus. Cryptococcal meningitis is a deep fungal infection caused by certain species or variants of Cryptococcus invading the central nervous system.

9.1.5.4 Treatment Principle

Orthopedic treatment is mainly aimed at bone and joint deformities caused by lower limb muscle spasm secondary to meningitis nervous system damage. The principle of treatment is to correct bone and joint deformities, restore lower limb joint line and gravity line, relieve spasm, stabilize joints, and improve standing and walking function.

9.1.6 Sequelae of Tetanus

9.1.6.1 Etiology

Tetanus is a specific infection of muscle spasm caused by Clostridium tetani, which invades the human body through skin or mucosal wounds, grows and reproduces in anoxic environment, and produces spasmodic toxins. Tetanus toxin mainly attacks motor neurons in the nervous system, mainly affecting muscle groups including masseter, dorsal spinalis, abdominal muscles, limb muscles, and so on. If permanent damage to the central neurons is caused, spastic paralysis of

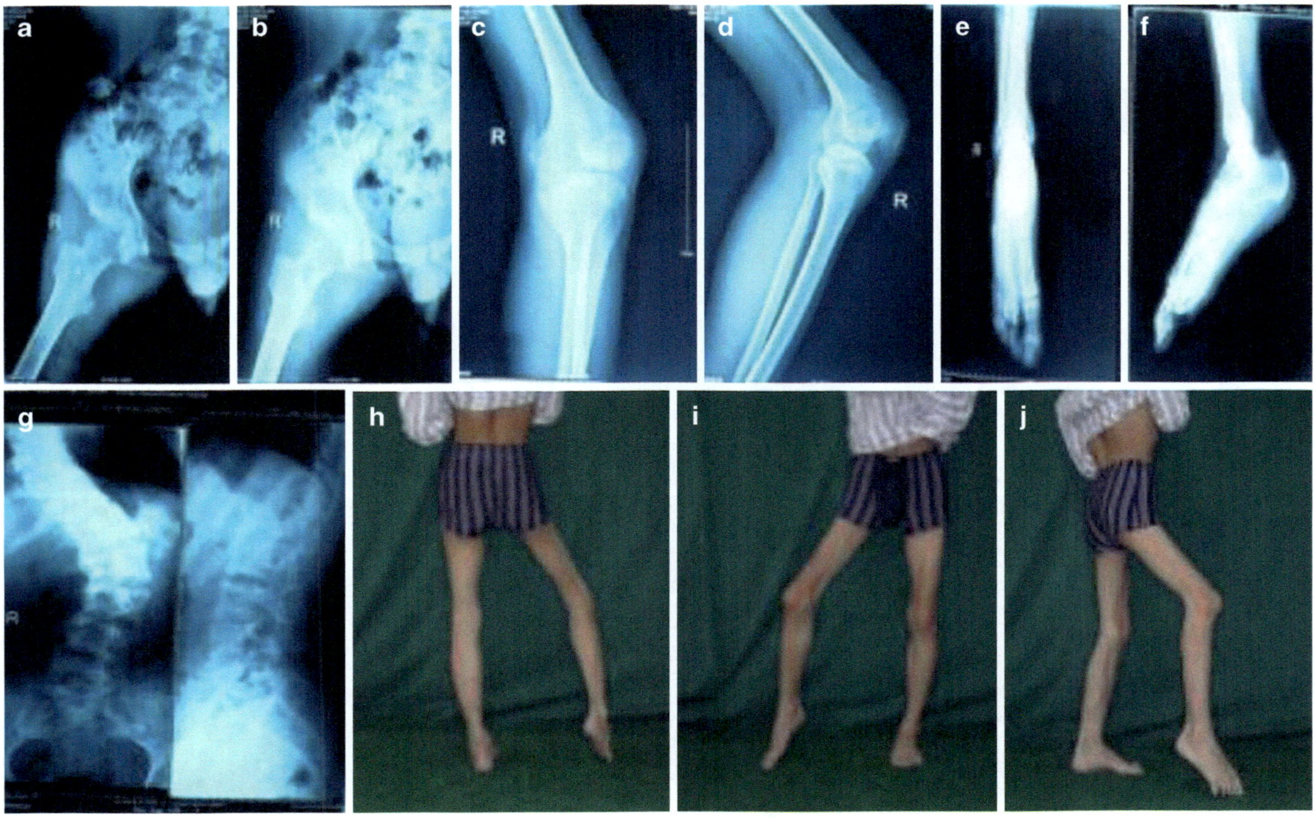

Fig. 9.5 Right lower limb deformity after meningitis. (**a**) Anteroposterior film of right hip joint; (**b**) X-ray: lateral film of right hip joint; (**c**) X-ray: anteroposterior film of right knee joint; (**d**) X-ray: lateral film of right knee joint. (**e**) X-ray: anteroposterior film of right ankle joint. (**f**) X-ray: lateral film of right ankle joint; (**g**) full-length anteroposterior and lateral film of spine; (**h**) Gross view from the back of both lower extremities; (**i**) Gross view from the front of both lower extremities; (**j**) Gross view of both lower extremities in profile

the corresponding limbs will be left behind, followed by spastic bone and joint deformities.

9.1.6.2 Clinical Manifestation

During the acute attack of tetanus, it is characterized by local muscle tightness, pulling pain, hyperreflexia, and other symptoms. The main manifestations of motor nervous system disinhibition include myotonia and muscle spasm. Usually the first muscle group affected is the masticatory muscles, followed by the facial expression muscles, the muscles of the neck, back, abdomen, and limbs, and finally the diaphragmatic muscles, i.e., trismus, opisthotonus, or opisthotonus. Most of the patients recovered after treatment without sequelae. A small number of patients have sequelae due to permanent damage to the affected motor neurons, mainly manifested as contracture paralysis of the affected muscles, increased muscle tension, tendon hyperreflexia, secondary muscle contracture after a long time, and deformity of adjacent joints caused by traction. Knee flexion, talipes equinovarus deformity, and high arch foot are more common in the lower limbs (Fig. 9.6).

9.1.6.3 Classification

1. Tetanus can be divided into three types: mild, moderate, and severe.
   (a) Mild latent period is more than 10 days, and the degree of systemic myotonia is mild. Muscle spasmodic contraction may occur 4–7 days after onset, but it lasts for a short time and usually stops in a few seconds.
   (b) The incubation period was 7–10 days and the initial spasmodic period was 2–4 days. Clinically, muscle rigidity is prominent, with typical trismus and opisthotonos. The duration of paroxysmal spasm was prolonged to more than 10 s, and the frequency of paroxysmal spasm increased, but no dyspnea and laryngospasm occurred.
   (c) The incubation period of severe patients was shorter than 7 days, and the initial spasmodic period was shorter than 48 hours. Systemic muscle rigidity is obvious, spasmodic muscle contraction occurs frequently and lasts for a long time, which often causes cyanosis and laryngospasm asphyxia. Patients often have high fever and lung infection, or cerebral edema

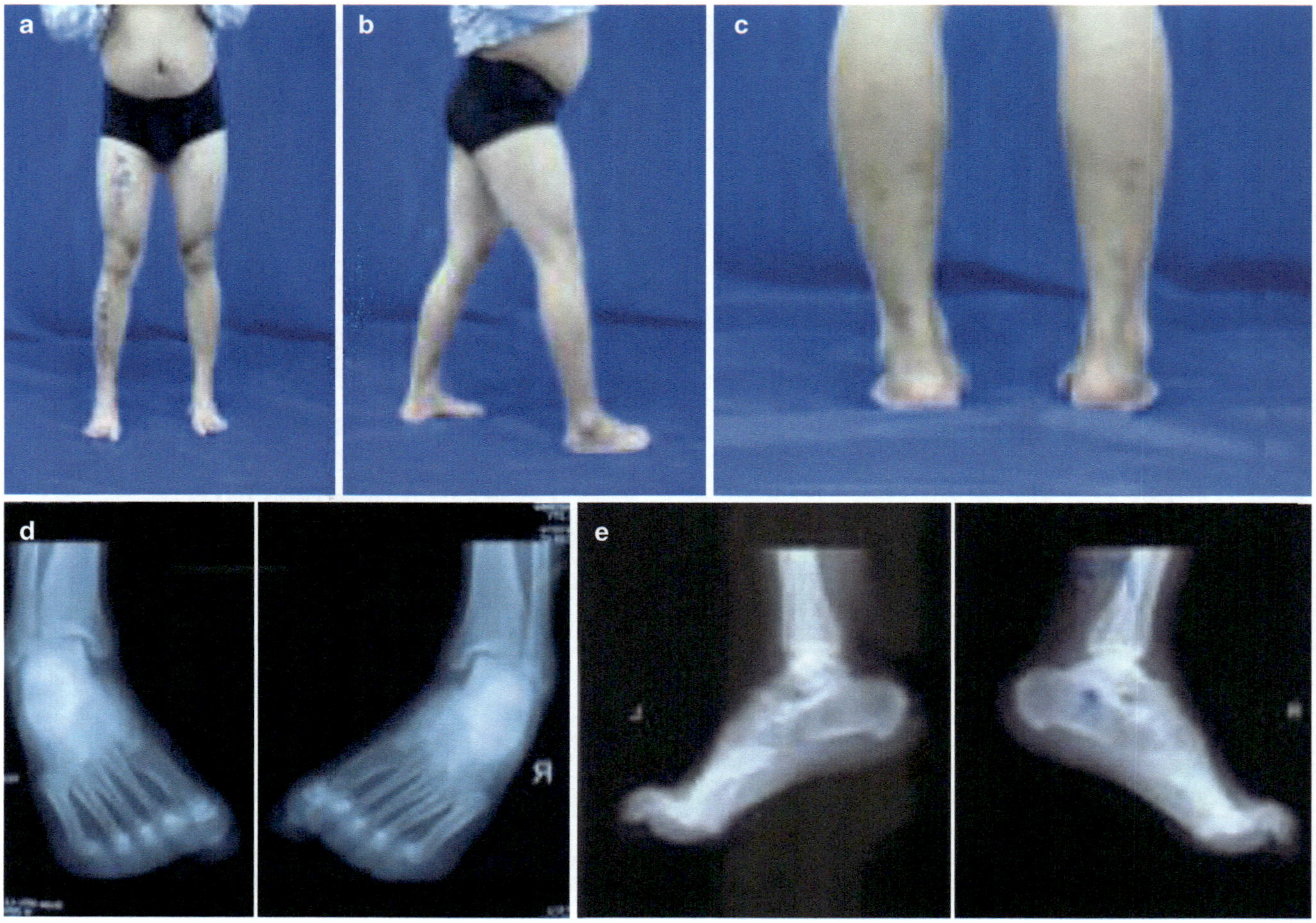

Fig. 9.6 Sequelae of tetanus. (**a**) Gross view from the front of both lower extremities; (**b**) Gross view of both lower extremities; (**c**) Gross photograph; Posterior view of both lower extremities; (**d**) X line; Ankle joint anteroposterior film; (**e**) Lateral X-ray film of ankle joint of both feet

due to frequent convulsions and hypoxia. In severe cases, coma occurred and eventually died of respiratory failure and systemic failure.

9.1.6.4 Treatment Principle

Orthopedic treatment is mainly aimed at limb deformities caused by muscle spasm caused by nerve damage after tetanus infection. The principle of treatment is to correct bone and joint deformities, relieve spasm, and improve standing and walking function.

9.1.7 Deformity of Lower Limbs after Septicemia

9.1.7.1 Etiology

Septicemia is an acute systemic infection caused by various pathogenic bacteria invading the blood circulation, growing and reproducing in the blood, and producing toxins. Pathogenic microorganisms include bacteria, fungi, viruses, and parasites. Bacteria in blood migrate to joints, bones, and other places with blood flow, and multiply in large numbers, infecting local tissues, resulting in the destruction of joints, bones, cartilage, and soft tissues and causing deformities.

9.1.7.2 Clinical Manifestation

Septicemia can be caused by any part of the infection, clinically common in pneumonia, peritonitis, cholangitis, urinary tract infection, cellulitis, meningitis, abscess, etc., showing the corresponding symptoms of infection. When the pathogen migrates to the bone and joint (which can occur in any joint of the hip, knee, and ankle), the deformity of the bone and joint can occur secondary to joint damage, with symptoms similar to suppurative osteoarthritis (Fig. 9.7).

9.1.7.3 Treatment Principle

The primary goal during the acute phase of infection is to control the inflammatory response. When bone and joint destruction leads to limb dysfunction, orthopedic surgery is needed to correct bone and joint deformity, restore the gravity line of lower limbs, and improve the function of standing and walking.

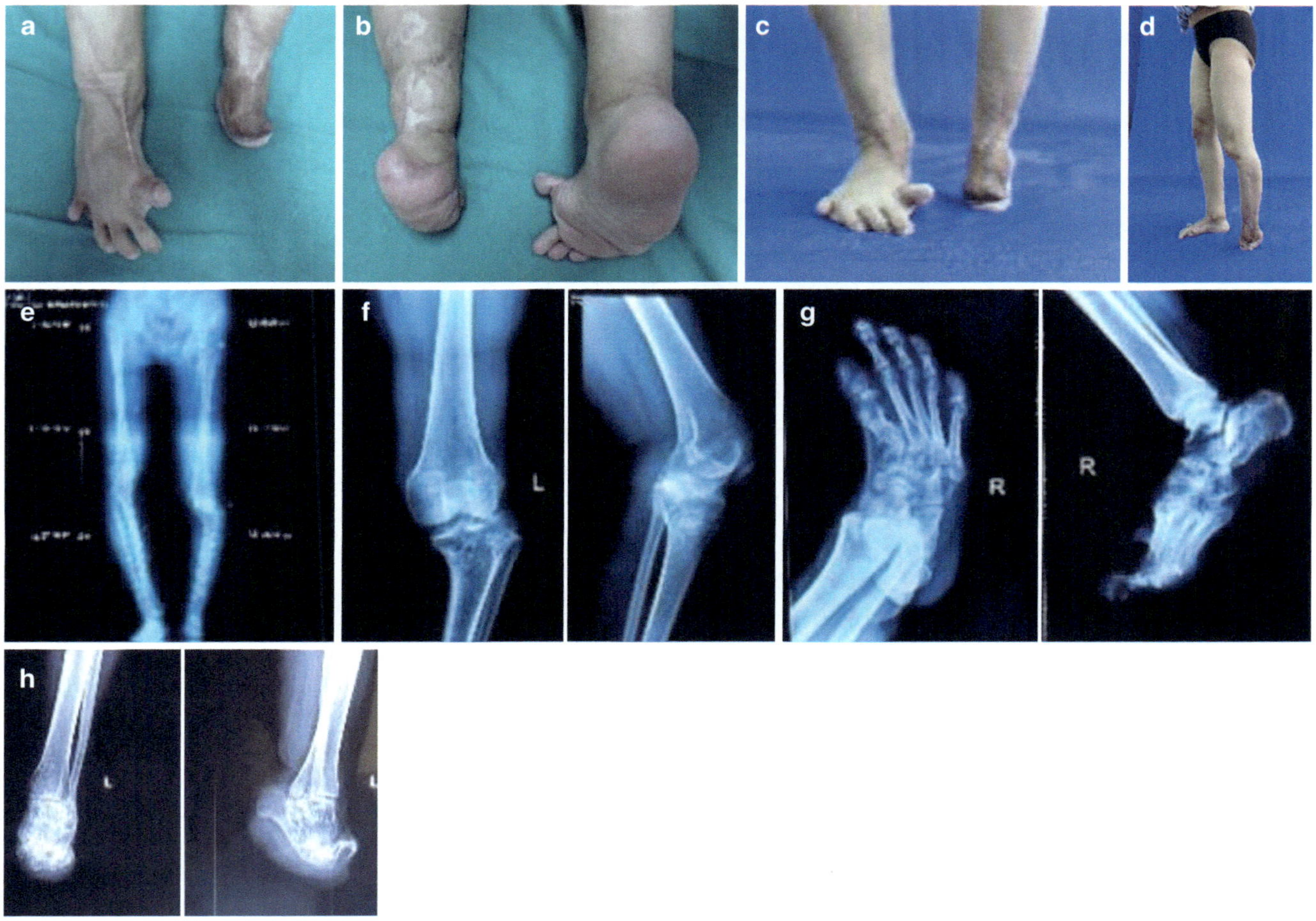

Fig. 9.7 Deformity of both lower limbs after septicemia. The patient, a 26-year-old female, suffered from septicemia at the age of 9 months, resulting in multiple abscesses and ulcerations in both lower limbs, resulting in limb defects and deformities. (**a**) Viewed roughly from the front of both feet; (**b**) Generally viewed from the back of both feet; (**c**) View roughly from the front of both feet (weight-bearing); (**d**) Lateral view of both lower extremities in gross view (weight-bearing); full-length anteroposterior radiographs of both lower extremities in (**e**) X line; anteroposterior and lateral radiographs of left knee joint in (**f**) X line; anteroposterior and lateral radiographs of right ankle in (**g**). X line; anteroposterior and lateral radiographs of left ankle in (**h**). X line

9.1.8 Infective Absence of Femoral Head in children's Hip Joint

9.1.8.1 Etiology

Hip joint septic arthritis is a kind of arthritis caused by pathogens invading the joint, resulting in joint destruction and loss of function. If not treated timely and effectively, it may lead to serious complications, such as ischemic osteonecrosis, osteomyelitis, chondrolysis, hip dislocation, unequal length of lower limbs, systemic sepsis and osteoarthritis, leaving joint function limited, fibrous stiffness, and even bone stiffness in the non-functional position, affecting limb function.

9.1.8.2 Clinical Manifestation

It is characterized by joint pain, joint dislocation, femoral head necrosis, even complete destruction and absorption, non-functional joint fiber stiffness, joint bony fusion, etc. (Fig. 9.8).

9.1.8.3 Treatment Principle

Orthopedic treatment is mainly aimed at limb deformities caused by muscle spasticity caused by nerve damage after tetanus infection. The treatment principle is to relieve spasticity, correct bone and joint deformities, and improve standing and walking function.

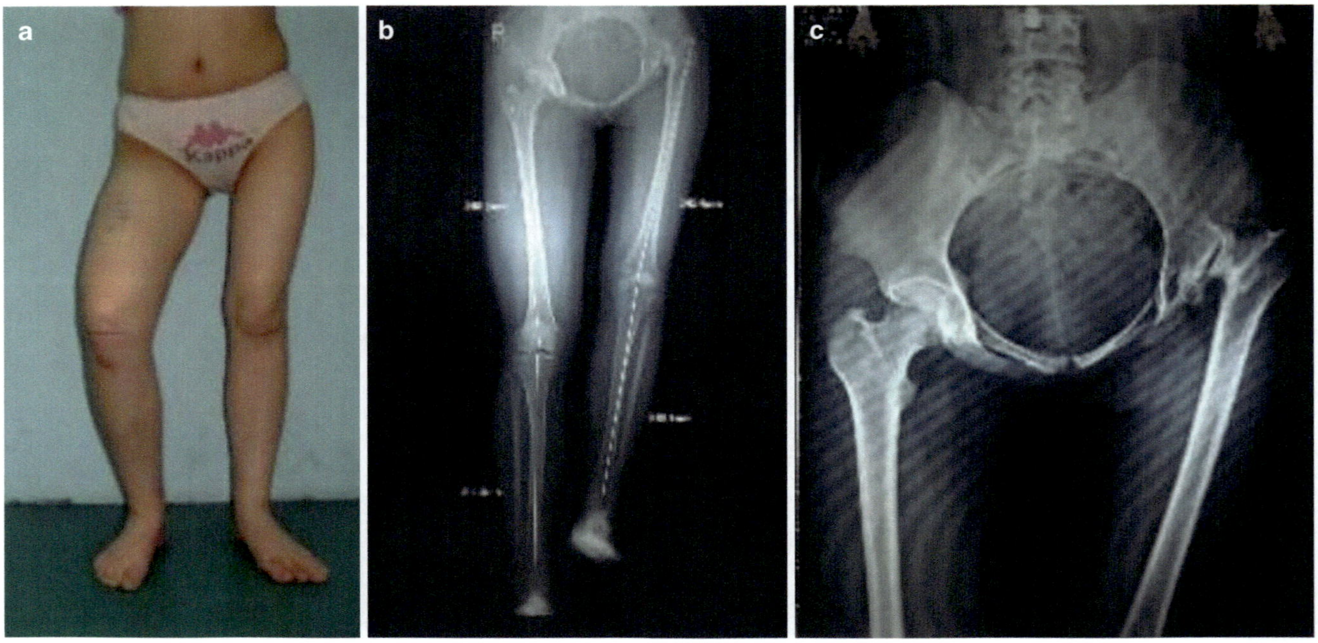

Fig. 9.8 (**a**) Absence of the femoral head caused by pyogenic infection of the left hip joint in infancy. Gross radiographs of both lower extremities; (**b**) Full-length anteroposterior radiographs of both lower extremities; (**c**) Anteroposterior radiograph of pelvis

9.2 Viral Infection

9.2.1 Sequelae of Poliomyelitis

9.2.1.1 Etiology

Post-poliomyelitis Sequelae is an acute infectious disease caused by poliovirus (a neurotropic virus), which infects the anterior horn cells of the spinal cord and some motor nuclei of the brainstem. It is characterized by flaccid paralysis of the limbs after fever, and some patients are left with lifelong disability. The virus is mainly transmitted by fecal-oral route. It mainly damages the motor nerve cells in the anterior horn of the spinal cord. From the cross section of the spinal cord, the anterior horn cells are gray, so it is called poliomyelitis. At the time of onset, more than 85% of infants are 3 months to 3 years old, so it is commonly known as polio. Two years after the onset of the disease, the remaining limb paralysis is no longer improved, and the limb deformity gradually appears, which is called the sequela of poliomyelitis or poliomyelitis.

9.2.1.2 Clinical Manifestation

In the acute stage of infection, the main manifestations are cold-like symptoms with fever, followed by sudden onset of limb paralysis, most common in the lower limbs, but also in the upper limbs. After treatment, the limb paralysis gradually began to recover to varying degrees. In the sequelae stage, limb paralysis recovers to a certain level after 2 years of onset, and there is no further improvement. Due to the imbalance of muscle strength, bone and joint deformities gradually appear and may gradually aggravate.

Common deformities include various degrees of muscle atrophy of the limbs, scoliosis, pelvic tilt, hip dislocation, knee flexion contracture, knee recurvation (Fig. 9.9), talipes equinovarus, talipes equinovarus (Fig. 9.10), talipes equinovarus, calcaneus, etc. The above deformities can occur alone or in combination (Fig. 9.11). And because of the different degree of muscle paralysis and the different parts of the combined deformity, there are different walking gaits, such as typical gaits such as point foot limp, thigh pressing gait (Fig. 9.12), unilateral limb suspension with double crutches, squatting (Fig. 9.13), crawling, and so on.

Common lower limb deformities in sequelae of poliomyelitis:

9.2.1.3 Treatment Principle

The main treatment principles of orthopedic surgery include: (1) correcting the deformity of lower limbs and restoring the gravity line of lower limbs; (2) Balancing muscle strength to prevent the recurrence of deformity caused by imbalance of muscle strength; (3) Balancing the length of both lower limbs and reducing the limping gait caused by unequal length of limbs; (4) The facet joints of the ankle were stabilized by arthrodesis to facilitate weight-bearing walking.

9.2.2 Limb Paralysis Caused by Hand-Foot-Mouth Disease

9.2.2.1 Etiology

Hand-foot-mouth disease (HFMD) is an infectious disease caused by enterovirus. There are more than 20 types of

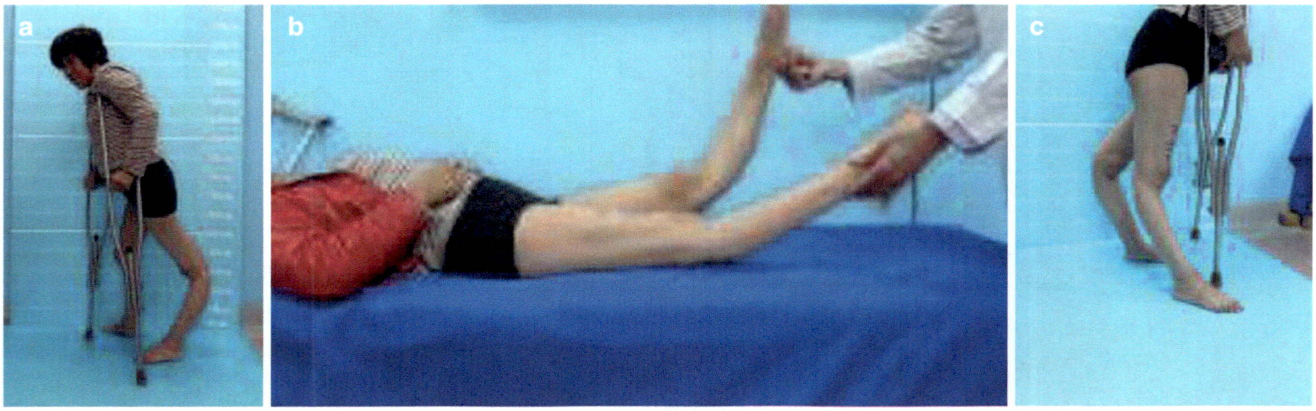

Fig. 9.9 Genu recurvatum deformity after poliomyelitis. (**a**) Gross view of both lower extremities (weight-bearing); (**b**) Gross view of both lower extremities; (**c**) Gross view of both lower extremities in profile (weight-bearing)

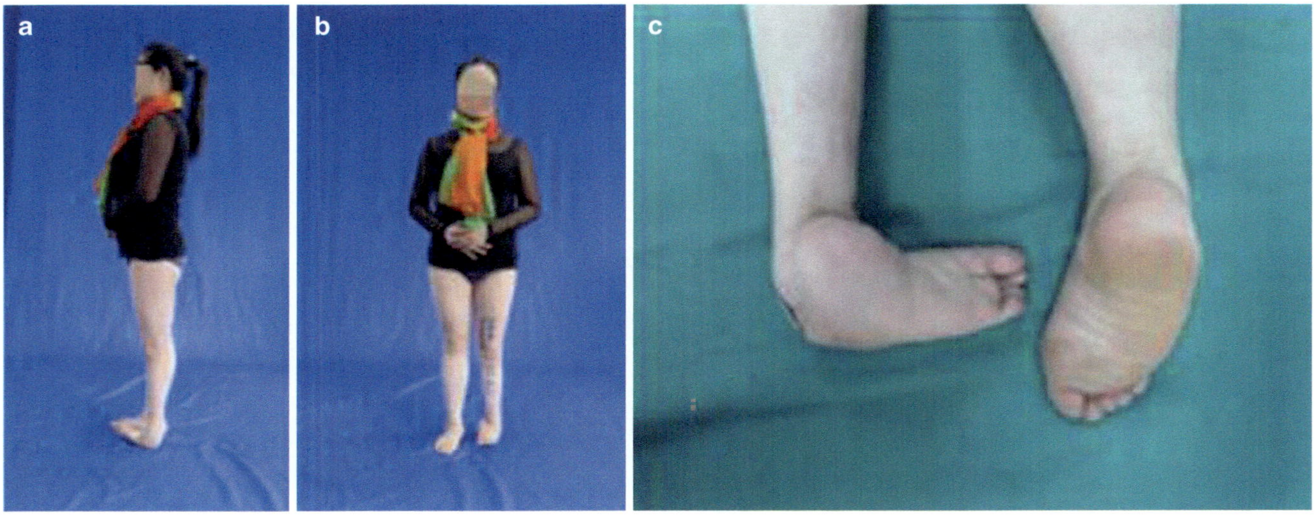

Fig. 9.10 Left varus deformity after poliomyelitis. (**a**) Gross view of both lower extremities (weight-bearing); (**b**) General view of the front of both lower limbs (weight-bearing); (**c**) Generally viewed from the back of both feet

enterovirus causing HFMD, among which Coxsackievirus A16 (Cox A16) and Enterovirus 71 (EV71) are the most common. Most of them occur in children under 5 years old, manifested as mouth pain, anorexia, low fever, small herpes or ulcers in hands, feet, mouth, and other parts. A few cases are in critical condition, which can lead to death. A few cases may have central nervous system damage, which mostly occurs within 1–5 days of the course of the disease. Surviving cases may have sequelae.

9.2.2.2 Clinical Manifestation

Nervous system involvement is characterized by poor spirit, lethargy, weakness in sucking, fright, headache, vomiting, irritability, limb shaking, muscle weakness, neck stiffness, etc. A small number of neurological sequelae are left, and the main clinical manifestations are lower motor neuron injury, mainly including changes in muscle strength and muscle tension, muscle atrophy or rigidity (Fig. 9.14); spinal curvature and pelvic tilt may occur. Hip joint dislocation, femoral deformity, knee joint flexion deformity, retroflexion deformity, foot varus, and valgus deformity (Figs. 9.15 and 9.16) may occur in long-term weight-bearing walking. Long-term walking in abnormal state may aggravate the progress of deformity and cause compound deformity (Fig. 9.17).

9.2.2.3 Treatment Principle

The main treatment principles of orthopedic surgery include: (1) correcting the deformity of lower limbs and restoring the gravity line of lower limbs; (2) Balancing muscle strength to prevent the recurrence of deformity caused by imbalance of muscle strength; (3) Balancing the length of both lower limbs and reducing the limping gait caused by unequal length of limbs; (4) The facet joints of the ankle were stabilized by arthrodesis to facilitate weight-bearing walking.

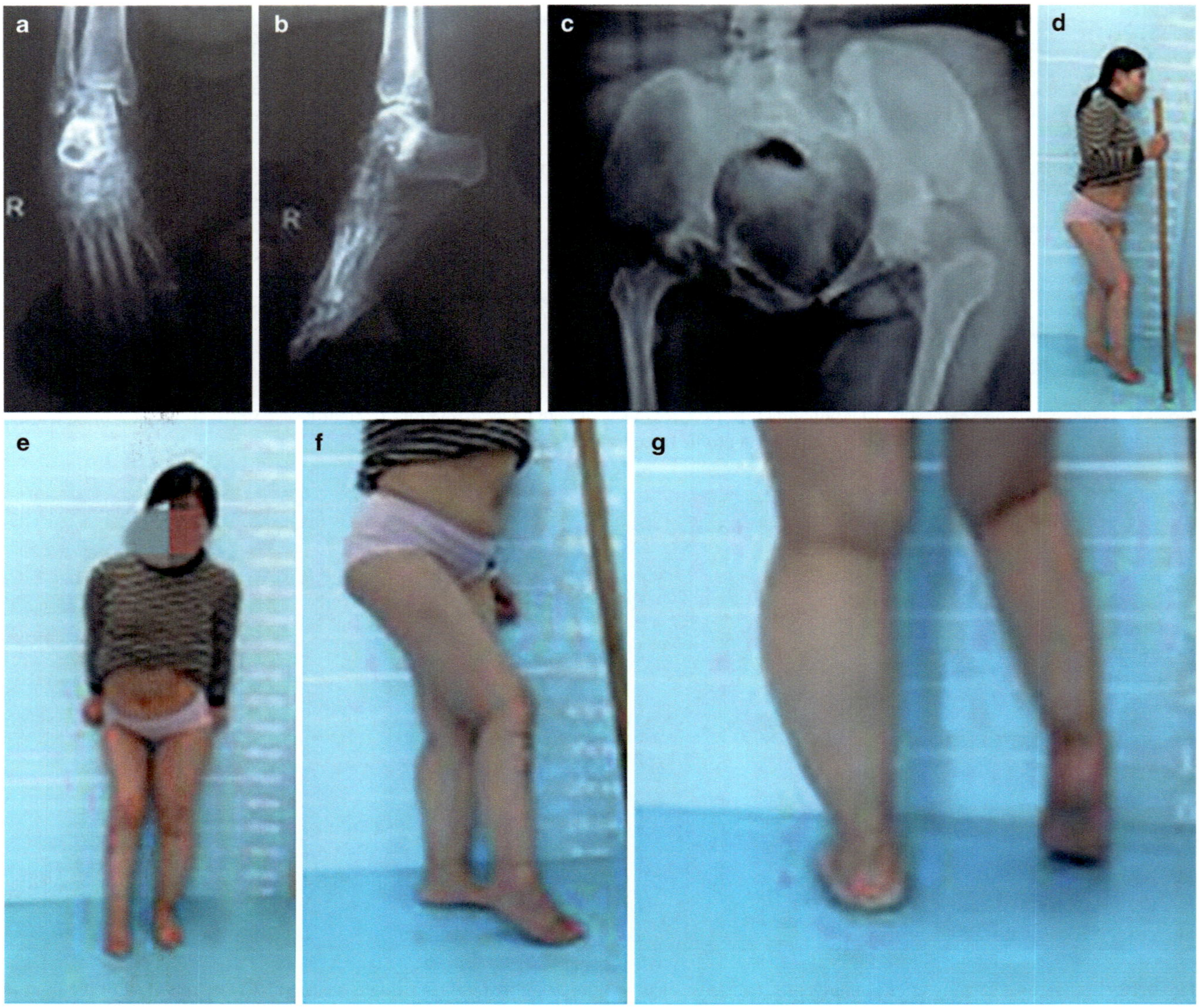

Fig. 9.11 Equinovarus deformity of right lower limb after poliomyelitis. Anteroposterior radiographs of right ankle joint of (**a**). X; lateral radiographs of right ankle joint of (**b**). X; anteroposterior radiographs of pelvis of (**c**). X; (**d**) Gross view of both lower extremities; (**e**) Front view of both lower extremities; (**f**) Gross view of both lower extremities in profile; (**g**) Gross view of the posterior aspect of both lower extremities

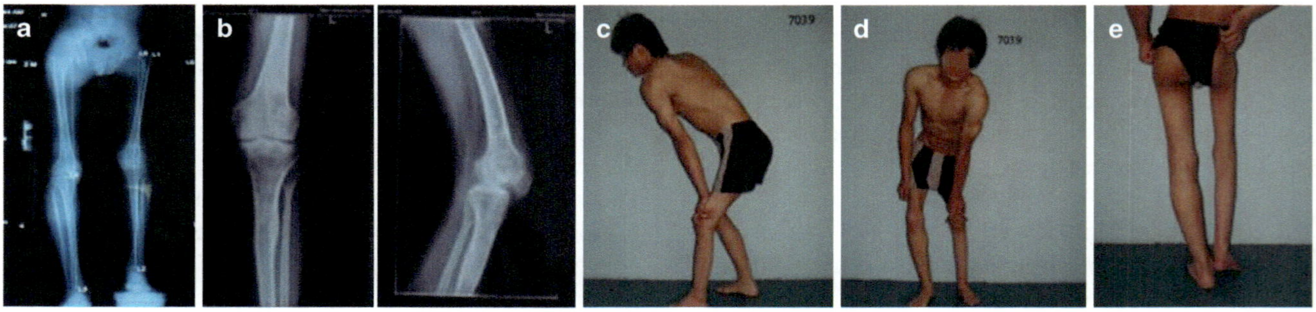

Fig. 9.12 Limp gait of left lower limb after poliomyelitis. Frontal radiographs of the whole length of both lower extremities of the (**a**). X; Frontal radiographs of the left knee joint of the (**b**). X; Lateral radiographs of the left knee joint of the (**c**). X; (**d**) Gross view of both lower extremities; (**e**) General view of the front of both lower limbs; (**f**) Gross view of the posterior aspect of both lower extremities

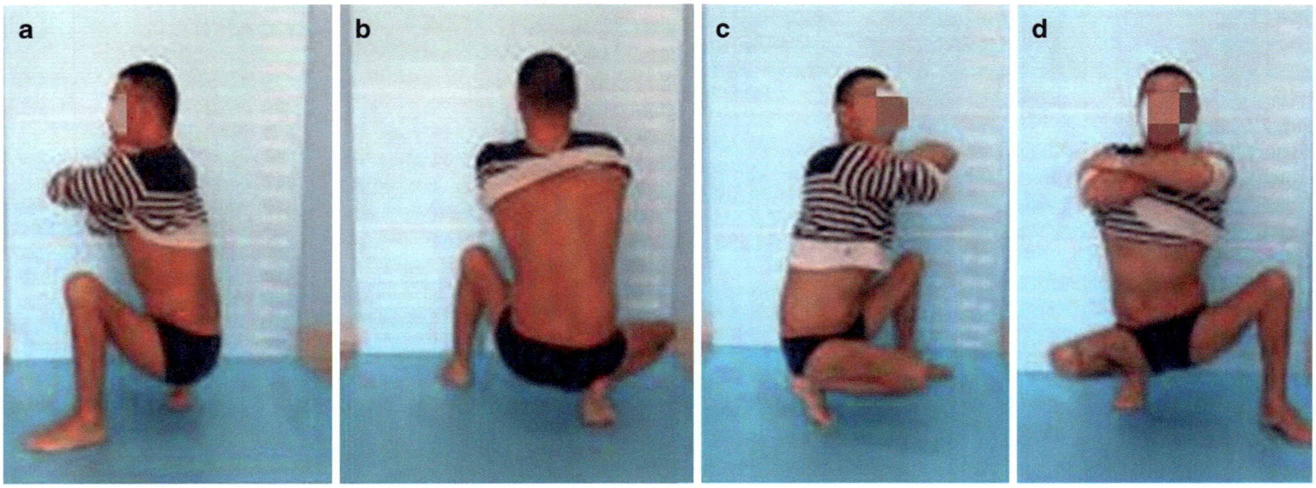

Fig. 9.13 Squat gait of deformity of both lower limbs after poliomyelitis. (**a**) Gross view of both lower limbs in squatting position; (**b**) General view from the back of both lower limbs in squatting position; (**c**) Macroscopically, the lower limbs were viewed from the side in squatting position. (**d**) The general view is the front view of both lower limbs in squatting position

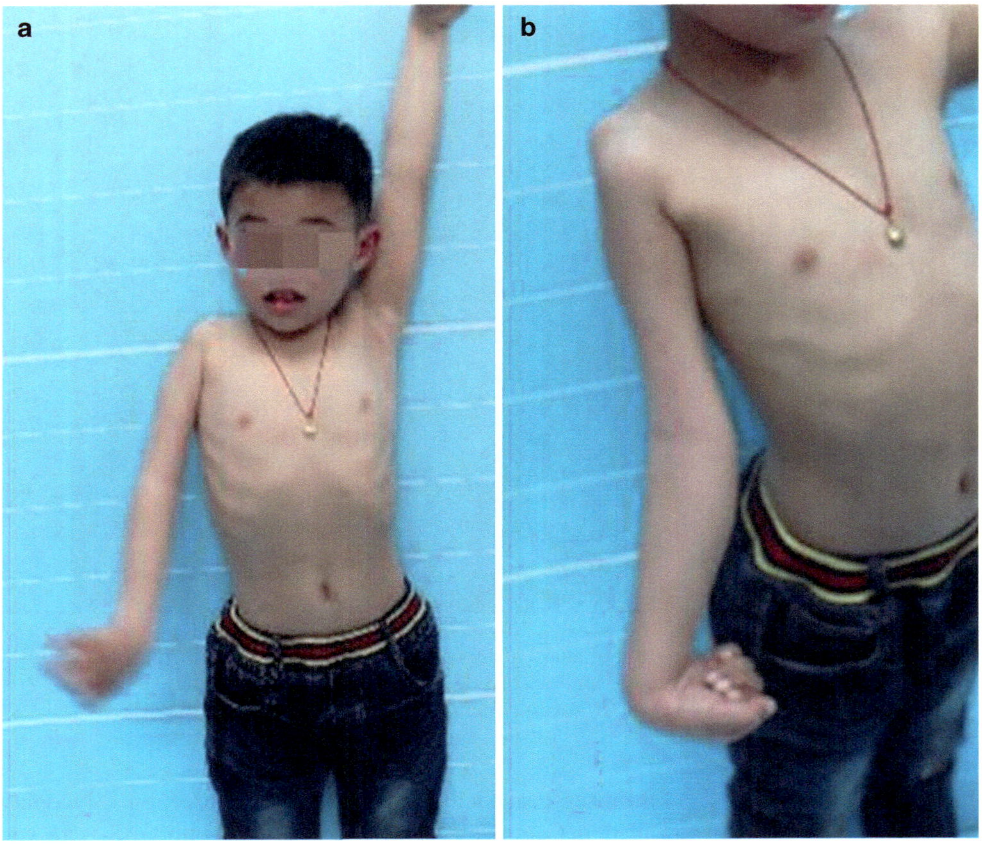

Fig. 9.14 Right upper limb deformity after hand, foot and mouth disease, male patient, 8 years old, 1 and half years old, suffered from hand, foot, and mouth disease, with incomplete paralysis of right upper limb: (**a**) Appearance: front view of right upper limb; (**b**) Exterior view of the right upper limb in profile

9.2.3 Guillain-Barre Sequelae

Guillain-Barré syndrome (GBS) is an autoimmune peripheral neuropathy pathologically characterized by demyelination of peripheral nerves and nerve roots and infiltration of inflammatory cells in small blood vessels. The classic GBS is called acute inflammatory demyelinating polyneuropathy (AIDP). The clinical manifestation was acute symmetrical flaccid paralysis.

9.2.3.1 Etiology

The etiology has not been fully elucidated. About 70% of patients with GBS had a history of prodromal infection within 8 weeks before the onset of the disease, usually

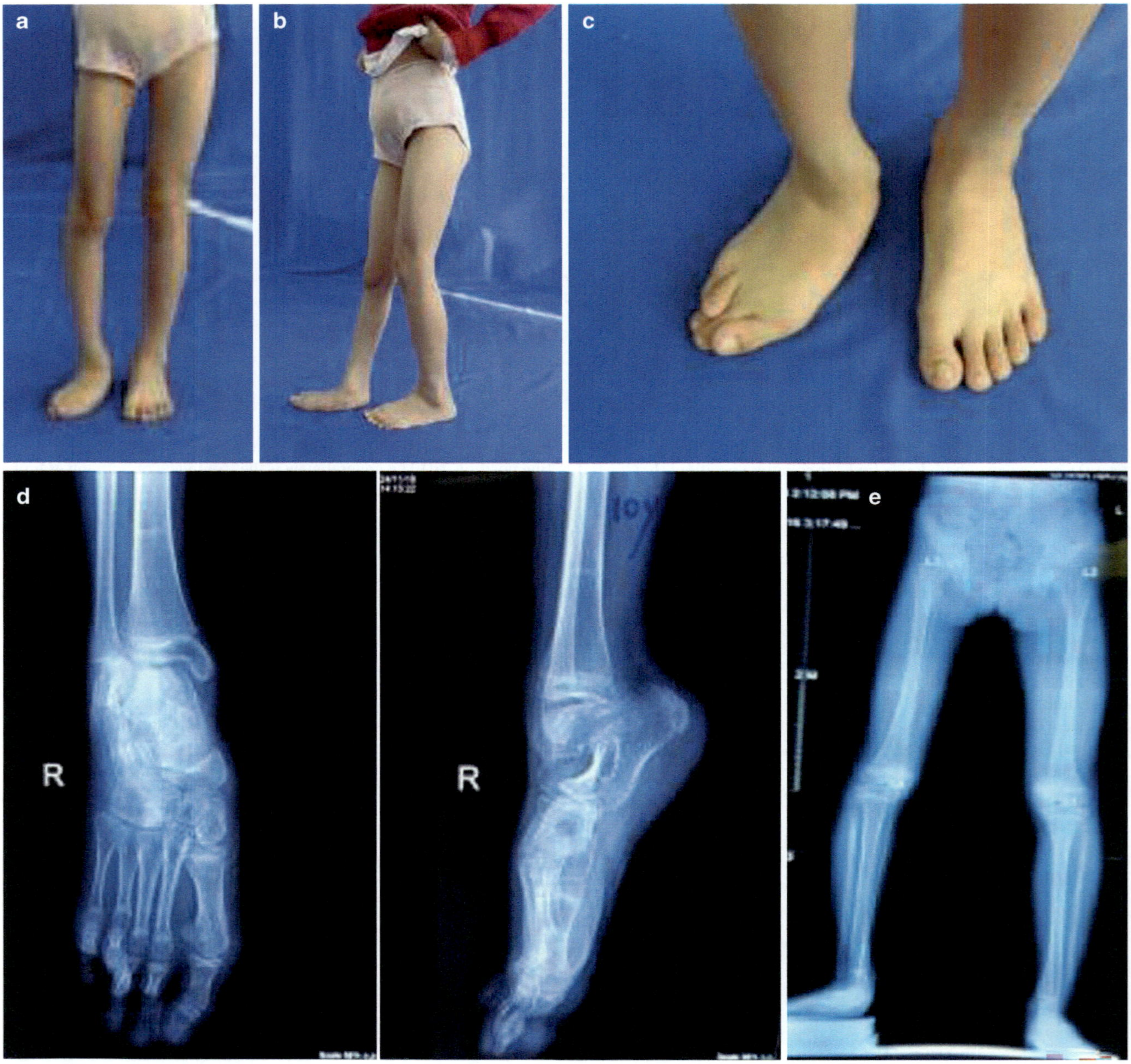

Fig. 9.15 Valgus deformity of right foot after hand-foot-mouth disease. (**a**) Anterior view of both lower extremities; (**b**) Side view of both lower limbs; (**c**) Bipedal anterior view; (**d**) Anteroposterior and lateral X-ray film of right ankle; (**e**) Full-length lateral radiograph of right lower extremity

1–2 weeks before the onset of the disease, and a few patients had a history of surgery or vaccination. Campylobacter jejuni (CJ) infection is the most common, accounting for about 30%. The infection rate of CJ in GBS patients with diarrhea as a prodromal symptom is as high as 85%, which is often related to acute motor axonal neuropathy (AMAN). Cytomegalovirus (CMV) infection is associated with severe sensory GBS, and a cluster of CMV-infected GBS has been observed. GBS occurring around the onset of infectious mononucleosis is often associated with Epstein–Barr virus (EBV) infection. Mycoplasma pneumoniae (MP)-infected patients with GBS were younger. The incidence of GBS in patients with HBV infection was significantly higher than that in patients without HBV infection.

9.2.3.2 Clinical Manifestation

The main symptoms are acute progressive symmetrical limb flaccid paralysis, subjective sensory disturbance, and weakening or disappearance of tendon reflexes. Limb tardive paralysis is the most important symptom of this disease,

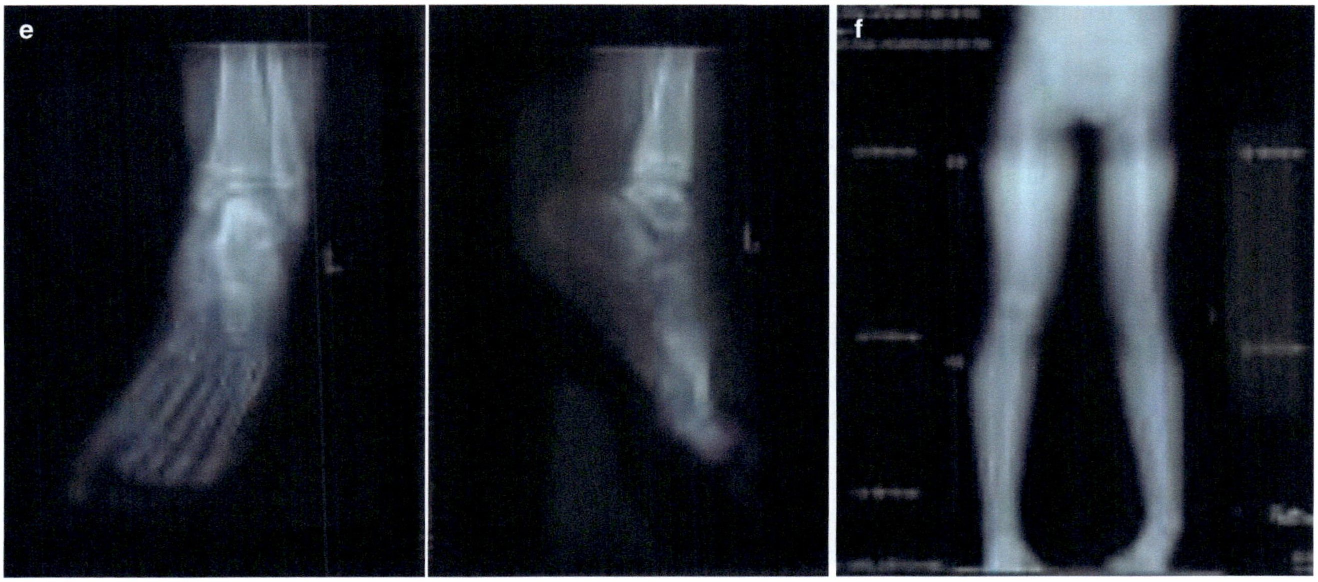

Fig. 9.16 Left foot varus deformity caused by sequelae of hand-foot-mouth disease. (**a**) Anterior view of both lower extremities; (**b**) Lateral view of both lower limbs; (**c**) Posterior view of both lower extremities; (**d**) Lateral view of left lower limb; (**e**) Anteroposterior and lateral X-ray film of left ankle; (**f**) Full-length anteroposterior radiographs of both lower extremities

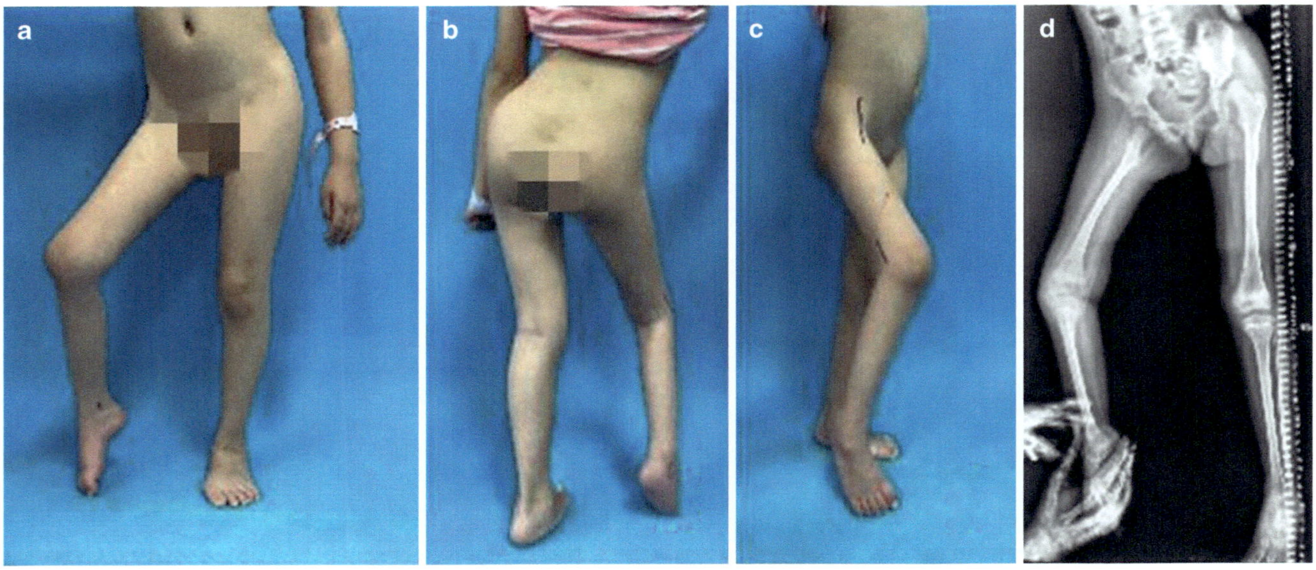

Fig. 9.17 A 5-year-old female patient with right lower limb deformity after hand-foot-and-mouth disease suffered from hand-foot-and-mouth disease at the age of 19 months, with secondary deformity of right hip flexion, knee flexion and talipes equinovarus: (**a**) Anterior view of both lower extremities; (**b**) Posterior view of both lower extremities; (**c**) Side view of both lower limbs; (**d**) Full-length lateral X-ray film of right lower limb

which generally starts from the lower limbs and gradually affects the trunk, upper limbs and cranial nerves, and the proximal end of hypotonia is often heavier than the distal end. In critical cases, complete paralysis of limbs, paralysis of respiratory and swallowing muscles, dyspnea, and swallowing disorders endanger life. Sensory disorders are generally milder than motor disorders, but common limb paresthesias, such as numbness, tingling, burning, etc., may precede or coincide with paralysis, and vibration and joint movement are usually preserved. Tendon reflexes of the four limbs were mostly symmetrically weakened or disappeared, cremaster reflexes of the abdominal wall were mostly normal, and a few patients had pathological reflex signs due to pyramidal tract involvement (Fig. 9.18).

According to the case of Qin Sihe orthopedic surgery database (time: 1978.05.25–2018.12.31; Total number of cases: 35075 cases) statistics, a total of 83 patients with Guillain-Barré syndrome were treated, including 55 male patients and 28 female patients, with a mean age of 20.2 years.

9.2.3.3 Classification

The most common subtypes of GBS are acute inflammatory demyelinating polyradiculoneuropathy (AIDP) and acute motor axonal neuropathy (AMAN). The second was Miller-Fisher syndrome (MFS), which was characterized by ophthalmoplegia, ataxia, and loss of deep tendon reflexes.

9.2.3.4 Treatment Principle

Orthopedic treatment is mainly aimed at the lower limb dysfunction caused by delayed paralysis and joint instability caused by GBS. The treatment principle is to correct defor-

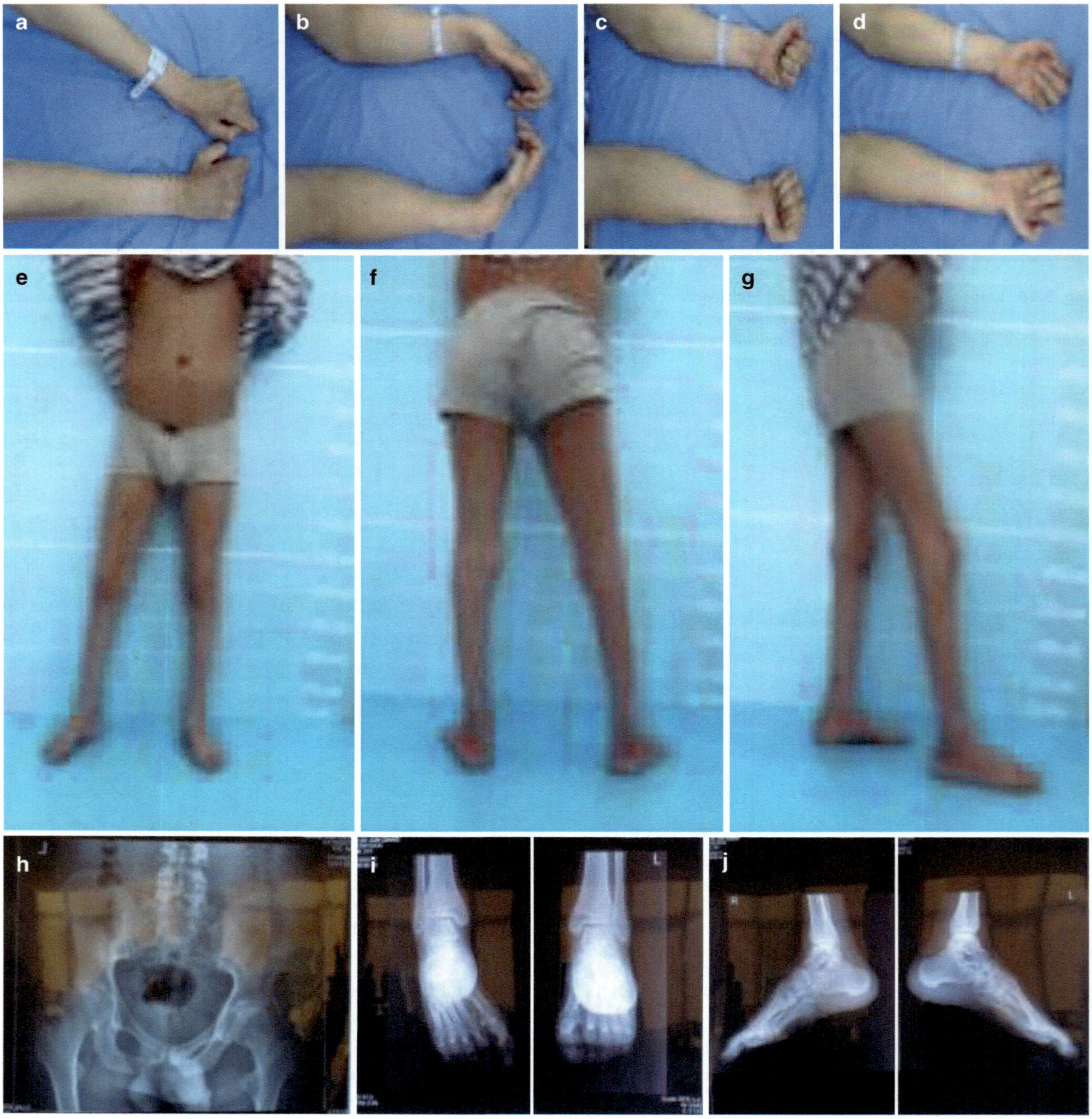

Fig. 9.18 Guillain-Barre Sequelae. (**a**) Gross dorsal view of both wrist joints; (**b**) Gross observation of bilateral wrist flexion position; (**c**) General view of flexion of metacarpophalangeal joints of both hands; (**d**) General view of metacarpophalangeal joints of both hands in extension position; (**e**) Gross view from the front of both lower extremities; (**f**) Gross posterior view of both lower extremities; (**g**) General view of lower limbs; Pelvic anteroposterior radiographs of (**h**). X; Anteroposterior radiographs of (**i**). X; (**j**) Lateral X-ray films of both feet and ankles

mity, balance muscle strength, stabilize joints, restore the gravity line of lower limbs, and improve standing and walking function.

9.2.4 Sequelae of Epidemic Encephalitis B

9.2.4.1 Etiology

Japanese B encephalitis (also called Japanese B encephalitis epidemic encephalitis B) is a central nervous system infectious disease caused by Japanese encephalitis virus infection. The pathogen was discovered in Japan in 1934, also known as Japanese B encephalitis. The disease is mainly distributed in the Far East and Southeast Asia, transmitted by mosquitoes, mostly in summer and autumn.

9.2.4.2 Clinical Manifestation

Clinically, the disease is acute onset, with high fever, disturbance of consciousness, convulsion, tonic spasm, meningeal irritation sign, etc. It belongs to blood infectious disease. Severe patients often have sequelae after illness, with spastic deformity of limbs (Fig. 9.19), similar to limb deformity of cerebral palsy.

9.2.4.3 Classification

According to the severity of the disease, Japanese encephalitis can be divided into four types:

Mild: The patient's consciousness is always awake, but there are varying degrees of lethargy, generally without convulsions (individual children with convulsions due to high fever). The body temperature is between 38 °C and 39 °C, and most of them recover within 1 week. The diagnosis is often confirmed by cerebrospinal fluid and serological examination.

Common model: Consciousness disorders occur, such as coma or light coma, disappearance of abdominal wall reflex and cremaster reflex, and there may be short-term convulsions. The body temperature is generally about 40 °C, the course of disease is about 10 days, and there are no sequelae.

Severe: Body temperature continues to be above 40 °C, coma, and repeated or persistent convulsions. Superficial reflexes disappear, deep reflexes disappear first and then hyperfunction, and there are pathological reflexes. There are often localized symptoms and signs. Central respiratory failure may occur. The course of the disease is often more than 2 weeks, and the recovery period often has different degrees of mental disorders and paralysis, and some patients have sequelae.

Fulminant type: body temperature rises rapidly, showing high fever or excessive high fever, accompanied by repeated or persistent strong convulsions, deep coma occurs within 1–2 days, with pupil changes, cerebral hernia and central respiratory failure, and other manifestations, if not rescued in time, often due to respiratory failure and death. Survivors have severe sequelae.

9.2.4.4 Treatment Principle

Orthopedic treatment is mainly aimed at limb spasms, dyskinesia, and limb deformities similar to cerebral palsy caused by Japanese encephalitis virus invading the nervous system. The principle of treatment is to correct deformity, restore the gravity line of lower limbs, relieve spasticity, stabilize joints, and improve standing and walking function.

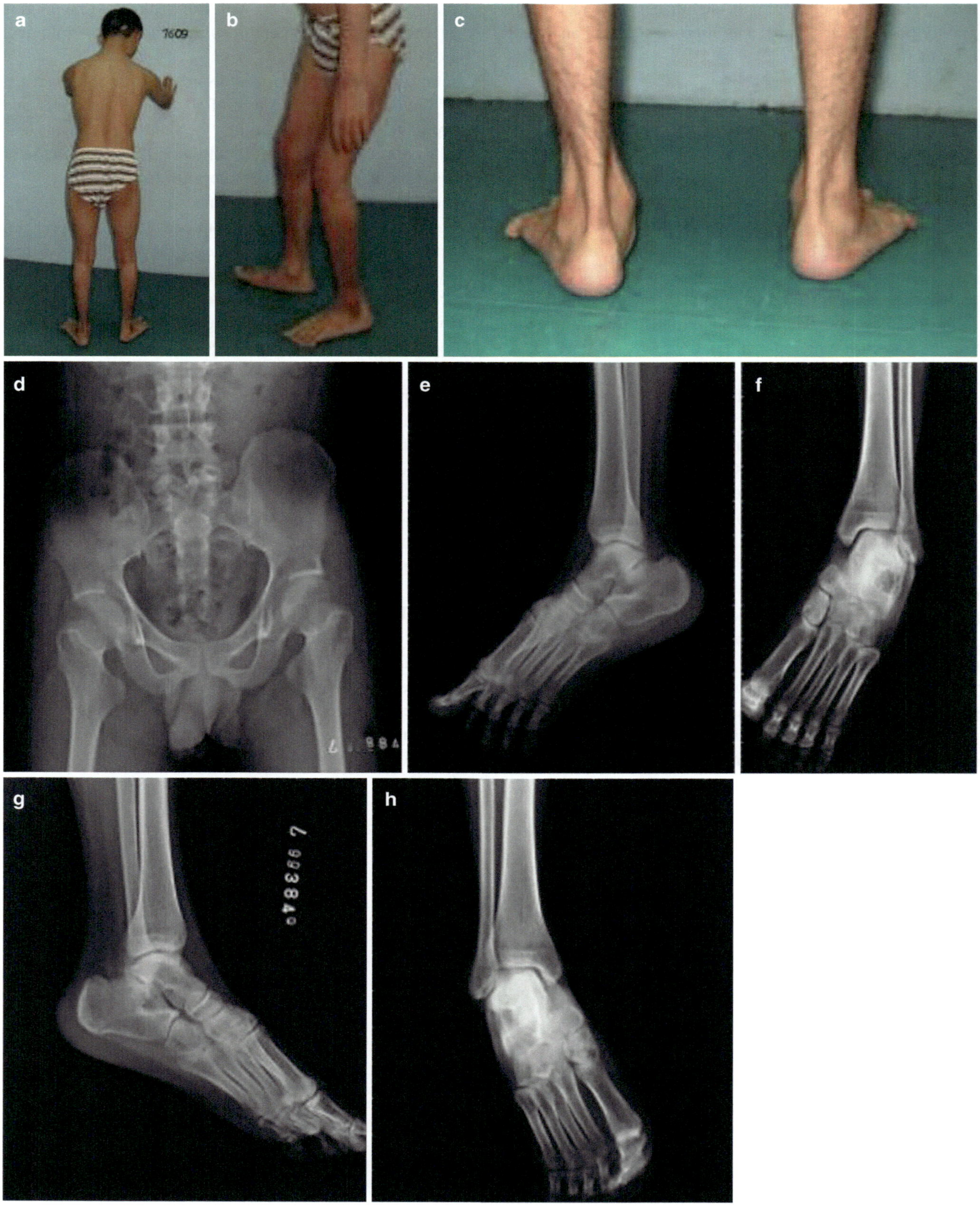

Fig. 9.19 Spastic deformity of lower limbs after epidemic encephalitis B. (**a**) Posterior view of both lower extremities; (**b**) Lateral view of both lower limbs; (**c**) Bipedal posterior view; (**d**) Anteroposterior radiograph of pelvis; (**e**) Lateral X-ray film of left ankle; (**f**) Anteroposterior radiograph of left ankle; (**g**) Lateral X-ray film of right ankle; (**h**) Anteroposterior X-ray of right ankle

10 Post-Traumatic Limb Deformity

Sihe Qin, Shaofeng Jiao, and Baofeng Guo

10.1 Limb Deformity after Nerve Injury

10.1.1 Craniocerebral Injury

10.1.1.1 Sequelae of Brain Trauma (Traffic Accident, Fall Injury)

Etiology

Brain trauma can be seen in high-energy injuries such as traffic accidents or falling from high places, central paralysis, increased muscle tension of limbs, or long-term coma and bed rest, leading to limb deformities.

Clinical Manifestations

The muscle tension of the limbs is increased, and the motor function is weakened or mostly lost. Some patients have fixed deformity of the limbs due to delayed rehabilitation training after injury, resulting in muscle contracture. The lower limbs are often secondary to hip flexion, knee flexion or equinus deformity. Those with severe multi-joint deformity lose the condition of independent walking and can only rely on wheelchairs (Fig. 10.1).

Treatment Principles

Correct deformity of lower limbs, release contracture of soft tissue, reduce muscle tension, stabilize joints, restore gravity line of lower limbs, combine rehabilitation training and orthosis, restore standing and walking function.

S. Qin (✉)
Department of Orthopaedics, Rehabilitation Hospital of the National Research Center for Rehabilitation Technical Aids, Beijing, China

S. Jiao
Department of Orthopaedics, Rehabilitation Hospital, National Research Center for Rehabilitation, Beijing, China

B. Guo
Department of Orthopedics, Chuiyangliu Hospital affiliated to Tsinghua University, Beijing, China

10.1.1.2 Sequelae of Brain Tissue Injury Caused by Craniocerebral Operation

Etiology

Craniocerebral surgery may cause brain tissue injury, involving the motor center or motor conduction pathway, resulting in limb motor dysfunction, increased muscle tension, weakened muscle strength, and secondary bone and joint deformities in the corresponding parts of the limbs.

Clinical Manifestations

After craniocerebral surgery, limb motor dysfunction, increased muscle tension, weakened or lost muscle strength occurred. In the process of rehabilitation, the fixed deformities of the limbs gradually appeared. The most common deformities of the lower limbs were hip adduction, knee flexion deformity, and equinovarus or valgus deformity of the foot and ankle (Fig. 10.2).

Treatment Principles

Improve muscle spasm of lower limbs, reduce muscle tension, release contracture of fascia and tendon, stabilize hind foot joints, and improve walking function combined with rehabilitation training.

10.1.2 Spinal Cord Injury

10.1.2.1 Incomplete Paraplegia after High Spinal Cord Injury

Etiology

Spinal trauma above the thoracic spine, intraspinal tumors, abscesses, and other diseases can cause cervicothoracic spinal cord injury, resulting in spastic paralysis of limbs below the injured segment, and long-term development of limb deformities.

S. Qin et al. (eds.), *Atlas of Limb Deformity*, https://doi.org/10.1007/978-981-97-0999-1_10

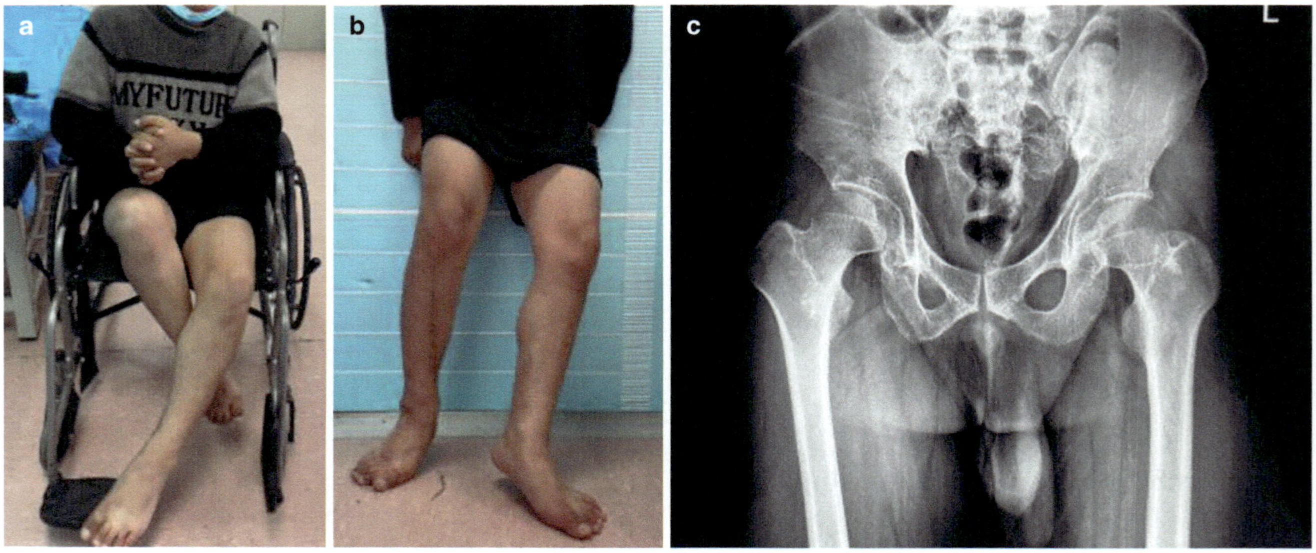

Fig. 10.1 Deformity of lower limbs caused by sequelae of traumatic brain injury. (**a**) In wheelchair, muscle tension of limbs increased, bilateral hip flexion and knee flexion femoral adduction contracture; (**b**) Barely standing against the wall, hip and knee flexion, horseshoe deformity; (**c**) The bony relationship of the hip joint was normal on the anteroposterior X-ray of the pelvis

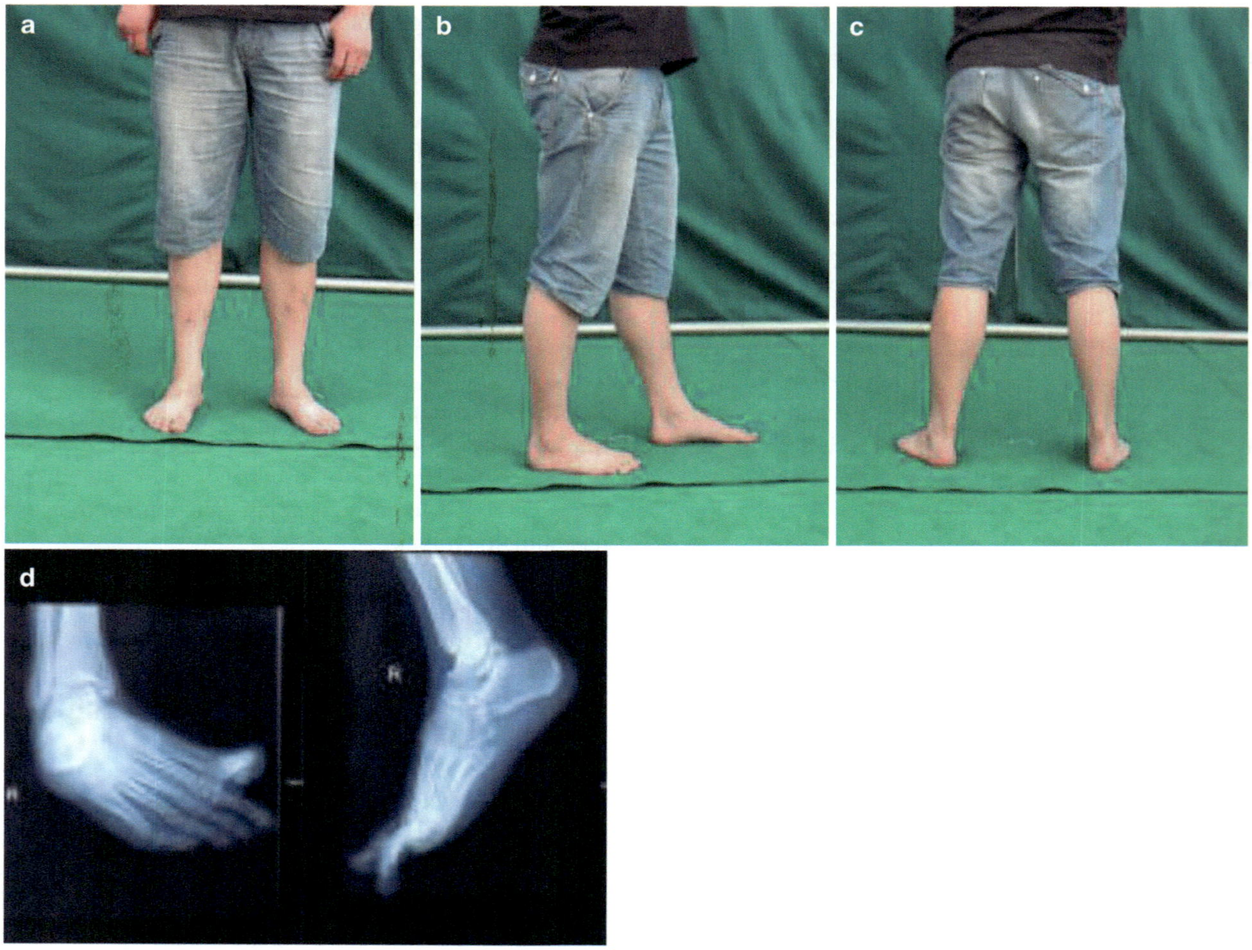

Fig. 10.2 The patient underwent intracranial germ cell tumor resection. After the operation, the patient developed spastic varus deformity of the right foot. However, after standing still for a period of time, the varus deformity of the foot could be corrected naturally. (**a**) Front view of both lower limbs standing; (**b**) Standing lateral view of the lower extremity (**c**) View from the back of standing lower limbs; (**d**) X-ray examination of the right ankle showed varus foot

Clinical Manifestations

The levels of motor, sensory, reflex, and autonomic nerve dysfunction were different in different levels of spinal cord injury. The sensory of the innervated area below the level of spinal cord injury was weakened or even completely lost. Some muscles of the lower limbs have hard or soft paralysis, increased muscle tension, weakened or lost muscle strength, and secondary deformities of the lower limbs, such as foot and ankle deformities, such as talipes equinovarus, talipes valgus, and calcaneus (Fig. 10.3).

Treatment Principles

Correct the deformity of the ankle, balance the muscle strength, and if necessary, perform ankle arthrodesis to restore the plantar foot and increase the weight-bearing stability of the foot.

10.1.2.2 Sequelae of Lumbar Spinal Cord Injury

Etiology

In the process of high-energy traffic accident, incomplete or complete injury of lumbar spinal cord is caused by hyperextension, hyperflexion, rotation, and separation of lumbar spine, which leads to severe dysfunction of limbs below the injured segment and long-term development of limb deformity.

Clinical Manifestations

The sense of the innervated area below the level of spinal cord injury is weakened or completely lost, some muscles of the lower limbs are paralyzed or paralyzed, the muscle tension is increased, the muscle strength is weakened or lost, and the deformity of the lower limbs is secondary, which is more common in the ankle deformity, such as talipes equinovarus, talipes valgus, calcaneus, etc. (Fig. 10.4).

Treatment Principles

The treatment is aimed at the limb deformity caused by incomplete paralysis after spinal cord injury, so as to correct the deformity, balance the muscle strength of joints, stabilize joints, restore the gravity line of lower limbs, and improve the standing and walking function in combination with rehabilitation training. If the deformity is extremely serious, it is recommended to install artificial limbs after amputation.

10.1.2.3 Incomplete Paralysis of both Lower Limbs Caused by Shotgun Injury to the Lumbar Spinal Cord

Etiology

Incomplete or complete injury of the lumbar spinal cord is caused by a shotgun shot in the waist, resulting in severe sensory and motor dysfunction of the limbs below the spinal cord injury segment, and long-term secondary bone and joint deformities.

Clinical Manifestations

The sense of the innervated area below the level of spinal cord injury is weakened or completely lost, some muscles of the lower limbs are paralyzed or paralyzed, the muscle tension is increased, the muscle strength is weakened or lost, and the deformity of the lower limbs is secondary, which is more common in the ankle deformity, such as talipes equinovarus, talipes valgus, calcaneus, etc. (Fig. 10.5).

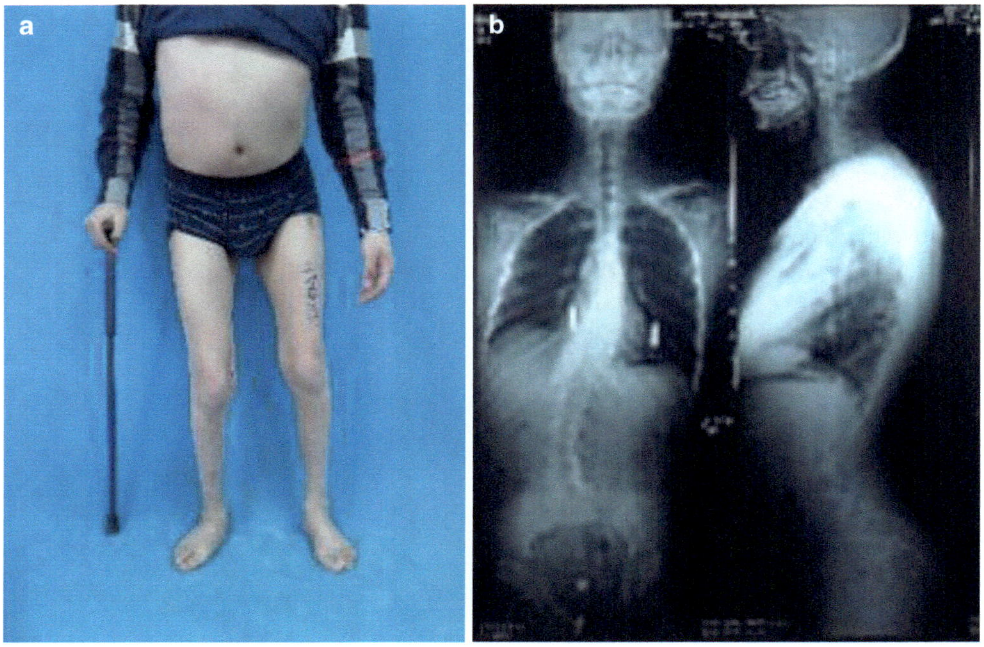

Fig. 10.3 High spinal cord injury and incomplete paraplegia caused by traffic accident. (**a**) Both lower limbs standing in front view; (**b**) Full-length anteroposterior and lateral radiographs of the spine

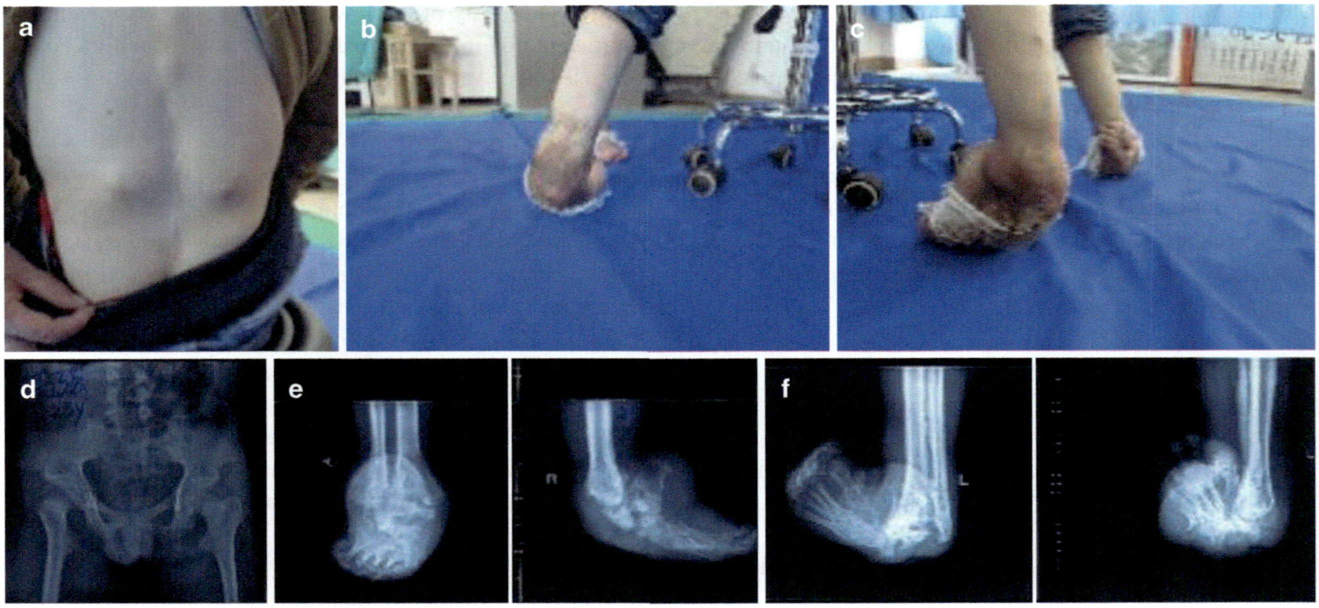

Fig. 10.4 Sequelae of lumbar spinal cord injury caused by traffic accident. (**a**) Lumbodorsal posterior view showing spinal injury site; (**b**) Complete retroversion deformity of the standing foot; (**c**) Lateral view of the affected foot; (**d**) Anteroposterior radiograph of pelvis; (**e, f**) Bilateral ankle radiographs showed the degree of bony deformity of the ankle

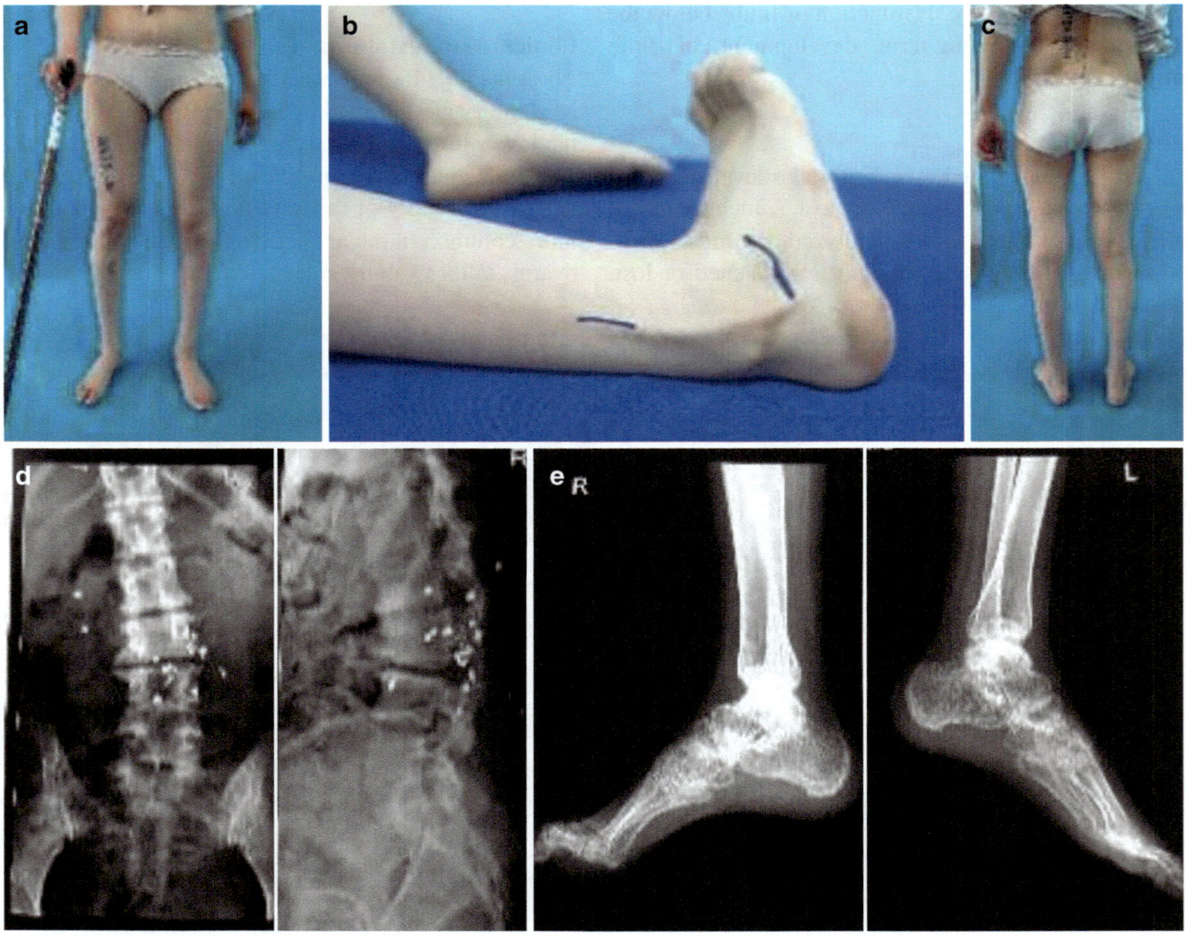

Fig. 10.5 Incomplete paralysis of both lower limbs caused by shotgun injury to lumbar spinal cord. (**a**) Standing and viewing from the front; (**b**) The right foot shows a calcaneal varus foot; (**c**) Back and lower extremity posterior view; (**d**) Thoracolumbar spine anteroposterior and lateral X-ray films showed that a large number of metal sand particles remained in the body. (**e**) Lateral X-ray film of bilateral ankle joint

Treatment Principles

The treatment is aimed at the limb deformity caused by incomplete paralysis after spinal cord injury, in order to correct the deformity, release the contracture of soft tissue, stabilize joints, restore the gravity line of lower limbs, and establish the basic function of standing and walking of lower limbs in combination with rehabilitation training.

10.1.2.4 Sequelae of Accidental Nerve Injury after Spinal Surgery

Etiology

Spinal cord or nerve roots are damaged to varying degrees due to misoperation or accidental side injury during spinal surgery, resulting in motor, sensory, reflex, and autonomic nerve dysfunction of limbs below the injured segment, and long-term development may lead to limb deformities.

Clinical Manifestations

The sensation of the area innervated by the nerve below the level of spinal cord injury was weakened or even completely lost. Rigid paralysis or flaccid paralysis occurs in some muscle groups, with secondary deformities. The paralysis of the hand is claw-shaped. Malformations of the foot and ankle are common in the lower limbs, such as talipes equinovarus, talipes valgus, and calcaneus (Fig. 10.6).

Treatment Principles

Correct deformity, balance muscle strength, restore plantar foot, increase foot weight-bearing stability, and improve walking function.

10.1.3 Peripheral Nerve Injury of Lower Limbs

10.1.3.1 Sequelae of Sciatic Nerve Injury

Etiology

The causes of injury are mostly caused by thigh or buttock stab and firearm injury, and sometimes hip dislocation and pelvic fracture can also be combined with sciatic nerve injury.

Clinical Manifestations

High sciatic nerve injury causes paralysis of the posterior femoral muscles and all the muscles of the leg and foot, resulting in complete loss of knee flexion, ankle and toe movement, and foot drop. Incomplete injury of sciatic nerve can cause muscle dynamic imbalance, knee joint or (and) ankle deformity. Such as clubfoot deformity, claw toe deformity, long-term walking under abnormal muscle strength can lead to fixed deformity and bony changes (Fig. 10.7).

Treatment Principles

Release the contracture of soft tissue, balance the muscle strength, and perform osteotomy and arthrodesis to stabilize the joint, correct the deformity of the foot and ankle, and restore the shape and function.

10.1.3.2 Sequelae of Tibial Nerve Injury

Etiology

Trauma or mechanical compression of the posterior part of the lower thigh, popliteal fossa, iatrogenic injury, etc. leads to partial or complete rupture or injury of the tibial nerve.

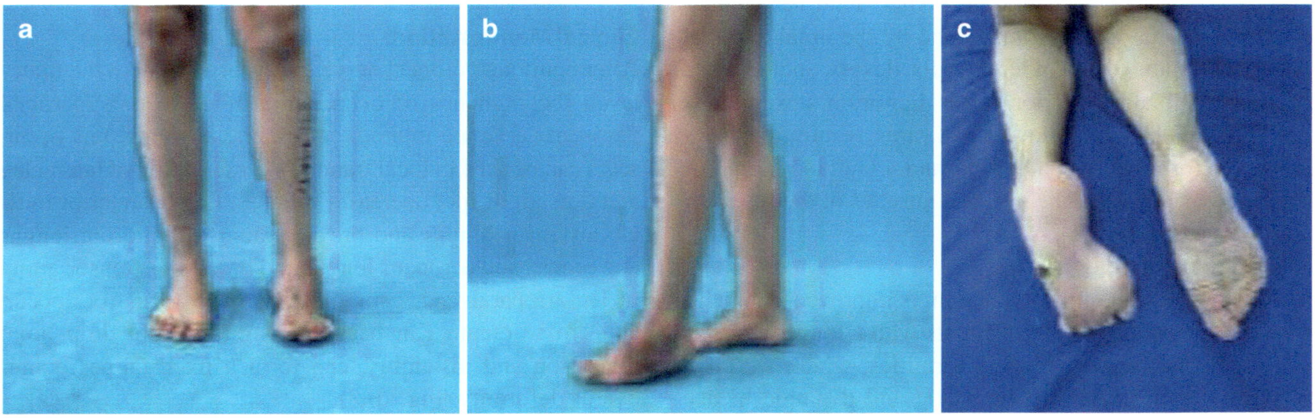

Fig. 10.6 Male, 15 years old. Spinal cord ependymoma resection was performed at the age of 10, complicated by nerve root injury, secondary to left talipes equinovarus deformity, and ulcer in the lateral weight-bearing area of the foot. (**a**) Standing and viewing from the front; (**b**) Lateral view of standing lower limbs; (**c**) Biplantar appearance

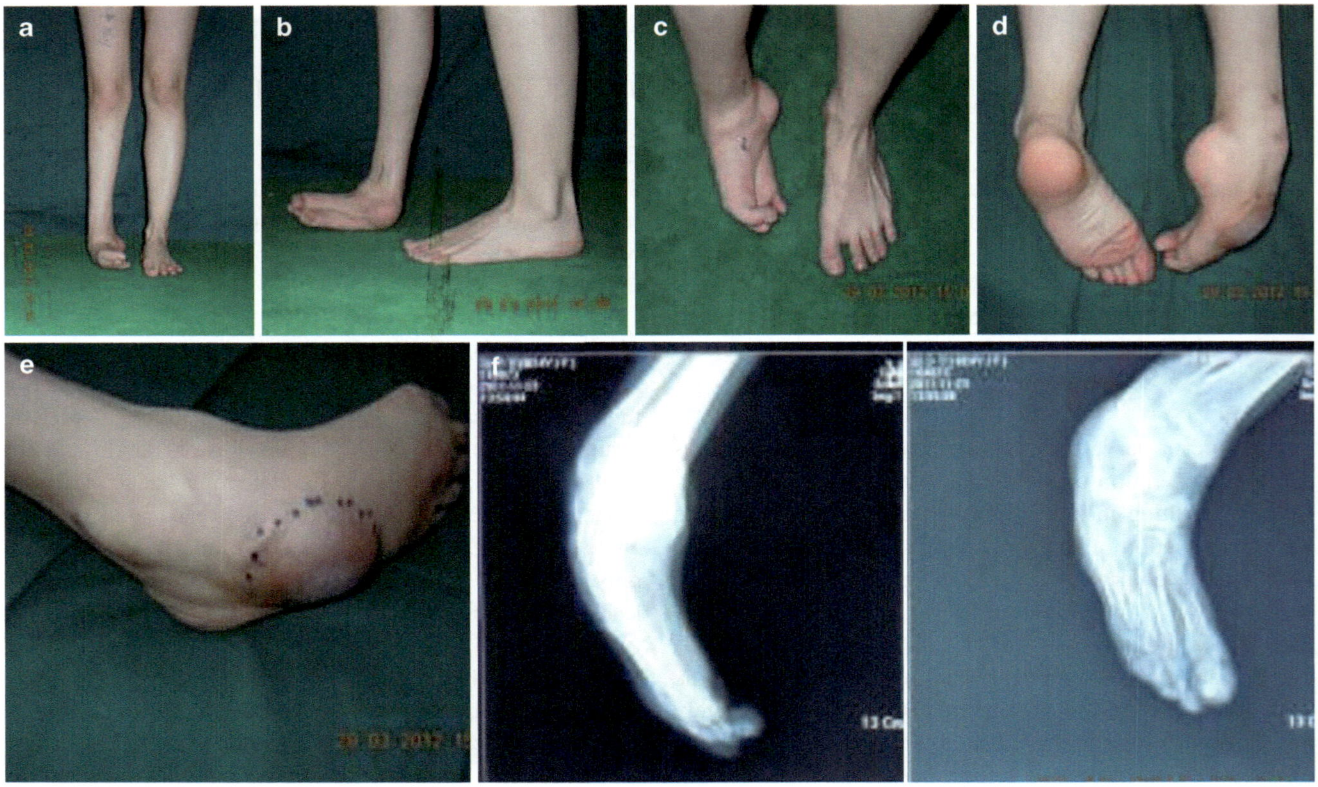

Fig. 10.7 Right talipes equinovarus caused by incomplete sciatic nerve injury. (**a**) Standing and viewing from the front; (**b**) Standing lateral view of the lower extremity (**c**). Bipedal frontal view; (**d**) Double plantar appearance; (**e**) Appearance of the lateral weight-bearing area of the right foot; (**f**) Anteroposterior and lateral radiographs of right ankle joint

Clinical Manifestations

The tibial nerve descends vertically from the sciatic nerve and descends through the popliteal fossa along the posterior middle of the leg, along which it branches to innervate the posterior leg and plantar muscles. After tibial nerve injury, all or part of the muscles innervated by the tibial nerve are paralyzed, mainly the ankle and foot flexors, including triceps surae, tibialis posterior, flexor digitorum, flexor, and so on. They cannot plantar flexion and varus, resulting in hallux valgus deformity. Arcuate foot and claw toe deformity caused by paralysis of the intrinsic muscles of the foot.

Treatment Principles

The plantar flexion of the ankle joint is improved as much as possible by tendon transfer. Patients with a longer course of disease had secondary bony deformities, which were corrected by osteotomy. Achieve static and dynamic balance and restore the function of standing and walking.

10.1.3.3 Sequelae of Common Peroneal Nerve Injury

Etiology

The common peroneal nerve is in the neck of the fibula, the location is superficial, and on the surface of the bone, the surrounding soft tissue is less, the mobility is poor, trauma, inflammation, iatrogenic, and other reasons can cause the injury of the common peroneal nerve, resulting in sensory and motor disorders in the ankle.

Clinical Manifestations

After common peroneal nerve injury, according to the injury level, the branches of deep peroneal nerve or superficial peroneal nerve are injured, corresponding symptoms occur, scars can be seen in local trauma, skin sensation of lateral leg and dorsum of foot decreases or loses, tibialis anterior muscle, extensor longus and brevis, extensor digitorum longus and brevis, and peroneus longus and brevis of extensor group of leg are paralyzed, paralytic droop and varus foot occur, and cross-domain gait occurs. Long-term foot drop, joint relaxation and instability, can form a fixed talipes equinovarus deformity (Fig. 10.8).

Treatment Principles

To correct the deformity of the foot and ankle, the tendon transposition was carried out according to the residual muscle strength, and the dorsiflexion function of the foot was reconstructed. At the same time, the calcaneal-talar joint was stabilized to achieve the static and dynamic balance of the foot and ankle and to restore the standing and walking function.

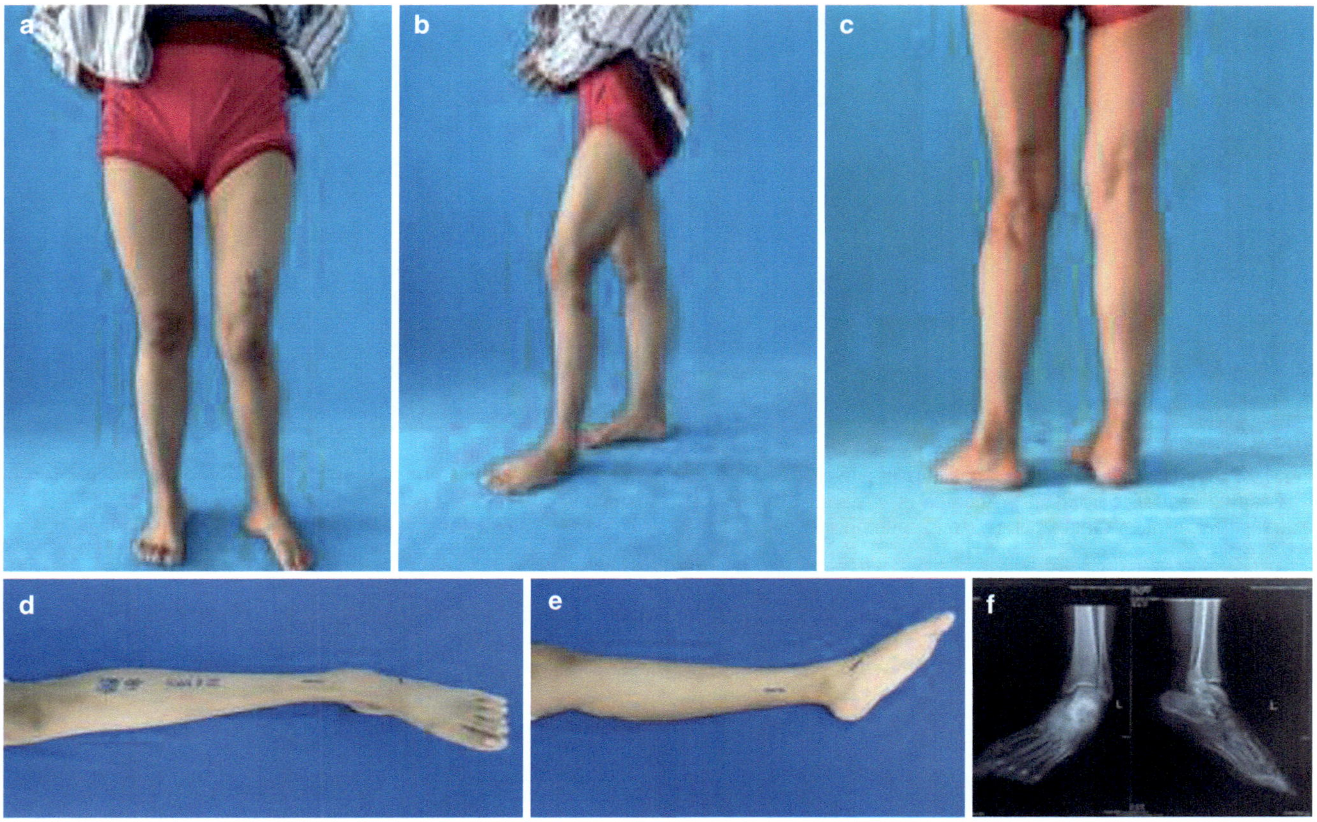

Fig. 10.8 Paralytic ankle ptosis due to common peroneal nerve injury. (**a**) Standing and viewing from the front; (**b**) Lateral view of lower extremity; (**c**) Posterior view of lower limbs; (**d**) Front view of non-weight-bearing affected limb; (**e**) Lateral view of non-weight-bearing affected limb; (**f**) X-ray film of affected ankle joint

10.2 Limb Deformity after Pelvic and Thigh Trauma

10.2.1 Traumatic Pelvic Deformity

10.2.1.1 Etiology

After severe trauma, multiple pelvic fractures, sacroiliac joint dislocation, anterior and posterior pelvic injuries occur, resulting in pelvic ring deformation, pelvic malposition healing deformity, resulting in a series of deformity changes in the hip, lower limbs, and spine.

10.2.1.2 Clinical Manifestation

Severe deformation of pelvic fracture leads to unequal length of both lower limbs, resulting in claudication and spinal deformity over time. The deformity involving the weight-bearing roof of the acetabulum results in loss of joint function or partial loss of joint function. Malunion of the pelvis in the women of childbearing age may result in birth canal deformation, stenosis, and deformity, which may affect natural delivery, causing physical and mental injury to the patient (Fig. 10.9).

10.2.1.3 Treatment Principle

Correct the deformity, reconstruct the stability of the pelvic ring, restore the flatness of the acetabular articular surface and the normal relationship between the head and the acetabulum, and reconstruct the balance of the lumbar spine and the pelvis through proximal femoral osteotomy and pelvic osteotomy.

10.2.2 Malunion of Femoral Fracture

10.2.2.1 Etiology

Femoral fractures are common, mostly caused by high-energy trauma or severe combined injuries, which can easily lead to malunion and nonunion of fractures.

10.2.2.2 Clinical Manifestation

Malunion of femoral fracture may be manifested as flexion and shortening of the thigh, and overgrowth may occur after fracture in childhood. Coxa vara deformity is common in proximal fractures, and malunion of middle and distal fractures can be manifested as overlapping, angulation, and rotation deformity, accompanied by different degrees of knee

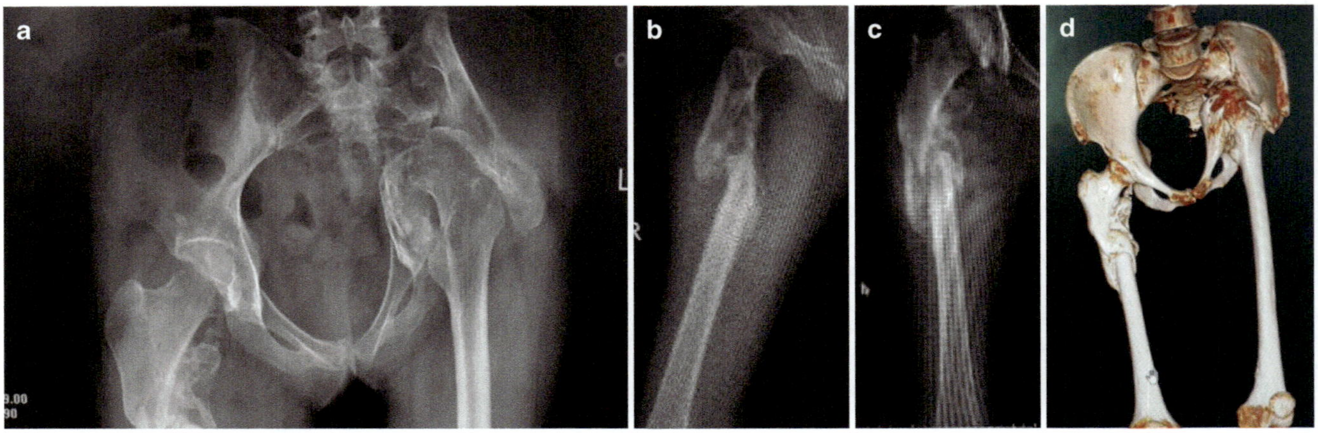

Fig. 10.9 Female, 29 years old. The fracture of pelvis and right femur was caused by traffic accident at the age of 27, with malunion. (**a**) Anteroposterior plain film of pelvis; (**b**, **c**) Anteroposterior and lateral radiographs of right proximal femur; (**d**) Three-dimensional reconstruction CT images of pelvis and femur

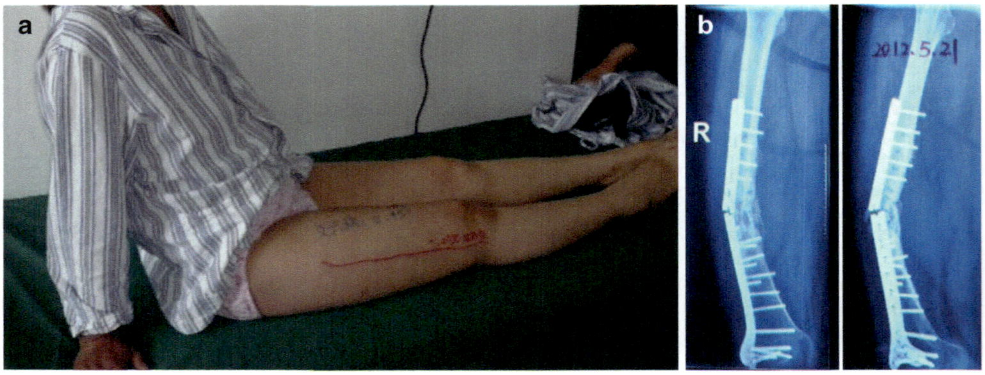

Fig. 10.10 Nonunion of right femur. (**a**) The appearance of the right thigh shows the scar of the previous surgical incision. (**b**) X-ray of the right femur showed femoral nonunion and a broken plate

flexion and extension dysfunction. Malunion of proximal femoral fractures is characterized by malunion (see Fig. 10.9b).

10.2.2.3 Treatment Principle

Correct deformity, restore the gravity line of lower limbs, restore the joint line of hip and knee joints, increase the range of motion of joints, equal-length limbs, and improve walking function.

10.2.3 Bone Nonunion and Bone Defect

10.2.3.1 Bone Nonunion

Etiology

The most common causes of nonunion are infection, insufficient local blood supply, separation of fracture ends, and insufficient fracture stability.

Clinical Manifestations

Bone nonunion is manifested by local pain, discomfort, swelling, slight movement at the fracture end, abnormal movement, and pseudarthrosis after open or closed fracture of limbs for more than 9 months. After internal fixation, patients are often accompanied by breakage of internal fixation (Fig. 10.10). X-ray film shows that the fracture line is clear and no continuous callus passes through.

Classification

Classification of nonunions: Nonunions can be divided into hypertrophic, sclerotic, and atrophic types, but most patients present with mixed nonunions (Fig. 10.11).

1. In hypertrophic nonunion, the broken ends are mainly connected by cartilage. It is generally believed that the cartilage cap of the broken end has the characteristics of epiphyseal cartilage. The speed of cartilage formation and the speed of cartilage ossification form a dynamic balance, so the fracture fissure exists for a long time. The broken end of hypertrophic nonunion often expands to both sides, forming an "elephant foot sign" or a spherical change (Fig. 10.12).
2. In sclerotic nonunion, the medullary cavity was closed and the broken end was sclerotic (Fig. 10.13).
3. The broken ends of atrophic nonunion were atrophied and thinned, mainly with fibrous connection (Fig. 10.14).
4. Mixed bone nonunion often presents with hypertrophy, sclerosis or atrophy and sclerosis (Fig. 10.15).

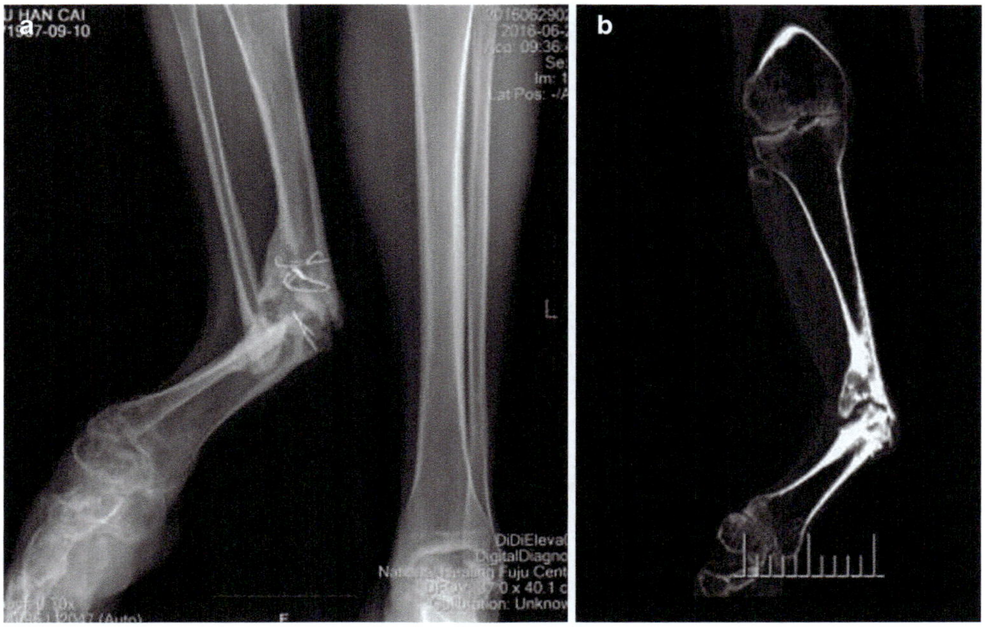

Fig. 10.11 Hypertrophic nonunion. (**a**) Tibial X-ray showed hypertrophic nonunion in the middle and lower segments. (**b**) Three-dimensional CT reconstruction of the tibia showed a ball-holding change at the broken end

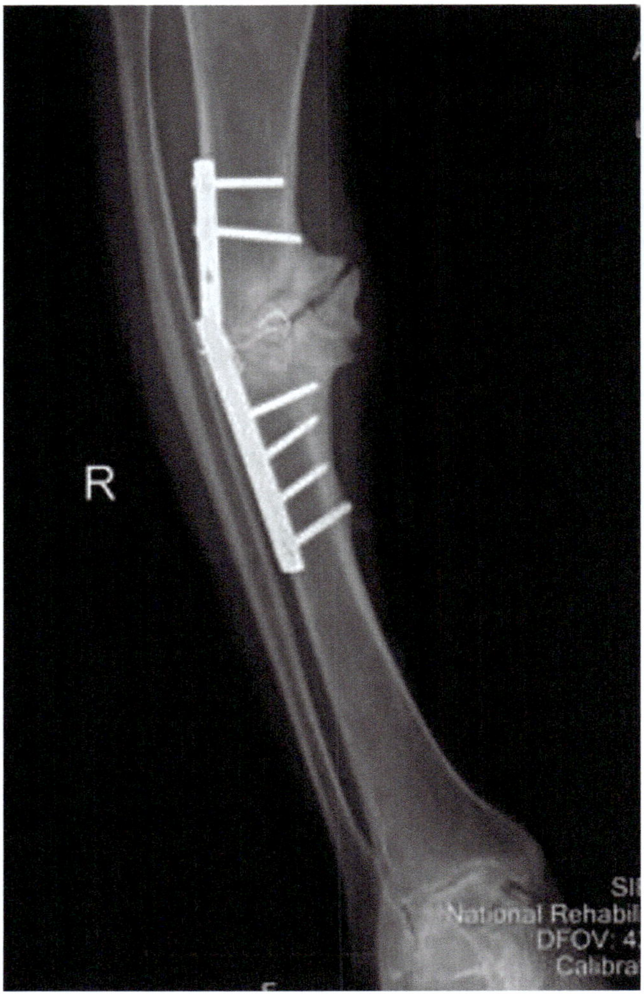

Fig. 10.12 Sclerotic nonunion

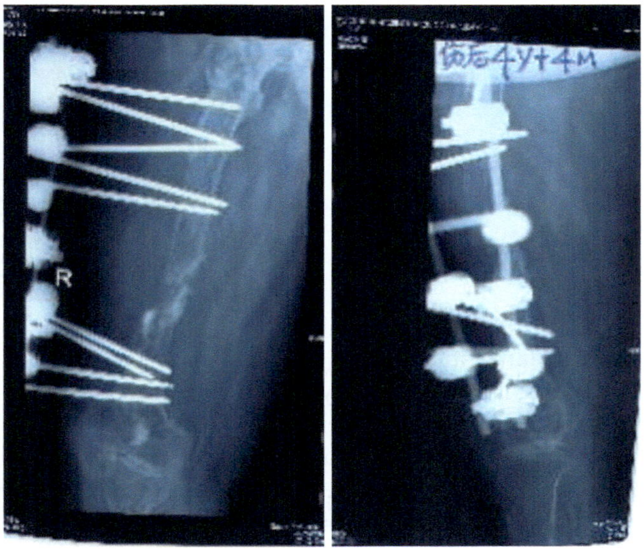

Fig. 10.13 Atrophic nonunion

Treatment Principles

Increasing the local stability of the broken end, protecting the local blood supply, grafting the bone, and activating the local bone healing potential; if there is deformity at the broken end of bone nonunion, the deformity should be corrected at the same time.

10.2.3.2 Bone Defect

Etiology

Trauma, infection, bone disease, surgery, and other factors can cause bone defect.

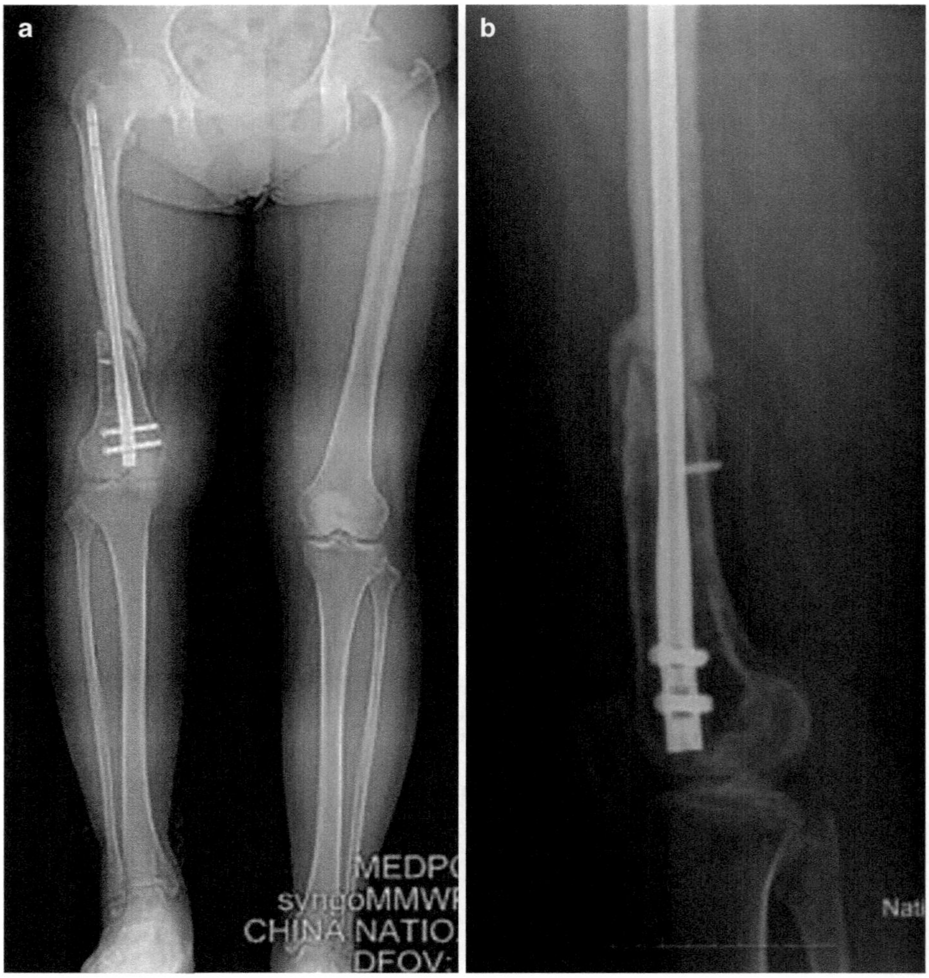

Fig. 10.14 Mixed type nonunion. (**a**) mixed nonunion of the middle and lower segments of the right femur; (**b**) Lateral radiograph of right femur

Clinical Manifestations

Bone defect is characterized by pain, swelling, abnormal activity, continuous middle segment, soft tissue depression, limb weakness, and inability to bear weight according to the defect location, degree, and infection. After treatment, external fixator can be retained to maintain limb continuity, accompanied by sinus or internal fixation, and exposure of bone cement. The X-ray film showed that the fixator remained and the bone was partially or segmentally absent from the bone defect (Fig. 10.15).

Treatment Principles

To repair bone defects and restore bone continuity and limb length, infection control and thorough debridement are needed for infected bone defects. The main methods include bone transplantation, bone removal, and so on.

10.2.4 Post-Traumatic Myositis Ossificans

10.2.4.1 Etiology

The etiology is not clear, and it is often related to severe trauma. After trauma, the deposition of bone structure in muscle and connective tissue causes muscle sclerosis, which can be disabled by joint stiffness.

10.2.4.2 Clinical Manifestation

Musculus biceps brachii, musculus triceps brachii, musculus quadriceps femoris, and musculus adductor femoris are prone to myositis ossificans, which usually forms 3–6 months after injury. A hard mass appears in the soft tissue of the injured site, which gradually increases and is accompanied by pain. The pain disappeared after the mass stopped growing, which affected the movement of adjacent joints. Serum alkaline phosphatase may be elevated. The ossification shadow can be seen on the X-ray film, which begins to show cloud-like calcification, and then gradually becomes clear in outline and bright in the center. After maturity, the peripheral ossification is obviously dense, with bone trabeculae inside, and a transparent boundary line between adjacent bones (Fig. 10.16).

10.2.4.3 Treatment Principle

Early treatment of fracture and dislocation of traumatic site and removal of hematoma; once ossification is formed, it

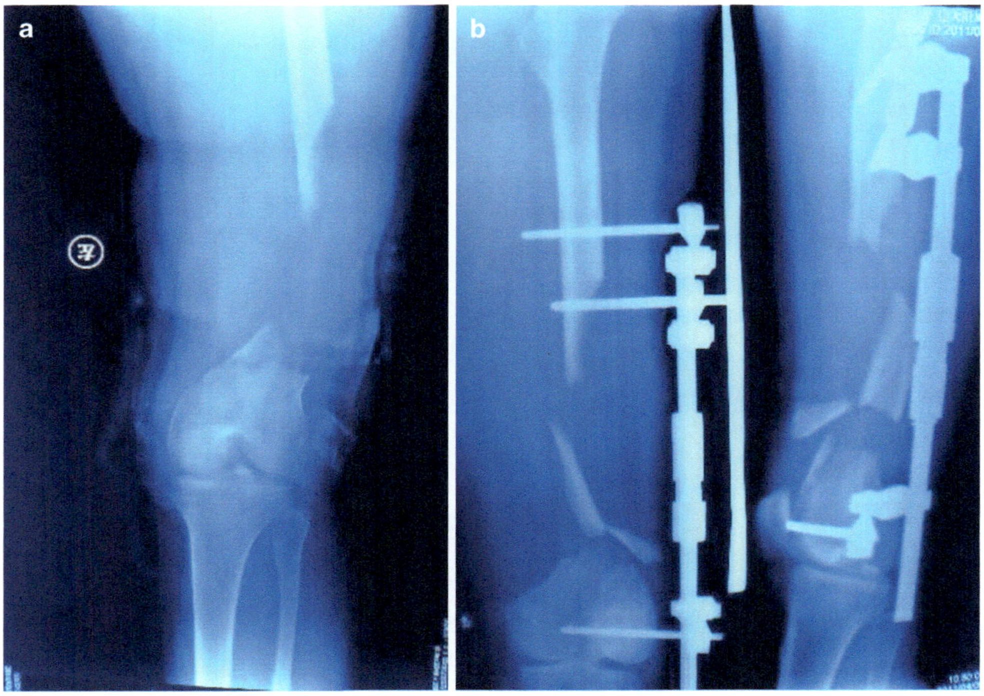

Fig. 10.15 Large bone defect of middle and lower segment of left femur caused by traffic accident. (**a**) The anteroposterior X-ray film of the left femur showed bone defect in the middle and lower segments of the femur. (**b**) Temporary external fixator fixation

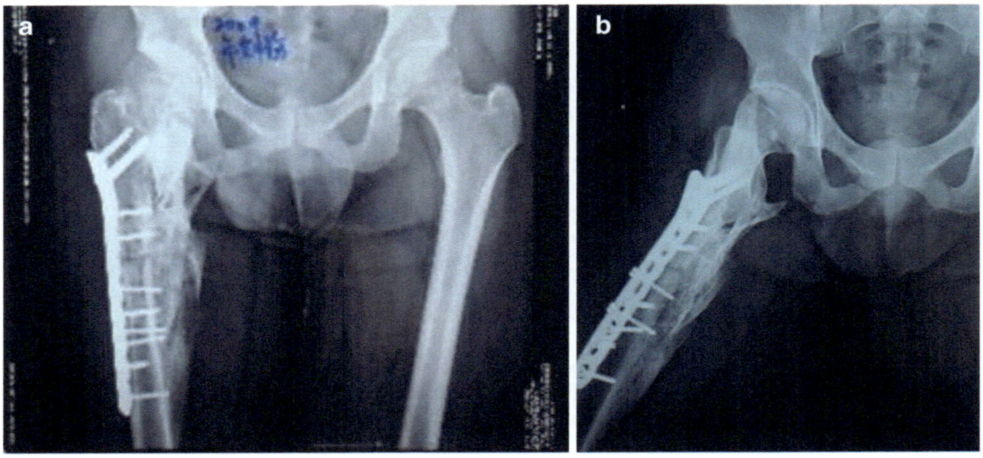

Fig. 10.16 Male, 28 years old, 20 years old, suffered from right proximal femur fracture and myositis ossificans. (**a**) Bilateral anteroposterior radiographs of proximal femur; (**b**) Lateral radiograph of right proximal femur

should be removed after maturity in order to maximize the recovery of limb function. At the same time, radiotherapy or indomethacin and other drugs can be used for symptomatic treatment.

10.2.5 Severe Osteoporosis Secondary to Failure of Multiple Fracture Operations

10.2.5.1 Etiology

After the fracture,there were many failed surgeries, the blood supply of the injured surgical site was destroyed, the affected limb could not bear weight, disuse muscle atrophy, osteoporosis.

10.2.5.2 Clinical Manifestation

Multiple surgical scars, muscle atrophy, joint movement disorders, flexion contracture, stiffness, limb cannot take the initiative to move because of fear of pain, cannot stand and walk with weight, may be accompanied by limb angulation, rotation, shortening deformity; X-ray examination showed that the bone density decreased, the bone trabeculae decreased, thinned, the branches disappeared, or even completely disappeared, the tubular bone cortex became thinner, the medullary cavity enlarged, and the internal fixation remained (Fig. 10.17).

Treatment Principles

Provide stable fixation for the affected limb, avoid stress shielding, through bone grafting, restoration of limb grav-

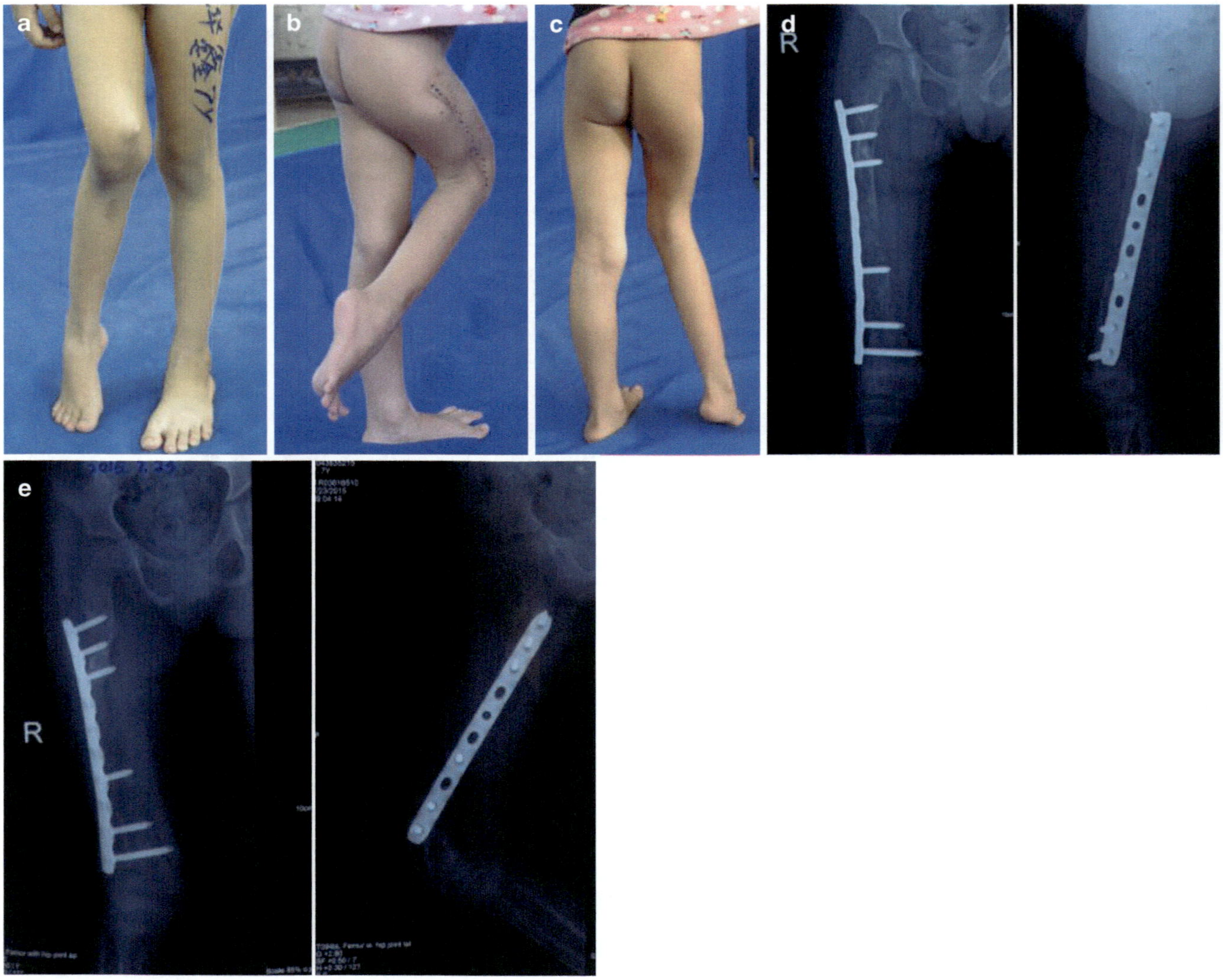

Fig. 10.17 Female, 7 years old, severe osteoporosis secondary to repeated failure of fracture operation. (**a**) Front view of both lower limbs standing; (**b**) Standing lateral view of the lower extremity (**c**) View from the back of standing lower limbs; (**d**) X-ray film of right femur, anteroposterior and lateral (bone was not absorbed); (**e**) X-ray film of right femur (bone absorption, osteoporosis)

ity line, intramedullary fixation and other means, as far as possible is limb weight-bearing exercise, increase nutrition, light.

10.3 Post-Traumatic Deformity of Knee, Calf, Foot, and Ankle

10.3.1 Ankle Deformity Left after Replantation of Amputated Leg

10.3.1.1 Etiology

Leg amputation caused by mechanical extrusion or traffic accident, shortening deformity after successful replantation, nerve injury, muscle fibrosis, contracture, traction of ankle joint, secondary talipes equinovarus deformity.

10.3.1.2 Clinical Manifestation

The main manifestations were shortening of the lower leg, trauma scar, and surgical incision scar. It may be accompanied by varus, valgus or rotational deformity of the lower leg and talipes equinovarus deformity of the ankle. There are disorders of active movement in the ankle joint and toes, and sensory disorders of the skin. The X-ray film showed that the lower limbs were shortened and the force line was abnormal, and the ankle joint was deformed (Fig. 10.18).

10.3.1.3 Treatment Principle

Lengthen the shortened legs and isometric limbs, correct bony deformities, restore the gravity line of lower limbs, correct foot and ankle deformities, balance muscle strength, stabilize joints, and improve standing and walking functions.

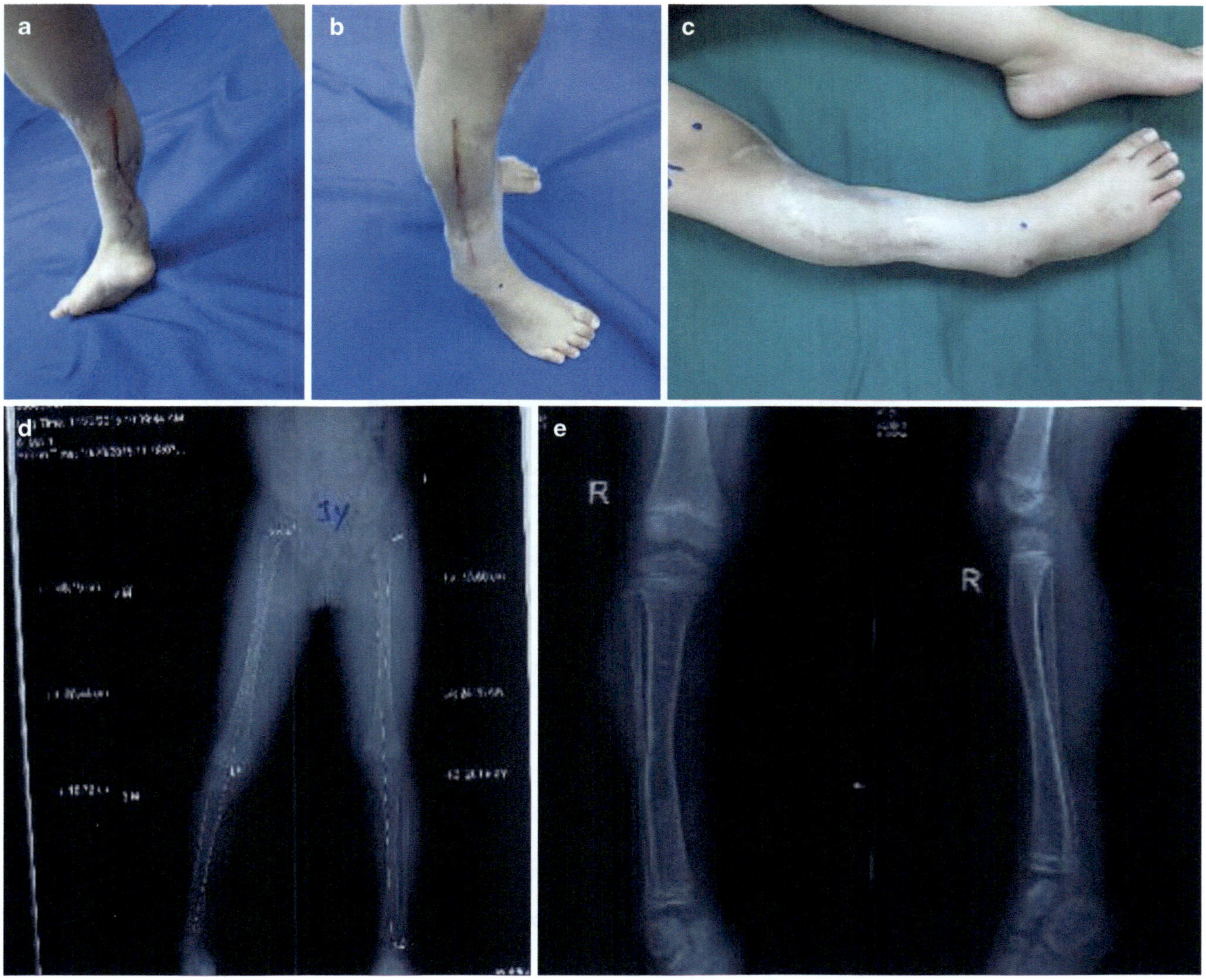

Fig. 10.18 Male, 5 years old. When he was 2 and half years old, the right leg was crushed by the escalator, resulting in amputation. After successful replantation of the amputated limb, the right leg was shortened and the equinovarus deformity occurred. (**a**) Medial view of standing right foot; (**b**) Standing anterolateral view of right foot; (**c**) Right leg and foot decubitus view; (**d**) Full-length anteroposterior radiographs of lower extremities in standing position; (**e**) Anteroposterior and lateral radiograph of right tibia and fibula

10.3.2 Stiffness of Knee Joint after Trauma

10.3.2.1 Etiology

Thigh and knee joint trauma, including distal femoral fracture, patellar fracture, tibial plateau fracture, can cause knee joint stiffness.

10.3.2.2 Clinical Manifestation

The flexion and extension function of knee joint was impaired, and the range of motion was reduced to varying degrees. The knee joint of most patients was stiff in the extension position, and the flexion movement was limited. A small number of patients with knee stiffness in knee flexion, knee flexion deformity angle and knee range of motion vary according to the degree of injury. X-ray showed old fractures of distal femur, patella and proximal tibia, and narrow knee joint space (Fig. 10.19).

10.3.2.3 Treatment Principle

Individualized treatment, muscle and tendon release, knee joint release, if necessary, femoral supracondylar osteotomy, restoration of joint range of motion, preservation of muscle strength, restoration of standing and walking function.

10.3.3 Tibia and Fibula Defect after Trauma

10.3.3.1 Etiology

Open comminuted fracture of tibia caused by severe trauma is often accompanied by soft tissue defect, nerve injury, bone

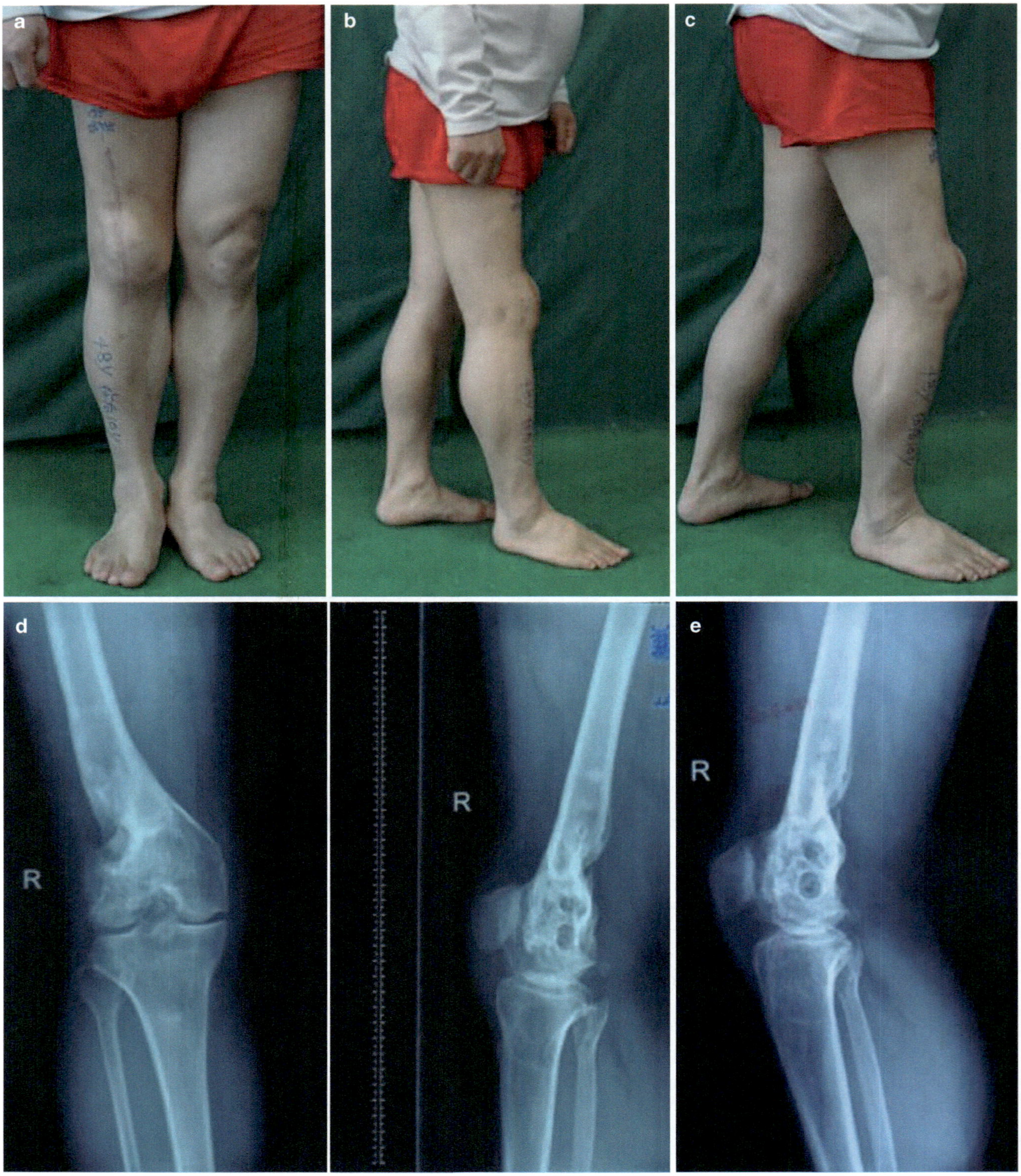

Fig. 10.19 Male, 48 years old, knee joint stiffness after fracture of right distal femur. (**a**) Front view of both lower limbs standing; (**b**) Lateral view of standing right knee joint in extension (**c**) Lateral view of the right knee joint in maximum flexion in standing; (**d**) Anteroposterior X-ray film of right knee joint at maximum extension; (**e**) Lateral radiograph of right knee joint at maximum flexion

defect, bone infection, and other serious complications, resulting in bone defect of tibia and severe deformity of the injured limb after long-term development.

10.3.3.2 Clinical Manifestation

Post-traumatic skin scar can be seen on the lower leg, with or without limb deformity. Patients with tibial defect need to walk with crutches because they cannot bear weight (Fig. 10.20); patients with simple fibular defect generally do not affect the weight-bearing walking function of limbs (Fig. 10.21). Radiographs of the lower leg showed varying degrees of defect in the tibia or fibula.

10.3.3.3 Treatment Principle

According to the type of bone defect, bone grafting and bone transfer were performed to repair bone defect, promote bone healing, restore limb length and lower limb strength line, correct foot and ankle deformity, and restore walking function.

10.3.4 Ischemic Muscle Contracture Caused by Juvenile Trauma and Infection

10.3.4.1 Etiology

Leg soft tissue trauma, infection or iatrogenic causes ischemia, hypoxia, edema, and increased pressure, thus forming osteofascial compartment syndrome, leading to muscle ischemia and necrosis, neurological dysfunction, and late formation of fixed joint deformity and dysfunction.

10.3.4.2 Clinical Manifestation

Large areas of skin scars, muscle atrophy, soft tissue defects, and even large areas of bony scars can be seen in the lower leg, ankle horseshoe stiffness, foot varus or valgus deformity, claw toe deformity, etc. Juvenile trauma can lead to bone development disorders, limb shortening, X-ray bone atrophy, ankle severe horseshoe, talus forward dislocation, arch enlargement, metatarsophalangeal hyperextension and claw (Fig. 10.22).

10.3.4.3 Treatment Principle

According to the condition of deformity, an individualized surgical plan was formulated. Release the contractured soft tissue, release and lengthen the tendon, balance the muscle strength, and perform osteotomy or arthrodesis to correct the deformity of the foot and ankle, stabilize the joint, and restore the shape and function of the limb.

10.3.5 Calcaneal Bone Defect after Trauma

10.3.5.1 Etiology

Many factors such as trauma and infection lead to calcaneal compression, malunion and bone defect, often accompanied by local soft tissue defect and local scar, leaving functional disorders.

10.3.5.2 Clinical Manifestation

Because of bone defect, abnormal stress on the sole of the foot leads to pain and skin ulcer caused by friction at the

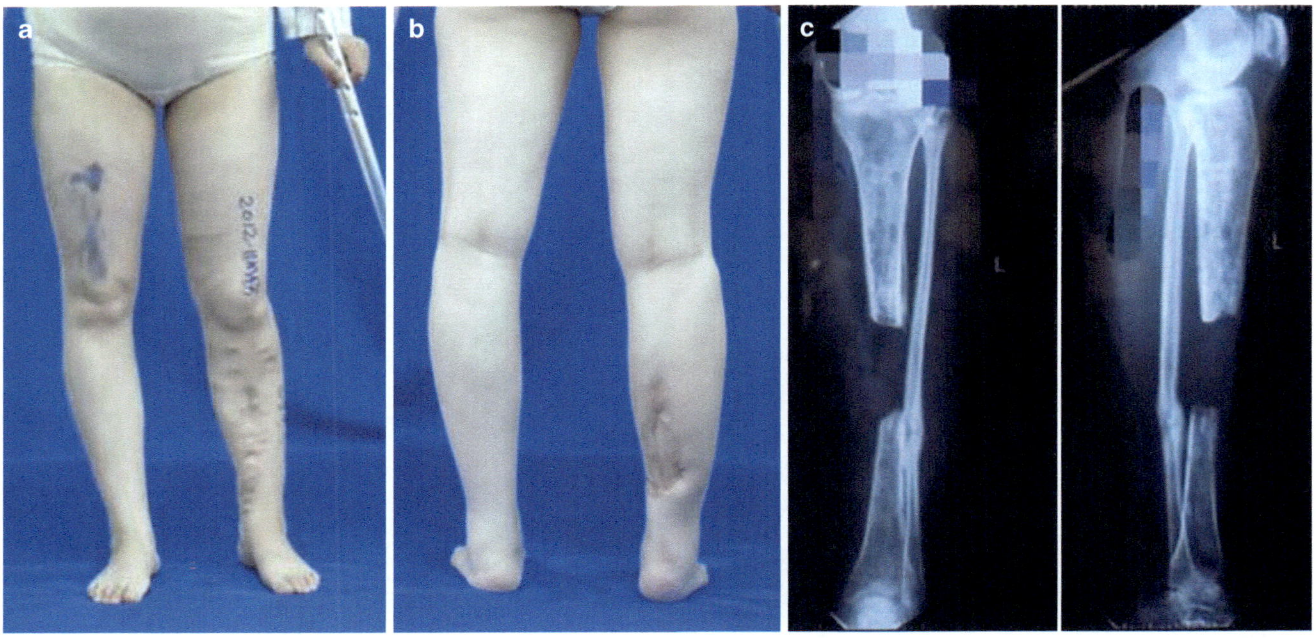

Fig. 10.20 Female, 38 years old, left leg trauma, comminuted fracture of middle tibia, after six times of surgical treatment, resulting in a defect of about 10 cm in the middle tibia. (**a**) is viewed from the front in standing position; (**b**) is viewed from the back in standing position; (**c**) Anteroposterior and lateral X-ray film of left lower leg

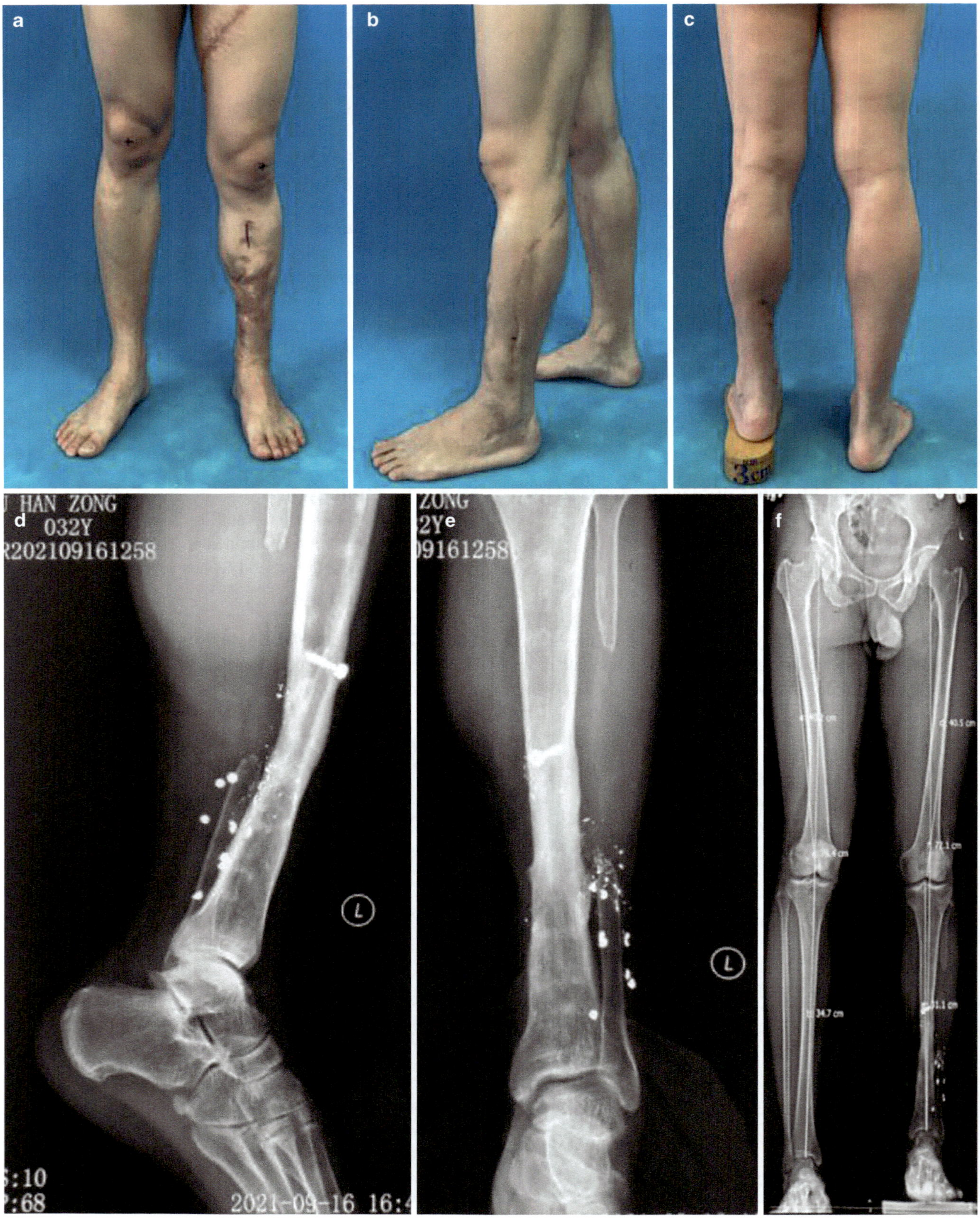

Fig. 10.21 Male, 34 years old, at the age of 16, the tibia defect was caused by gunshot wound in the leg, and the fibula was transplanted after debridement, resulting in the defect of the left fibula and the deformity of the leg. (**a**) Frontal view of lower limbs in standing position; (**b**) Lateral view of lower extremity in standing position (**c**). Posterior view of lower extremities in standing position; (**d**) Lateral radiograph of left tibia; (**e**) Anteroposterior X-ray film of left tibia; (**f**) Full-length radiograph of lower extremity in standing position

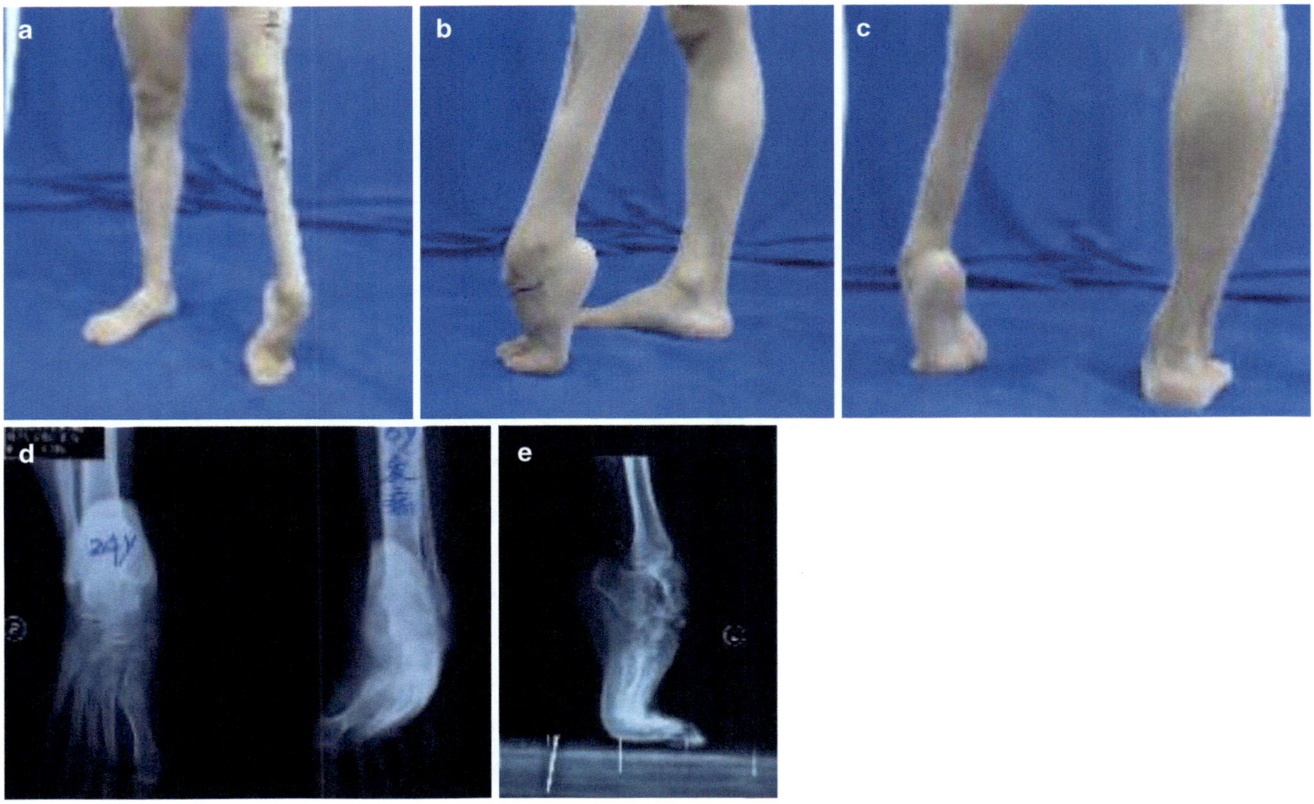

Fig. 10.22 Male, 24 years old. When he was 6 years old, he suffered from leg trauma and infection, resulting in talipes cavus deformity. (**a**) Front view of both lower limbs standing; (**b**) Standing lateral view of the lower extremity (**c**) Posterior view of standing lower limbs; (**d**) Anteroposterior and lateral X-ray films of ankle joint; (**e**) Lateral X-ray film of ankle joint under weight-bearing

bone protrusion. Local skin scar or soft tissue defect of heel, bone exposure; X-ray film showed that the calcaneus was incomplete, the calcaneal body was partially missing and shortened, and foreign bodies such as internal fixators or bone cement could be left after acute trauma treatment, resulting in calcaneal varus or valgus deformity (Fig. 10.23).

Treatment Principles

According to the infection and the condition of soft tissue, the individual treatment plan was adopted to effectively cover the soft tissue, repair the bone defect, and restore the shape of the calcaneus. The main methods included autogenous bone (or musculocutaneous flap) transplantation, Ilizarov bone transfer, Masquelet membrane induction, and so on.

10.3.6 Post-Traumatic Ankle-Foot Deformity Due to Extensive Bony Cicatricial Deformity of the Lower Leg

Severe traffic accident injury, resulting in extensive necrosis of calf muscle, surgical resection, extensive scar skin covering the calf after wound repair, only scar skin wrapping the tibia and fibula, and secondary talipes equinovarus deformity (Fig. 10.24).

According to the principle of treatment, the simplest and most effective way for such patients is to install artificial limbs after amputation, but the thinking of Chinese culture is more about correcting ankle deformity and improving walking function on the premise of limb salvage.

10.3.7 Poor Stump after Lower Leg Amputation

10.3.7.1 Etiology

After lower limb amputation, the muscle of the stump of the affected limb has different degrees of disuse atrophy, the treatment, embedding and length of the tibiofibular stump are not appropriate during amputation, and the skin of the stump is accompanied by scar contracture, which brings difficulties to the adaptation and installation of the prosthesis and increases the pain of patients.

10.3.7.2 Clinical Manifestation

Compared with the skin temperature of the healthy side, it is usually about 3 C lower, more patients are accompanied by phantom limb pain, and their joints are usually stiff. At the same time, scar contracture causes joint stiffness,

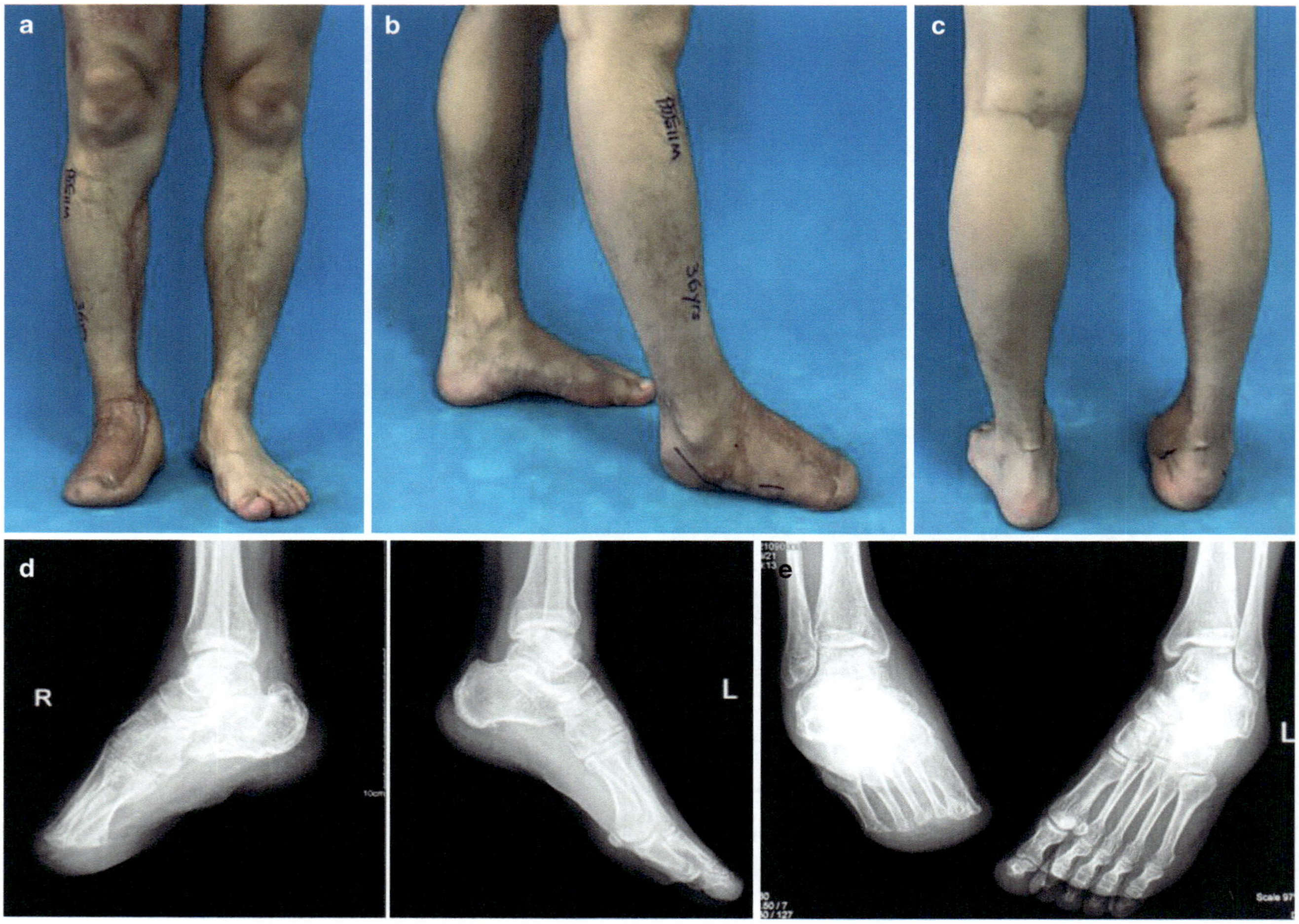

Fig. 10.23 Male, 35 years old, compression defect and varus after calcaneal fracture caused by traffic accident injury of right foot, loss of forefoot. (**a**) Frontal view of lower limbs in standing position; (**b**) Lateral view of lower extremity in standing position; (**c**) Posterior view of lower extremities in standing position; (**d**) Keywords Amputation of lower leg; Anteroposterior X-ray film of knee joint; (**e**) Lateral radiograph of knee joint of amputated lower leg

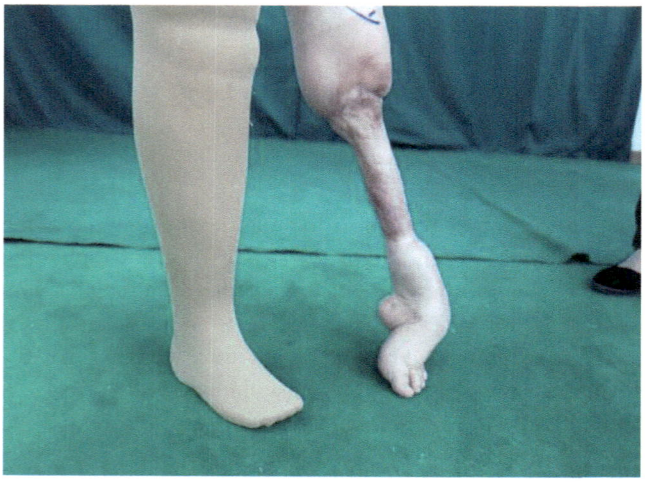

Fig. 10.24 Female, 28 years old, right leg amputation caused by traffic accident, left leg skin and bone with equinovarus deformity

stump pain, repeated ulceration of the stump to form sinus, exudation, stump deformity and inability to wear artificial limbs also bring great pain to patients, and also bring many adverse effects on the installation of artificial limbs. In a small number of patients with stump syndrome, the condition is aggravated, resulting in severe mental disorders (Fig. 10.25).

10.3.7.3 Treatment Principle

Treatment varies from person to person, the principle of symptomatic treatment, conservative and feasible rehabilitation physiotherapy, suitable for artificial limbs; a good contact surface can be obtained by trimming that feasible stump; it is feasible to lengthen the stump and increase the length of the stump to facilitate the fitting of the prosthesis.

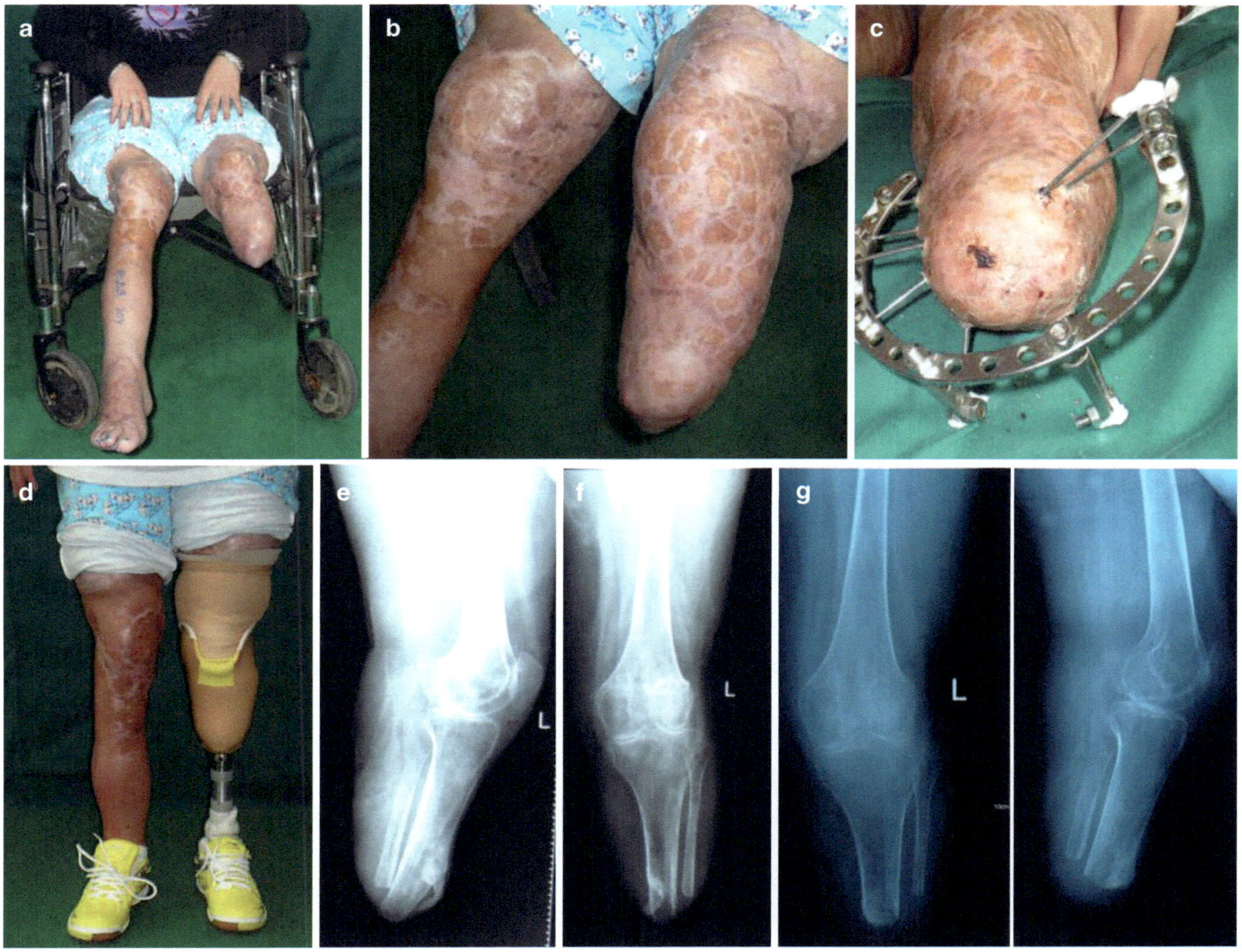

Fig. 10.25 Poor stump after amputation of right lower leg. (**a**) Wheelchair, standing with both lower limbs, frontal view; (**b**) Poor appearance of knee flexion contracture stump after amputation of left lower leg (**c**). Appearance of left leg stump after fascia repair and Kirschner wire fixation; (**d**) Left leg stump repaired, standing with prosthesis, frontal view; (**e**, **f**) Anteroposterior and lateral X-ray film of knee joint with amputation stump of lower leg; (**g**) Anteroposterior and lateral radiographs of knee joint after repair of amputation stump of lower leg

10.4 Lower Limb Deformity Caused by Epiphyseal Injury in Children

10.4.1 Knee Joint Deformity Caused by Epiphyseal Injury of Distal Femur

10.4.1.1 Etiology

In childhood or adolescence, the injury of distal femoral epiphysis caused by falls and traffic accidents leads to premature closure of some epiphyses. During the growth and development of children, the uneven growth of distal femur can cause genu varum, genu valgum, genu flexion, or genu recurvatum deformity, of which genu varum and genu valgum are the most common.

10.4.1.2 Clinical Manifestation

The early closure of the medial epiphysis of the distal femur can cause genu varus deformity, the early closure of the lateral epiphysis can cause genu valgus deformity, the early closure of the anterior epiphysis can cause genu recurvatum deformity, and the early closure of the posterior epiphysis can cause genu flexion deformity, accompanied by femoral torsion and thigh shortening deformity. Lumbar scoliosis can cause discomfort in the waist and hip (Fig. 10.26).

10.4.1.3 Treatment Principle

To correct the deformity of distal femur, restore the normal mechanical axis of lower limbs and knee joint line, lengthen

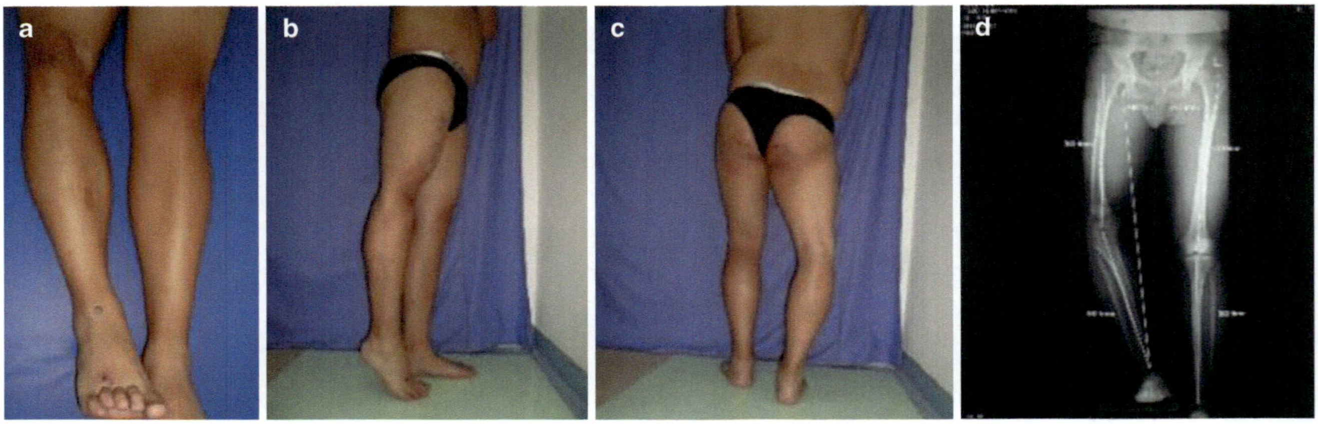

Fig. 10.26 Male, 23 years old, suffered medial trauma of the right knee when he was 3 years old, and gradually developed varus deformity of the right knee. (**a**) Frontal view of lower limbs in standing position; (**b**) Lateral view of lower extremity in standing position; (**c**) Posterior view of lower limbs in standing position; (**d**) Full-length anteroposterior radiograph of lower extremity in standing position

the femur at the same time or by stages, make the length of both lower limbs equal, and improve the walking function.

10.4.2 Deformity of Proximal Tibial Epiphyseal Injury

10.4.2.1 Etiology

The injury of proximal tibial epiphysis in children or adolescents caused by external forces, such as falls and traffic accidents, can cause early closure of the epiphysis at the injury site, resulting in uneven growth of the proximal tibia in the process of growth and development, and gradually secondary deformity of the proximal tibia.

10.4.2.2 Clinical Manifestation

The medial epiphyseal premature closure of the proximal tibia can cause genu varus deformity, the lateral epiphyseal premature closure can cause genu valgus deformity, the anterior epiphyseal premature closure can cause genu recurvatum deformity, and the posterior epiphyseal premature closure can cause genu flexion deformity. It may be accompanied by the phenomenon of high fibular head due to the shortening deformity of the leg and the relative overgrowth of the fibula (Fig. 10.27).

10.4.2.3 Treatment Principle

Proximal tibial osteotomy can correct tibial deformity, lengthen the leg at the same time, restore the negative gravity line of the lower limb, equal-length limbs, and improve walking function.

10.4.3 Ankle Deformity Caused by Epiphyseal Injury of Distal Tibia

10.4.3.1 Etiology

Before the closure of the distal tibial epiphysis in children or adolescents or uneven injury of the distal tibial epiphysis caused by trauma leads to partial closure of the epiphysis. During the growth and development of children, the deformity of ankle varus or valgus gradually occurs, accompanied by leg shortening.

10.4.3.2 Clinical Manifestation

Three months to six months after ankle injury, the deformity of ankle and foot varus or valgus gradually appeared, and the deformity gradually aggravated with growth and development, and the calf was shortened, and the length of both lower limbs was unequal. Radiographs show closure of the medial or lateral epiphyseal plate of the distal tibia and inclination of the ankle facet (Fig. 10.28).

10.4.3.3 Treatment Principle

Children with unclosed epiphyseal plate were treated with epiphyseal block and supra-malleolar osteotomy to correct varus deformity of the ankle, and at the same time, subtibial osteotomy was performed to restore limb length.

10.4.4 Sequelae of Multiple Epiphyseal Injuries

10.4.4.1 Etiology

Before epiphyseal closure in children or adolescents, epiphyseal hypoplasia or uneven injury caused by genetic factors, multiple trauma, and other factors leads to partial epiphyseal closure, and limb deformities gradually occur in the process of growth and development of children.

10.4.4.2 Clinical Manifestation

Severe trauma leads to a large area of scars on the limbs, mostly close to the bone. The joint deformity of epiphyseal injury is varus or valgus, which is gradually aggravated with the growth and development of the deformity, and the limbs are shortened and unequal in length. X-ray film showed that the epiphyseal plate was closed and the articular surface was inclined at the site of epiphyseal injury (Fig. 10.29).

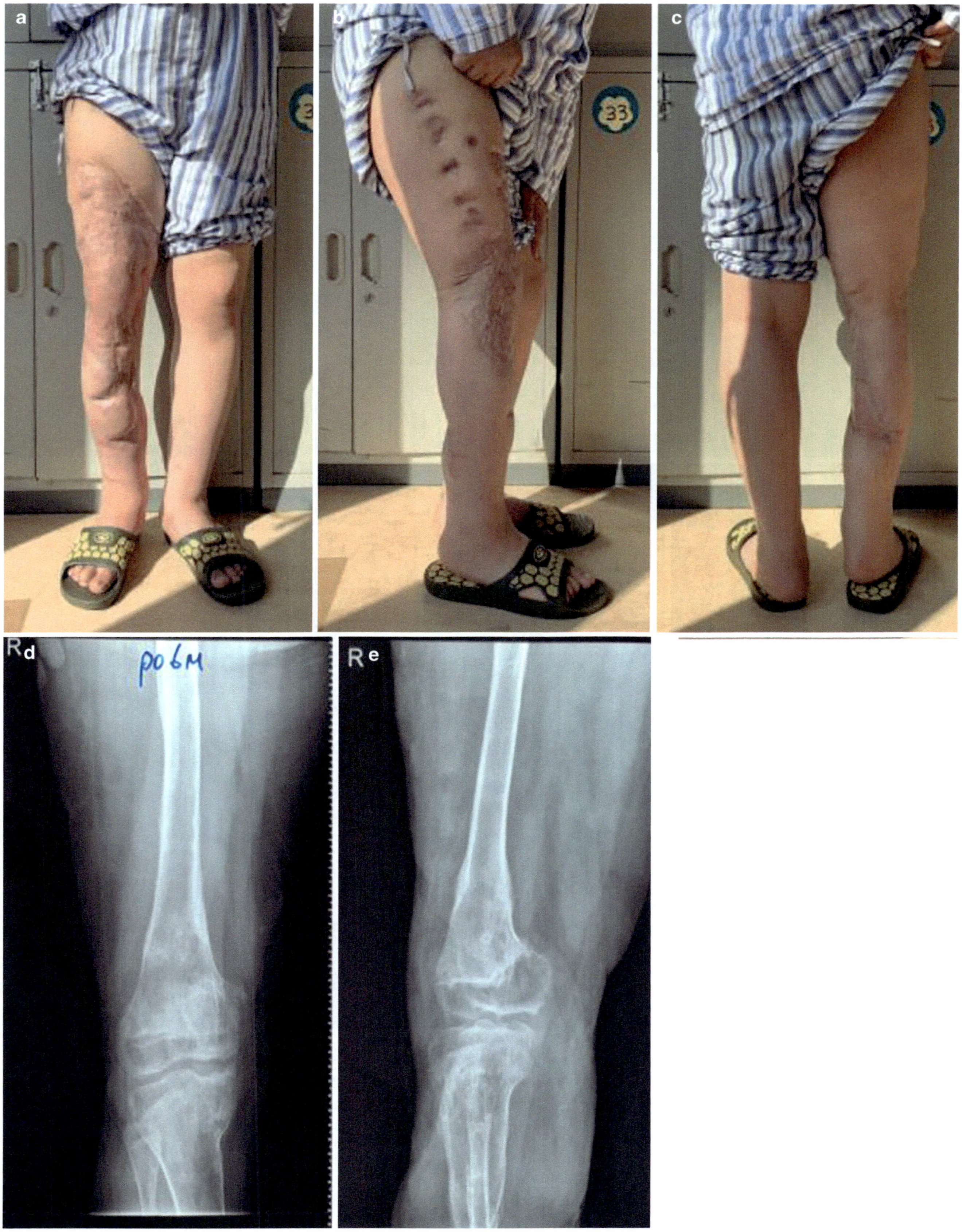

Fig. 10.27 Male, 12 years old. The fracture of distal femur and proximal tibia was caused by traffic accident at the age of 9, resulting in varus deformity of leg and stiffness of knee joint. (**a**) Frontal view of lower limbs in standing position; (**b**) Lateral view of lower extremity in standing position; (**c**) Posterior view of lower extremities in standing position; (**d**) Anteroposterior X-ray of right knee joint; (**e**) Lateral radiograph of right knee joint

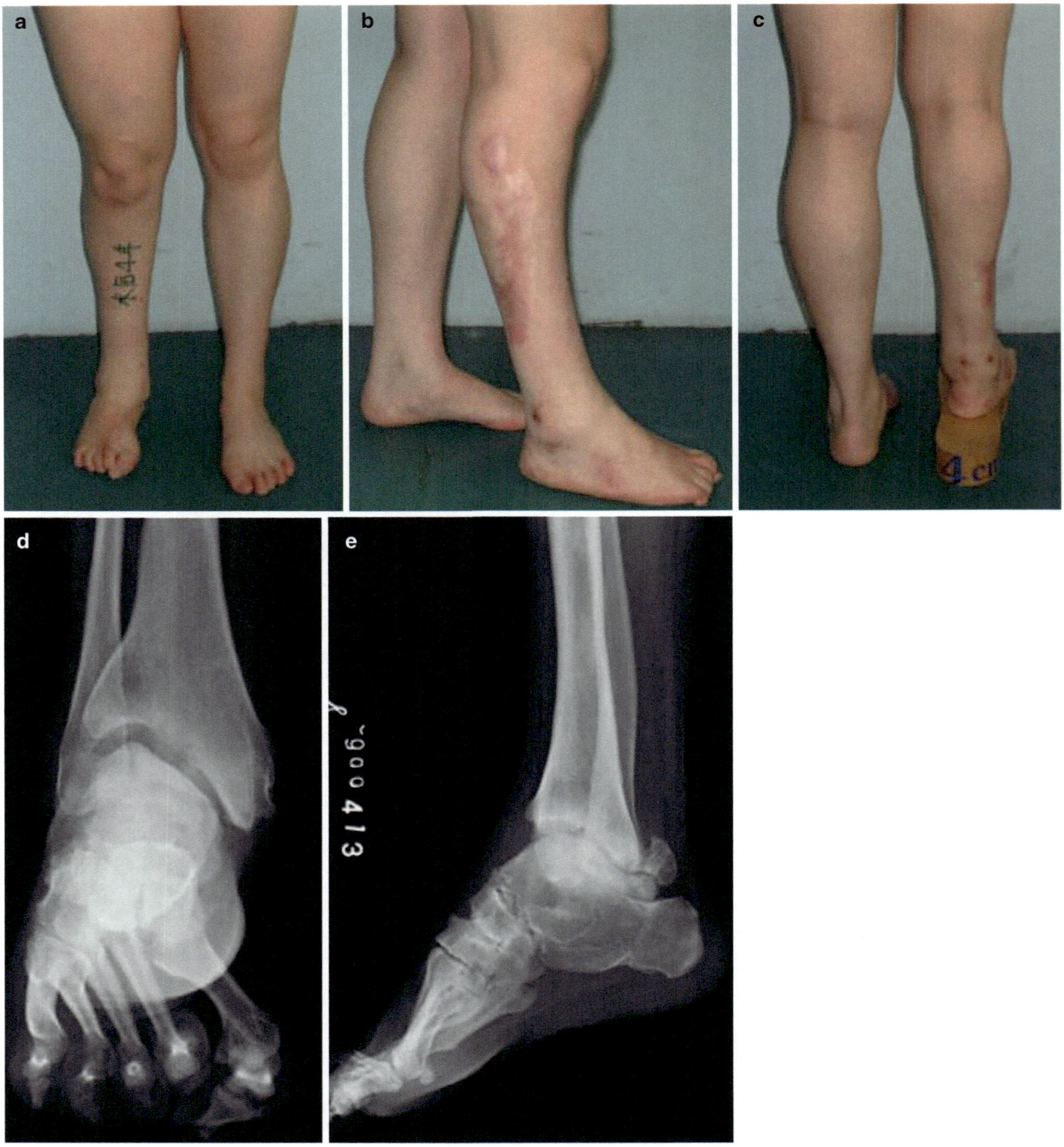

Fig. 10.28 Valgus deformity of ankle joint caused by injury of distal epiphysis of tibia. (**a**) Frontal view of lower limbs in standing position; (**b**) Lateral view of lower extremity in standing position; (**c**) Posterior view of lower limbs in standing position; (**d**, **e**) Anteroposterior and lateral radiographs of right ankle joint

10.4.4.3 Treatment Principle

Pediatric patients with unclosed epiphyseal plate were treated with epiphyseal block, osteotomy to correct varus deformity, and osteotomy to lengthen and restore limb length.

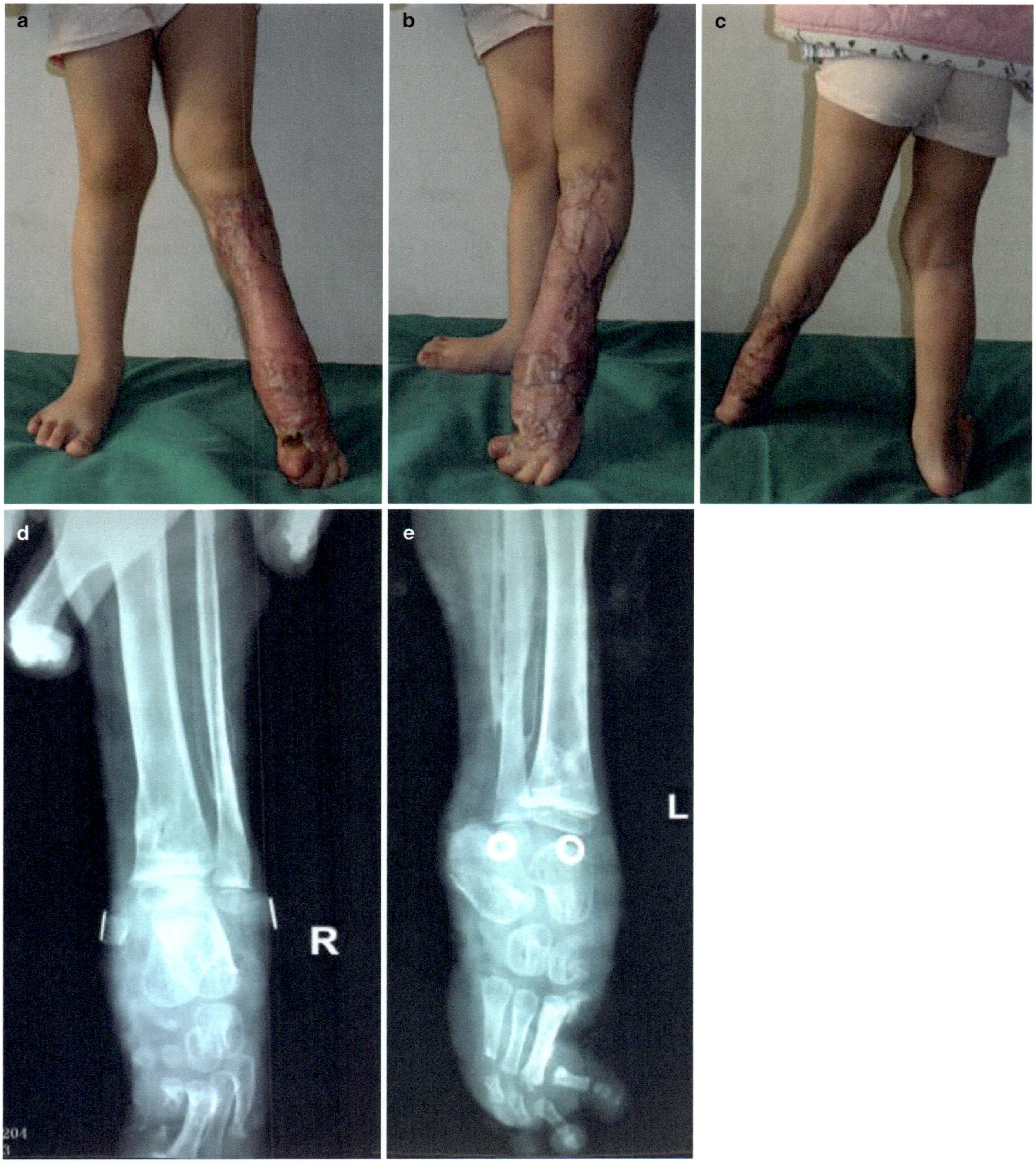

Fig. 10.29 Malformation caused by multiple epiphyseal injuries of foot and ankle. (**a**) Frontal view of lower limbs in standing position; (**b**) Lateral view of lower extremity in standing position; (**c**) Posterior view of lower limbs in standing position; (**d**, **e**) Anteroposterior and lateral radiographs of ankle joint

10.5 Burn Cicatricial Contracture Deformity of Limbs

Large area of burn and scald of second degree and above, insufficient donor site of skin transplantation, scar healing contracture, and continuous traction of joint lead to fixation deformity.

10.5.1 Scar Contracture Deformity of Burns and Scalds of Upper Limbs and Hands

10.5.1.1 Etiology

Hand burns and scalds cause contracture of skin and joint capsule, which affects nerves, bones, tendons, and blood vessels, and causes disuse deformity of hand with the development of time.

10.5.1.2 Clinical Manifestation

Clinical skin scar contracture, joint stiffness, fixed flexion or dorsiflexion deformity of wrist and fingers, scar wing web formation on the flexion side of fingers, joint movement disorder, unable to complete opposition and grasping movements, X-ray film shows that the joint is fixed in the contracture position, and there may be excessive osteoporosis (Figs. 10.30 and 10.31).

10.5.1.3 Treatment Principle

Individualized treatment, scar release, skin graft, skin flap repair, Irizalov technique scar stretching and softening, correction of joint contracture deformity, combined with appropriate orthodontics, to maximize the recovery of hand opposition, grasping function and appearance.

10.5.2 Joint Deformity Caused by Burn and Scald Scar Contracture of Knee Joint

10.5.2.1 Etiology

Because of the burn and scald of the knee, the early treatment is improper, and with the development of time, the adhesion of the tissue around the burn site and the contracture of the joint capsule occur, resulting in the deformity of knee flexion, varus and valgus.

10.5.2.2 Clinical Manifestation

Scar contracture and skin depression can be seen at the injured part of the joint. Scar traction of the joint leads to deformity. In childhood injury, scar can restrict the growth of the epiphysis, resulting in varus and valgus of the distal femur and proximal tibia, rotation, shortening deformity, joint movement disorder, claudication, and narrowing of the knee joint space on X-ray film. Varus, valgus, knee flexion, hyperextension, rotation, shortening, and other deformity changes (Fig. 10.32).

10.5.2.3 Treatment Principle

Individualized treatment, according to the deformity, scar soft tissue release, osteotomy correction of bony deformity, restoration of lower limb gravity line, restoration of joint line, reconstruction of joint dynamic and static balance, isometric limbs, increase of joint range of motion, restoration of walking function.

10.5.3 Ankle Deformity Caused by Burn Scar Contracture of Leg

10.5.3.1 Etiology

Ankle and foot II degree and above burns and scalds, improper early treatment, wound scar healing, scar contracture traction joints, resulting in ankle and foot deformities.

10.5.3.2 Clinical Manifestation

Because of the large number of ankle and foot joints and the complex movement trajectory, the deformities caused by burn and scald scar contracture in different parts are complex and diverse. Burns and scalds occur on the dorsal side, often causing dorsiflexion contracture of the foot and forming calcaneal deformity. Occurs on the lateral side, causing foot valgus and abduction deformity; it occurs on the medial side, causing foot varus and adduction deformity (Fig. 10.33); Because of the low probability of burns and scalds on the posterior side of the foot, horseshoe feet caused by them are rare.

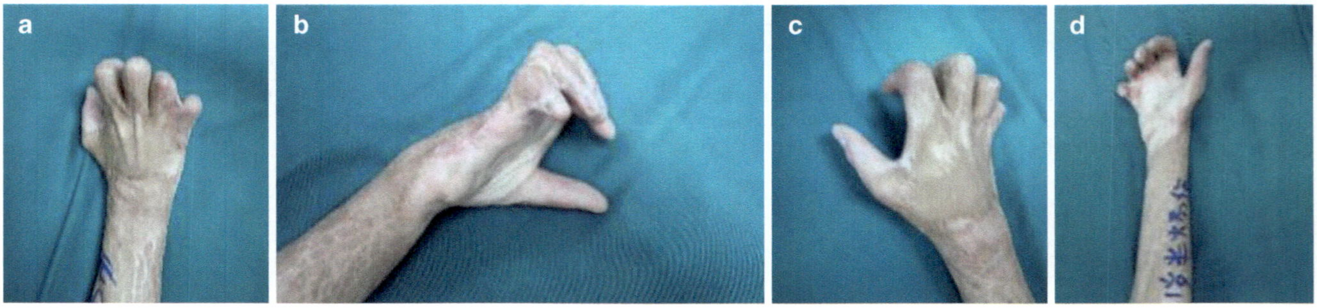

Fig. 10.30 A female, 7 years old, with flexion deformity secondary to burns on her right hand and forearm at the age of one and a half years. (**a**) Dorsal view of the hand; (**b**) Lateral view of the hand; (**c**) Hand profile view; (**d**) Palmar view of the hand

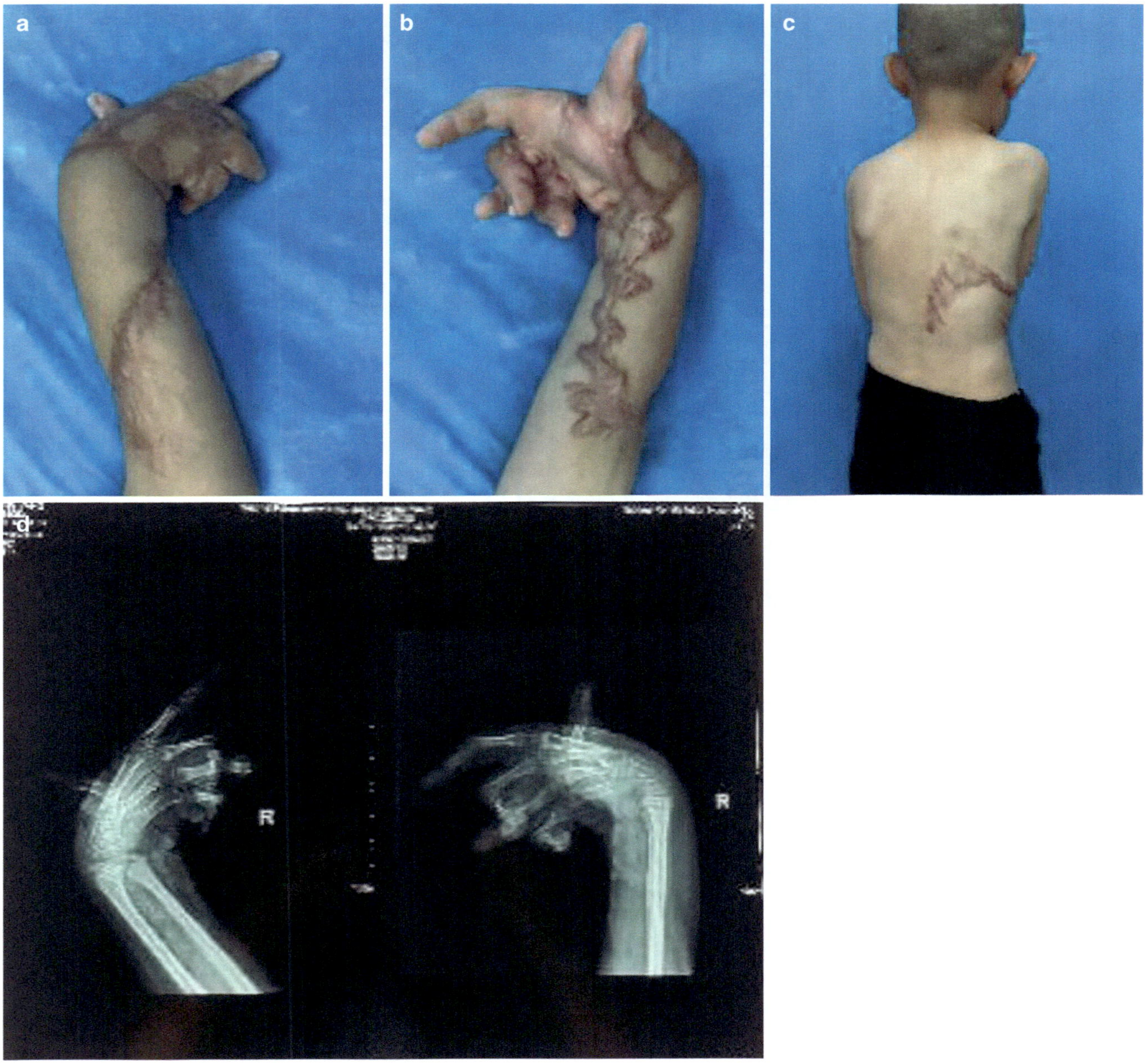

Fig. 10.31 Male, 8 years old, 10 months old, right hand burn caused finger flexion contracture deformity. (**a**) Dorsal view of the hand; (**b**) A lateral view of the hand; (**c**) Appearance of dorsal skin graft donor site; (**d**) X-ray film of wrist and knuckle

10.5.3.3 Treatment Principle

Individualized treatment, according to the deformity, scar soft tissue release, osteotomy correction of bony deformity, restoration of lower limb gravity line, restoration of joint line, reconstruction of joint dynamic and static balance, isometric limbs, increase of joint range of motion, restoration of walking function.

10.5.4 Lower Limb Deformity after Electric Injury

Electrical injury in the lower extremities causes necrosis of the skin, fascia, and muscle of the lower extremities, replacement of fibrous scar, contracture of scar tissue, traction of distal joints, and secondary deformity of bone and joint.

10.5.4.1 Etiology

Local tissue necrosis and fibrosis in the electric shock area. After healing, fibrous scar contracture pulls the joint, which can lead to joint contracture deformity in adults and epiphyseal development retardation in children, resulting in bony deformity changes in the process of growth and development.

10.5.4.2 Clinical Manifestation

Survivors of electric injury showed burn scars on the skin at the entry and exit points of the electric current in the limbs,

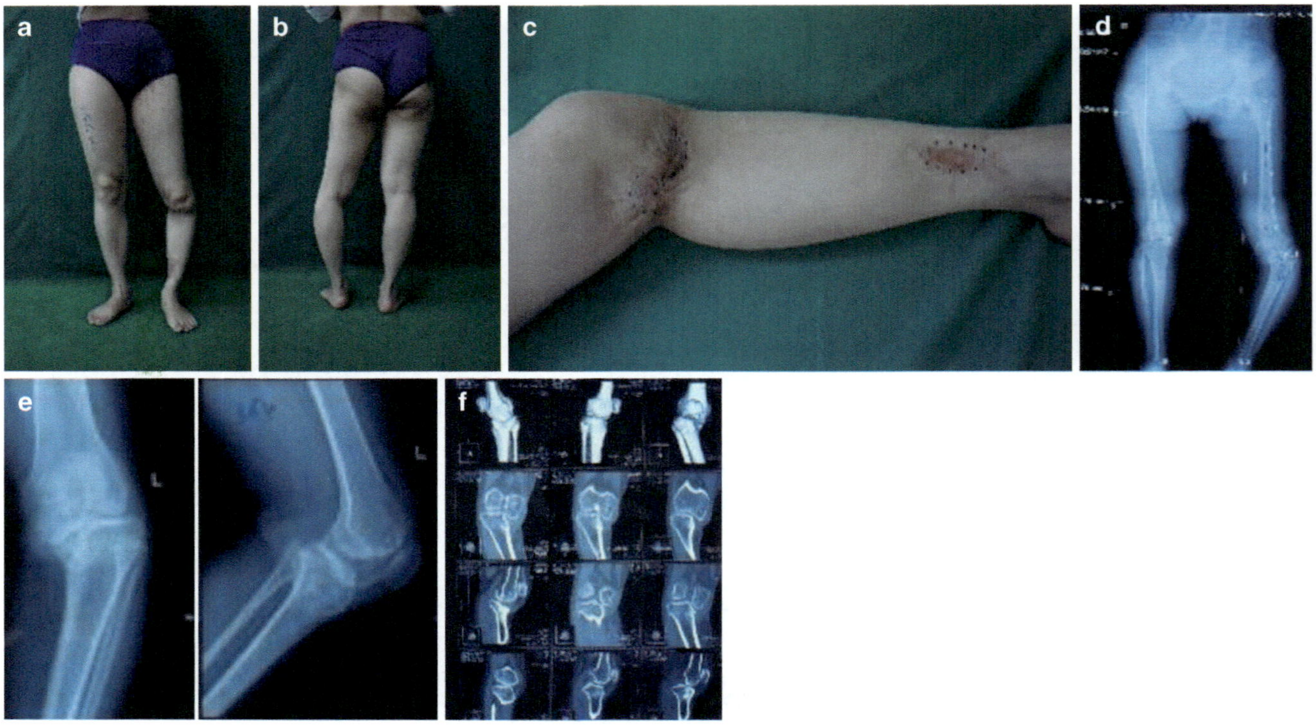

Fig. 10.32 Male, 36 years old, 6 years old, left upper leg burn with genu varum deformity. (**a**) Frontal view of lower limbs in standing position; (**b**) Posterior view of standing lower limbs (**c**). Medial view of knee and leg; (**d**) Full-length standing radiographs of the lower extremities; (**e**) Anteroposterior and lateral X-ray film of knee joint; (**f**) Three-dimensional CT reconstruction of knee joint

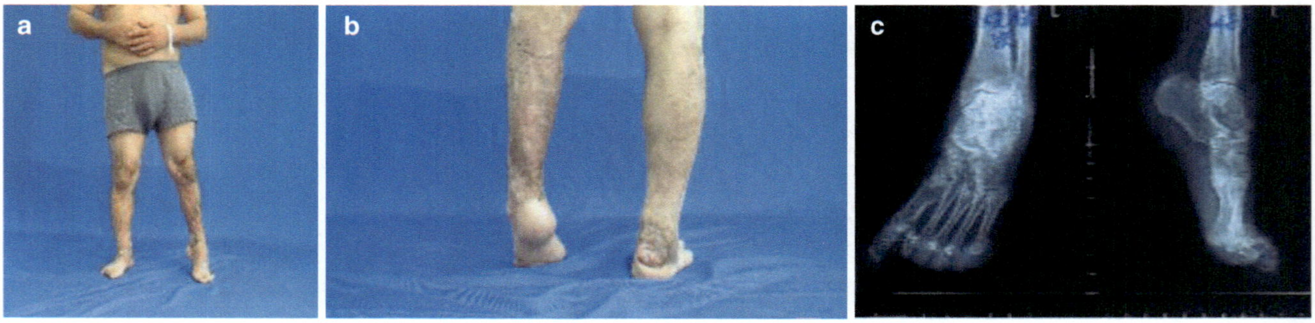

Fig. 10.33 Male, 48 years old, left talipes equinovarus deformity secondary to left leg burn at the age of 18. (**a**) Front view of lower limbs in standing position; (**b**) Posterior view of lower extremities in standing position (**c**) X-ray film of left ankle joint

stiffness, contracture, and movement disorder of the joint fibers near the scars. If injured in childhood, it may lead to epiphyseal development retardation, bony malformation changes in the process of growth and development, unequal limb length, and walking dysfunction. The female patient, 29 years old, was injured by electric shock when she was 7 years old. During the growth process, she developed right ankle varus, retroflexion, and leg shortening deformity. She underwent supra-ankle osteotomy and ring fixation orthopedic lengthening in the local hospital (Fig. 10.34).

10.5.4.3 Treatment Principle

Release the scar tissue of contracture, correct the deformity of bone and joint, restore the gravity line of lower limbs and the running line of joints, improve the blood supply of limbs, promote the healing of bone nonunion, and improve the walking function.

10.5.5 Infant Burn Scar Contracture-Bulbous Foot Deformity with Ulcer in Weight-Bearing Area

The skin, fascia, and muscle of the severely burned calf, foot, and ankle in childhood are extensively necrotic and replaced by fibrous scars. If the early treatment is not appropriate and the skin flap transplantation is not carried out in the later stage after injury, the bone and joint structure of the ankle and foot

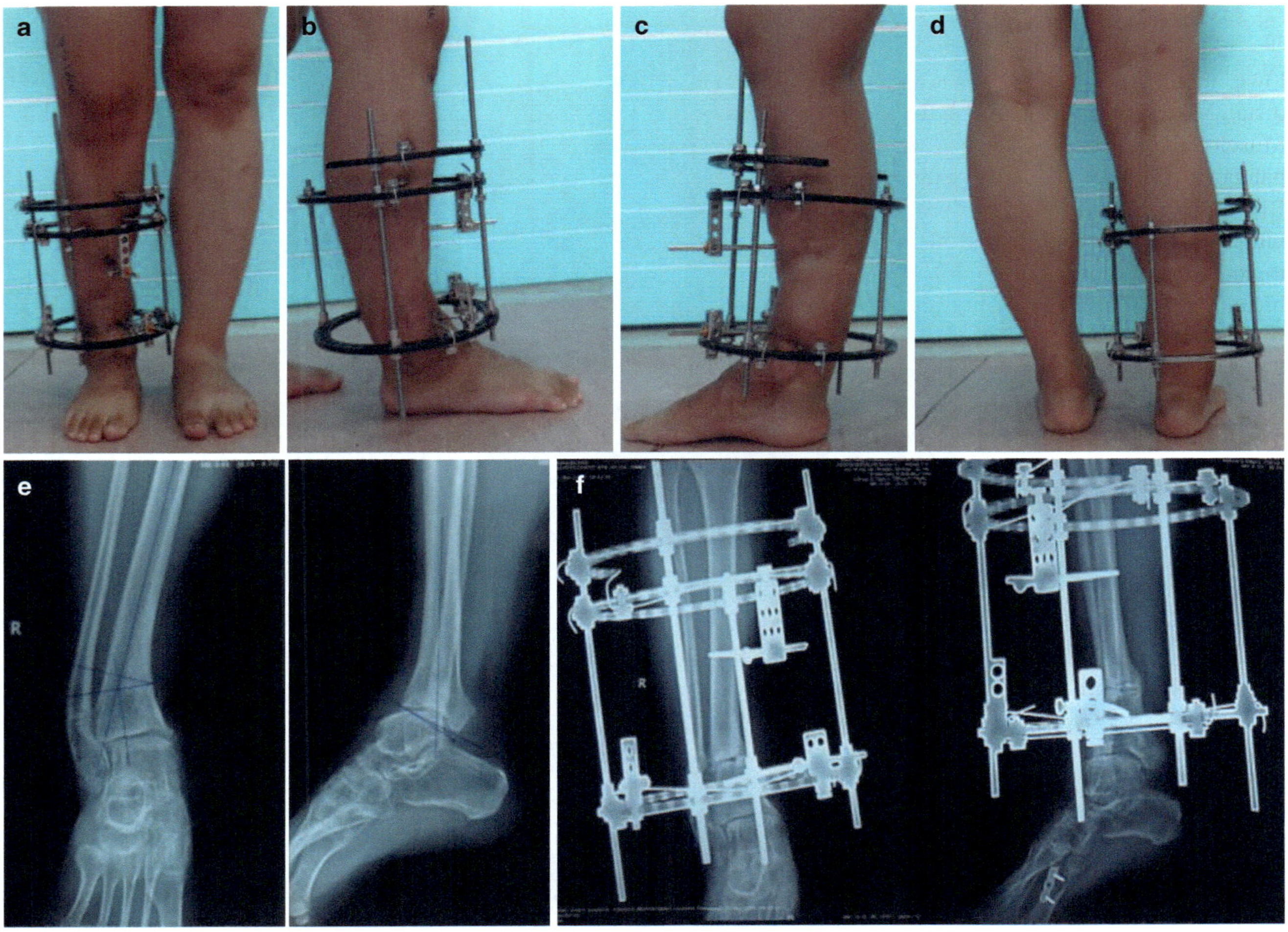

Fig. 10.34 Deformity of foot and ankle joint in sequela of electric injury. (**a**) Frontal view of lower limbs in standing position; (**b**) Lateral view of lower extremity in standing position; (**c**) Medial view of lower extremity in standing position; (**d**) Posterior view of weight-bearing leg and ankle; (**e**) Preoperative X-ray film of varus deformity of ankle joint after electric injury; (**f**) An anteroposterior and lateral radiograph of the right ankle joint after orthopedic supra-malleolar osteotomy

will inevitably be entangled in the growth and development of children, resulting in a special ball ankle and foot deformity. The author met a 30-year-old female who did not accept the effective surgical method of amputation and artificial limb.

10.5.5.1 Etiology

The 1-year-old patient had extensive burns on both legs and ankles and was not treated with skin grafting in the early and middle and late stages. The fibrous scar tissue slowly wrapped and squeezed the ankle-foot bone joints.

10.5.5.2 Clinical Manifestation

A 30-year-old female presented with extensive scar contracture of both legs and ankles, left midfoot, and good ankle flexion and extension function. The outside of the right foot is shaped like a football, and there is an ulcer that does not heal for a long time in the weight-bearing area. X-ray showed that the right toe was present and completely encased in the scarred skin (Fig. 10.35).

10.5.5.3 Treatment Principle

The patient did not receive a post-prosthetic treatment, and the Ilizarov technique was used to slowly stretch and expand the scarred skin, then repair the apophysis and eliminate the ulcer.

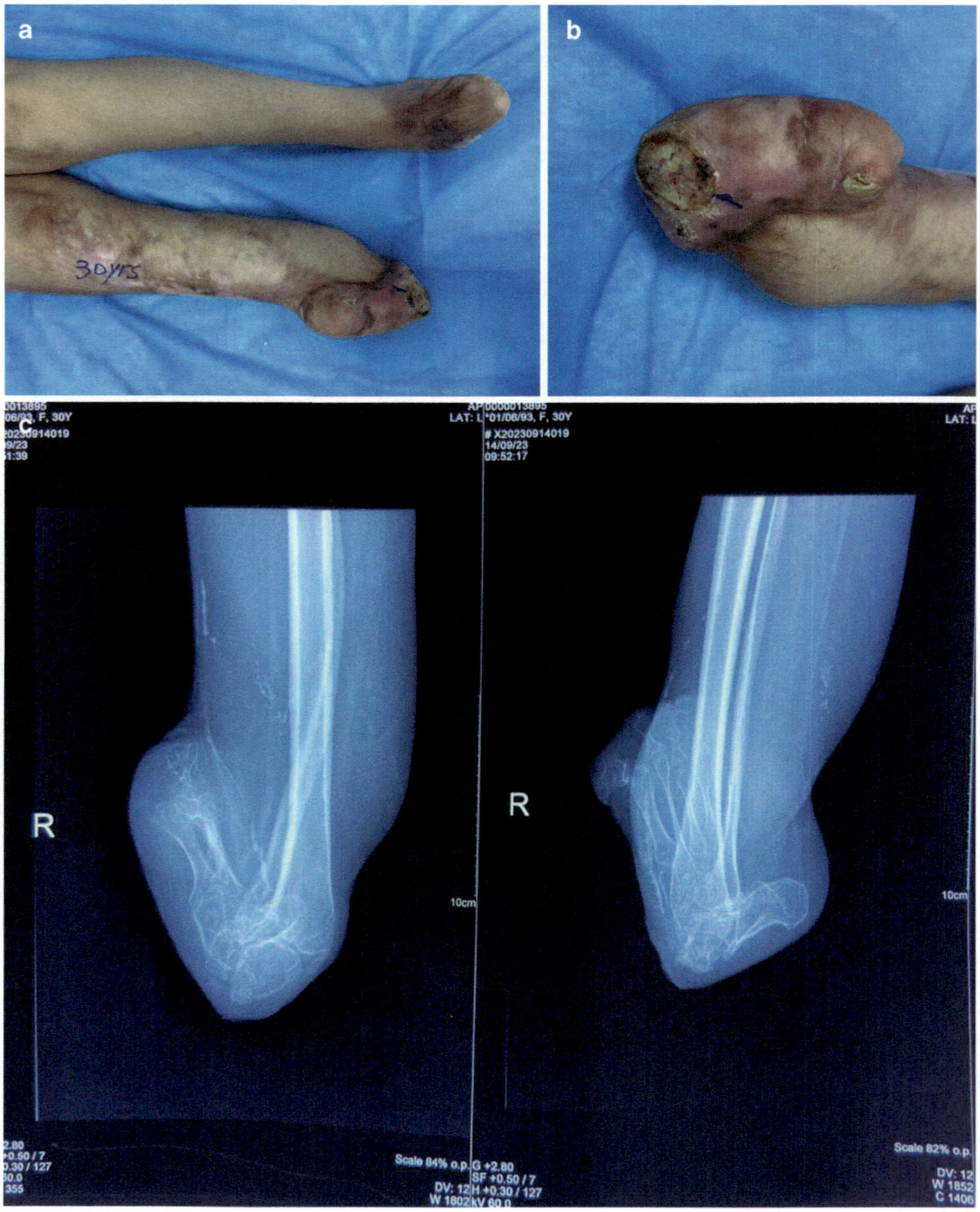

Fig. 10.35 (**a**) Female, 30 years old, 1 year old, burn, extensive scar contracture of both feet, left midfoot remnant, (**b**) The scar contracture of the right foot was football-shaped, and the weight-bearing area was ulcerated. By UNK1 X-ray examination, the tarsus and toes of the right foot were wrapped and compressed in the scar tissue

10.6 Limb Deformity Caused by Rare Injury

10.6.1 Beasts Attack

10.6.1.1 Etiology

Beasts attack can cause damage to human muscles, nerves, blood vessels, ligaments and even bones, leaving limb deformities, and dysfunction.

10.6.1.2 Clinical Manifestation

According to the severity of the injury and the corresponding symptoms of the injured part, the patient was scratched by a bear on the buttock when he was a teenager, and the local skin, muscle, fascia, and other soft tissues were missing, leaving a large area of scar and the appearance of the buttock soft tissue defect. Resulting in foot skin sensory disturbance, calcaneal varus deformity, and walking disorder (Fig. 10.36).

10.6.1.3 Treatment Principle

Give priority to prevention, carry out thorough debridement and proper functional exercise when injured; if the early treatment is wrong and the deformity has been formed, the wound should be excised, the free flap should be transplanted, the scar tissue should be repaired, and then the deformity should be corrected, the joint should be balanced and the function should be restored.

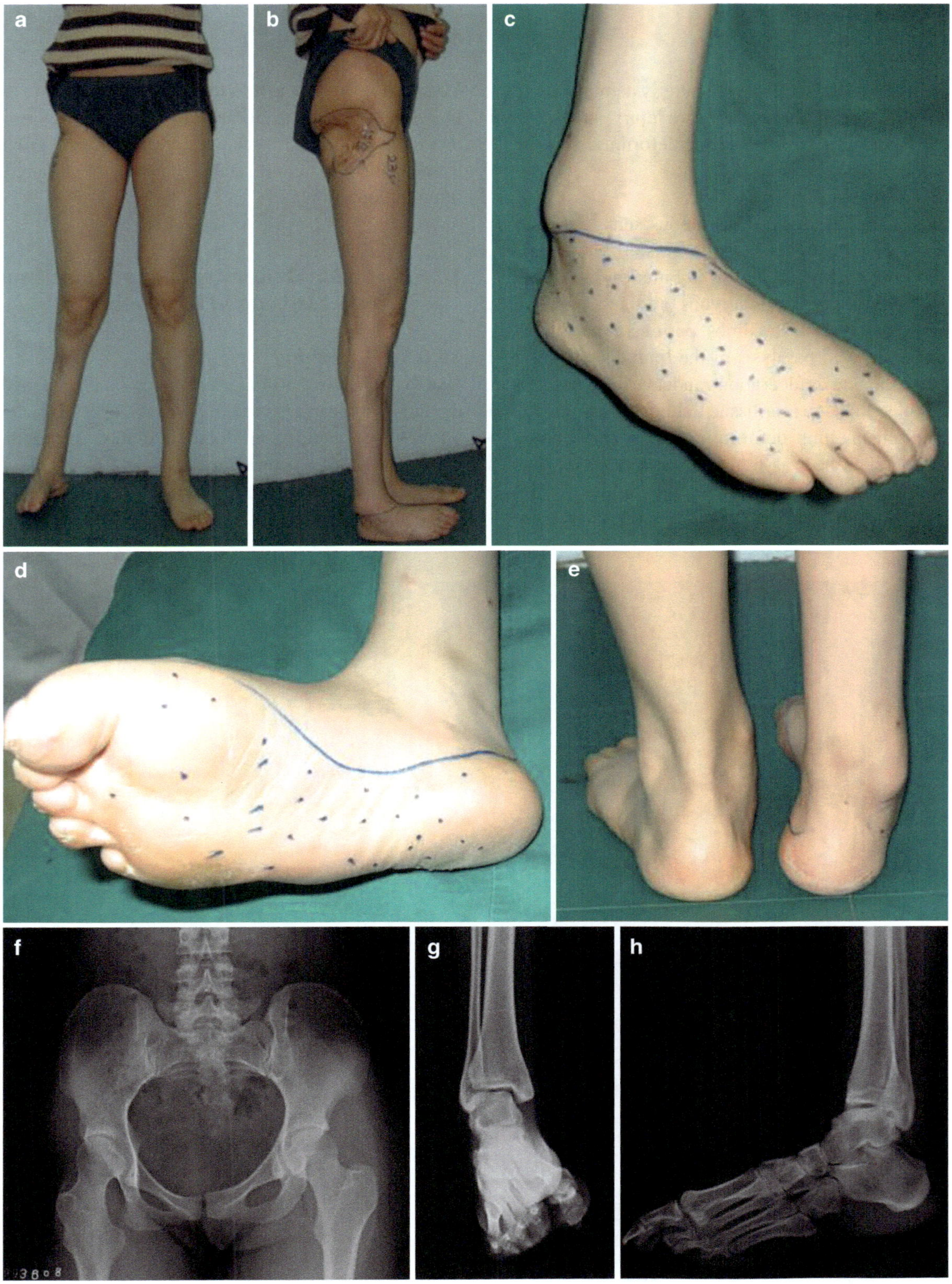

Fig. 10.36 The bear scratches the buttock and causes sciatic nerve injury, followed by heel varus deformity. (**a**) Standing position Lower limb standing frontal view; (**b**) Lateral view of lower extremity in standing position; (**c**) Lateral view of right foot; (**d**) Right plantar appearance; (**e**) Bipedal posterior ankle view in standing position; (**f**) Anteroposterior X-ray of pelvis; (**g**, **h**) Anteroposterior and lateral radiographs of right ankle joint

10.6.2 Venomous Snake Bite

10.6.2.1 Etiology

Bite by venomous snake can cause acute systemic toxic reaction, local skin necrosis and ulcer, nerve injury, and local soft tissue scar contracture can cause limb deformity.

10.6.2.2 Clinical Manifestation

The clinical manifestations of venomous snake bite can be divided into three categories: nerve poison, blood poison, and mixed poison. After a person is bitten by a venomous snake and survives, central nervous system damage can cause spastic paralysis of the limbs, peripheral nerve paralysis can cause delayed paralysis of the limbs, local skin and soft tissue of the bite or ulceration can leave deep scars, injuries in childhood, due to scar tissue traction to limit bone and joint development, limb deformities can occur, leading to dysfunction. When he was 6 and a half years old, he was bitten by a venomous snake on the dorsum of his foot, resulting in a large area of local skin ulceration, deep tissue necrosis, severe scar, and foot valgus deformity during growth and development (Fig. 10.37).

10.6.2.3 Treatment Principle

Individualized treatment, according to limb deformity, correct deformity, release scar, restore lower limb gravity line, balance muscle strength, stabilize joints, equal-length limbs, improve limb function.

10.6.3 Flexion Deformity of Knee Joint Caused by Cross-Legged Meditation

10.6.3.1 Etiology

Due to compulsive postures such as cross-legged meditation, the hip and knee joints are in a state of excessive curling for a long time, resulting in blood circulation disorders around the joints, tendon contracture, muscle atrophy, nerve compression and nutritional disorders, resulting in limb deformities.

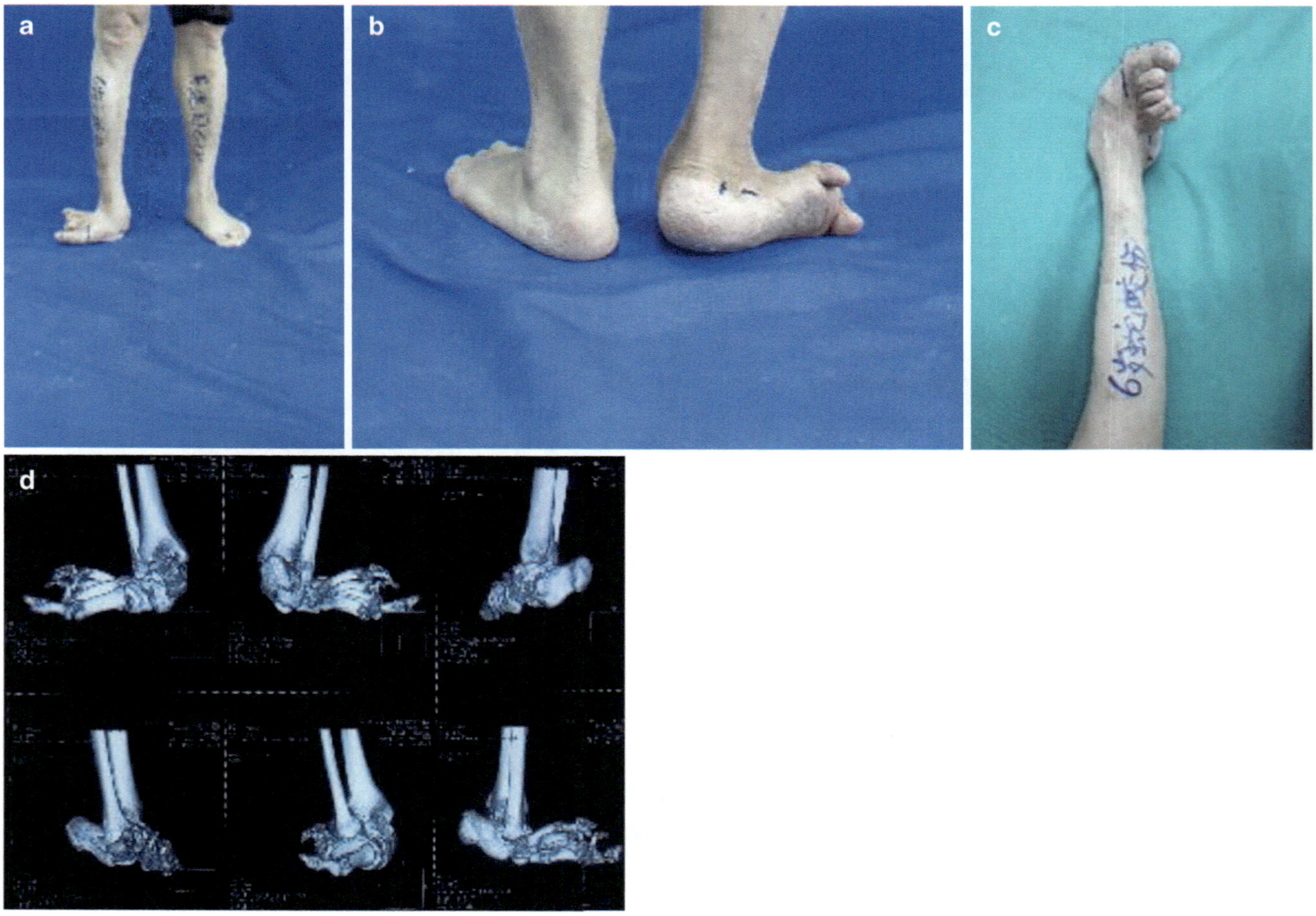

Fig. 10.37 Foot valgus deformity caused by venomous snake bite. (**a**) Frontal view of lower limbs in standing position; (**b**) Posterior view of lower extremities in standing position; (**c**) Non-weight-bearing frontal view of right ankle; (**d**) Three-dimensional reconstruction CT images of right ankle joint

10.6.3.2 Clinical Manifestation

Because the joint is forced to be in an unnatural state for a long time, tendon strain, contracture, nerve injury, joint stiffness and limited movement, knee flexion contracture cannot be straightened, walking is difficult, dysfunction; There may be no obvious abnormal bony deformity on the knee joint X-ray (Fig. 10.38).

10.6.3.3 Treatment Principle

Elimination of teratogenic external causes, joint rehabilitation functional exercise, physical and mental treatment, orthopedic surgery if necessary, release of contracture soft tissue, restoration of lower limb gravity line, and joint balance and stability.

10.6.4 Lower Limb Deformity Caused by Intrauterine Fetal Injury

10.6.4.1 Etiology

Intrauterine treatment or examination during pregnancy, irregular operation or errors, resulting in fetal intrauterine injury, affecting development, resulting in limb deformities.

10.6.4.2 Clinical Manifestation

Because of the different injuries, the clinical manifestations are irregular, so the medical history of intrauterine examination and injection during pregnancy should be carefully inquired and analyzed, combined with clinical physical examination and judgment, to clarify the causes and mechanisms of limb deformities. As shown in the figure, the patient is a 21-year-old female with a self-reported medical history. Her mother was treated with intrauterine injection at the eighth month of pregnancy (the details are unknown). After birth, she was found to have right calf injury. With the growth and development, she gradually developed right calf muscle atrophy and scar cord formation. After adulthood, she had calf shortening and varus, severe horseshoe deformity on her right foot, and walking disorder (Fig. 10.39).

10.6.4.3 Treatment Principle

The principle of individualization is to analyze the specific situation, correct the deformity according to its characteristics, rebuild the balance of soft tissue and joint, restore the weight line of lower limbs and the shape of limbs, restore the function of joints as much as possible, and improve the walking ability.

10.6.5 Knee Joint Stiffness Caused by Umbilical Cord Infection and Septicemia in Infants

10.6.5.1 Etiology

Due to the improper handling of the umbilical cord at birth, septicemia, bone and joint suppuration and infection lead to deformity.

10.6.5.2 Clinical Manifestation

The clinical manifestations are irregular and have their own characteristics, so we should carefully inquire about the medical history, combine with clinical examination and judgment, and clarify the causes and mechanisms of limb deformities. For example, in the legend, the female patient, 31 years old, complained of fever caused by "umbilical cord wind" at birth. The deformity was not obvious in infancy. With the growth and development, the left knee joint gradually appeared retroflexion. The adult left knee joint was stiff in retroflexion posi-

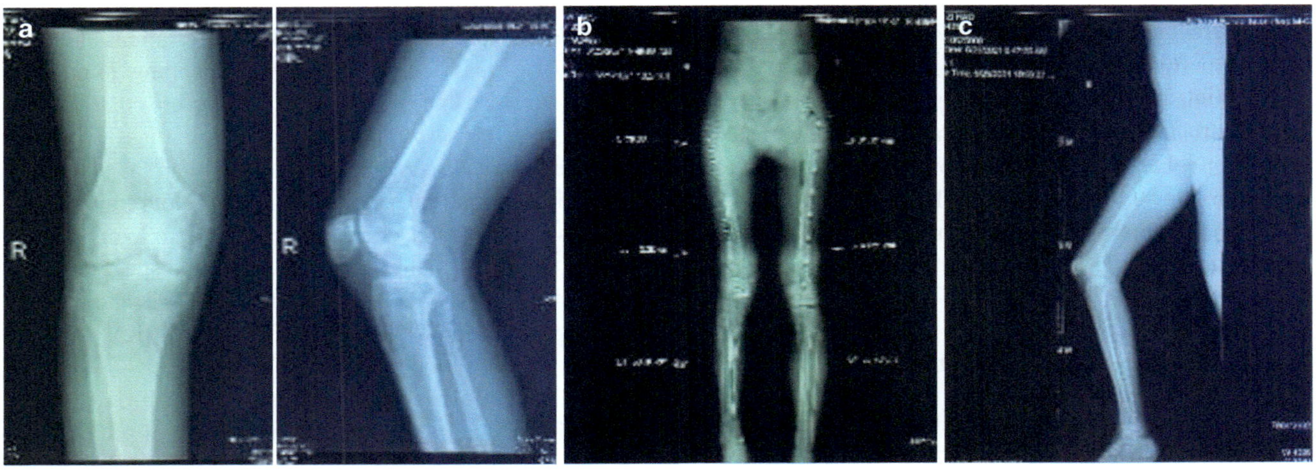

Fig. 10.38 Male, 26 years old. When he was 25 years old, he practiced cross-legged meditation, resulting in flexion deformity of knee joint and limitation of extension. (**a**) Anteroposterior and lateral X-ray films of right knee joint; (**b**) Full-length standing anteroposterior X-ray film of lower limbs; (**c**) Full-length standing lateral radiograph of right lower limb

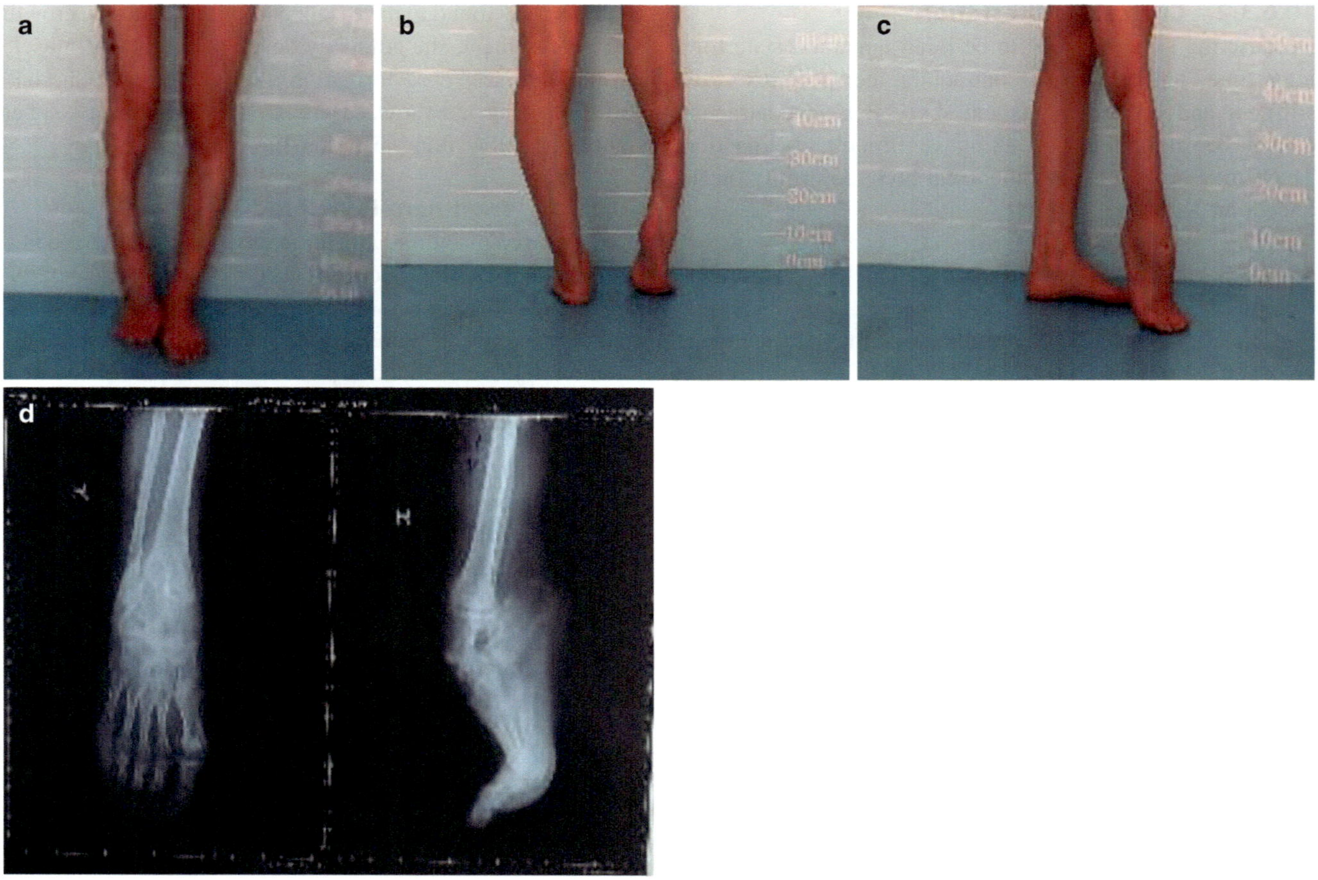

Fig. 10.39 Equinus deformity caused by intrauterine injection. (**a**) Frontal view of lower limbs in standing position; (**b**) Posterior view of lower extremities in standing position; (**c**) Lateral view of lower limbs in standing position; (**d**) Anteroposterior and lateral radiographs of right ankle joint

tion, squatting and walking obstacles, which seriously affected daily life. X-ray film shows that the knee joint is structurally abnormal, the patella is obviously moved upward, the front of the distal femur and the proximal tibia form a joint, the space is narrow, and the bone is hyperosteogeny (Fig. 10.40).

10.6.5.3 Treatment Principle

The principle of individualized treatment is to analyze the specific situation, correct the deformity according to its characteristics, rebuild the balance of soft tissue and joint, restore the weight line of lower limbs and the shape of limbs, restore the function of joints as much as possible, and improve the walking ability.

10.6.6 Infantile Buttock Injection Infectious Scar Contracture

10.6.6.1 Etiology

Local aseptic inflammation or infection, degeneration and contracture of gluteal muscles and fascia, limitation of hip joint function and limb deformity are mainly caused by repeated intramuscular injection of benzyl alcohol solvent drugs such as penicillin into the buttocks of infants or preschool children.

10.6.6.2 Clinical Manifestation

According to the degree of gluteal muscle contracture, there are different manifestations. Mild manifestations are only inability to cross legs, splayed gait, snapping joints, and inability to close knees when squatting. Severe contracture is characterized by scar adhesion, depression, muscle atrophy, palpable contracture of gluteal muscle as hard as plate, limited adduction and internal rotation of hip joint, inability to sit and squat normally, and positive Ober sign. X-ray showed that the hip joint could not be adducted, the space was narrow, and the proximal femoral neck-shaft angle and anteversion angle were abnormal (Figs. 10.41 and 10.42).

10.6.6.3 Treatment Principle

According to the location, degree and depth of gluteal muscle contracture, open surgery or arthroscopic release of contracture tissue should be performed. Proximal femoral osteotomy should be performed for joint structural changes, supplemented by postoperative functional exercise to restore hip function.

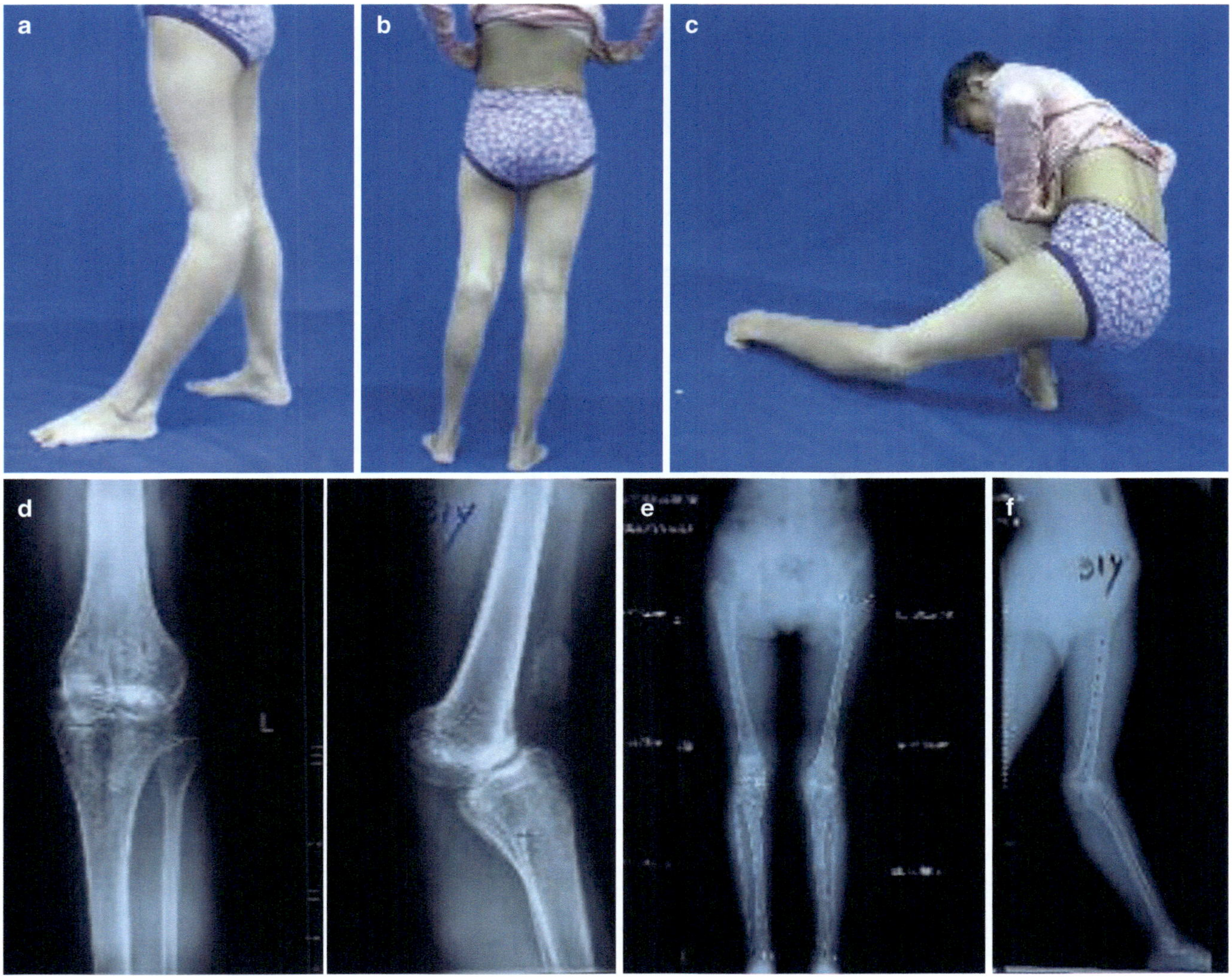

Fig. 10.40 Knee regurgitation and stiffness caused by infection and septicemia of umbilical cord. (**a**) Lateral view of the lower extremity in standing position; (**b**) Posterior view of lower extremities in standing position; (**c**) Side view of squat position; (**d**) Anteroposterior and lateral radiographs of knee joint; (**e**, **f**) Full-length standing anteroposterior and lateral radiographs of both lower extremities

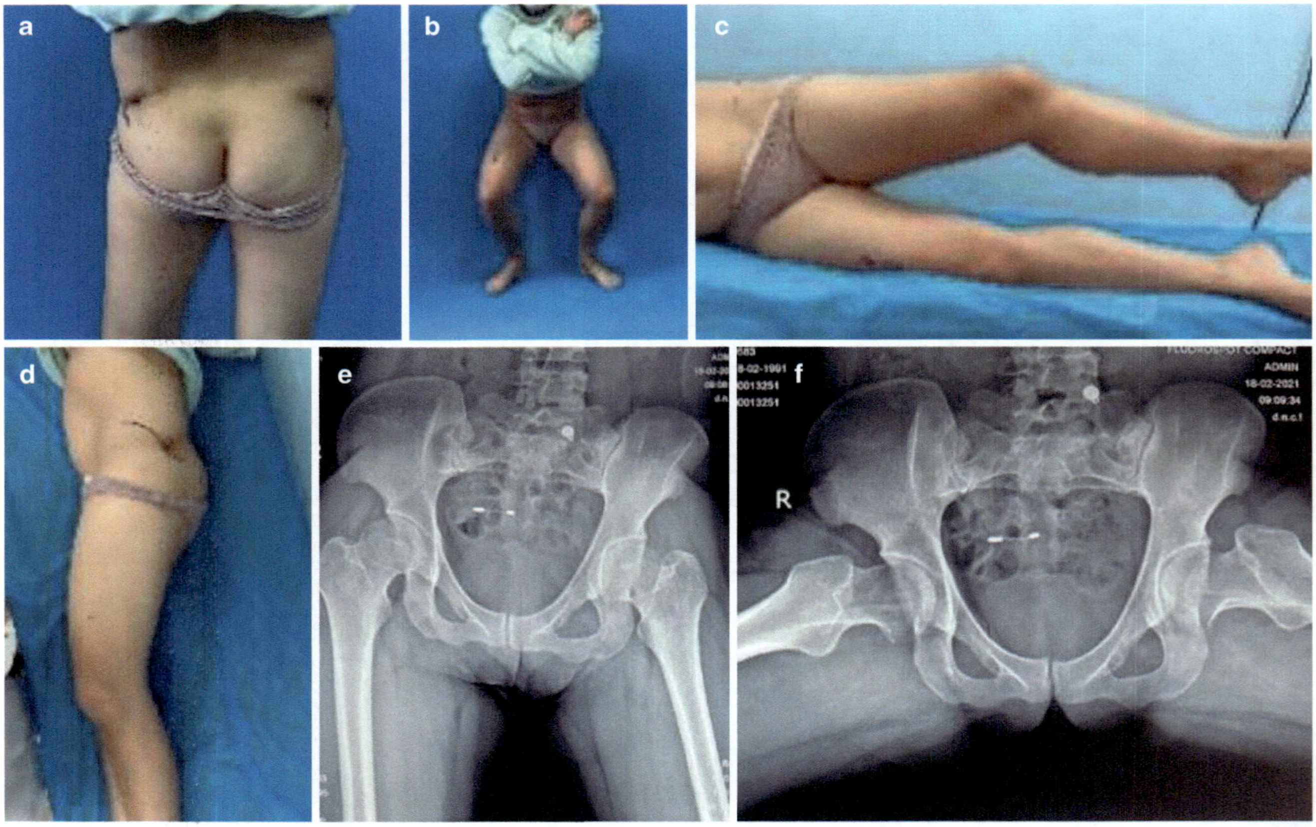

Fig. 10.41 A 30-year-old female with bilateral gluteal muscle contracture caused by injection infection in young buttocks. (**a**) Appearance of lower extremity buttocks in standing position; (**b**) Front view when squatting; (**c**) The affected limb is in the upper lateral decubitus position; (**d**) Lateral view of the affected limb in the upper lateral decubitus position; (**e**) Anteroposterior X-ray film of pelvis in adduction position of both hips; (**f**) Anteroposterior radiograph of pelvis of bilateral hip abduction position

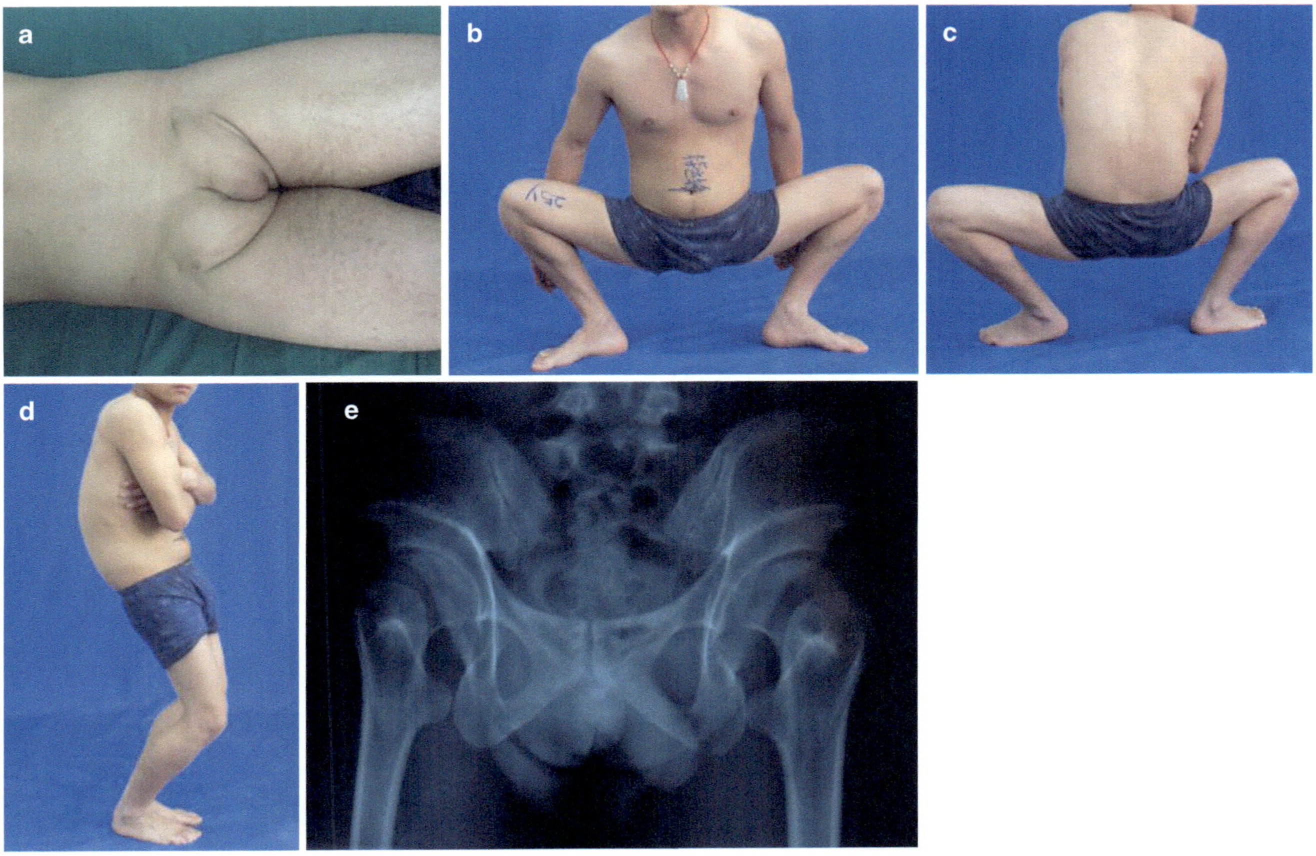

Fig. 10.42 Male, 27 years old, severe contracture of bilateral gluteal muscles caused by injection into the buttocks in childhood. (**a**) Appearance of the buttocks in the prone position; (**b**) Front view when squatting; (**c**) View from behind while squatting; (**d**) Side view in standing position; (**e**) Anteroposterior radiograph of pelvis

Limb Deformity Caused by Comprehensive Causes

11

Sihe Qin

11.1 Myofascial Contracture Deformity of Lower Limb

11.1.1 Contracture of Gluteal Muscles and Fascia

11.1.1.1 Bilateral Gluteal Muscle Contracture

Gluteal muscle contracture is a kind of fibrotic contracture of gluteal muscles and fascia, which causes abduction and external rotation deformity of hip joint, and flexion disorder of hip joint in severe cases.

1. Etiology
   (a) A history of repeated gluteal intramuscular injections in childhood, especially repeated injections of penicillin antibiotics. It mainly includes the mechanical injury of needles and the chemical injury of drugs.
   (b) Genetic and idiopathic factors. Nearly 10% of patients have no history of repeated gluteal intramuscular injections, and some cases have never received gluteal intramuscular injections. However, they have a family history of high incidence of the disease, which makes people think that the incidence of these patients is related to heredity. There are also a small number of children who have no history of gluteal muscle injection and no family history, which is called idiopathic.
   (c) Susceptible factors gluteal muscle contracture occurs in children, and children are susceptible to the disease. However, only a part of the children who received long-term repeated intramuscular injection suffered from the disease, indicating that there are great differences in the susceptibility of children to the disease. Patients with scar constitution are more likely to develop the disease after receiving gluteal muscle injection.
2. Clinical manifestations
   (a) Posture and gait: In the patient's standing position, when the lower limbs are close together, it appears to be laborious. In severe cases, the toes of both feet cannot be touched together, and when walking, it is a splayed gait. When stepping forward, the knee joint points to the anterolateral side, unable to lift the knee joint to the front, showing a circular gait. When squatting, the knees of the light squatters are separated first, and then they are closed together after squatting (circle sign). Severe cases can only squat in the abduction and external rotation position. When squatting, the hip joints are in the abduction and external rotation position, and the knees cannot be close to each other, showing a frog style (Fig. 11.1). Severe patients are particularly difficult to wear their own pants or socks and need to sit on pillows or quilts to wear their own pants or socks.
   (b) Examination of the buttocks: The patient's buttocks were sunken on the lateral side, losing the bulging and smooth shape of the normal buttocks. The posterior part of the iliac crest and the greater trochanter of the greater femur were more prominent. The upper 1/4 of the buttocks were sunken most seriously, where the hard fibrous cords under the skin could be touched, losing the normal elasticity of the buttocks muscles. When the hip is adducted and rotated passively, the fiber cord on the outside of the buttock is more tough and obvious.
   (c) Examination of the range of motion of the hip joint: (1) The knee squat test was positive: both knees together could not complete the squat action; (2) When sitting, the action of crossing legs cannot be completed; (3) Positive hip flexion test: unable to complete hip flexion in neutral position; (4) When the contracture of one side gluteal muscle or the contracture of both sides gluteal muscle is different in

S. Qin (✉)
Department of Orthopaedics, Rehabilitation Hospital of the National Research Center for Rehabilitation Technical Aids, Beijing, China

S. Qin et al. (eds.), *Atlas of Limb Deformity*, https://doi.org/10.1007/978-981-97-0999-1_11

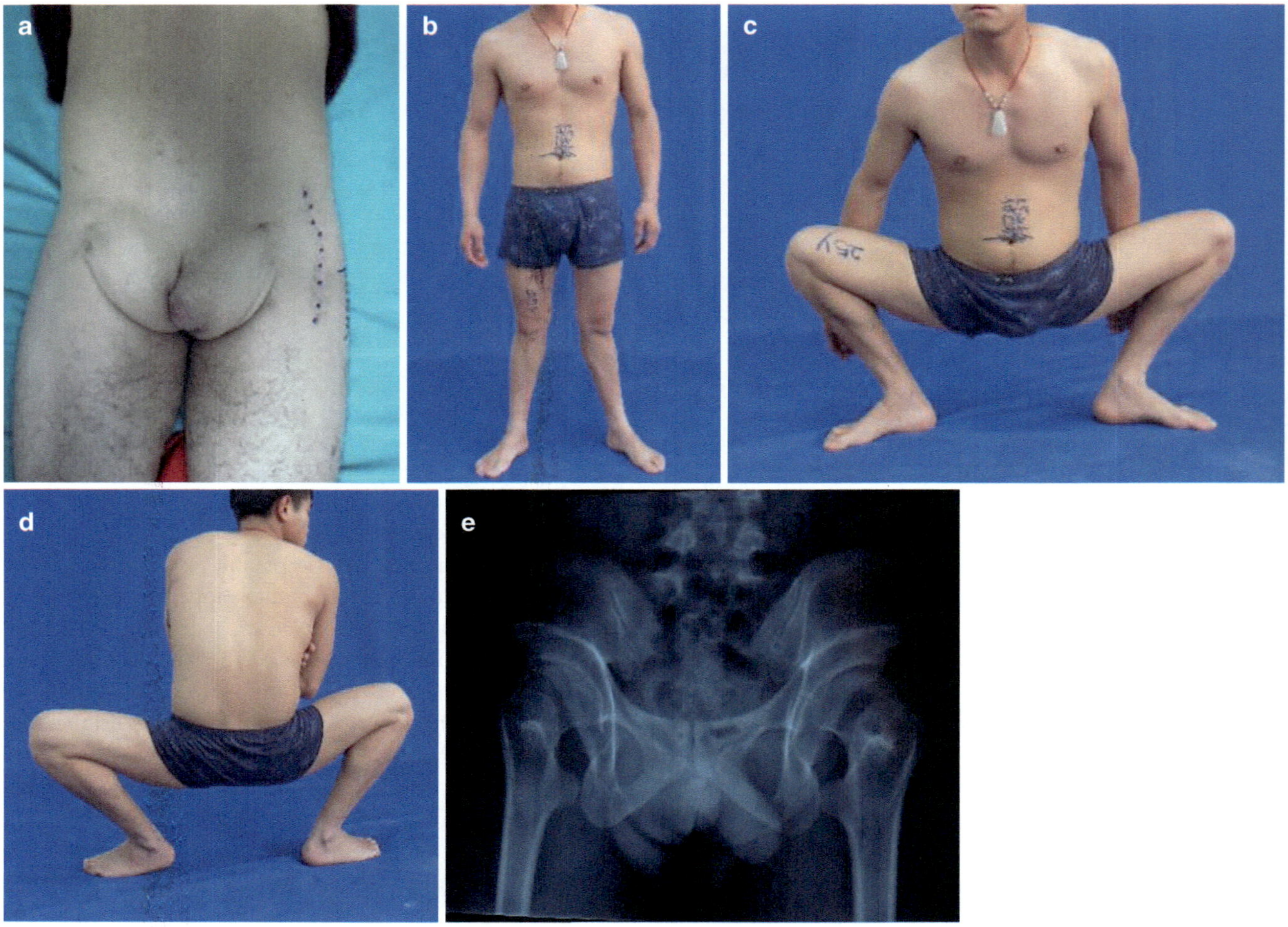

Fig. 11.1 Male, 24 years old, repeated intramuscular injection of buttocks in childhood, secondary bilateral gluteal muscle contracture: (**a**) appearance of buttocks, bilateral gluteal muscle contour disappeared, pointed buttocks deformity, surgical incision scar on the right buttocks; (**b**) appearance of standing position, external rotation of both lower limbs; (**c**) extreme external rotation of both hip joints during squatting; (**d**) dorsal view of squatting position; (**e**) anteroposterior radiograph of the pelvis showed outward rotation of the femur and upward displacement of the femoral head

degree and contracture degree, it may be manifested as unequal length of lower limbs.

(d) Other examinations: X-ray examination was generally normal, but in a few cases, there were secondary bony changes in the pelvis and hip joint. X-ray showed that the acetabular index increased. The neck-shaft angle and anteversion angle increased. Subluxation of hip joint was secondary to severe gluteal muscle contracture.

3. Classification

Shrestha et al. divided gluteal muscle contracture into four types according to the hip adduction angle at 90° flexion and 90° flexion: type I (hip adduction −5° to −20°), type II (hip adduction −20° to −40°), type III (hip adduction −40° to −60°), and type IV (hip adduction > −60°).

4. Treatment principles

Once the diagnosis is confirmed, if there is no clear surgical contraindication, surgical treatment should be carried out as soon as possible. Surgical release of gluteal muscle contracture is an effective treatment measure. If the femoral deformity changes significantly, subtrochanteric osteotomy should be added.

11.1.1.2 Unilateral Gluteal Muscle Contracture-Pelvic Obliquity

1. Etiology

Gluteal trauma, intramuscular injection, sequelae of poliomyelitis, and other factors can cause unilateral gluteal muscle contracture.

2. Clinical manifestations

Unilateral gluteal muscle contracture is characterized by varying degrees of pelvic obliquity and pseudo-inequality of the lower extremities. Contracture of the gluteal muscle on the affected side, traction of the hip joint with abduction deformity, adduction of the hip joint, and downward inclination of the pelvis when standing (Fig. 11.2). In walking gait, when the affected side is

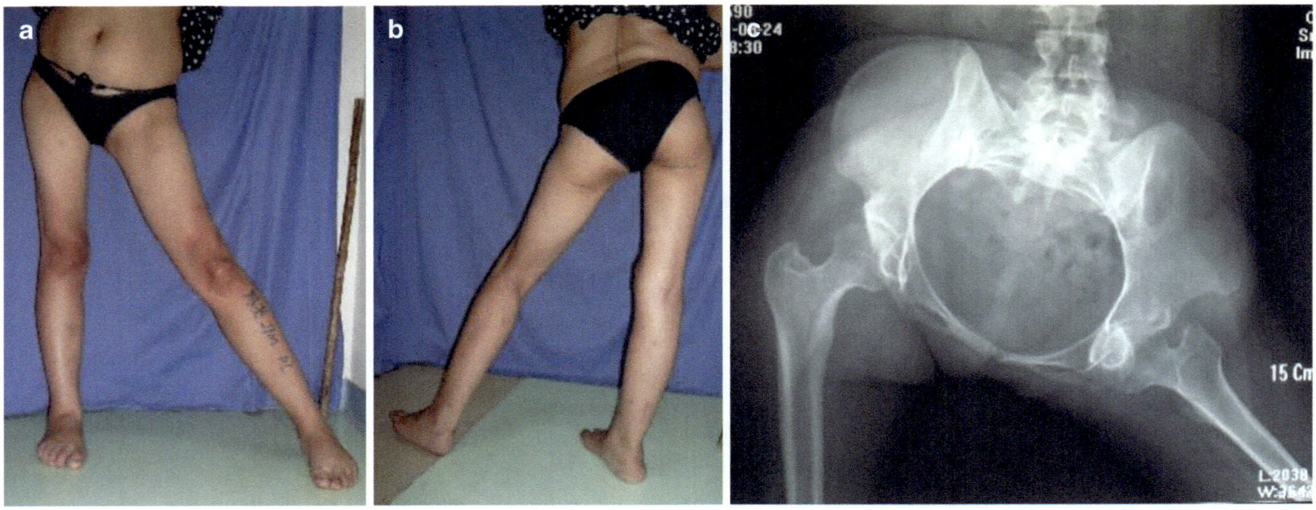

Fig. 11.2 Female, 27 years old, sequelae of poliomyelitis, left gluteal muscle contracture, pelvic obliquity. (**a**) View from the front in standing position; (**b**) view from the back in standing position; (**c**) anteroposterior radiograph of pelvis

weight-bearing, the downward inclination of the pelvis leads to the relative lengthening of the affected limb, which is similar to the limping gait of unequal limb length. Pelvic X-ray showed abduction deformity of the hip joint on the affected side, and pelvic tilt could be seen in the full-length film of both lower limbs, but the length of both lower limbs was equal, and even the length of the patient's lower limbs was slightly shorter.

3. Treatment principles

   Release the contracture of gluteal fascia, and in severe cases, combine with subtrochanteric osteotomy to correct pelvic tilt.

11.1.2 Gastrocnemius Contracture

Gastrocnemius contracture refers to a clinical syndrome of special gait and signs caused by the decrease of elasticity of gastrocnemius muscle and its fascia caused by various reasons, which makes it in a short state or a specific position for a long time, and then causes the limitation of ankle dorsiflexion.

11.1.2.1 Etiology

Gastrocnemius contracture caused by trauma, infection, neuromuscular diseases such as cerebral palsy, sequelae of poliomyelitis, hemangioma, etc.

11.1.2.2 Clinical Manifestation

Equinus deformity, ankle dorsiflexion is limited in knee extension, unable to reach neutral position, ankle dorsiflexion is not limited in knee flexion, able to reach neutral position. Silverskiold's test is positive, that is, in the state of extending the knee joint and flexing the knee joint, the ankle joint is passively extended to the neutral position. If the ankle joint can be extended to the neutral position when the knee is flexed, while the equinus deformity occurs when the knee is extended, and the ankle joint cannot be extended to 0°, it indicates that the gastrocnemius muscle has contracture. If the equinus deformity does not improve with or without knee extension and flexion, it indicates Achilles tendon contracture (Fig. 11.3).

11.1.2.3 Treatment Principle

After the diagnosis was confirmed, gastrocnemius aponeurosis lengthening was performed to correct the foot drop deformity moderately.

11.1.3 Myositis Ossificans Progressiva

Myositis Ossificans Progressiva (MOP), also known as fibrodysplasia Ossificans Progressiva, is a rare hereditary, progressive connective tissue disorder characterized by congenital thumb deformities and progressive myositis ossificans.

11.1.3.1 Etiology

The etiology has not yet been thoroughly understood, and the basic factor is the secondary calcification and ossification caused by genetic defects in some components of connective tissue, which belongs to dominant inheritance.

11.1.3.2 Clinical Manifestation

It is more common in males, mostly before the age of 6. Occasionally, the lesions in fascia and tendon exist before birth. Most of the sick children have various congenital abnormalities, especially the small thumb or toe deformity.

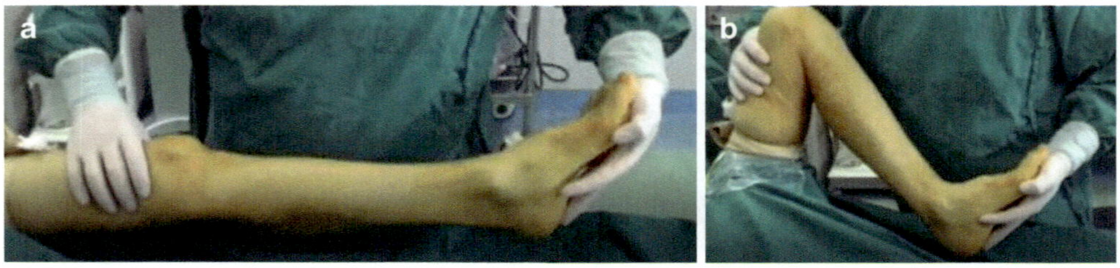

Fig. 11.3 Gastrocnemius contracture. (**a**) Talipes equinus deformity occurs in the knee extension position, and the ankle joint cannot be extended to the neutral position; (**b**) in the knee flexion position, the ankle can be extended to the neutral position

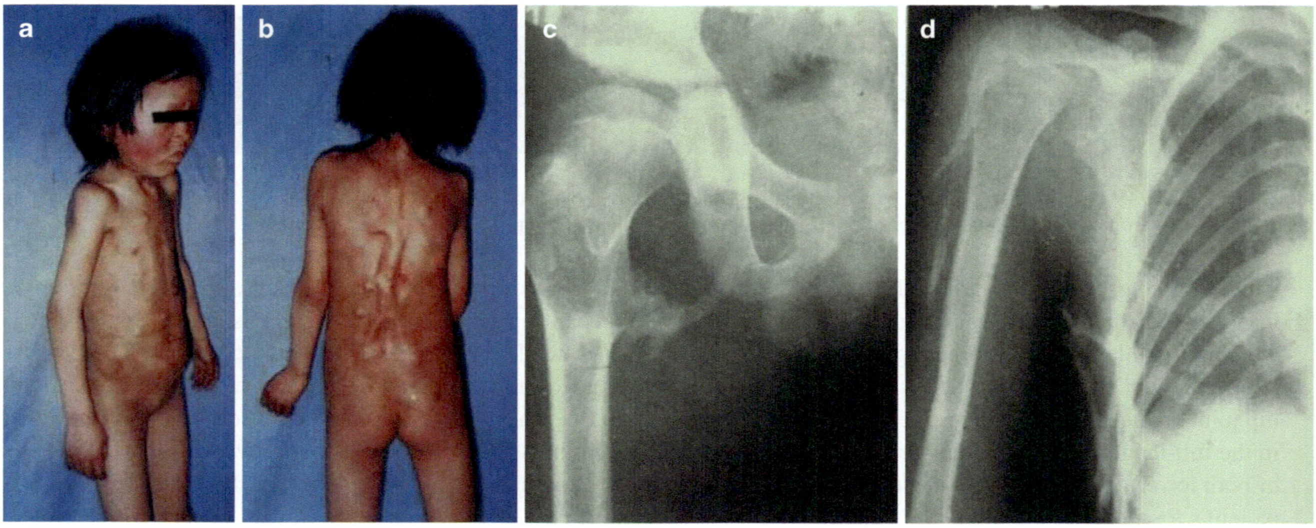

Fig. 11.4 Myositis ossificans progressiva with soft tissue ossification in many parts of the body. (**a**) Lateral view in standing position; (**b**) posterior view in standing position, multiple ossification foci on the back can be seen; (**c**) anteroposterior X-ray film of right hip joint; (**d**) the anteroposterior film of the right humerus showed "strip-like" ossification foci on the lateral side of the humerus

Typical lesions first appear in the neck, the back of the trunk and shoulder, and finally in the proximal end of the limbs. The lesion area is swollen, the scope is small, sometimes up to the size of an egg. In the early acute stage, the local area is muddy swelling, pain, tenderness and mild fever, accompanied by systemic low fever. The mass often clings to the deep fascia, the local skin can be loosened, and the flushing and swelling of the skin are optional. After several days or weeks, the local swelling subsides, leaving a relatively firm nodule, and after 2–8 months, the local bone tissue forms (Fig. 11.4).

11.1.3.3 Treatment Principle

If there are no obvious symptoms, they cannot be treated. If pain and discomfort occur and affect joint movement, surgical resection is feasible to improve limb function.

11.1.4 Charcot Painless Arthropathy

Neuropathic arthropathy was first described by Charcot in 1868, so it is also called Charcot arthropathy. This kind of disease is caused by painlessness, also known as painless arthropathy.

11.1.4.1 Etiology

Sensory nerve injury caused by central nervous system syphilis, syringomyelia, diabetic neuropathy, myelomeningocele, congenital absence of pain (painless anhidrosis), and other reasons, resulting in the weakening or disappearance of pain, shoulder, elbow, cervical spine, hip, knee, ankle, toe, and other joints due to the lack of pain protection mechanism. Eventually, joint destruction and deformity occur.

11.1.4.2 Clinical Manifestation

In neuropathic arthropathy, the joints are gradually swollen, unstable, and effusion, and the joints may be punctured with blood-like fluid. Most of the swollen joints had no pain or only slight swelling pain, and the limitation of joint function was not obvious. This disease is characterized by joint pain and functional limitation inconsistent with joint swelling and destruction. In the late stage, the joint destruction develops further, which can lead to pathological fracture or dislocation of the joint (Fig. 11.5).

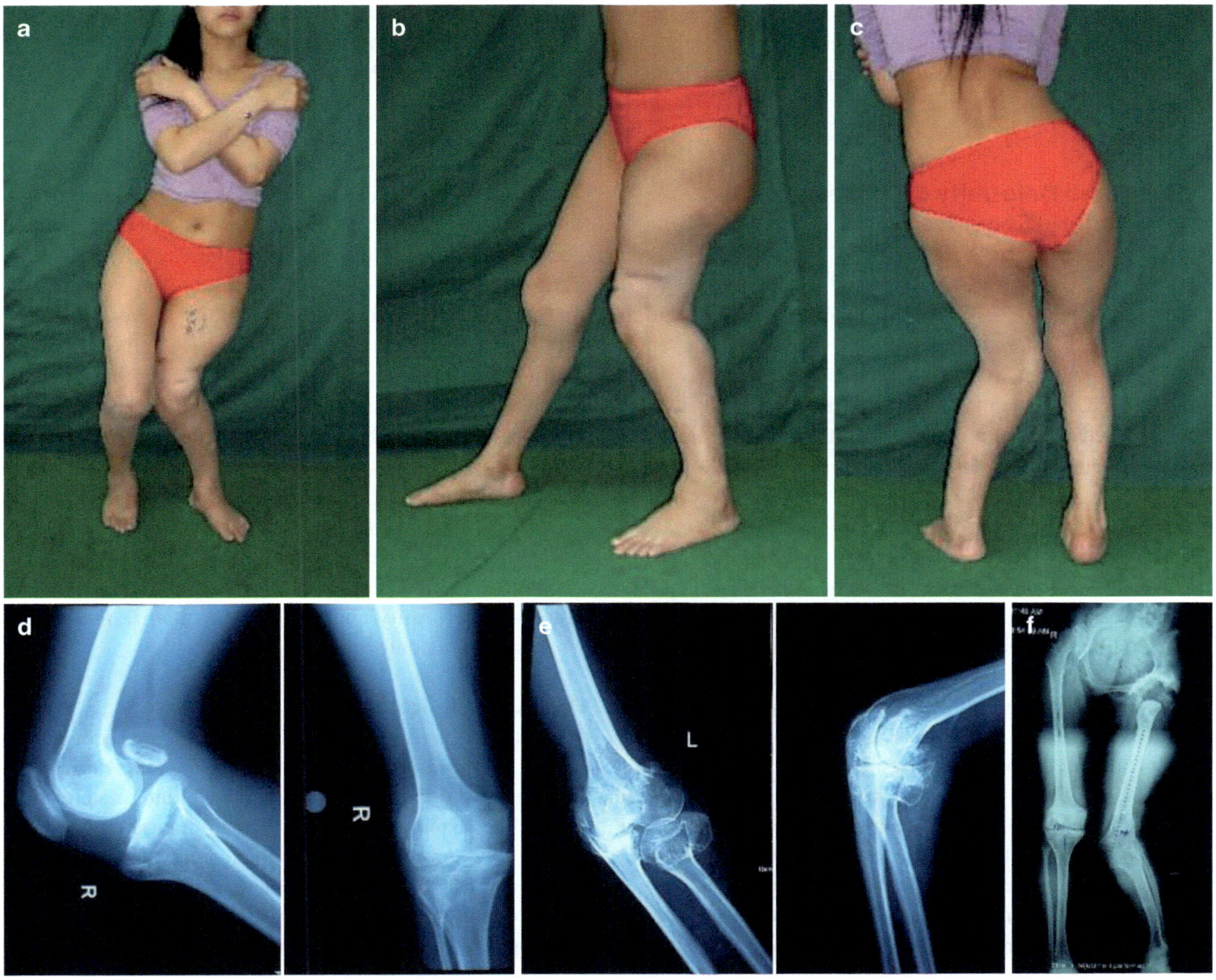

Fig. 11.5 Female, 19 years old, joint deformity caused by Charco arthropathy. (**a**) Frontal view in standing position; (**b**) left lateral view in standing position; (**c**) dorsal view in standing position; (**d**) anteroposterior and lateral X-ray film of right knee joint, giant corpus liberum can be seen on the posterior side of knee joint; (**e**) anteroposterior and lateral X-ray film of left elbow joint, joint destruction can be seen; (**f**) Full-length X-ray film of both lower extremities in standing position showed severe destruction of the left hip joint and fusion of the left knee joint in valgus position

11.1.4.3 Treatment Principle

(1) Diseased joints, upper limbs should avoid hard work, and lower limbs should try to reduce weight. (2) The seriously damaged joints (such as knee, elbow, and spine) can be protected by brackets. (3) If the foot is seriously ill and the ulcer is not healed, it can undergo amputation. Knees of young and middle-aged patients, Ankle If the damage is severe, arthrodesis may be performed, but the disease may recur in the adjacent joints. Reducing activity and bracket protection are effective methods for multiple purposes. (4) For patients with subluxation of the joint or collapse of the articular surface, osteotomy and orthopedic surgery can be used to restore the gravity line of the lower limb, which can slow down the progress of joint destruction.

11.2 Iatrogenic Limb Deformity

Iatrogenic limb deformity refers to the sequelae secondary to medication, medical methods, and surgical errors, such as ischemic muscle contracture caused by prolonged tourniquet time, arthroscopic injury, external fixation needle injury, improper splint fixation or plaster fixation after fracture, and limb ischemia and necrosis caused by prolonged tourniquet time during operation. Improper operation or misoperation can cause irreversible injury of large blood vessels and nerves, and improper postoperative treatment can lead to malunion of osteotomy end.

11.2.1 Limb Deformity of Obstetrical Palsy (Injury) Sequelae

11.2.1.1 Etiology

Obstetrical injury refers to the injury to the newborn caused by mechanical factors during delivery. In recent years, antenatal examination and obstetric technique have been strengthened, and the incidence of birth injury has been significantly reduced, but it is still one of the causes of neonatal death and long-term disability.

11.2.1.2 Clinical Manifestation

There are many kinds of obstetrical injuries, which can involve soft tissues (such as scalp), bones such as skull, clavicle, humerus, femur, and nerves such as cranial nerves and peripheral nerves. Different types of birth injuries have different clinical symptoms. Limb deformities caused by obstetrical injury mainly include three types: (1) obstetrical injury causes brain, spinal cord, and other central nerves, which can lead to spastic paralysis of limbs, and the symptoms are similar to the clinical manifestations of cerebral palsy (CP); (2) peripheral nerve injury caused by obstetrical injury is commonly brachial plexus injury, which is characterized by different degrees of upper limb muscle paralysis and secondary deformity such as drooping wrist (Fig. 11.6); (3) obstetrical injury fracture. The predilection sites of obstetrical injury fracture are clavicle, humeral shaft, femoral shaft, skull, humerus or femoral epiphyseal separation. If obstetrical injury fracture is found in time and handled properly, there are few sequelae, and it generally does not cause limb dysfunction.

11.2.1.3 Treatment Principles

To correct secondary limb deformities, the goal of treatment is to improve hand function in upper limbs and to restore plantar foot and improve walking function in lower limbs.

11.2.2 Foot and Ankle deformity of Ischemic Muscle Contracture Caused by Improper Plaster Fixation

11.2.2.1 Etiology

Ischemic muscle contracture caused by plaster immobilization often occurs in the forearm and leg. After acute traumatic fracture of the leg, plaster fixation, especially tubular plaster fixation, causes traumatic reactive swelling of the soft tissue of the leg, increases the volume, the internal space of the plaster cannot increase with the swelling, the swollen tissue is compressed, the blood circulation is impaired, and the swelling of the tissue is aggravated, forming a vicious circle. If the soft tissue compression cannot be relieved in time, muscle necrosis will occur. It continues to develop and even causes limb necrosis and has to be amputated. If the compression is relieved in time during the period of muscle necrosis, limb necrosis can be avoided, but the necrotic muscle will be fibrotic, contracture, traction of ankle and foot joints will cause deformity changes, mostly manifested as talipes equinovarus deformity.

11.2.2.2 Clinical Manifestation

Ischemic muscle contracture of the leg is often secondary to talipes equinovarus deformity, which is characterized by thinning of the leg, scar incision on the anterolateral side, rigid talipes equinovarus deformity, limitation of dorsiflexion and eversion of the foot, complete paralysis of the dorsiflexion and eversion muscles in severe cases, and numbness or loss of sensation of the lateral skin of the dorsum of the foot in patients with common peroneal nerve injury. A contracture of the flexor pollicis longus muscle causes a claw foot deformity (Fig. 11.7).

11.2.2.3 Treatment Principle

The contracture of the plantar flexor varus tendon was released and Ilizarov technique was used to correct the deformity of the ankle and foot. The subtalar joint or triple arthrodesis was performed at the same time for the patients with bony deformity caused by long course of disease.

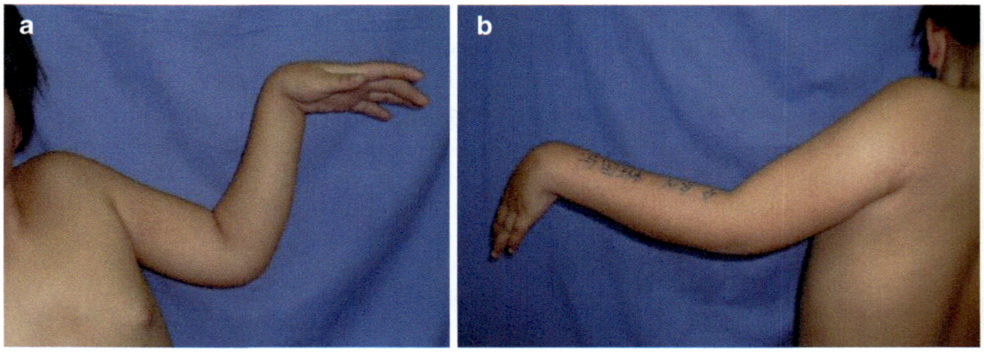

Fig. 11.6 Female, 10 years old, left upper limb dysfunction caused by obstetric palsy. (**a**) Shoulder abduction and wrist dorsiflexion dysfunction; (**b**) back view

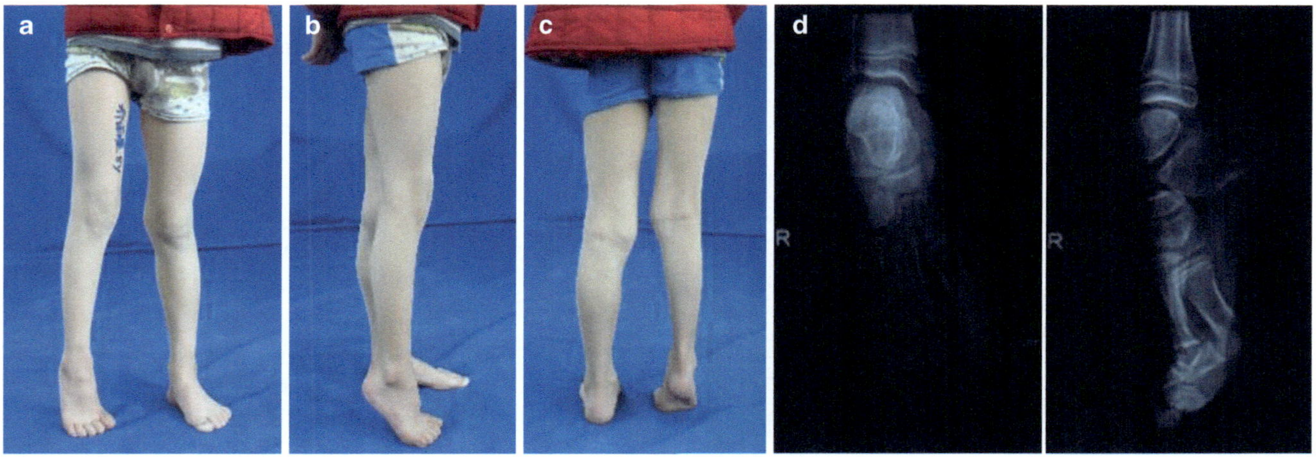

Fig. 11.7 Male, 8 years old. When he was 3 years old, the lower part of the left leg was fractured. After plaster fixation, the plaster was too tight and limb ischemia occurred. The plaster was removed in emergency, and then the talipes equinovarus deformity was gradually secondary. (**a**) Standing appearance, left equinus deformity; (**b**) lateral view, left toe touching the ground; (**c**) dorsal view; (**d**) X-ray film of left foot

11.2.3 Bone Infection and Bone Defect After Internal Fixation of Fracture

The infection after internal fixation of fracture refers to the infection of bone tissue caused by the contamination of pathogenic microorganisms or the low autoimmunity of patients after the placement of internal fixation of fracture, which is in contact with the internal fixation, with or without the infection of surrounding soft tissue.

11.2.3.1 Etiology

(1) Internal fixation of open fracture, (2) Internal fixation of non-open fractures causes severe damage to soft tissue due to long operation time. The patient's body is weak and the immune function is decreased. (4) Hematogenous infection of fracture site.

11.2.3.2 Staging and Clinical Manifestations

Early infection is mostly caused by highly virulent pathogens, mainly manifested as local redness, swelling, heat, pain, poor wound healing, and may be accompanied by systemic symptoms, such as fever. In the chronic phase of infection, there will be skin ulceration, sinus, etc. (Fig. 11.8).

11.2.3.3 Treatment Principle

After thorough debridement, the internal fixation was removed, and the infected bone segment was cleared, the Ilizarov technique was used to repair the bone defect.

11.2.4 Muscle Necrosis and Degeneration Caused by Injection of Drugs

11.2.4.1 Etiology

After injection of drugs into the buttocks due to illness in childhood (details unknown), muscle necrosis, fibrosis, and contracture in the injection area occurred, resulting in hip deformity.

11.2.4.2 Clinical Manifestation

The skin of the buttocks is sunken, the muscle elasticity is lost, the hip joint is deformed in abduction and external rotation, and the function of adduction and internal rotation is impaired (Fig. 11.9).

11.2.4.3 Treatment Principle

Loosen the soft tissue of hip contracture and improve hip joint movement.

11.2.5 Multiple Osteonecrosis Caused by Corticosteroids

11.2.5.1 Etiology

The pathogenesis of steroid-induced osteonecrosis (SION) is still not very clear. It is generally believed that the long-term accumulation of hormones in the body causes increased blood viscosity, increased blood lipids, fat embolism and

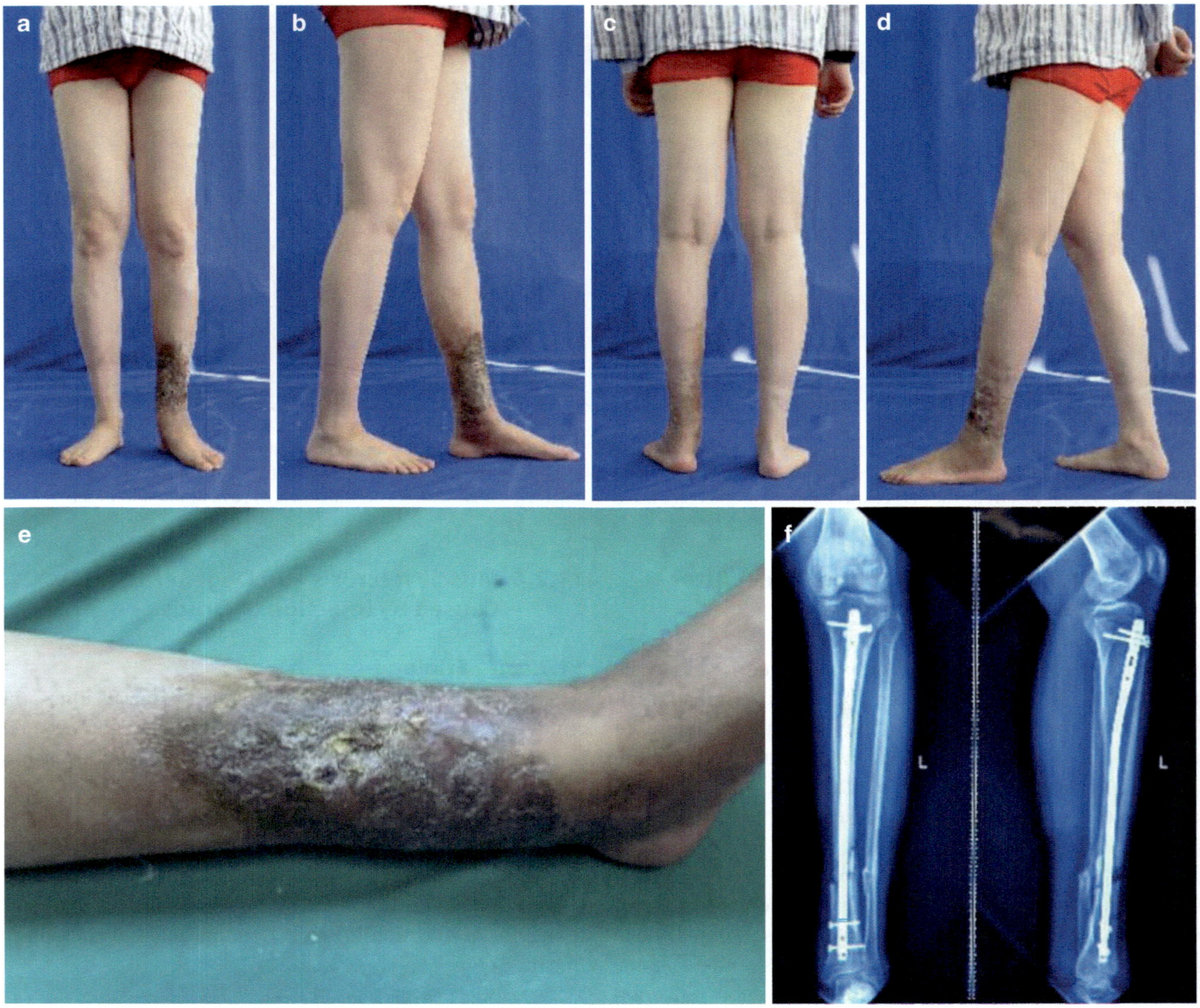

Fig. 11.8 Bone infection and defect after intramedullary nail fixation of left middle and lower tibial fracture. Male, 37 years old, 1 year after injury. (**a**) Appearance in standing position, skin pigmentation, sinus and bone exposure in the anteromedial part of the middle and lower part of the right leg; (**b**) medial view of the left lower limb in standing position; (**c**) dorsal view of the lower part of the left leg in standing position; (**d**) left side view; (**e**) wound, sinus, and bone exposure of the left leg; (**f**) anteroposterior and lateral X-ray films of left lower leg

fatty liver. It causes microvascular obstruction, ischemia, reduction of bone synthesis, calcium absorption disorders, osteoporosis, and accumulation of micro-fractures, and finally leads to steroid-induced osteonecrosis.

11.2.5.2 Clinical Manifestation

Steroid-induced osteonecrosis mostly occurs in the femoral head, the early clinical symptoms are not obvious, only seen in thigh muscle weakness and adductor pain, individual patients have limb pain far away from the site, some patients may have intermittent hip pain after fatigue, alternating hip pain or mild claudication. On clinical examination, slight tenderness in the hip and groin area can be seen, and the "4" test and Thomas's sign can be positive. Because there are no typical clinical symptoms, signs and X-ray manifestations in the early stage, the misdiagnosis rate is high. Symptoms in the middle and late stages: steroid-induced osteonecrosis of the femoral head is mostly intermittent and insidious. With the evolution of the disease in the middle and late stages, the main clinical symptoms are hip pain with slow development, which is aggravated during activities and not obvious during rest. About 1/4 of the patients have intermittent attacks, which are characterized by sudden severe pain and sudden disappearance. During the onset of hip pain, conventional analgesics are ineffective in individual patients. The onset of hip pain has the following characteristics: (1) Location of pain: In most patients, the onset of pain is mainly in the groin and the medial side of the thigh, followed by a certain part of the anterior thigh and the posterior buttock, and some patients have more than two parts, so it is often difficult to distinguish

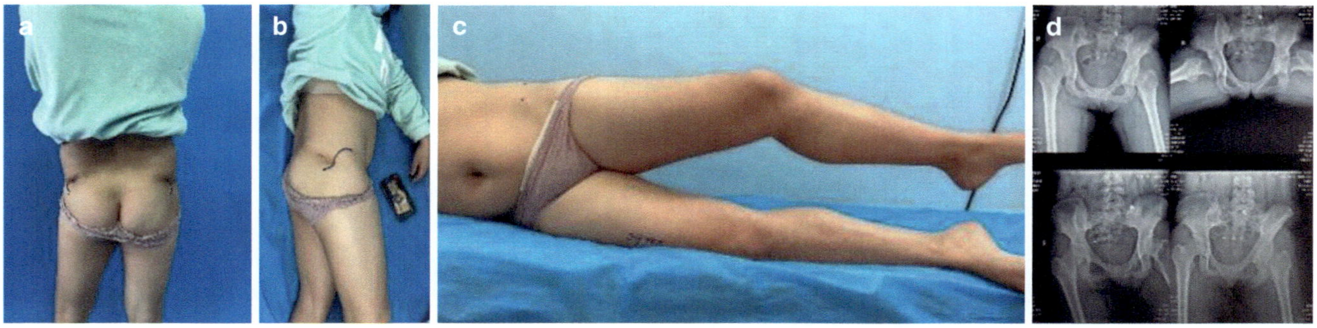

Fig. 11.9 Female, 30 years old, muscle necrosis caused by intramuscular injection in young buttocks, secondary to bilateral hip abduction contracture. (**a**) The appearance of the buttocks, the skin depression can be seen on the outer upper edge of the buttocks on both sides; (**b**) the appearance of the right buttocks; (**c**) the hip joint cannot be adducted, and the right lower limb cannot be put down naturally; (**d**) pelvic radiograph

from radiating pain or referred pain. (2) Nature of pain: The common clinical pain attacks may be acute severe pain or chronic dull pain. The typical pain attacks are needle-like radiation pain, some of which are confined to the hip, and some of which radiate to the knee joint.

Early X-ray film may not be positive, but with the progress, bone trabecula disorder, and interruption occur in the weight-bearing area, followed by cystic degeneration and sclerosis of subchondral bone of femoral head. CT examination showed that in the early stage, the bone trabeculae on the weight-bearing surface of the femoral head were disordered, partially absorbed, mixed with thickening, fusion, cystic absorption, and partial sclerosis. CT can show that the crescent sign is a three-layered structure: the center is a sequestrum surrounded by a clear bone absorption zone, and the outermost is a new osseous bone. In the late stage, the femoral head collapses and deforms, there is a large low-density area in the center, a shell-like fracture piece appears under the articular cartilage, the acetabular glenoid labium protrudes, and there may be joint deformation (Fig. 11.10). MRI can detect bone necrosis early and make a diagnosis before finding abnormalities on X-ray and CT films.

11.2.5.3 Treatment Principle

(1) Early detection, early diagnosis, and early treatment. (2) Improve the local microcirculation, reduce the local stress, and avoid the collapse and deformation of the necrotic area. (3) If the necrotic area has collapsed and deformed, bone reconstruction or joint replacement should be performed according to the patient's age and the degree of bone and joint deformation.

11.2.6 Deformity of Lower Limbs After Spinal Cord Injury Caused by Drug Poisoning

11.2.6.1 Etiology

Drug poisoning leads to high level injury of spinal cord, resulting in incomplete paralysis of the injured level, and gradually secondary deformity of lower limbs.

11.2.6.2 Clinical Manifestation

Spastic paralysis of both lower limbs, increased muscle tension, hyperreflexia of tendons, deformity of bilateral hip flexion, knee flexion, heel and foot valgus, and difficulty in walking (Fig. 11.11).

11.2.6.3 Treatment Principle

Release the contracture of soft tissue, correct the deformity of hip and knee flexion, and restore the negative gravity line of lower limbs. Osteotomy was performed to correct the bony deformity.

11.2.7 Deformity Caused by Accidental Injury of Great Vessels and Nerves in Lower Limb Surgery

11.2.7.1 Etiology

Arthroscopic treatment of knee joint disease resulted in accidental injury of popliteal artery and failure to detect it in time, resulting in ischemic muscle contracture of the leg and subsequent rigid talipes equinovarus deformity.

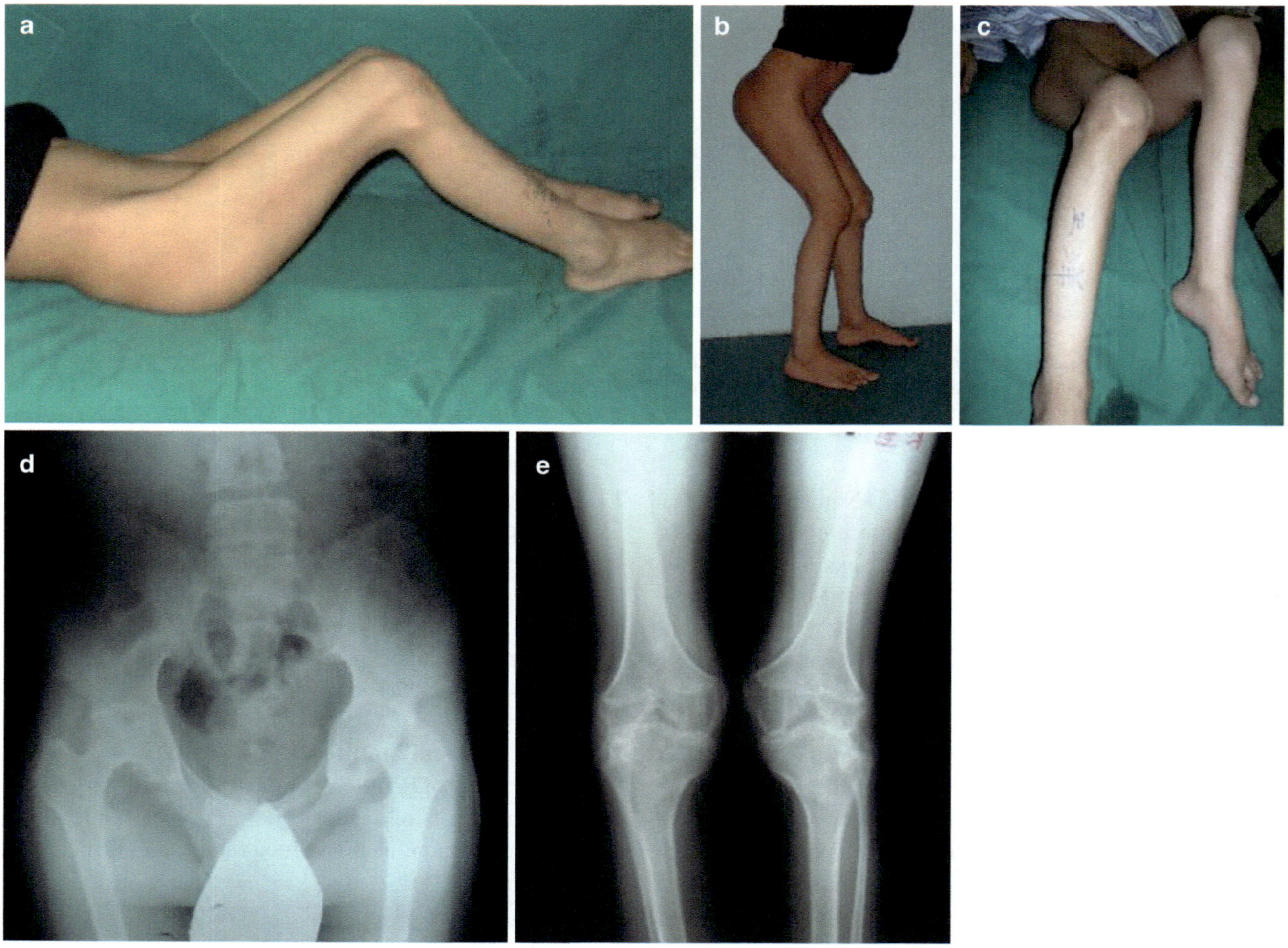

Fig. 11.10 An 18-year-old male, who had been taking corticosteroids for more than 10 years due to rheumatism, developed bilateral femoral head necrosis. (**a**) Bilateral hip flexion and knee flexion deformity; (**b**) appearance of standing under support; (**c**) appearance of both lower limbs in supine position; (**d**) anteroposterior X-ray film of pelvis; (**e**) anteroposterior X-ray film of both knee joints

11.2.7.2 Clinical Manifestation

The main manifestations are rigid talipes equinovarus or talipes equinovarus deformity, limitation of foot dorsiflexion and eversion function, skin sensory disturbance in the posterior part of the distal leg and the area innervated by the tibial nerve of the sole. According to the degree of muscle ischemia injury, there may be different degrees of muscle weakness (Fig. 11.12).

11.2.7.3 Treatment Principle

Soft tissue release, balance of muscle strength, correction of clubfoot deformity.

11.2.8 Fibrous Stiffness of the Knee Due to Long-Term Immobilization

11.2.8.1 Etiology

After femoral fracture, tibiofibular fracture, patellar fracture, meniscus or cruciate ligament, collateral ligament, and other soft tissue injuries around the knee joint, inappropriate long-term fixation of the knee joint during surgery or conservative treatment, failure to timely and correctly guide patients to exercise knee flexion and extension function, resulting in a significant reduction in knee flexion and extension activity, seriously affecting knee flexion, and extension function. The direct causes of decreased range of motion of the knee can be divided into intra-articular and extra-articular causes. Intra-articular causes included synovial adhesions, cruciate ligament adhesions or contractures, and collateral ligament adhesions or contractures. Extra-articular causes include quadriceps adhesions, contractures, and fibrosis.

11.2.8.2 Classification and Clinical Manifestation

The normal range of motion of the knee joint is about 0–130°, and the range of motion of the knee joint is less than 120°. It is considered that there is knee joint stiffness, which is mainly manifested by the decrease of the range of motion of the knee joint in different degrees (Fig. 11.13). When the

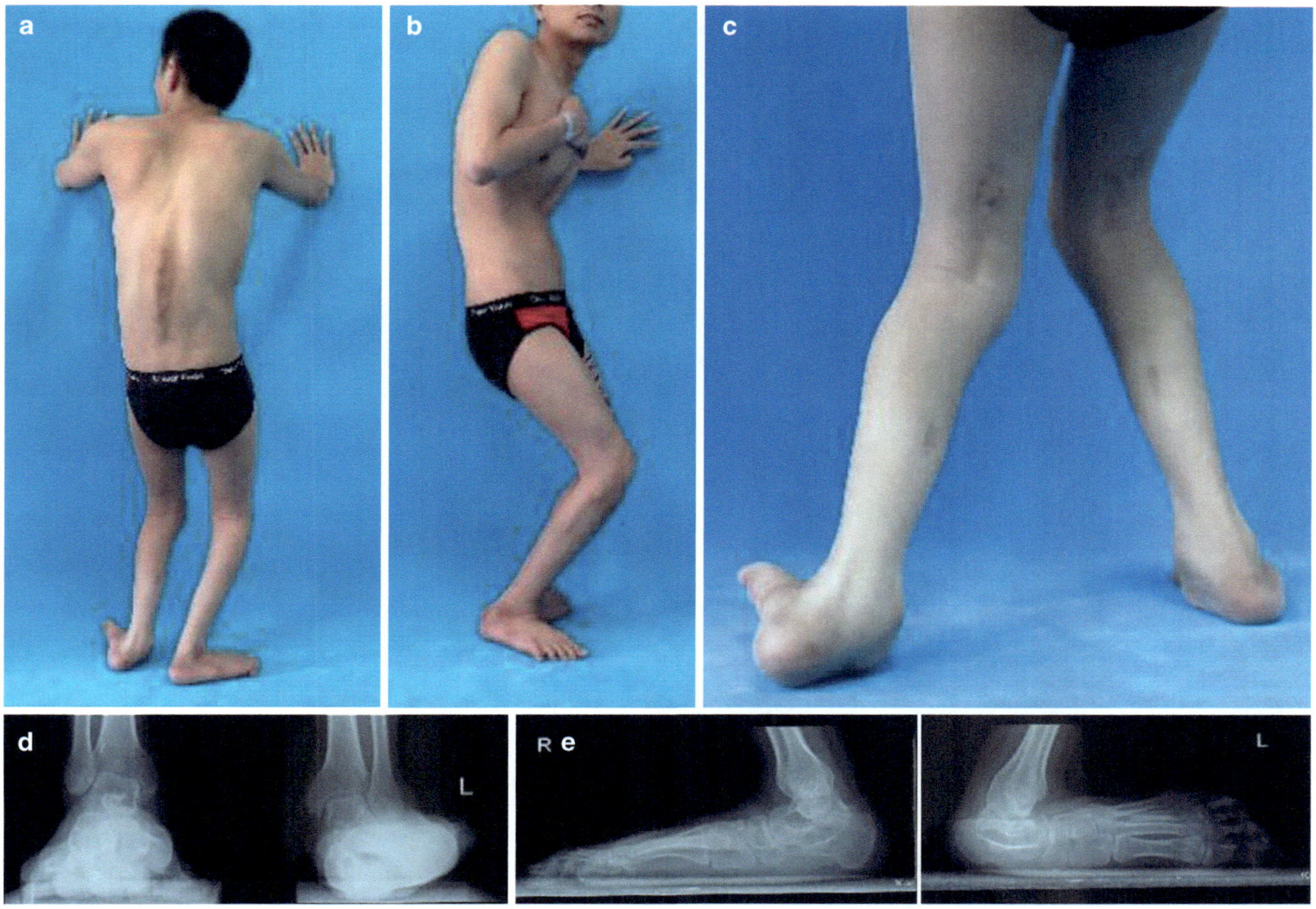

Fig. 11.11 Spastic paralysis of lower limbs secondary to high level injury of spinal cord caused by drug poisoning: Male, 26 years old, spinal cord was injured by drugs when he was 4 years old. (**a**) Standing position dorsal view, bilateral hip flexion, knee flexion, calcaneus valgus deformity; (**b**) lateral view; (**c**) dorsal view; (**d**) weight-bearing position ankle and foot anteroposterior X-ray film; (**e**) lateral X-ray film of ankle and foot in weight-bearing position

flexion and extension angle of the knee joint is less than 0–30° (the maximum flexion angle is less than 30°), abnormal gait can occur when walking at normal speed, which is severe knee stiffness. The maximum flexion angle of the knee joint is 30–70°. The gait of the patient is basically normal when walking at normal speed, but the speed and gait will be affected when running, which is moderate knee stiffness. The maximum flexion angle of the knee joint was 70–90°, which had little effect on the gait of the patients, but affected the squatting and sitting on a low stool, which was mild knee stiffness. If the maximum flexion angle is greater than 90° but less than 120°, it has little effect on the daily life of patients and cannot be attributed to knee fibrous stiffness, but only to mild flexion limitation of the knee.

11.2.8.3 Treatment Principle

Conservative treatment is the first choice for knee fibrous stiffness, and correct guidance is given to patients for knee flexion and extension exercises. Patients with moderate or severe stiffness after conservative treatment for more than 2 years should be treated with quadriceps plasty or quadriceps limited release combined with Ilizarov technique according to the cause and degree of knee stiffness.

11.2.9 Lumbosacral Plexus Injury Caused by Lumbar Spondylolisthesis Surgery

11.2.9.1 Etiology

Because of lumbar spondylolisthesis, the left sacral plexus was injured carelessly during the operation, resulting in incomplete paralysis of the left lower limb.

11.2.9.2 Clinical Manifestation

On the right foot, the muscle strength of the ankle and foot was weakened, especially the dorsiflexion and eversion of the foot. The muscle strength of the anterior tibial muscle was grade 0, and the muscle strength of the extensor thumb, extensor toe, and peroneus longus and brevis was grade 2.

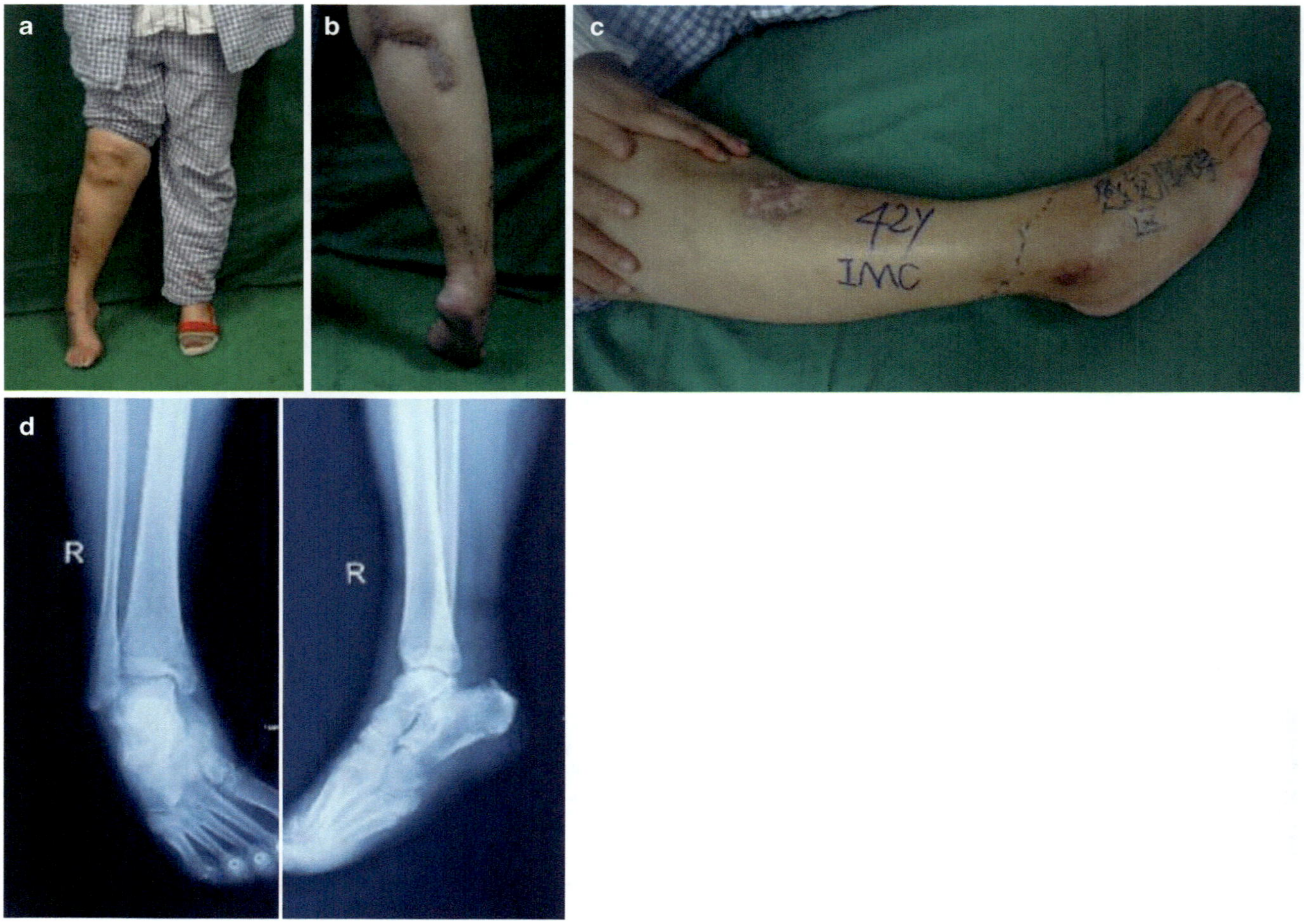

Fig. 11.12 Female, 40 years old, the popliteal artery was accidentally injured during the arthroscopic operation of the right knee, resulting in ischemic muscle contracture of the right leg and secondary talipes equinovarus deformity. (**a**) Standing appearance, right foot talipes equinovarus deformity; (**b**) dorsal view, popliteal fossa can be seen to repair the popliteal artery incision; (**c**) dorsalis pedis skin sensory disturbance; (**d**) X-ray film of the right foot showed the change of equinovarus deformity of the right foot bone joint

Other muscle strength grade 4; The sensation of the plantar skin is slightly reduced (Fig. 11.14).

11.2.9.3 Treatment Principle

Stabilize the ankle joint and reconstruct the dorsiflexion function of foot.

11.2.10 Ischemic Contracture of Lower Leg

After the occurrence of extremity compartment syndrome (ECS), the remaining muscle necrosis and ankle deformity were not treated in time.

11.2.10.1 Etiology

Fracture of tibia and fibula, vascular injury of leg, severe contusion of soft tissue or iatrogenic injury, improper treatment, can cause soft tissue ischemia, hypoxia, edema, and pressure increase in the bone-fascia compartment of limbs, forming osteofascial compartment syndrome. If it is not found and treated correctly in time in the early stage of the disease, it will lead to ischemic necrosis, fibrosis, contracture, fibrosis, and contracture of leg muscles. The ankle and foot joints are pulled to form fixed deformities and functional disorders of the ankle and foot joints.

11.2.10.2 Clinical Manifestation

In severe ischemic muscle contracture, all tissues in the affected area, including blood vessels, nerves, joint capsules, and ligaments, have different degrees of pathological changes, and nerve fibers accompanied by muscles have different degrees of degeneration due to ischemia and hypoxia. In the later stage, they are compressed by scar tissue on nerves and blood vessels, resulting in poor blood circulation and neurotrophic status of the affected foot. The elasticity of the skin is reduced, and even skin ulcers that are not easy to heal appear in the weight-bearing area of the foot; fibrotic and contracted muscles pull on the ankle and foot joints, causing talipes equinovarus deformity (Fig. 11.15).

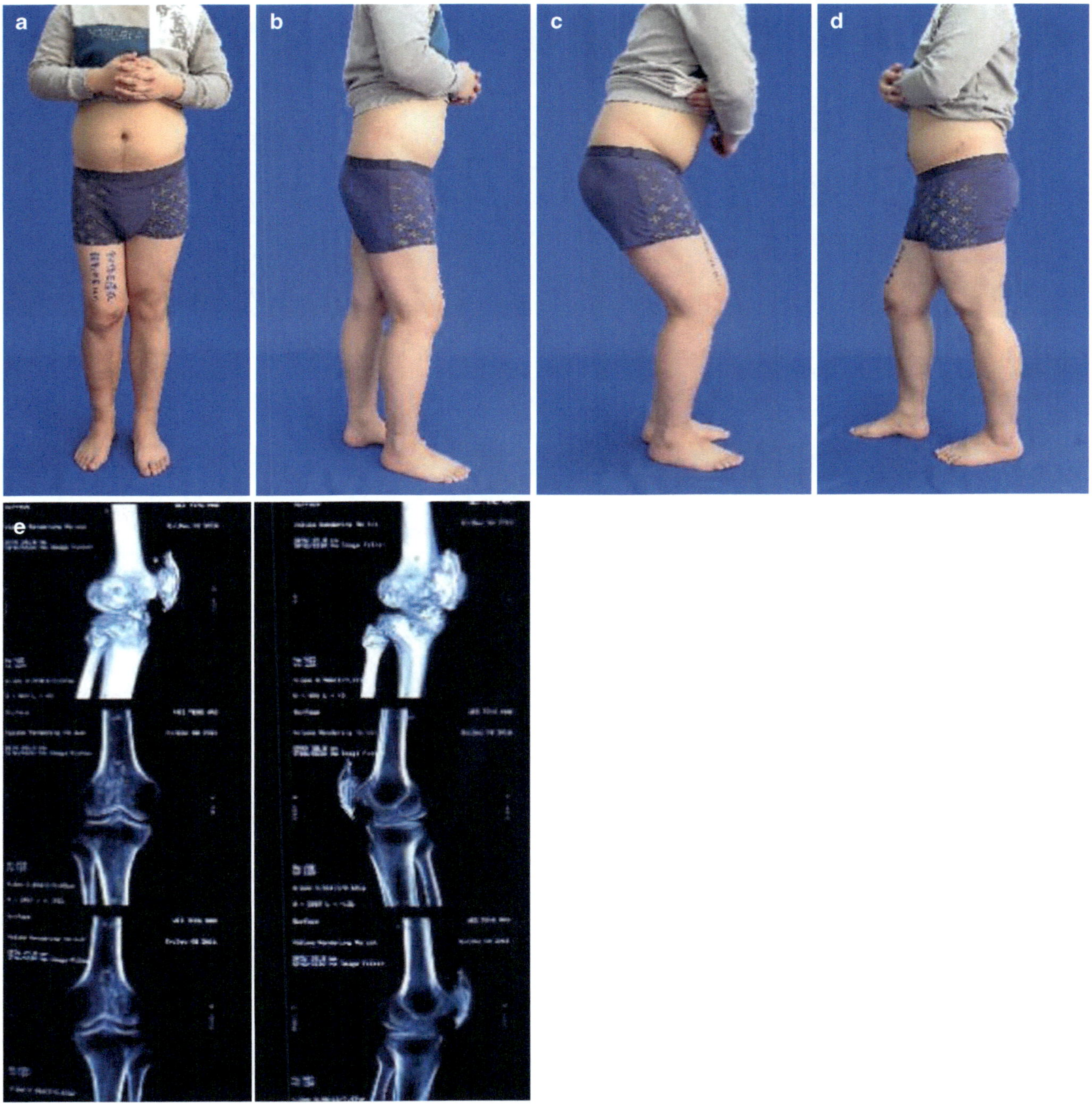

Fig. 11.13 A 19-year-old man suffered from fibrous stiffness of the right knee 14 months after surgery for a right patellar fracture. (**a**) Front view of standing position; (**b**) right side view, right knee maximum extension position, mild knee flexion deformity; (**c**) right knee maximum flexion position, only about 30° of flexion; (**d**) left side view of right knee maximum flexion; (**e**) three-dimensional CT reconstruction of right knee joint

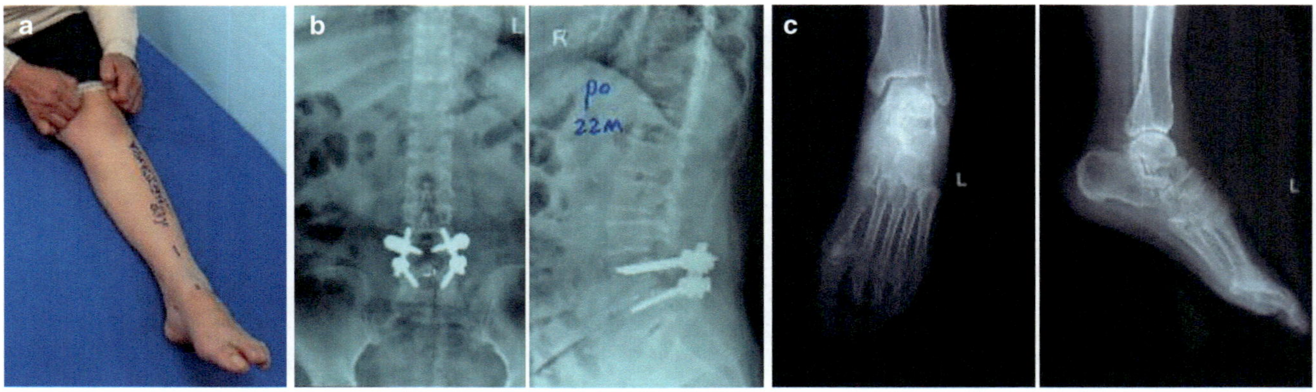

Fig. 11.14 A 64-year-old female patient was operated on for lumbar spondylolisthesis at the age of 62. The lumbosacral plexus nerve was accidentally injured, and the left equinovarus deformity was gradually developed. (**a**) Left foot drop, dorsiflexion weakness; (**b**) lumbar anteroposterior and lateral X-ray film, lumbosacral internal fixation; (**c**) anteroposterior and lateral X-ray films of foot and ankle

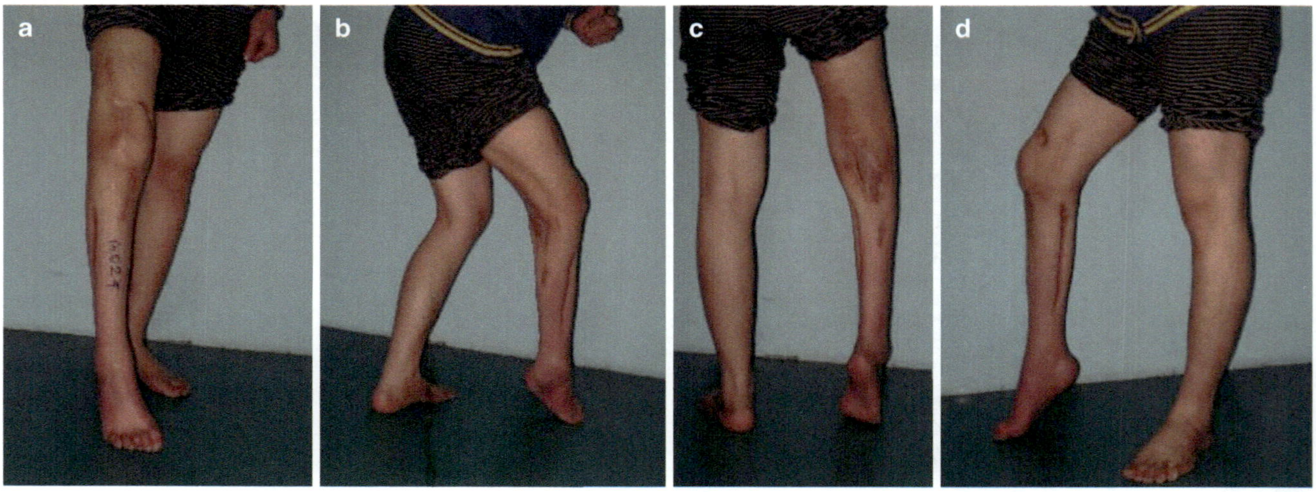

Fig. 11.15 Ischemic muscle contracture of the right leg: Male, 19 years old, suffered from distal femoral fracture caused by a traffic accident 2 years ago, compressed the popliteal artery, and developed compartment syndrome of the left leg. Compartment incision decompression was performed, and then talipes equinovarus deformity was gradually developed. (**a**) Standing appearance, left foot talipes equinovarus deformity; (**b**) lateral view, left foot outer edge touching the ground; (**c**) dorsal view, left foot varus, skin scar on the posterior side of the proximal end of the left leg; (**d**) left foot local view, talipes equinovarus deformity

11.2.10.3 Treatment Principle

The contractured tendon was released, and the subtalar joint or triple arthrodesis was performed to stabilize the foot joint, and the Ilizarov technique was used to gradually pull and correct the ankle deformity.

11.2.11 Hallux Varus Deformity Caused by Excessive Correction of Hallux Valgus

11.2.11.1 Etiology

Because of hallux valgus deformity, the choice of orthopedic surgery is inappropriate, or the osteotomy and soft tissue release are excessive, and the postoperative fixation in the over-orthopedic position is too long to be found and corrected in time. A combination of one or more of the above factors causes hallux varus deformity.

11.2.11.2 Clinical Manifestation

It was characterized by varus deformity of the metatarsophalangeal joint of the great toe, joint stiffness, reduced range of motion, especially limited abduction. Secondary varus deformity of 2–4 toes; the forefoot is widened, which affects the wearing of shoes; when walking, the force of forward propulsion is weakened, and some patients have pain in metatarsophalangeal joints (Fig. 11.16a). Radiographs showed shortening of the first metatarsal bone, narrowing of the metatarsal head, medial subluxation of the metatarsophalangeal joint, and narrowing of the joint space (Fig. 11.16b).

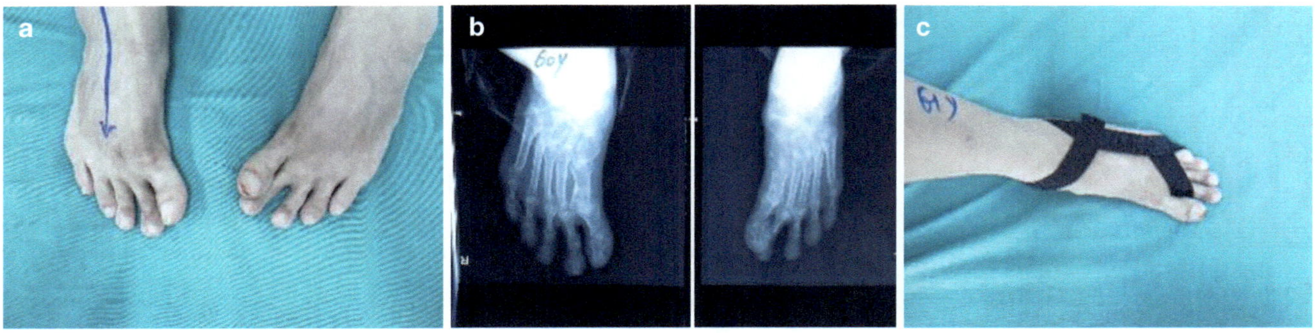

Fig. 11.16 A 60-year-old man with hallux varus deformity due to overcorrection of hallux valgus. (**a**) Appearance of both feet, bilateral hallux varus deformity; (**b**) anteroposterior X-ray film of both forefeet; (**c**) correction of varus deformity of toes with elastic cloth belt

11.2.11.3 Treatment Principle

Mild hallux varus deformity that does not affect walking function should be treated conservatively (Fig. 11.16c). If the deformity is serious or the walking function is affected, orthopedic surgery should be performed again.

11.3 Toxic Limb Deformity

11.3.1 Poisoning Sequelae of Tri-o-cresyl Phosphate

11.3.1.1 Etiology

Tri-o-cresyl phosphate (TOCP) is an ortho-isomer of tricresyl phosphate in the class of organic phosphoric acids. In addition to acute poisoning symptoms caused by inhibition of cholinesterase, ingestion poisoning mainly produces delayed neurotoxicity, or delayed polyneuropathy.

11.3.1.2 Clinical Manifestation

The clinical manifestations of delayed neuropathy caused by TOCP poisoning were as follows: (1) There was a latent period (12–20 days) before the onset of neurological symptoms, and the shorter the latent period, the more severe the toxic manifestations. (2) The initial symptom of all patients was gastrocnemius pain, and the tenderness of gastrocnemius was obvious. (3) In the acute stage, the activity of cholinesterase decreased, but returned to normal soon. The symptoms of nerve damage do not recover with the recovery of vitality. (4) Lower limb paralysis was more serious than upper limb paralysis, and distal limb paralysis was more serious than proximal limb paralysis. (5) Dyskinesia was severe and sensory disturbance was mild. Sensory disturbance was manifested by superficial sensory disturbance of gloves and socks, while deep sensory disturbance was not impaired. (6) Central paralysis caused by upper motor neuron damage and pyramidal tract damage, with increased muscle tension of lower limbs, hyperreflexia of tendons, positive pathological signs, scissors gait, long course of disease, and secondary fixed deformities such as adduction, knee flexion and talipes equinovarus (Fig. 11.17).

11.3.1.3 Treatment Principle

Patients with fixed spastic deformity were treated with soft tissue release, osteotomy or arthrodesis to correct lower limb deformity and improve gait.

11.3.2 Ankle Deformity After Organophosphorus Pesticide Poisoning

11.3.2.1 Etiology

Organophosphorus pesticides mainly include dichlorvos, parathion (1605), phorate (3911), demeton (1059), dimethoate, trichlorfon, malathion (4049), and so on, which are the most widely used pesticides in China. Acute organophosphorus pesticide poisoning refers to a series of injuries, mainly nervous system damage, caused by organophosphorus pesticides entering the human body in large quantities for a short time.

11.3.2.2 Clinical Manifestation

Clinically, it mainly includes cholinergic excitation or crisis in patients with acute poisoning, followed by intermediate syndrome and delayed peripheral neuropathy. Acute organophosphorus pesticide poisoning generally has no sequelae. Delayed neuropathy may occur in individual patients 2–3 weeks after the disappearance of acute poisoning symptoms, mainly involving the extremities, and neurological symptoms such as lower limb paralysis and limb muscle atrophy may occur. Delayed peripheral neuropathy can lead to changes in limb muscles, resulting in limb deformities and dysfunction, such as talipes equinovarus (Fig. 11.18).

11.3.2.3 Treatment Principle

Correcting limb deformities and improving the walking function of patients.

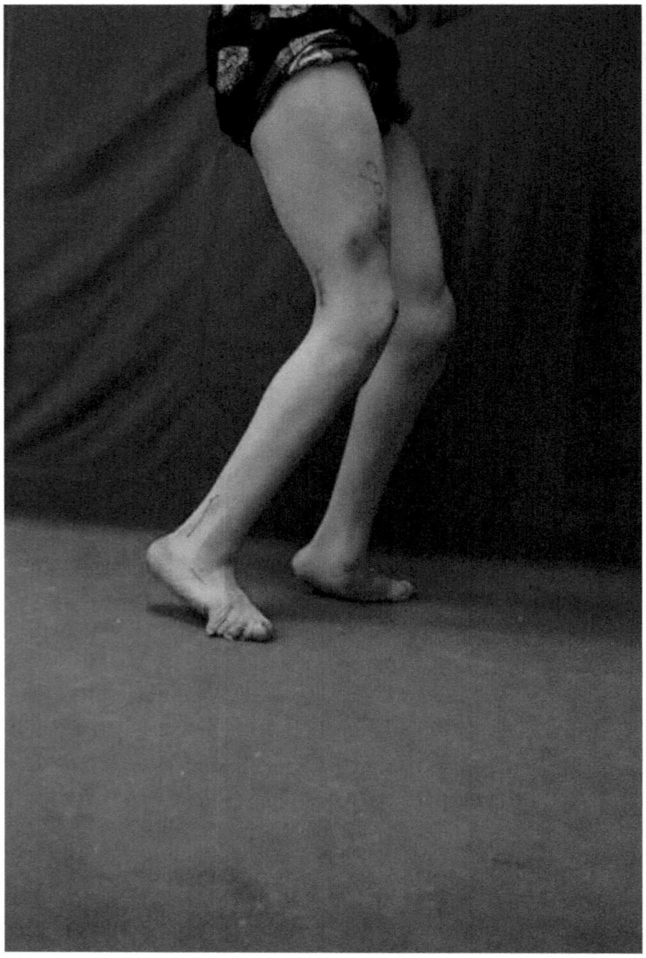

Fig. 11.17 Appearance photo of standing on the side of the lower limbs

11.3.3 Sequelae of Carbon Monoxide (Gas) Poisoning

11.3.3.1 Etiology

The affinity of carbon monoxide (CO) and hemoglobin is 200–300 times higher than that of oxygen and hemoglobin. Carbon monoxide combines with hemoglobin to form carboxyhemoglobin, which makes hemoglobin lose its ability and function of carrying oxygen, resulting in tissue asphyxia. It has toxic effects on tissues and cells of the whole body, especially on the cerebral cortex.

11.3.3.2 Clinical Manifestation

The main clinical manifestation of poisoning is hypoxia, and its severity is proportional to the saturation of HbCO. HbCO saturation is 30–40%. Severe cases showed deep coma, accompanied by high fever, increased muscle tension of limbs and paroxysmal or tonic spasm, HbCO saturation >50%. Most patients have cerebral edema, pulmonary edema, myocardial damage, arrhythmia, and respiratory depression, which can cause death. Some patients with acute carbon monoxide poisoning will be in coma again after 2–30 days of false recovery, and will suffer from dementia, stupor psychosis, paralysis agitans syndrome, sensorimotor disorders or peripheral neuropathy, also known as delayed encephalopathy of acute carbon monoxide poisoning. In the later stage, patients will suffer from limb deformities and dysfunction, and enter the sequelae period.

The manifestations of sequelae are closely related to the severity of nervous system damage, which are characterized by increased muscle tension, decreased muscle strength, hyperreflexia of tendons, and secondary limb deformities. Elbow flexion, forearm pronation, wrist dropping, and other deformities can be seen in the upper limbs (Fig. 11.19); Knee flexion, talipes equinovarus, and other deformities were common in the lower limbs.

11.3.3.3 Treatment Principle

Release contracture of soft tissue, reduce muscle tension, correct limb deformity, and improve limb function.

11.3.4 Sequela of Lead Poisoning

11.3.4.1 Etiology

Lead can easily pass through the blood–brain barrier of the placenta and developing brain, so the damage of lead to the developing central nervous system is particularly obvious. In the early stage of brain development, lead can inhibit the proliferation and differentiation of neurons, leading to the early differentiation of glial cells, and the interaction between glial cells and neurons cannot be carried out normally. Lead can also directly damage the blood-brain barrier, and also damage astrocytes, so that endothelial cells lose their barrier function. Lead also affects synapse formation. When lead poisoning occurs, the concentration of TTR in cerebrospinal fluid decreases, which affects the acquisition of thyroxine by the developing brain, thus affecting the development and damage of the brain and spinal cord, causing corresponding neuromuscular changes, resulting in corresponding limb deformities and dysfunction.

11.3.4.2 Clinical Manifestation

The central nervous system is damaged, resulting in increased muscle tension of limbs, hyperreflexia of tendons, secondary adduction of the thigh, flexion of the knee, talipes equinovarus and other deformities, affecting walking function.

11.3.4.3 Treatment Principle

Release contracture of soft tissue, reduce muscle tension, correct lower limb deformity, and improve walking function.

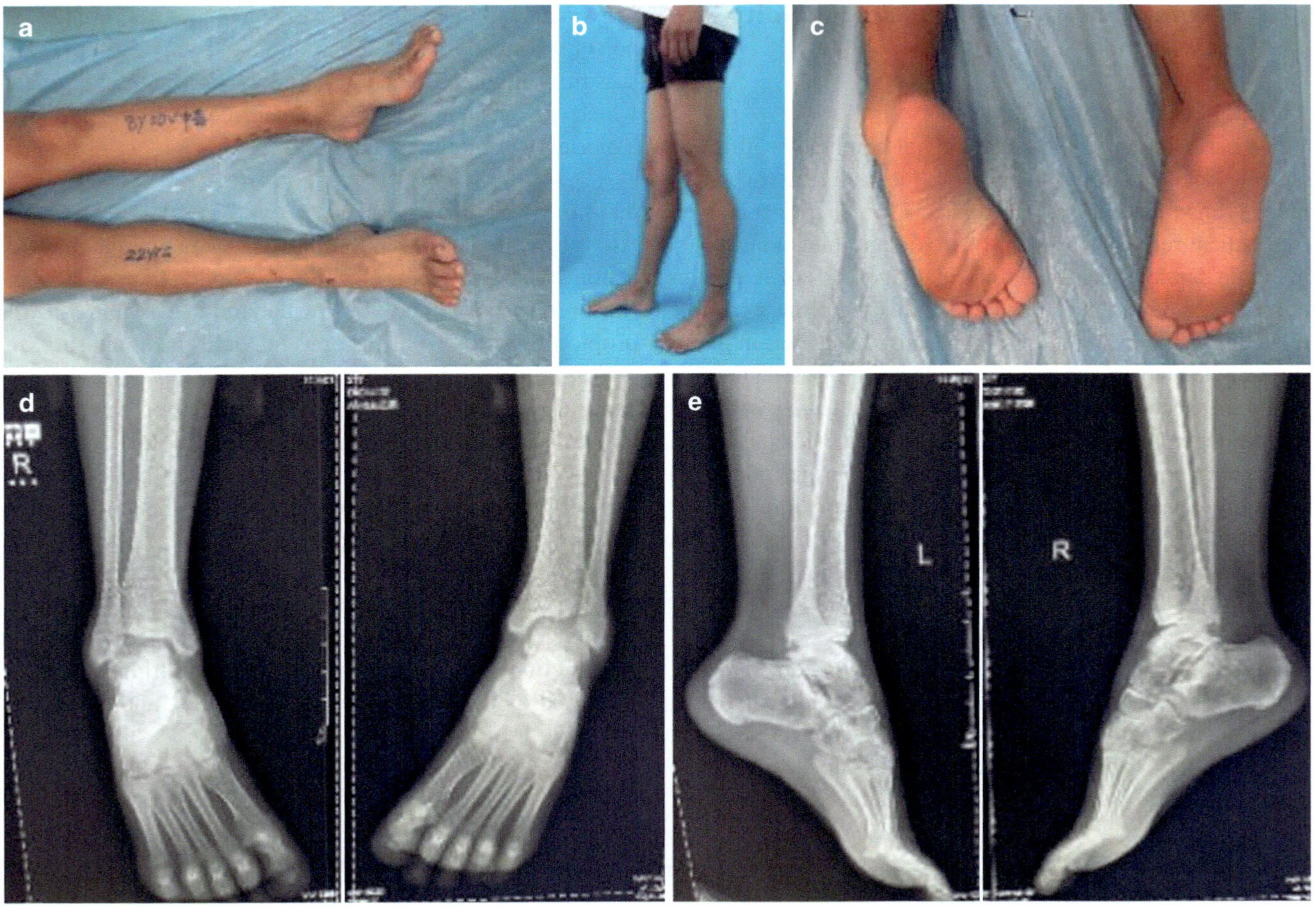

Fig. 11.18 Male, 22 years old, took organophosphorus pesticide by mistake at the age of 8, and then gradually developed bilateral talipes equinovarus deformity. (**a**) Appearance of both feet, slight talipes equinovarus deformity; (**b**) lateral view of standing position; (**c**) dorsal view, deformity of left foot is slightly heavier than that of right side; (**d**) anteroposterior X-ray of both ankles; (**e**) Lateral radiographs of both ankles

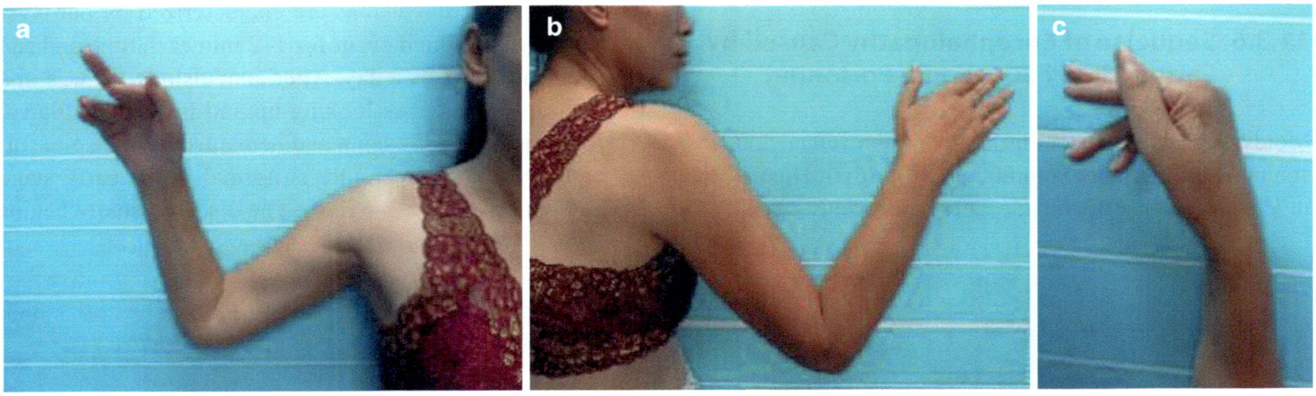

Fig. 11.19 Female, 47 years old, developed spastic paralysis of right upper limb due to carbon monoxide poisoning at the age of 41, and gradually developed right elbow flexion and forearm pronation deformity. (**a**) Frontal view of the right upper limb; (**b**) dorsal view of the right upper limb; (**c**) right-hand deformity change

11.3.5 Heroin Encephalopathy Limb Rigidity Deformity

11.3.5.1 Etiology

When heroin enters the human body, it combines with some enzymes and receptor proteins to produce active nitrogen free radicals and other types of free radicals, which trigger oxygen free radical reactions and lipid peroxidation reactions, causing brain damage, and brain tissue damage leads to demyelination. Some researchers also believe that the disease may be related to the impurity of heroin, because many heroin impurities contain toxic substances that have obvious damage to the brain, such as compound camphor tincture, pyribenzamine, talcum powder, and barbiturates. Both mechanisms are believed to be that heroin itself or other impurities contained in heroin cause damage to the brain tissue of drug addicts, resulting in corresponding clinical symptoms, resulting in deformity and dysfunction of the corresponding limbs.

11.3.5.2 Clinical Manifestation

The main symptoms are central nervous system damage, including increased limb muscle tension, tendon hyperreflexia, positive pathological signs, decreased muscle strength, and secondary limb deformities, such as hip flexion, knee flexion, femoral adduction, talipes equinovarus, and other deformities (Fig. 11.20).

11.3.5.3 Treatment Principle

Release contracture of soft tissue, reduce muscle tension, correct lower limb deformity, and improve walking function.

11.3.6 Sequelae of Encephalopathy Caused by Eating Moldy Sugarcane Poisoning

Moldy sugarcane poisoning is a common fungal food poisoning, which is more common in the north of Huaihe River in China. Because sugarcane eaters are mainly people aged 3–16 years old, their discrimination and alertness are low, so poisoning mostly occurs in children and young people. The season of high incidence is February to March every year, which can endanger life or leave neurological sequelae, with a mortality rate of more than 10%.

11.3.6.1 Etiology

At present, it is believed that the mold causing the deterioration of sugarcane is Arthrospira sp., which is a plant saprophyte distributed worldwide, and its toxin is 3-nitropropionic acid. 3-Nitropropionic acid is a neurotoxin, which is the main toxic substance causing moldy sugarcane poisoning. It is absorbed rapidly after entering the human body, causing extensive damage to the central nervous system in a short time, interfering with the metabolism of intracellular enzymes, enhancing the permeability of capillaries, thus causing cerebral edema, cerebral hernia, and so on. Severe cases lead to ischemic necrosis and various related focal symptoms, some of which are irreversible. If the brain motor center is damaged, the motor dysfunction of the limbs will occur, resulting in spastic paralysis of the limbs to varying degrees, and secondary bone and joint deformities.

11.3.6.2 Clinical Manifestation

1. In acute stage: After eating moldy sugarcane, temporary gastrointestinal dysfunction (nausea, vomiting, abdominal pain, etc., without diarrhea) may occur, and nervous system symptoms (headache, dizziness, blackening in front of the eyes, diplopia) may occur. In severe cases, frequent nausea, vomiting, and lethargy may occur, and in severe cases, convulsions and coma will soon occur. Convulsions are characterized by paroxysmal spasms, which occur for 1–2 min each time and can occur many times a day. After convulsions, he was in a coma, with his eyes looking up and his pupils dilated. Acute pulmonary edema and hematuria may also occur, and the body temperature is normal in the early stage and may rise after 3–5 days. The disease usually begins

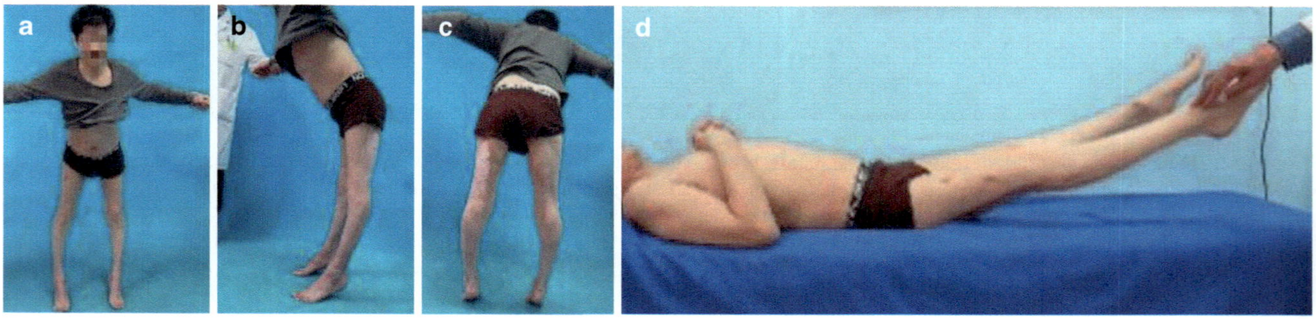

Fig. 11.20 Male, 59 years old, began to take drugs at the age of 36. Toxic encephalopathy was caused by heroin overdose, and bilateral hip flexion deformity, fibrous stiffness of knee joint and equinus deformity were gradually developed. (**a**) Cannot stand alone, only can barely stand with the help of others; (**b**) view from the side of the standing position, with bilateral hip flexion and horseshoe foot; (**c**) view from the back of the standing position; (**d**) supine position, bilateral hip flexion, both lower limbs cannot be put down

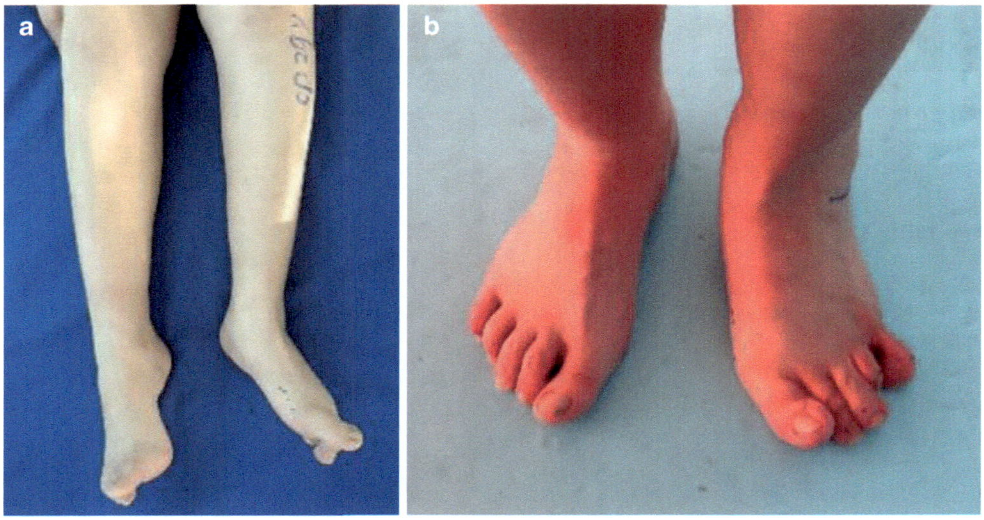

Fig. 11.21 Female, 29 years old. When she was 3 years old, she was poisoned by eating moldy sugar cane. She was in a coma with high fever, and then gradually developed deformity of the left lower limb. (**a**) Appearance of both legs and feet showed that the muscle tension of both lower limbs increased, and the left foot showed spastic flat foot valgus changes. (**b**) Standing appearance of both feet, left foot valgus, hallux valgus deformity

to recover after 5–10 days. There may be neurological sequelae such as generalized spastic paralysis, decortication syndrome, etc.

2. In the sequelae period: After active treatment, the muscle tension of the remaining limbs is increased, the movement is not flexible, the muscle strength is reduced to varying degrees, and due to the imbalance of muscle strength, the bone and joint deformities of the limbs are secondary, such as knee flexion deformity, ankle and foot deformity, and other deformities (Fig. 11.21).

11.3.6.3 Treatment Principle

(1) Acute stage: emetic, catharsis, and other detoxification treatment, supplement of water and electrolyte, elimination of cerebral edema, improvement of cerebral circulation, and other symptomatic treatment. (2) Sequelae stage: reduce muscle tension, functional exercise, prevent limb deformity; After the occurrence of fixed deformity of limbs, orthopedic surgery can be performed to improve the motor function of limbs.

Spine and Spinal Cord Malformation

12

Qianyu Zhuang, Jianguo Zhang, Yue Peng, Zhuosong Bai, Sihe Qin, and Yijian Liang

12.1 Superior Cervical Deformity

12.1.1 Basilar Invagination

Basilar invagination (BI) is a kind of occipitocervical deformity caused by the upward displacement or invagination of the atlantoaxial or basilar region bone tissue around the foramen magnum into the cranial cavity, resulting in the narrowing of the foramen magnum, the reduction of the volume of the posterior cranial fossa, and the compression of the brainstem, ventral aspect of the rostral cervical spinal cord, cerebellum, lower cranial nerves, and peripheral blood vessels, giving rise to a spectrum of symptoms and signs.

Basilar invagination (BI) is an occipitocervical deformity characterized by the upward displacement or invagination of bone tissue in the atlantoaxial or basilar region around the foramen magnum, leading it to extend into the cranial cavity. This results in the constriction of the foramen magnum, a reduction in the volume of the posterior cranial fossa, and the compression of vital structures such as the brainstem, ventral aspect of the rostral cervical spinal cord, cerebellum, lower cranial nerves, and peripheral blood vessels. These manifestations give rise to a spectrum of symptoms and signs.

Q. Zhuang
Peking Union Medical College Hospital, Beijing, China

J. Zhang · Z. Bai
Department of Orthopaedics, Peking Union Medical College Hospital, Beijing, China

Y. Peng
Department of Orthopedic Surgery, Peking Union Medical College Hospital, Chinese Academy of Medical Sciences and Peking Union Medical College, Beijing, China

S. Qin (✉)
Department of Orthopaedics, Rehabilitation Hospital of the National Research Center for Rehabilitation Technical Aids, Beijing, China

Y. Liang
Department of Orthopaedics, The Third People's Hospital of Chengdu, Southwest Jiao Tong University, Chengdu, Sichuan, China

12.1.1.1 Etiology

Since Homer's initial report in 1901, scholars worldwide have conducted extensive research on basilar invagination. However, to date, the academic community still lacks a comprehensive understanding of its pathogenesis.

12.1.1.2 Clinical Manifestations

Patients with basilar invagination may remain asymptomatic in the initial stages, which can pose challenges for diagnosis. Some individuals are identified through X-ray examinations, where malformation of the foramen magnum or a concave cranial base is observed. Others come to attention during routine medical examinations or in outpatient settings due to physical characteristics such as short stature, short neck, torticollis, limited neck mobility, Sprengel shoulder, low hairline, abnormal skull shape, facial or auricular asymmetry, among others. As patients age, symptoms tend to manifest progressively. Trauma to the neck and extreme flexion-extension movements can also act as precipitating or exacerbating factors for basilar invagination.

The clinical presentation of patients with basilar invagination can vary depending on the site of spinal cord and nerve compression. Common local manifestations encompass headache, neck and shoulder pain, radicular pain, neck stiffness, limited neck movement, instability in standing and walking, dysuria, dizziness, tinnitus, and more. When the pyramidal tract is under pressure, milder cases may exhibit fatigue, while severe instances can lead to spasmodic limb paralysis, hypertonia in all four extremities, tendon hyperreflexia, and the presence of positive pathological signs. Patients with cranial nerve involvement may experience bulbar palsy symptoms such as dysphagia, dysarthria, choking, weakened pharyngeal reflex, along with cerebellar ataxia and horizontal nystagmus.

Syringomyelia often emerges as a common complication of basilar invagination. Its development is linked to the extrusion of the fourth ventricle, the communicating branch of the central aqueduct of the medulla oblongata, and the exacerbated obstruction of cerebrospinal fluid reflux due to

S. Qin et al. (eds.), *Atlas of Limb Deformity*, https://doi.org/10.1007/978-981-97-0999-1_12

herniation of the cerebellar tonsil. In cases where patients simultaneously present with Chiari malformation and syringomyelia, compression of the medulla oblongata and upper cervical cord by the herniated cerebellar tonsils can result in symptoms like limb fatigue, dyspnea, fine motor impairment in the fingers, loss of position sense, and dissociative sensory disturbances. Vertebral artery blood supply disruption and increased intracranial pressure symptoms can also manifest.

Radiological examinations play a pivotal role in diagnosing basilar invagination. In 1939, Chamberlain first described the classic imaging features associated with this condition. While the lateral craniovertebral X-ray remains a fundamental diagnostic tool, it does have inherent imaging limitations, which somewhat restrict its clinical application. Multiplanar CT reconstruction, on the other hand, can provide a clear visualization of the osseous structures at the basilar region junction, offering valuable insights for pathological diagnosis. Additionally, MRI, with its impressive soft tissue resolution, excels in depicting soft tissue structures in the craniovertebral region and abnormalities within the neurological system, including conditions like Chiari malformation and syringomyelia.

Key imaging markers for diagnosing basilar invagination encompass the Chamberlain line, McGregor line, bull angle, basal angle, digastric sulcus line, medulla oblongata cervical spinal angle, and others (Figs. 12.1 and 12.2).

12.1.1.3 Classification

In 2004, the classification proposed by Goel and colleagues emerged as the most widely accepted system, both nationally and internationally. This classification categorizes basilar invagination based on the stability of the cranial base junction. Type A, also known as odontoid basilar invagination, is characterized by an increased atlanto-odontoid distance without a significant change in the angle and volume of the posterior fossa slope. It often coincides with atlantoaxial fusion. On the other hand, Type B, referred to as the slope type of basilar invagination, involves an upward movement of the odontoid process, resulting in a reduced volume of the posterior cranial fossa. However, there is no significant increase in the distance between the odontoid and atlas. Type B cases are often associated with syringomyelia.

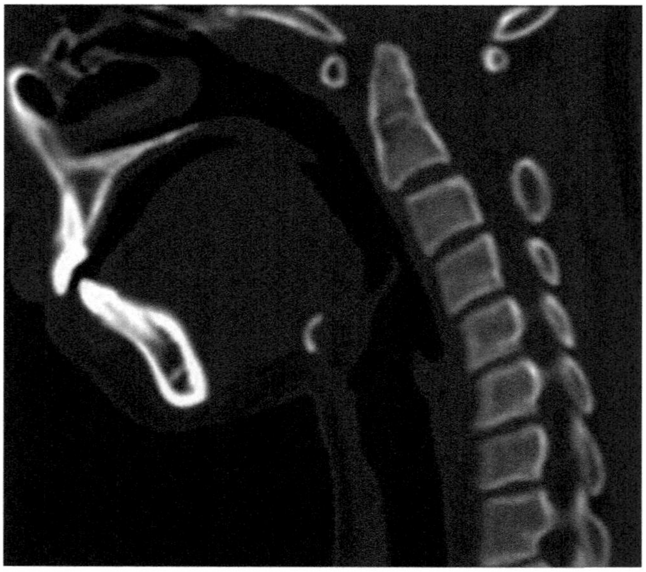

Fig. 12.1 CT image of basilar invagination sign

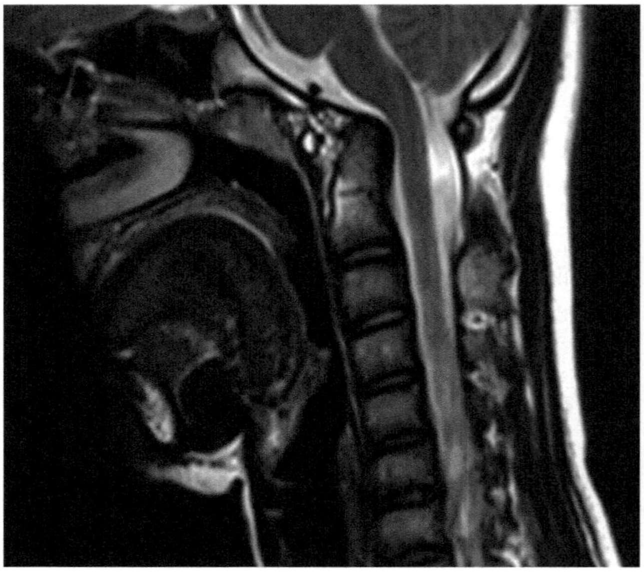

Fig. 12.2 MRI image of basilar invagination sign

12.1.1.4 Treatment Principles

At present, there is consensus regarding the treatment principles for basilar invagination. This entails the effective decompression of the spinal cord and nerve roots, along with the reconstruction of sequential structural stability in the cervical-cranial region and the restoration of normal cerebrospinal fluid circulation. While there is not a universally established standard for the surgical approach, clinical treatment should be tailored to the specific site of spinal nerve compression and the underlying pathogenic mechanism.

12.1.2 Chiari Malformation

Chiari malformation (CM), also known as cerebellar tonsillar herniation malformation, is a congenital developmental anomaly in which the cerebellar tonsils extend downward and protrude into the cervical canal through the foramen magnum. It represents a common malformation of the craniocervical junction.

12.1.2.1 Etiology

At present, the pathogenesis of CM remains obscure. The majority of scholars posit that CM Type II, Type III, and Type IV are caused by defects in neuroectoderm development. However, a consensus on the pathogenesis of CM Type I has yet to be achieved.

12.1.2.2 Clinical Manifestations

The clinical manifestations of this disease are diverse and complex. Patients may exhibit physical alterations, such as a shortened neck, and some may also experience dyspnea and voice changes. There are primarily five types as follows:

1. Neurocompression Type: This arises due to cerebellar tonsil herniation, fourth ventricular herniation, or association with a concave cranial base. Consequently, the posterior cranial nerves and upper cervical segmental nerves become angulated, resulting in symptoms like neck and occipital pain, neck and shoulder pain, facial numbness, blurred vision, dulled corneal reflex, hoarseness, and dulled pharyngeal reflex.
2. Central Spinal Cord Impairment Type: This subtype is characterized by compression of the upper cervical segment and the formation of a spinal cord syrinx. It prominently manifests as sensory disturbances with dissociated sensation in the scapular region, hemiparesis, quadriplegia, and predominant muscular atrophy.
3. Pyramidal Tract Type: Its symptoms and signs include muscle stiffness and/or spasticity, hyperreflexia, etc.
4. Cerebellar Impairment Type: This type presents with symptoms like gait instability, ataxia, nystagmus, etc.
5. Increased Intracranial Pressure Type (Paroxysmal): Elevated intracranial pressure due to compression of cerebral tissue leads to cerebral edema, resulting in symptoms such as headaches, vomiting, dizziness, and nuchal rigidity (exacerbated during movement or coughing).

The clinical symptoms of this condition can vary significantly due to individual factors.

MRI stands as the premier method for the imaging diagnosis of CM. Conventional T1 and T2-weighted imaging can yield high-quality images depicting brain anatomy and its physiological changes. Moreover, MRI can be employed to assess the extent of spinal cord compression in patients with CM Type I. T2-weighted imaging can clearly reveal spinal cord edema, while T1-weighted imaging can highlight abnormalities in the craniocervical junction (Figs. 12.3 and 12.4).

Anteroposterior, lateral, double oblique, and dynamic X-ray radiographs of the neck can reveal related abnormalities of the basilar region and cervical spine, enabling the evaluation of craniocervical junction stability prior to surgery. CT scan illustrates the low position of cerebellar tonsils, though its sensitivity is lower compared to MRI. Nonetheless, its advantage lies in its precision in showcasing osseous structures, providing invaluable support

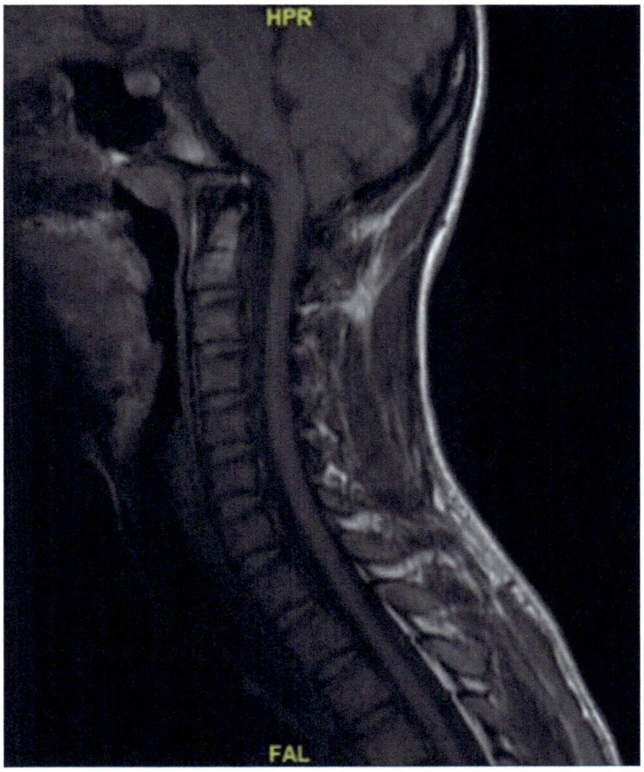

Fig. 12.3 MRI T1WI image of Chiari malformation

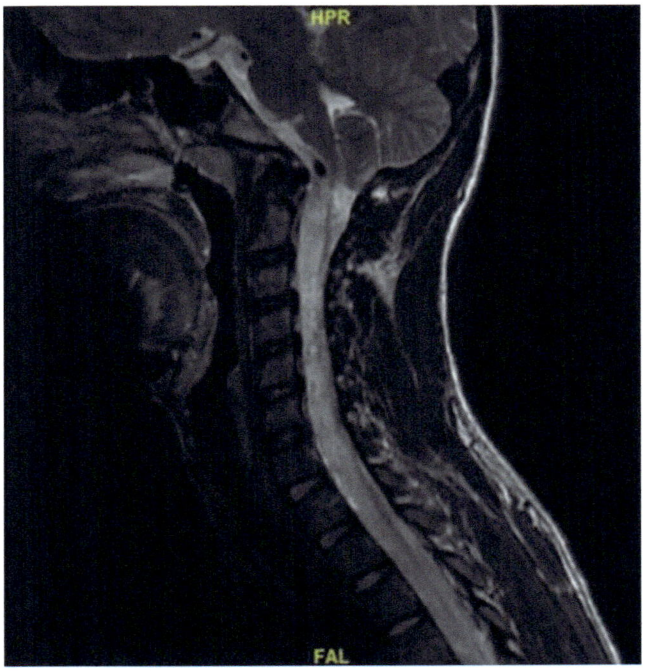

Fig. 12.4 MRI T2WI image of Chiari malformation

for preoperative planning through multifaceted reconstructions and three-dimensional reconstruction.

12.1.2.3 Classification

Type I is the most prevalent, with diagnostic criteria consisting of the herniation of the cerebellar tonsils below the plane of the foramen magnum by 5 mm or more unilaterally, or 3 mm or more bilaterally, while the positions of the medulla and fourth ventricle remain normal.

Type II, building upon Type I, entails the downward displacement of the medulla and the lower part of the brainstem, along with an elongation of the descent of the fourth ventricle; in most cases, patients exhibit concurrent syringomyelia and hydrocephalus.

Type III represents the most severe form, mainly manifesting as herniation of the cerebellum, medulla oblongata, and fourth ventricle into the occipital or bulging dural sac of the upper cervical segment, mostly affecting newborns and infants.

Type IV chiefly manifests as severe cerebellar hypoplasia or absence, small brainstem development, and the posterior fossa is filled with cerebrospinal fluid, but does not bulge downward. This type commonly appears in infancy.

Types III and IV are relatively rare clinical presentations.

12.1.2.4 Treatment Principles

The current Treatment approach for CM is a subject of considerable debate. Common surgical methods encompass posterior fossa decompression (PFD), PFD with posterior fossa decompression along with duraplasty (PFDD), PFD with cerebellar tonsil electrocautery or resection (PFDRT), removal of atlantooccipital fascia and opening of the epidural layer, release of the adhesion between the median foramen of the fourth ventricle and the upper mouth of the central canal of the spinal cord, internal fixation, neuroendoscopic atlantooccipital decompression, and syringomyelia subarachnoid shunt, among others.

In recent years, with advances in clinical and foundational research on CM, surgical techniques have also seen continual refinement. This is chiefly characterized by a shift from employing a single surgical approach to the combined application of multiple techniques, and from relying on a solitary monitoring method to incorporating a variety of monitoring technologies. The use of combined procedures has shown significant promise in alleviating patients' symptoms and signs, reducing the extent of syringomyelia, and lowering the incidence of adverse events and complications.

The incorporation of innovative technologies such as intraoperative neuromonitoring, intraoperative MRI, intraoperative ultrasound, and other emerging tools provides an added layer of assurance in enhancing the safety and effectiveness of the surgical intervention.

12.1.3 Odontoideum

Odontoideum, also referred to as odontoid free bone, was first reported by Giaromini in 1886. It constitutes a form of odontoid vertebra deformity and frequently leads to atlantoaxial joint instability. Diagnosis typically occurs when patients seek treatment for neck trauma, and some individuals may present with two or more anatomic variations. Clinical symptoms arise from the instability of the atlantoaxial joint, displacement, and compression of the spinal cord. This can result in partial or complete quadriplegia, and in severe cases, even lead to death.

12.1.3.1 Etiology

At present, it is widely believed that trauma and congenital malformations are the principal causes of odontoideum.

12.1.3.2 Clinical Manifestations

The clinical manifestations may become evident within the first 1–10 months after birth, presenting as follows:

1. Some cases may remain asymptomatic throughout their lives, with symptoms only discovered during routine medical examinations.
2. In other cases, individuals may experience neck discomfort, pain, neck rigidity, occipital pain with torticollis, paroxysmal dizziness, blurred vision, and sudden collapses.
3. Severe cases involving compression of the spinal cord can lead to quadriplegia.

According to reports, the disease presents in three distinct forms of attack:

1. Transient or paroxysmal radicular pain, numbness, or claudication of the lower or upper limbs may occur without an apparent cause or after minor trauma, but these symptoms can eventually subside and return to normal.
2. Spontaneous slow attack. While the initial symptoms may be mild, they persist and gradually worsen over time.
3. Sudden attack. This form is characterized by the abrupt onset of clear clinical symptoms, with severe cases even exhibiting tetraplegia.

The X-ray examination for diagnosing odontoideum includes obtaining cervical opening position, lateral position, and dynamic flexion-extension lateral position radiographs. In cases where necessary, tomographic images are captured to refine the diagnosis, focusing on the following aspects:

1. Whether the odontoideum merges with the upper cervical spine and if there is any malformation of the concave cranial base.
2. Assessing the degree of atlantoaxial instability and collecting morphological data.

On X-ray, the odontoideum typically appears as a distinct entity, separate from the vertebral body of the axis. Tomographic scans may reveal either two circular bone shadows within the vertebral ring of the atlas or numerous punctate calcifications (Figs. 12.5 and 12.6).

12.1.3.3 Classification

Based on the location of the odontoid tip, it can be categorized into two types: in situ type and ectopic type.

12.1.3.4 Treatment Principles

Once the diagnosis of odontoid process fracture is unequivocally established, the choice of treatment primarily hinges on the degree of atlantoaxial joint instability and the extent of spinal cord compression. In cases where only localized symptoms are present and radiological imaging indicates relative stability of the atlantoaxial joint, non-surgical interventions may be sufficient. However, if potential instability is evident, a proactive surgical approach should be pursued.

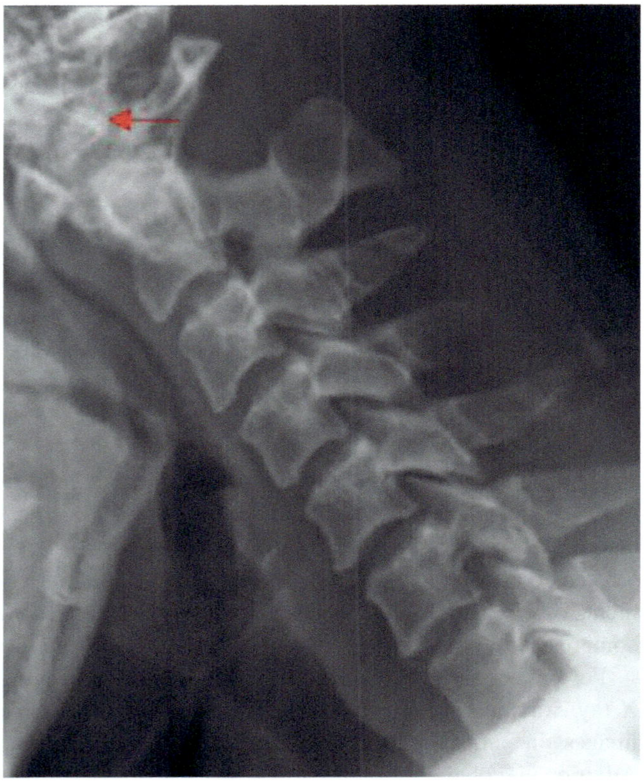

Fig. 12.5 X-ray radiograph of odontoideum deformity (showed by arrow)

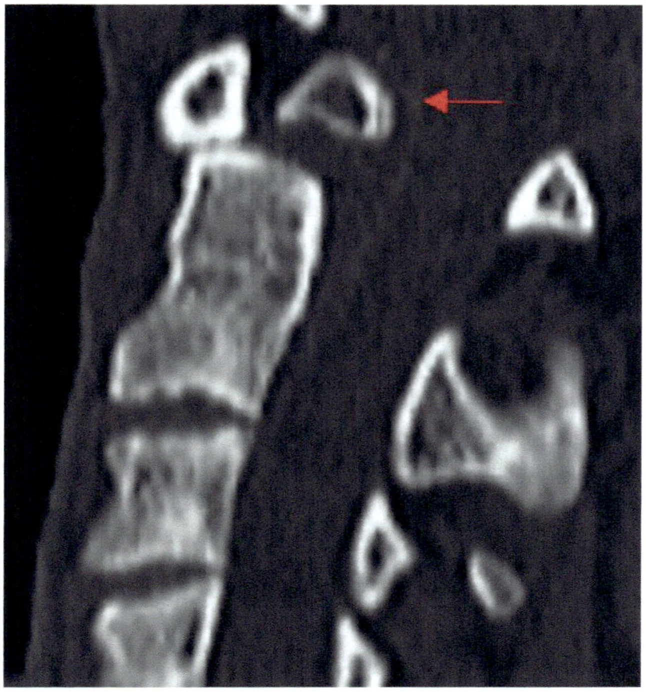

Fig. 12.6 CT image of odontoideum deformity (showed by arrow)

12.2 Cervical Deformity

12.2.1 Congenital Torticollis

Most cases of congenital torticollis are classified as congenital muscular torticollis (CMT). This type is characterized by hypertrophy, tautness, and shortening of the sternocleidomastoid muscle on the affected side, leading to a turning of the head and neck toward the affected side, with the face and mandible inclining in the opposite direction. Consequently, this leads to restricted mobility of the neck. In a minority of cases, congenital bony anomalies, such as cervical hemivertebrae, can also be a contributing factor to this condition.

12.2.1.1 Etiology

The etiology of pediatric torticollis is still unclear, with the majority of scholars positing that it arises from fetal malposition in utero, impeding the blood supply to the pectoral muscles on one side, resulting in muscle fiber edema, degeneration, inflammation, reactive granulation tissue proliferation, and subsequent gradual fibrosis, culminating in the manifestation of muscular torticollis. Some scholars also believe that it is related to trauma, such as compression or injury to the pectoral muscles during delivery, leading to hematoma formation and muscle contraction. However, the varying degrees of degeneration in the pectoral muscles of affected infants are unequivocally attributed to the progressive fibrotic transformation of neonatal neck masses, ultimately causing the loss of normal elasticity.

12.2.1.2 Clinical Manifestations

The etiology of pediatric torticollis remains unclear, with the majority of scholars suggesting that it arises from fetal malposition in utero. This can impede blood supply to the pectoral muscles on one side, resulting in muscle fiber edema, degeneration, inflammation, reactive granulation tissue proliferation, and subsequent gradual fibrosis. These processes ultimately lead to the manifestation of muscular torticollis. Some scholars also posit that it may be related to trauma, such as compression or injury to the pectoral muscles during delivery, which can lead to hematoma formation and muscle contraction. However, it is unequivocal that the varying degrees of degeneration in the pectoral muscles of affected infants are attributed to the progressive fibrotic transformation of neonatal neck masses, ultimately causing the loss of normal elasticity (Figs. 12.7 and 12.8).

12.2.1.3 Treatment Principles

Once diagnosed, it is crucial to initiate treatment for children as promptly as possible. Non-surgical interventions are employed in infancy, which can lead to complete recovery in select cases. However, in the case of adolescents and adults, surgical intervention is the primary treatment approach for the majority.

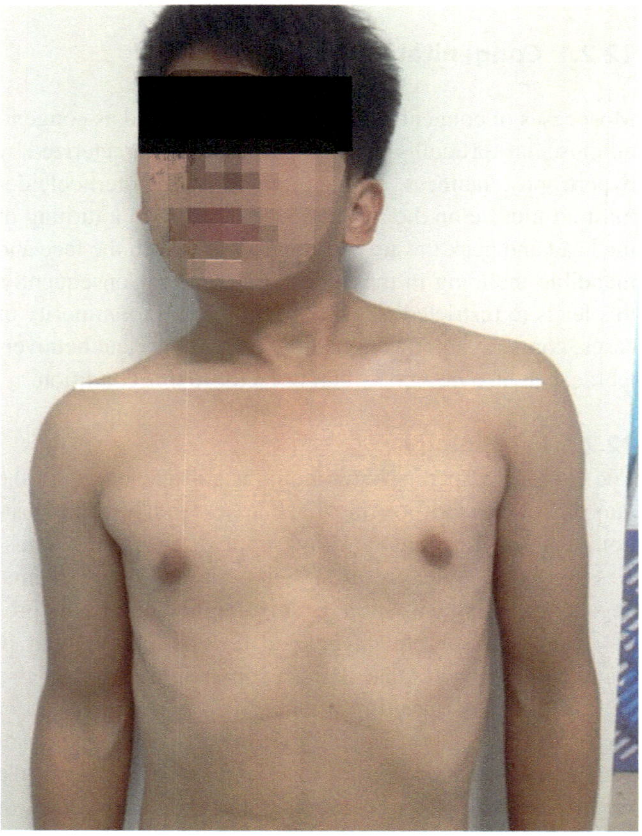

Fig. 12.7 General picture of congenital muscular torticollis

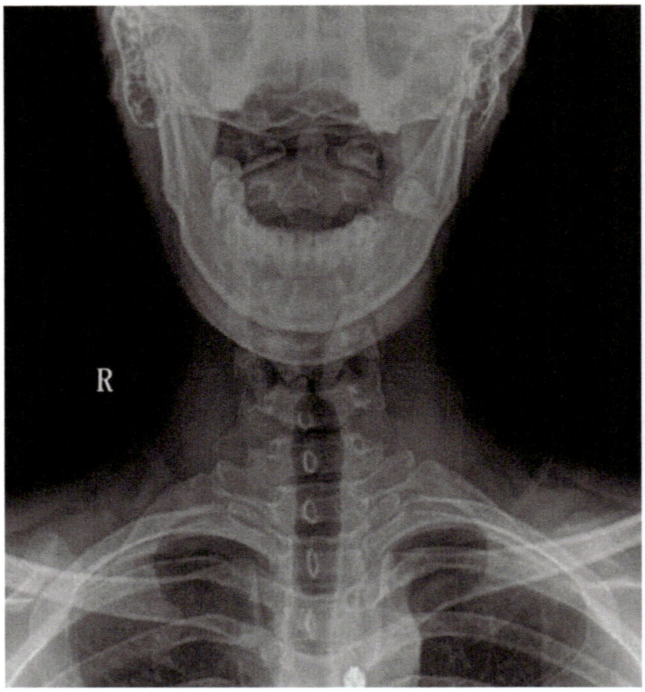

Fig. 12.8 X-ray of congenital muscular torticollis

12.2.2 Cervical Kyphosis

Cervical kyphosis, a clinical syndrome, stems from various underlying factors that lead to the loss of the physiological lordosis of the cervical vertebrae. This results in the formation of arcuate or angular kyphosis and disrupts the normal sequence of the cervical vertebrae, giving rise to localized symptoms, as well as neurological manifestations and signs.

12.2.2.1 Etiology

The etiologies of cervical kyphosis in children are multifaceted, encompassing congenital factors, infectious factors (such as tuberculosis), iatrogenic factors (following intraspinal tumor resection or laminectomy), traumatic factors, and syndromic factors. Each of these can potentially lead to varying degrees of cervical lordosis deformity.

12.2.2.2 Clinical Manifestations

In the pediatric population, cervical kyphosis is a rare deformity. This condition can diminish the volume of the spinal canal and exert pressure on the spinal cord, leading to symptoms such as pain, varying degrees of restricted limb movement, dysphagia, dyspnea, and other signs of spinal cord compression.

For patients with cervical lordotic deformity undergoing X-ray examination, it is advisable to capture cervical spine images in anteroposterior, lateral, and dynamic views. Additionally, obtaining full-length spinal X-ray scans is recommended. This comprehensive approach allows for a thorough assessment of the entire spinal curvature and flexibility.

CT imaging proves valuable in illuminating the osseous anatomical structures of the cervical spine. It enables observation of the morphology of the facet joint, lamina, and Luschka's joints. Furthermore, CT is instrumental in determining whether there is bone fusion and whether the path of the vertebral artery and the development of the pedicle are abnormal. In some cases, it may even facilitate the three-dimensional printing of vertebral bodies, offering invaluable assistance in intraoperative screw placement and bone resection strategies (Fig. 12.9).

MRI serves to visualize the compression of the spinal cord and nerve root by the kyphotic vertebral body. Generally speaking, the most severe compression of the posterior spinal cord occurs at the level of the apical vertebral body or the inferior intervertebral disc of the kyphotic vertebral body (Fig. 12.10).

12.2.2.3 Treatment Principles

When the posterior convex deformity progresses to the extent of causing postural disorders or secondary neurological symptoms, surgical intervention is often necessary. The objectives of surgery encompass nerve decompression, deformity correction, restoration of spinal stability, and reconstruction of spinal balance. The surgical principles for correcting cervical kyphosis are in line with those applied in the correction of spinal kyphosis in other regions. These principles entail using the posterior longitudinal ligament as a hinge to extend the anterior column and shorten the posterior column.

12.2.3 Klippel-Feil Syndrome

Klippel-Feil Syndrome (Klippel-Feil syndrome, KFS) is a congenital deformity characterized by cervical vertebral formation and segmental disturbances, leading to the fusion of two or more vertebral bodies and/or their appendages. Its estimated incidence is approximately 1 in 40,000 to 1 in 42,000 individuals.

12.2.3.1 Etiology

Epidemiological data reveals that cases of Klippel-Feil Syndrome (KFS) predominantly occur sporadically, although there are instances of familial clustering. In recent years, researchers have reported the pathogenic genes associated with the development of congenital cervical fusion deformity. This body of evidence unequivocally emphasizes the significant correlation between the occurrence of KFS and genetic factors, particularly gene mutations. The role of genetic factors in the pathogenesis of KFS is undeniably paramount.

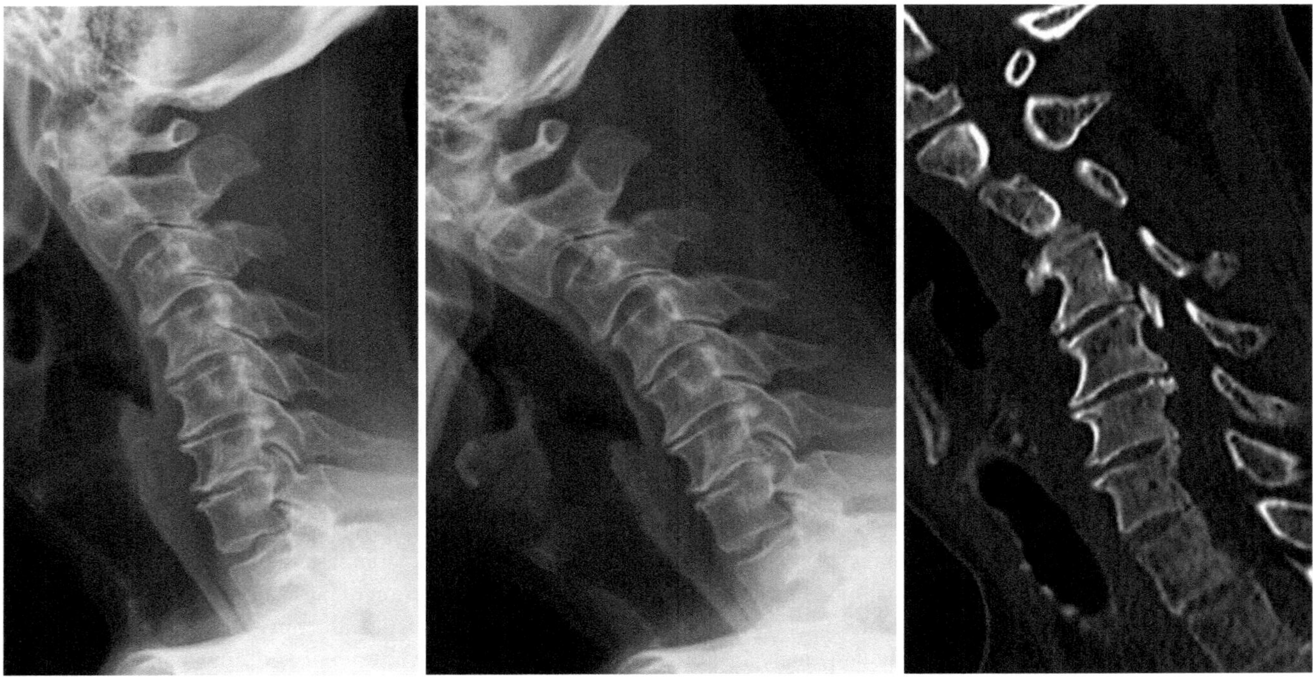

Fig. 12.9 X-ray and CT images of cervical kyphosis

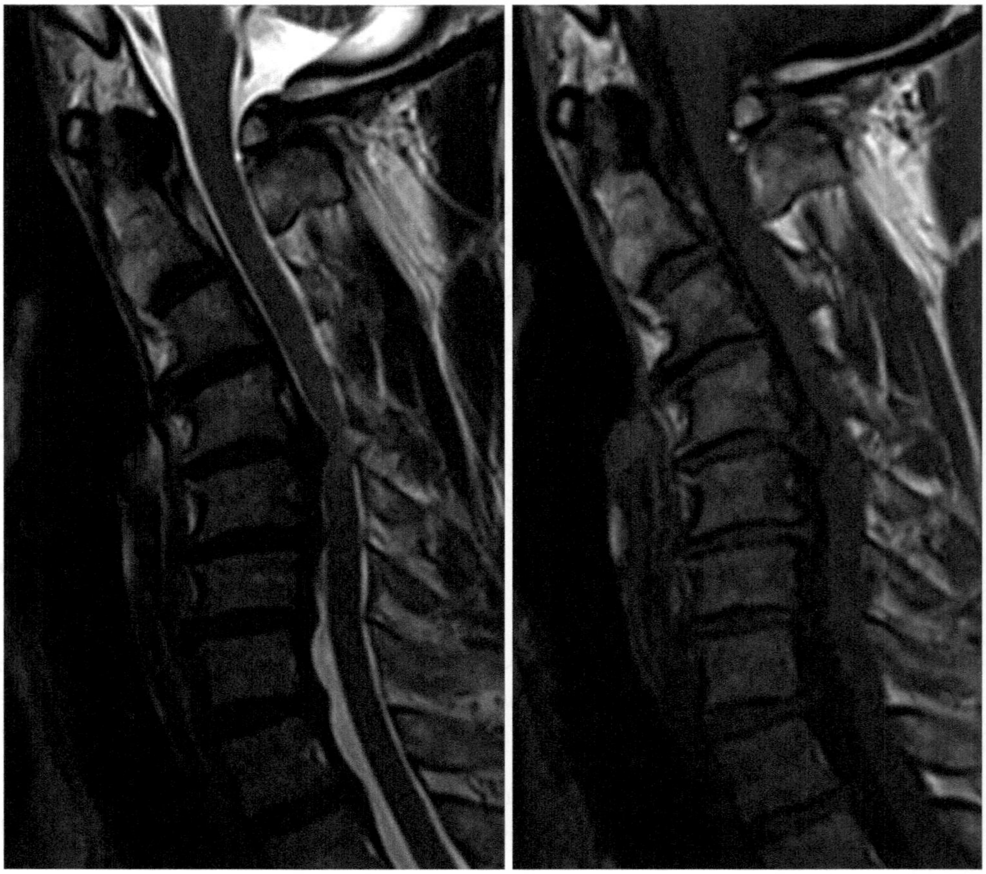

Fig. 12.10 MRI image shows cervical kyphosis and spinal cord compression

12.2.3.2 Clinical Manifestations

KFS, also known as cervical segmentation deficiency, often becomes evident in patients shortly after birth due to deformities. However, it is typically diagnosed when they start experiencing symptoms such as cervical and dorsal pain, morphological anomalies, or signs of neurological compression. While the disease typically presents with the clinical triad of short neck deformity, low posterior hairline, and limited neck activity, it's important to note that approximately 50% of KFS patients may not display these typical clinical characteristics. Therefore, the diagnosis of KFS primarily relies on radiological imaging (Fig. 12.11).

The imaging features of KFS are rather typical. Both X-ray and CT imaging can clearly depict the fusion of two or more cervical vertebrae. This fusion can occur in a contiguous manner, affecting consecutive vertebrae, or it may manifest in a discontinuous, intermittent fashion. Furthermore, the fusion can involve the vertebrae themselves, extend to their appendages, or indeed, occur simultaneously in both aspects (Fig. 12.12).

12.2.3.3 Classification

Klippel-Feil Syndrome is typically categorized into three distinct types:

Type I is characterized by the fusion of multiple cervical vertebrae.

Type II involves the fusion of only 1–2 adjacent intervertebral spaces.

Type III denotes the fusion deformity involving cervical vertebrae concurrent with thoracic or lumbar vertebrae.

12.2.3.4 Treatment Principles

For asymptomatic KFS patients, treatment is generally unnecessary. However, once neurological symptoms manifest, specific treatment interventions become imperative. These interventions encompass the alteration of daily activity patterns, the reduction of cervical mobility, localized cervical bracing, and traction therapy, all aimed at preventing cervical trauma. If symptomatic improvement remains elusive through conservative means, the recourse to appropriate

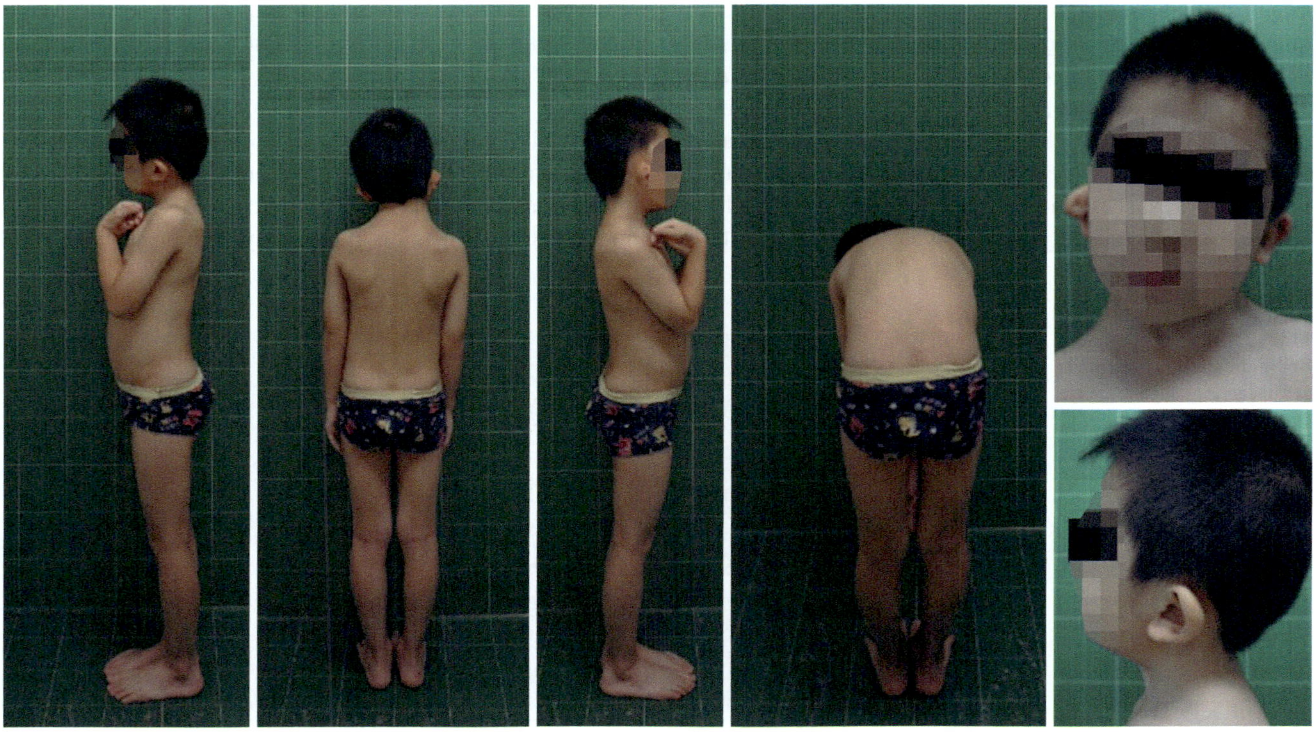

Fig. 12.11 General picture of children with Klippel-Feil syndrome

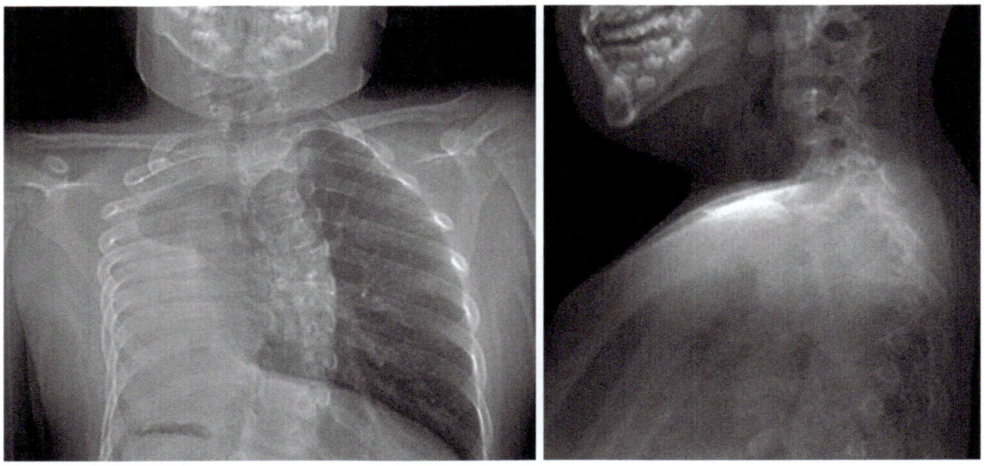

Fig. 12.12 X-ray of neck in children with Klippel-Feil syndrome

neuro-decompression and stabilization procedures becomes indispensable to forestall the further exacerbation of neurological symptoms.

12.3 Scoliosis

12.3.1 Congenital Scoliosis

Congenital scoliosis (CS) is a prevalent form of early-onset scoliosis, representing a common spinal deformity resulting from abnormal spine development during the embryonic stage.

12.3.1.1 Etiology

The exact cause of this condition remains unclear, with onset typically occurring during the embryonic phase or early postnatal stages.

12.3.1.2 Clinical Manifestations

CS is an early-onset form of scoliosis resulting from abnormal somite development during embryogenesis. It often manifests with marked severity and a progressive nature, frequently accompanied by malformations in other systems such as the kidney, heart, or intraspinal structures (Fig. 12.13).

For patients with CS, conducting X-ray examinations is imperative to ascertain the nature of the deformity. Features such as redundant vertebral arches, asymmetric or absent intervertebral spaces, and fusion or absence of ribs all contribute to the diagnostic process. Given that patients with CS often have associated spinal cord malformations, MRI examinations can offer a more precise assessment (Fig. 12.14).

12.3.1.3 Classification

The classification system of congenital scoliosis, revised by Winter and other scholars in 1968 and later accepted by the international Scoliosis Research Society (SRS), is known as the Winter Classification. It primarily categorizes congenital

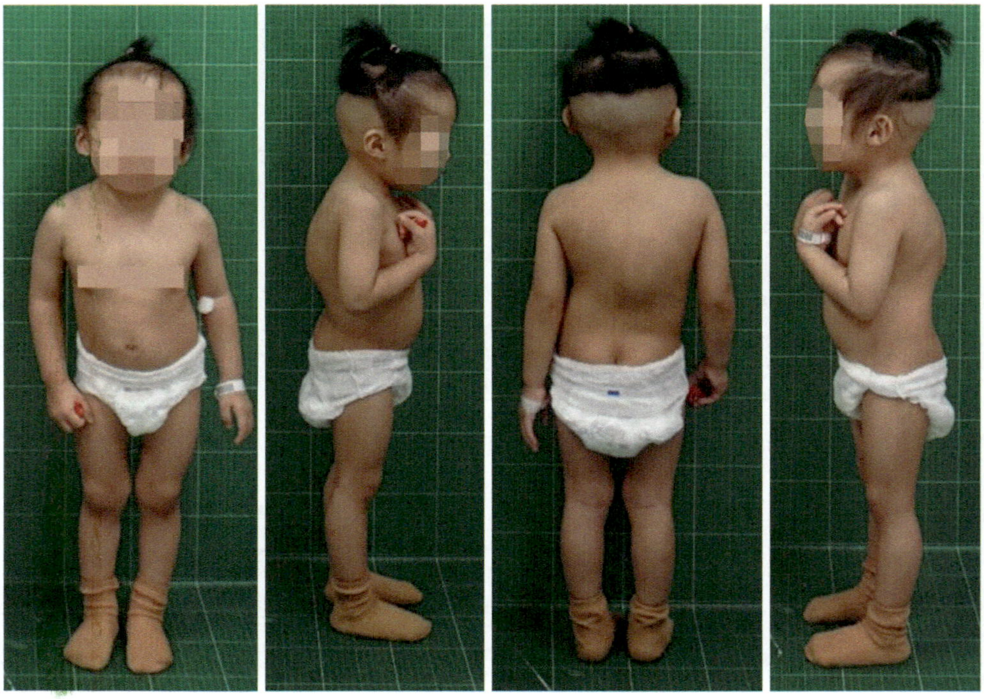

Fig. 12.13 General picture of children with congenital scoliosis

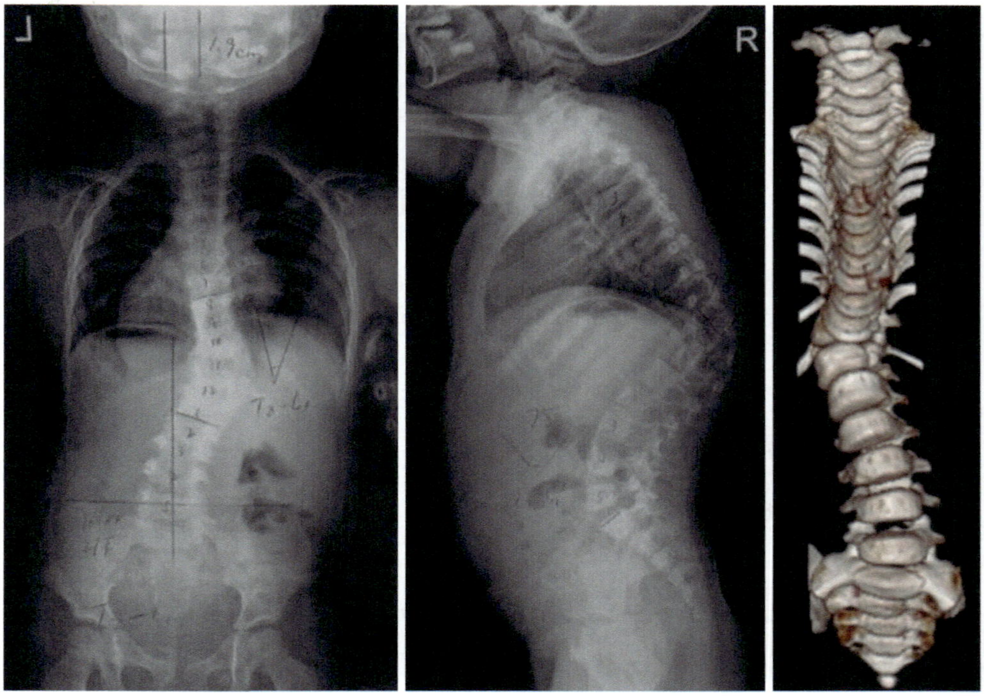

Fig. 12.14 X-ray and three-dimensional reconstruction of CT in children with congenital scoliosis, T10 and T11 hemivertebrae can be seen

scoliosis into three types: formation failure, segmentation failure, and mixed deformity.

- Formation failure outcomes encompass wedge-shaped vertebrae, hemivertebrae, and butterfly vertebrae.
- Segmentation failure includes the formation of block vertebrae or unilateral unsegmented bar.
- Mixed malformations often involve a combination of formation and segmentation failure.

This system further subdivides CS into six types:

1. Type I—Indivisible: This classification amalgamates diverse patterns, making it challenging to categorize definitively.
2. Type II—Rib Fusion Deformity.
3. Type III—Failure of Unilateral Partial Vertebral Body Formation: This leads to wedge-shaped vertebrae or trapezoidal vertebrae.
4. Type IV—Unilateral Complete Formation Failure of Vertebral Body: This results in hemivertebrae.
5. Type V—Bilateral Segmentation Failure of Vertebral Body: This leads to the complete absence of an intervertebral disc.
6. Type VI—Unilateral Segmentation Failure of the Vertebral Body: This results in the partial fusion of two or more vertebral bodies, which can lead to an unsegmented bar.

1. Type A—Unilateral isolated hemivertebrae with additional ribs and pedicles.
2. Type B1—Unilateral vertebral body complete formation failure, forming unilateral triangular hemivertebrae.
3. Type B2—Unilateral incomplete vertebral body formation failure, forming wedge-shaped hemivertebrae.
4. Type C—Round, oval, or wedge-shaped multiple hemivertebrae.
5. Type D1—Multiple isolated hemivertebrae with concave unsegmented bar.
6. Type D2—Multiple wedge-shaped vertebrae with unilateral unsegmented bar.
7. Type E—The vertebral column concurrently develops hemivertebrae on both its left and right sides, achieving a relative equilibrium of the spine.
8. Type F—The hemivertebrae are located in the posterior structure of the spine.

12.3.1.4 Treatment Principles

When determining the appropriate treatment approach for patients with congenital scoliosis, it is crucial to take into account factors such as the patient's age, growth potential, type of deformity, and overall prognosis. The available treatment options include both conservative (non-surgical) and surgical interventions.

For mild congenital spinal deformities with a low risk of progression, observation is the primary conservative treatment approach. However, most cases of congenital scoliosis tend to be progressive, often necessitating surgical intervention.

12.3.2 Adolescent Idiopathic Scoliosis

Adolescent idiopathic scoliosis (AIS) is a complex three-dimensional spinal deformity that occurs in adolescence.

12.3.2.1 Etiology

The etiology of AIS is still unclear. The etiological theory of AIS mainly includes genetic-related theories, hormonal and metabolic theories, biomechanical theories, bone marrow mesenchymal stem cell theories, neurological theories, and environmental theories, among others.

12.3.2.2 Clinical Manifestations

AIS is a complex three-dimensional deformity that constitutes coronal scoliosis, sagittal kyphosis/lordosis, and horizontal vertebral rotation. Due to spinal lateral curvature, torsion, and thoracic deformity, it directly impacts the patients' appearance, cardiopulmonary function, and quality of life.

12.3.2.3 Classification

PUMC classification (Fig. 12.15) is different from all previous classifications based on scoliosis aera. First, AIS is divided into three types according to the number of apexes: one apex point (single curve) is designated as PUMC Type I, two apex points (double curve) as PUMC Type II, and three apex points (triple curve) as PUMC Type III. Within the three types of scoliosis, they are divided into different 13 subtypes according to different three-dimensional deformity characteristics and the position of scoliosis apex. PUMC classification specifies the specific fusion scope and surgical approach for each subtype, which can provide guidance for surgical plan selection.

12.3.2.4 Treatment Principles

The current treatment methods are divided into conservative treatment and surgery. Conservative treatment is the best treatment choice for patients with early AIS. Conservative therapy stands as the optimal treatment selection for early-stage AIS patients. It is generally recommended for patients with a Cobb angle of less than 40°, as it effectively retards the progression of lateral curvature, ameliorating spinal deformity, thereby maximally preserving spinal functionality and circumventing the need for sur-

Modified PUMC classification

Major type	Apex numbers	Subtype	Characteristics	Schematic drawing	Selection fusion strategy
I Single curve	1	IA	Thoracic curve, apex between T2 and T11–T12 disc	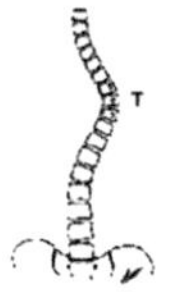	Single curve
		IB	Thoracolumbar curve, apex at T12, T12–L1 disc, and L1		
		IC	Lumbar curve, apex between L1–L2 and L4–L5 disc		
II Double curves	2	IIA	Double thoracic curves IIA1: Not meet all of the three criteria: 1) Left shoulder elevated or as high as right shoulder 2) Cobb angle of PT curve <30° 3) Cobb angle of PT curve on convex bending radiograph <20° IIA2: Meet one of the aforementioned criteria	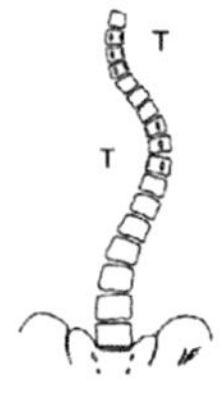	IIA1: Major thoracic curve IIA2: Double curves
		IIB	Thoracic curve plus thoracolumbar/lumbar curve, the former is at least 10° higher than the latter. IIB1: Fulfill all four criteria: 1) Without lumbar/thoracolumbar kyphosis (<10°) 2) Cobb angle of lumbar/thoracolumbar <45° 3) Apical rotation of lumbar/thoracolumbar curve <II° 4) Flexibility of lumbar/thoracolumbar curve >70% IIB2: Not meet any of the aforementioned criteria	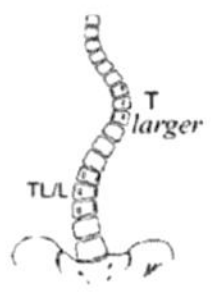	IIB1: Thoracic curve IIB2: Double curves
		IIC	Thoracic curve plus lumbar/thoracolumbar curve, the former is at least 10° smaller than the latter. IIC1: Cobb angle of the thoracic curve on convex bending radiograph <25° IIC2: Cobb angle of the thoracic curve on convex bending radiograph >25°	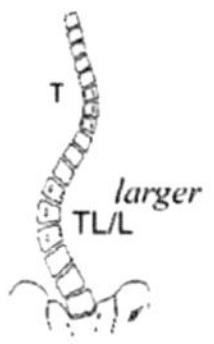	IIC1: Lumbar/thoracolumbar curve IIC2: Double curves
		IID	Thoracic curve plus lumbar/thoracolumbar curve, the curve magnitude difference <10°. IID1: Flexibility of thoracic curve <lumbar/thoracolumbar curve IID2: Flexibility of thoracic curve >lumbar/thoracolumbar curve	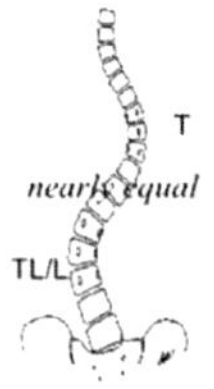	IID1: Refers to IIB IID2: Refers to IIC
III Triple curves	3	IIIA	Lumbar curve meets IIB1 criteria IIIA1: PT curve and shoulder balance meet IIA1 criteria IIIA2: PT curve and shoulder balance meet IIA2 criteria	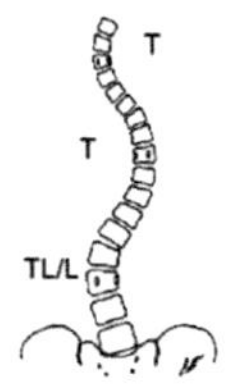	Lumbar/thoracolumbar curve not be fused PT curve refers to IIA
		IIIB	Lumbar curve meets IIB1 criteria IIIB1: PT curve and shoulder balance meet IIA1 criteria IIIB2: PT curve and shoulder balance meet IIA2 criteria		Lumbar/thoracolumbar curve be fused PT curve refers to IIA

Fig. 12.15 Modified PUMC classification of adolescent idiopathic scoliosis

gical intervention. It is generally believed that when the Cobb angle of AIS patients is ≥50°, surgery is recommended regardless of whether the patients are mature or not. Studies have shown that when the Cobb angle ≥50°, it will progress about 1° every year, and when the thoracic scoliosis angle reaches more than 70°, it adversely impacts pulmonary function. Surgical intervention is also a viable option when the Cobb angle falls within the range of 40–49° (Fig. 12.16).

12.3.3 Neuromuscular Scoliosis

Neuromuscular scoliosis (NS) is a coronal spinal deformity caused by a group of muscular neurological diseases.

12.3.3.1 Etiology

There are many reasons causing neuromuscular scoliosis, and the incidence varies among different patients and etiological factors. However, the most fundamental pathogenesis in all cases is the imbalance of muscular forces surrounding the spine, exerting their influence upon the vertebral endplates. These afflictions may manifest in various regions, including the cerebral, spinal, peripheral nervous, neuromuscular junctions, and muscular components, culminating in manifestations of cranial dysregulation, cervical and thoracic imbalance, and incoordination.

12.3.3.2 Clinical Manifestations

Neuromuscular scoliosis usually occurs at an early age, displaying rapid progression during the growth phase, and persists even after skeletal maturity is reached. Most of the curves are long, C-shaped, and involve the sacrum, often combined with pelvic tilt. Kyphosis is also common in NS. At times, spinal collapse occurs, necessitating the support of both hands to maintain an upright posture, often accompanied by back pain. Due to the limitation of patients' activities and the primary disease, most of them have malnutrition, cardiopulmonary dysfunction, gastrointestinal dysfunction, poor general condition, and are often combined with hip dislocation, lower limb deformity, and a loss of motor function (Figs. 12.17 and 12.18).

12.3.3.3 Classification

According to the etiology, it can be divided into: Type A. neurogenic; Type B. Myogenic.

12.3.3.4 Treatment Principles

It is similar to the treatment principle of adolescent idiopathic scoliosis.

12.3.4 Neurofibromatosis Type I with Scoliosis

Neurofibromatosis type I (NF1) is a genetic disease. In addition to disorders in skin, visual system and nervous system, approximately 26–50% of patients may present skeletal-related deformity, such as spinal curvature.

12.3.4.1 Etiology

Neurofibromatosis type I is an autosomal dominant disease. Thus, the etiology primarily stems from familial inheritance. The NF1 tumor suppressor gene in the patient is mutated, which in turn causes the inactivation of neurofibroma protein function and leads to abnormal proliferation of tumor cells. The skeletal abnormalities of NF1 are believed to be related to the changes in the bone microenvironment caused by tumors. Some scholars also believe that there are gene mutations in the bone cells of NF1 patients.

12.3.4.2 Clinical Manifestations

Clinical manifestations unrelated to the skeletal system in patients with NF1 encompass skin pigmented spots, peripheral nerve sheath tumors, gliomas (optic nerve, brainstem), cognitive dysfunction and behavioral difficulties, and Lisch nodules.

The skeletal-related clinical manifestations of NF1 include spinal deformity (about 30%) and deformity of long bones. The common spinal deformities include thoracolumbar kyphoscoliosis and cervical kyphosis (Figs. 12.19 and 12.20).

12.3.4.3 Classification

NF1-related scoliosis is mainly divided into dystrophic scoliosis and pseudo-idiopathic scoliosis. There are many characteristic clinical manifestations of skeletal abnormalities in patients with typical dystrophic NF1 spinal deformity, as shown in the table below. The patient's condition often progresses rapidly.

Various skeletal abnormalities in typical dystrophic NF1 spinal deformities.

Scallop like vertebral bodies (the posterior edge of the vertebral body is depressed, the posterior edge of the thoracic vertebral body is depressed to 3 mm, and the lumbar vertebral body reaches 4 mm)
Pencil like rib (the width of the rib is narrower than the narrowest part of the second rib)
Spindle like transverse process
Wedging degeneration of vertebral body
Paravertebral soft tissue
Scoliosis involving short segments and severe rotation
Enlarged intervertebral foramen
Pedicle dysplasia
Widening of pedicle distance

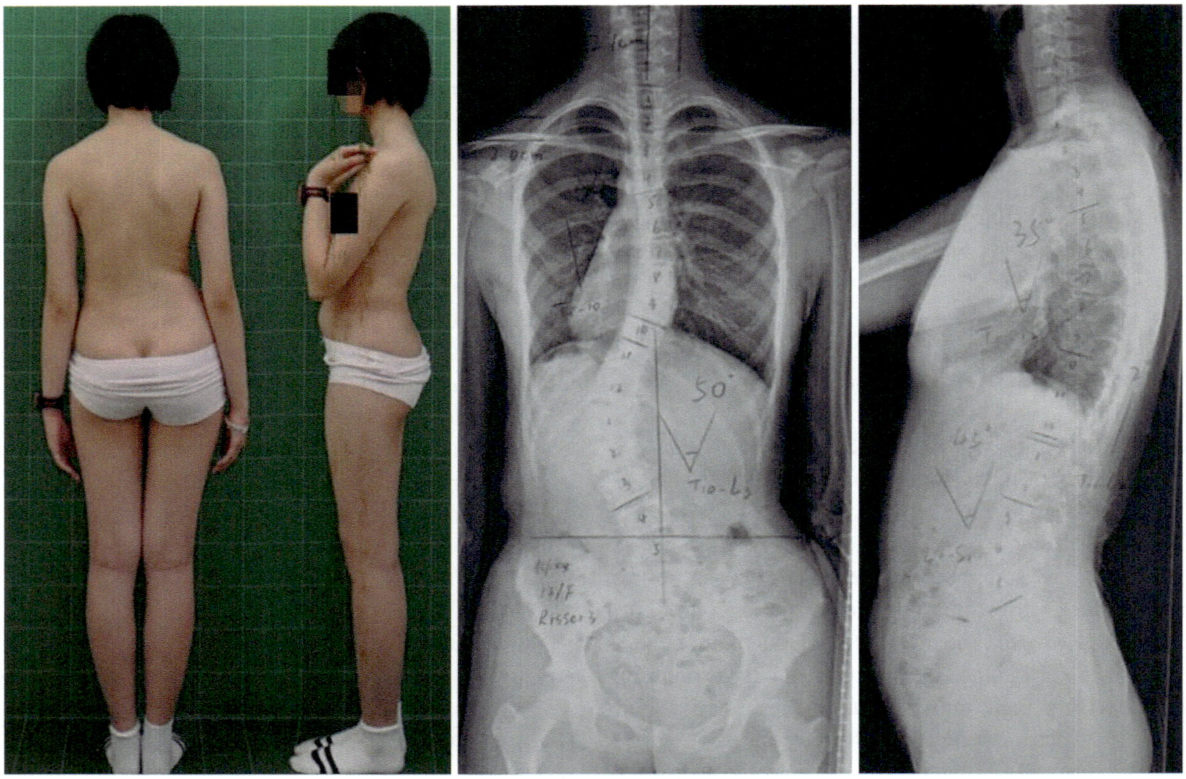

Fig. 12.16 Female, 12 years old, diagnosed with adolescent idiopathic scoliosis (PUMC IIC1, Lenke 5CN)

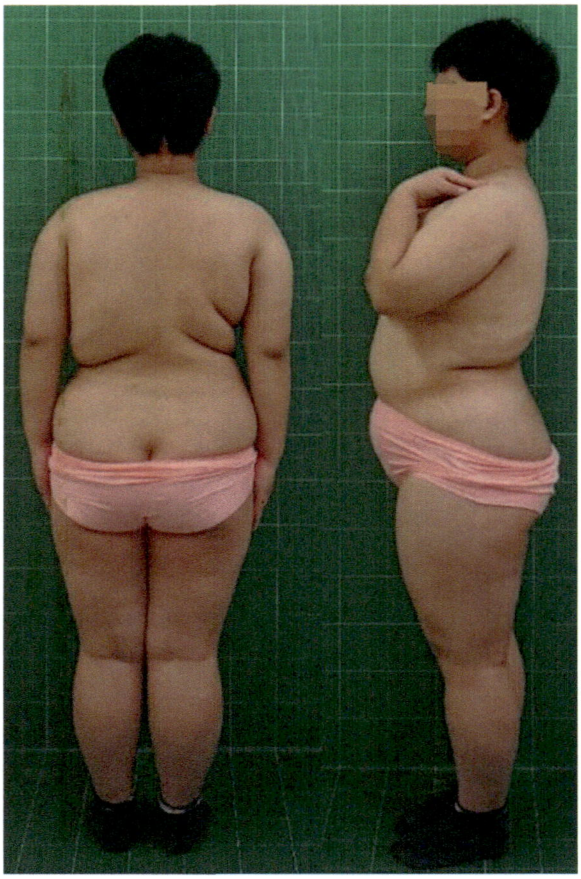

Fig. 12.17 Female, 14 years old, diagnosed with neuromuscular scoliosis

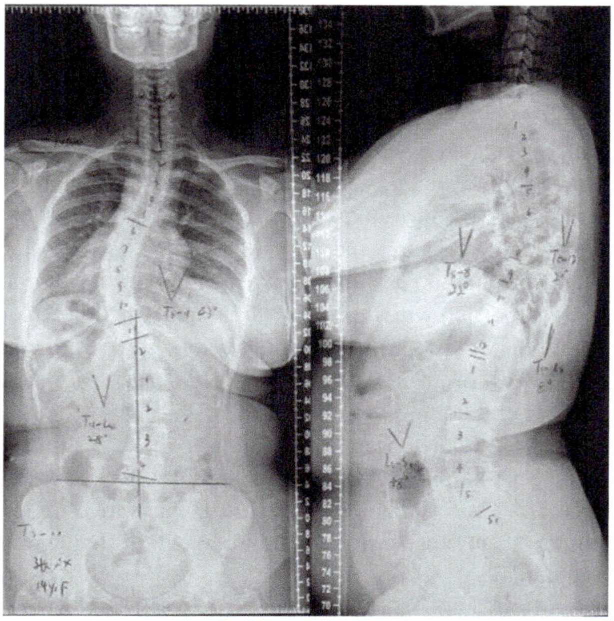

Fig. 12.18 X-ray of a 14-year-old female with neuromuscular scoliosis

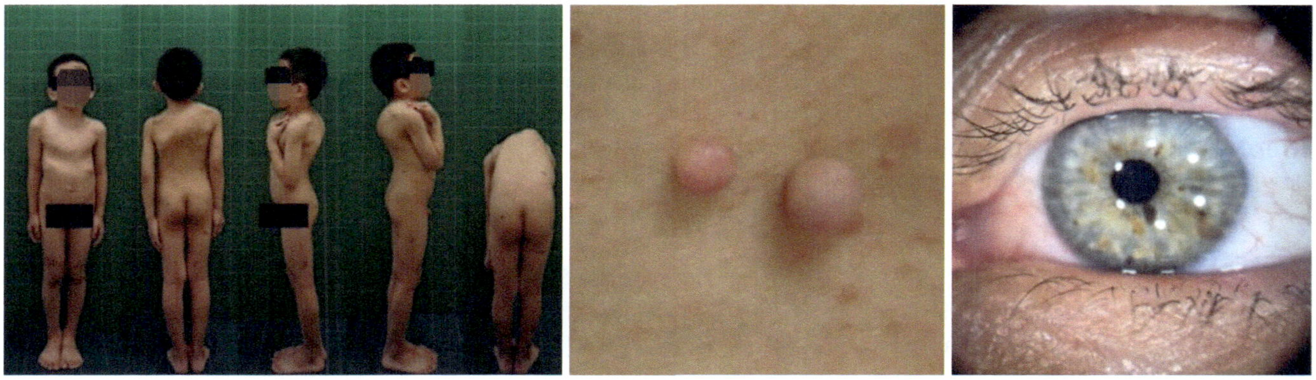

Fig. 12.19 Multiple cutaneous café-au-lait spots, cutaneous fibromas, and iris Lisch nodules in patients with neurofibromatosis type I. (Reproduced from Antoniolli et al. [1]; Cimino et al. [2])

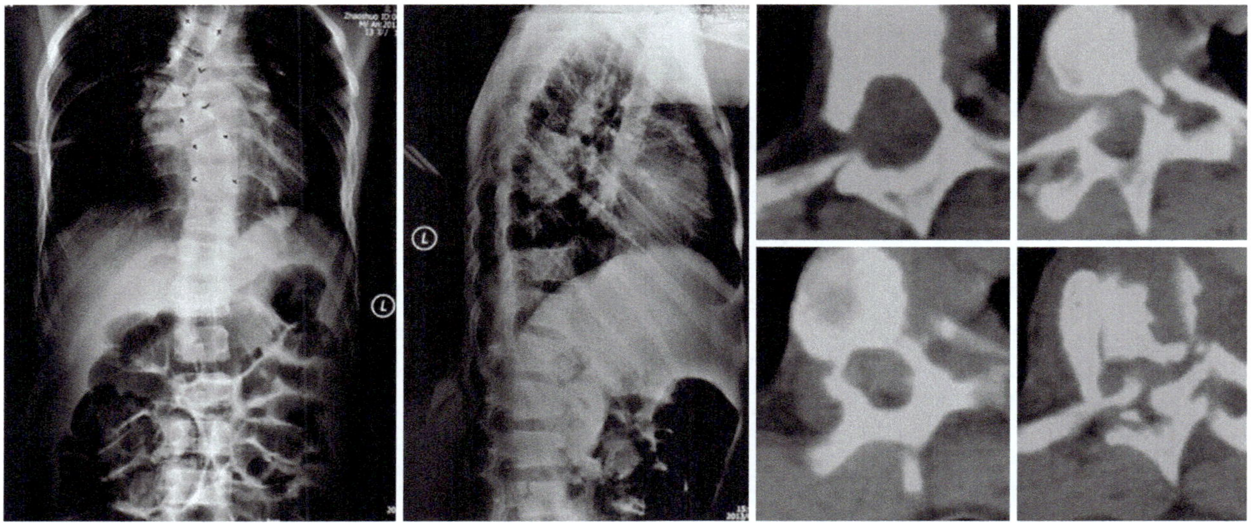

Fig. 12.20 Male, 20 years old, diagnosed with neurofibromatosis type I complicated with scoliosis. We can see vertebral morphological changes, pedicle dysplasia, pencil like ribs, and ribs enter the spinal canal

The clinical manifestations of idiopathic scoliosis and pseudo-idiopathic scoliosis are similar.

12.3.4.4 Treatment Principles

For NF1 related dystrophic scoliosis, conservative treatment can be taken when the degree of scoliosis is <20°, otherwise surgical intervention should be performed. When opting for the posterior fixation and fusion surgery, it is advisable to conduct follow-up examinations while monitoring complications associated with the spinal alignment. The implementation of growth rod techniques may potentially confer certain advantages in the treatment of early-onset cases among affected children.

For NF1 related pseudo-idiopathic scoliosis, its treatment method is similar to that of idiopathic scoliosis. When the degree of scoliosis is less than 40°, conservative treatment can be taken; otherwise, surgical intervention should be carried out.

12.3.5 Marfan Syndrome Scoliosis

Marfan syndrome (MFS) is a genetic connective tissue disease. It can affect various organs originating from the mesodermal layer, such as the skeletal system, cardiovascular system, visual organs, respiratory system, and more. Among individuals with Marfan syndrome, the incidence of spinal lateral convexity is estimated to be around 60%.

12.3.5.1 Etiology

Abnormal protein structure caused by fibrillin-1 gene (FBN1) mutation in patients with Marfan syndrome may be the cause of abnormal elastic fiber function in connective tissue. This connective tissue abnormality may involve the intervertebral disc and cause vertebral rotation, thus causing and aggravating scoliosis.

12.3.5.2 Clinical Manifestations

Marfan syndrome may affect the cardiovascular system, leading to dilation of the ascending aortic root, aortic dissection, mitral valve insufficiency, thereby causing associated symptoms; concerning visual organs, Marfan syndrome can result in crystalline lens dislocation, myopia, retinal detachment, and so forth.

In terms of skeletal system, patients with Marfan syndrome often present with long and thin body, spider fingers, flat feet, pectus excavatum/pectus carinatum, and joint ligaments relaxation. Spinal deformities of Marfan syndrome, characterized by early onset and rapid progression, can be manifested as scoliosis, cervical lordosis, lumbar spondylolisthesis, vertebral dysplasia, etc. (Figs. 12.21, 12.22 and 12.23).

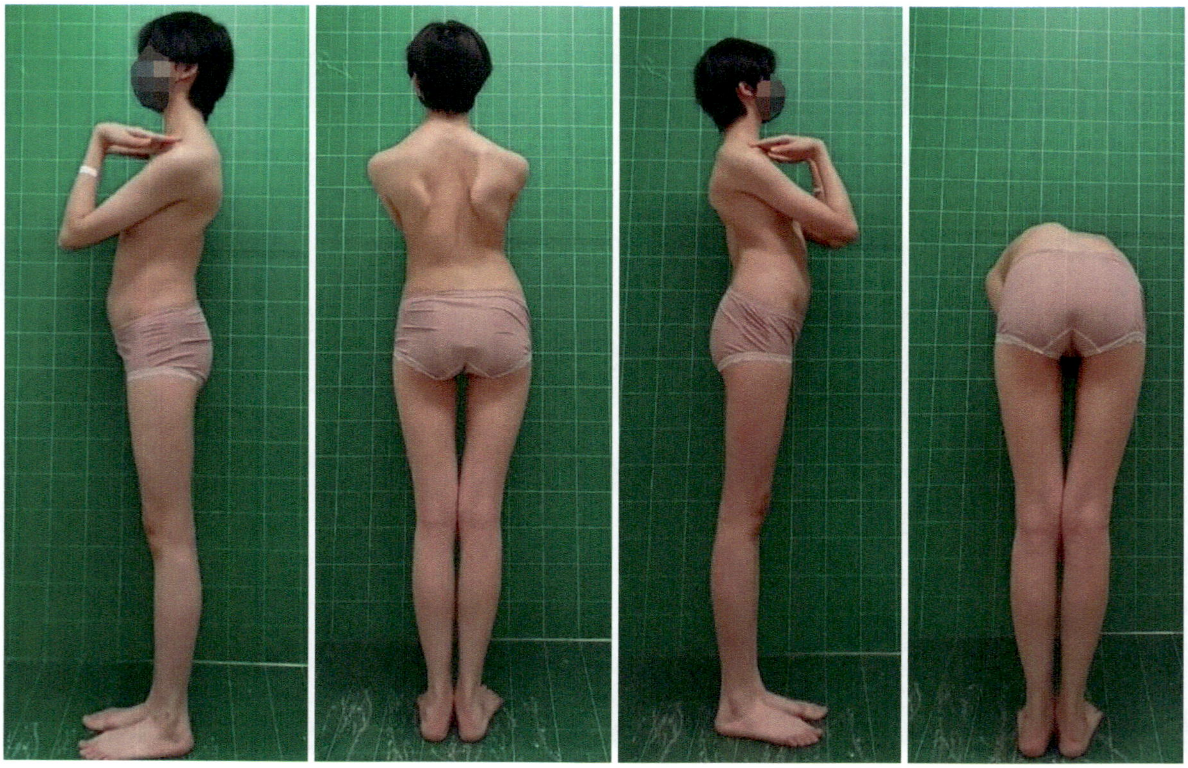

Fig. 12.21 Female, 12 years old, diagnosed with Marfan syndrome, with slender body and flat feet

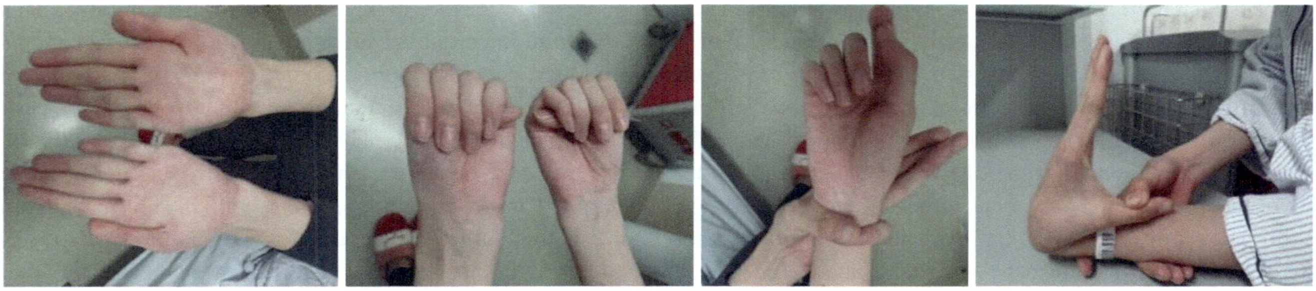

Fig. 12.22 Female, 12 years old, diagnosed with Marfan syndrome, with spider fingers, finger signs, wrist signs and joint hyperflexion and extension

Fig. 12.23 Anteroposterior and lateral X-ray radiographs of the full spine in patients with Marfan syndrome complicated with scoliosis

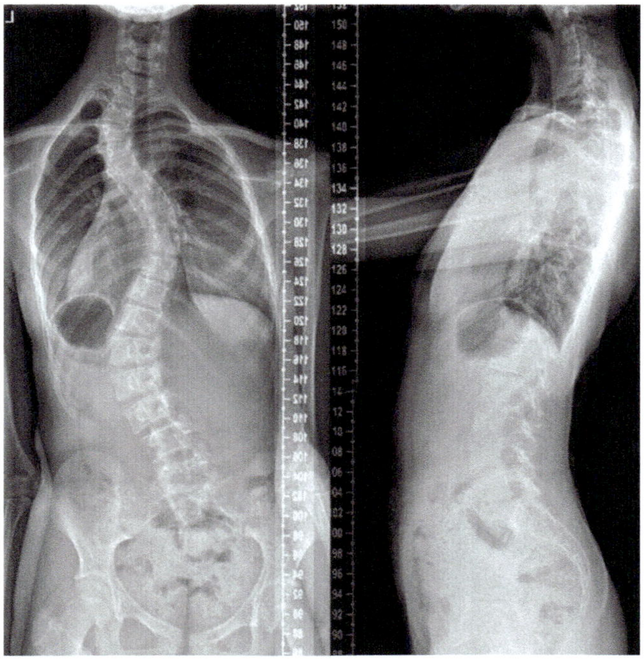

12.3.5.3 Treatment Principles

In terms of conservative therapy, some scholars believe that brace has poor Treatment effect on patients with Marfan syndrome. If the main curvature of scoliosis is greater than 40°or progresses rapidly, especially in patients with significant kyphosis, surgery is recommended.

12.3.6 Achondroplasia Scoliosis

Achondroplasia (ACH) is the most common disease of skeletal dysplasia (SD) combined with spinal deformity. It is a genetic disease with a prevalence of about 0.03–0.04‰. Patients often present thoracolumbar kyphosis and excessive lumbar lordosis.

12.3.6.1 Etiology

Achondroplasia is an autosomal dominant disease, mainly inherited from the father, caused by a kind of new gene mutation of fibroblast growth factor receptor-3 (FGFR3). FGFR3 is related to the maturation of chondrocytes in the growth plate. After mutation, it affects the maturation of chondrocytes in the growth plate, resulting in abnormal endochondral ossification and intramembranous ossification. Ultimately, it leads to abnormal skeletal development throughout the body, disrupting the longitudinal growth balance of the anterior and posterior columns of the spine, resulting in the wedging deformation of the thoracolumbar vertebral body to form local kyphosis.

12.3.6.2 Clinical Manifestations

The spinal deformities in patients with ACH mainly include thoracolumbar kyphosis, compensatory lumbar lordosis, and spinal stenosis. Thoracolumbar kyphosis often appears temporarily within 1 year after birth, and spontaneously ameliorates upon acquiring the ability to stand and walk. The deformities continue to adult in about 10–15% patients and develop into fixed angular kyphosis with vertebral wedge-shaped change. Then spinal cord injury and neurological dysfunction appears, such as lower limb weakness, numbness, bladder, and rectal dysfunction. The majority of patients gradually develop asymptomatic excessive lumbar lordosis following the acquisition of the ability to sit up and walk. Central type is the main type of spinal stenosis, most often involving the lumbar segment. Intermittent claudication, limb pain, limb numbness, and paresthesia, and defecation and urinary dysfunction can be seen in about 20–30% of patients. As the patient's age increases, the probability of presenting incidence of symptoms related to spinal stenosis also increases correspondingly. The progression of symptoms is rapid once they appear (Figs. 12.24, 12.25 and 12.26).

12.3.6.3 Treatment Principles

Nowadays, the main treatment methods for thoracolumbar kyphosis include behavioral intervention, brace treatment, and surgery. The choice of treatment methods needs to be comprehensively considered based on the analysis of the patient's age, degree of kyphosis, and other complications. Behavioral interventions are generally applicable to patients in infancy, providing support while sitting. Brace treatment is suitable for infants and children with a Cobb angle ≥30°, and thoracic lumbar sacral orthosis (TLSO) treatment should be initiated as soon as possible. The curative effect of a brace is limited when the Cobb angle is ≥40°. The mainstream view is that surgery is suitable for thoracolumbar kyphosis patients older than 10–12 years old; however, there are other opinions suggesting that patients should undergo surgical intervention as soon as possible if conservative treatment fails at 4–8 years old. When the Cobb angle is <30° with neurological symptoms occurring, spinal canal decompression and internal fixation with bone graft fusion can be considered. When patients persist with thoracolumbar kyphosis and the Cobb angle is ≥30°, thoracolumbar kyphosis correction is recommended, regardless of the presence of neurological symptoms. Osteotomy can be considered when the Cobb angle is ≥40°.

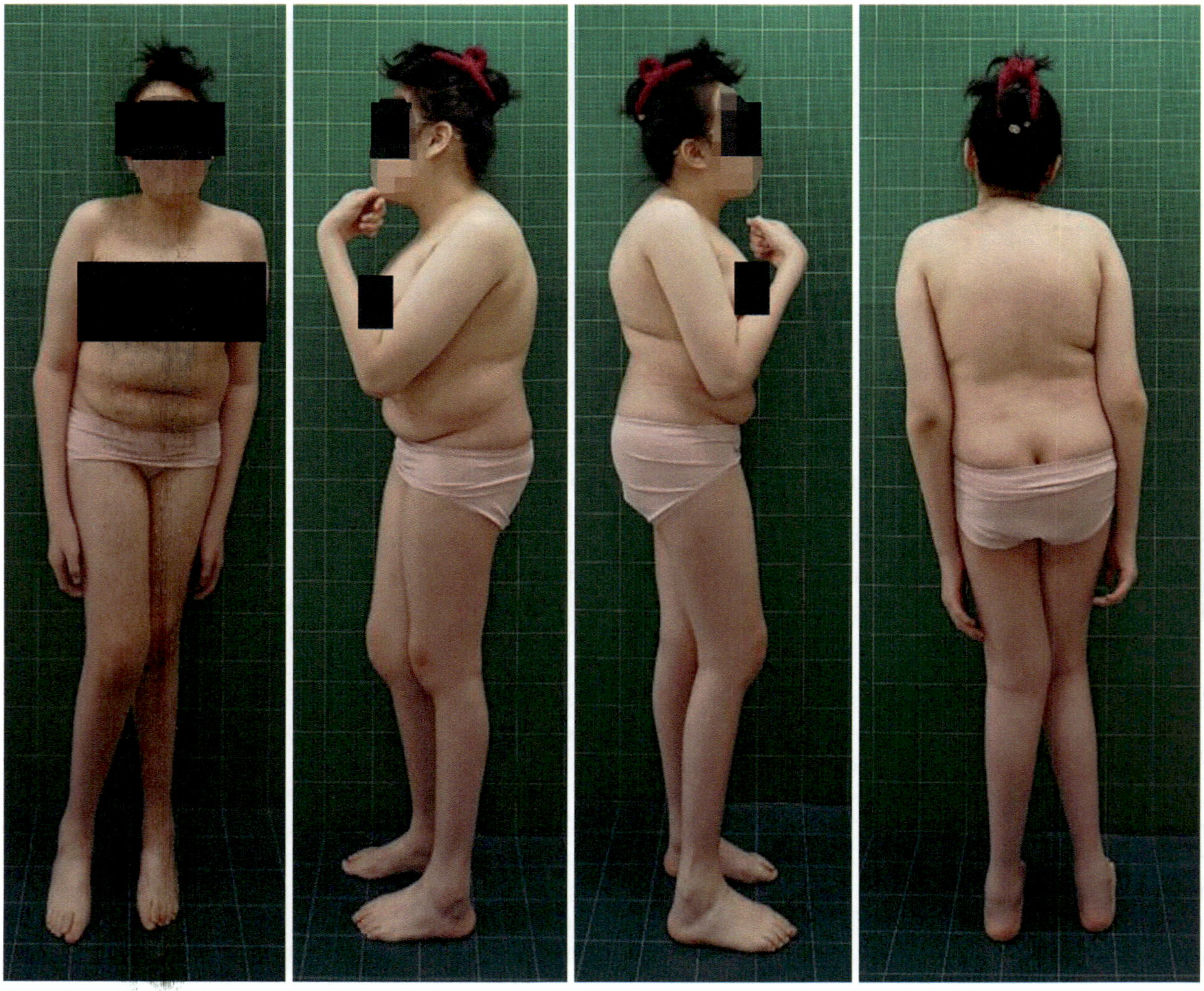

Fig. 12.24 General picture of the patient with achondroplasia. It can be seen that the limbs and fingers are short

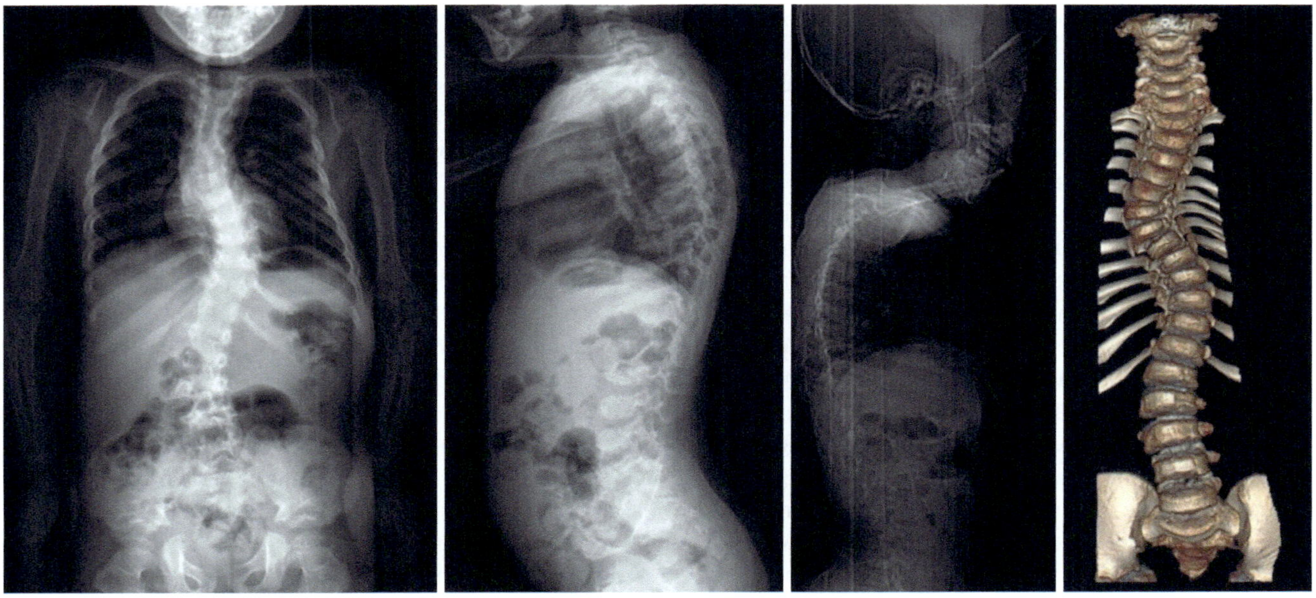

Fig. 12.25 A 4-year-old male with scoliosis, macrocephaly, and pectus excavatum, was diagnosed as achondroplasia scoliosis

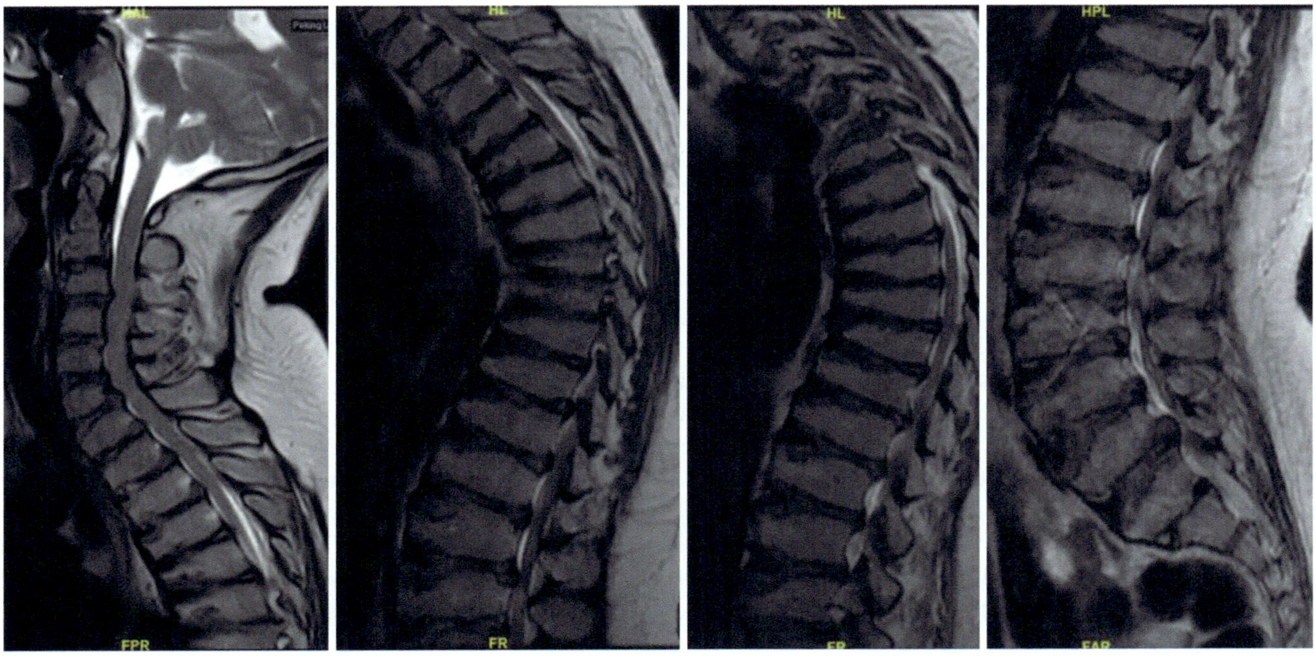

Fig. 12.26 MRI of the achondroplasia combined with spinal deformity shows thoracolumbar kyphosis and spinal stenosis

12.3.7 Scheuermann's Disease with Kyphosis

12.3.7.1 Etiology

The etiology of Scheuermann's disease remains unknown. It was first documented in 1920 by Danish physician Scheuermann. He initially postulated that the necrosis of blood vessels in the epiphyseal ring of the vertebral body halted the growth and development of the vertebral body, resulting in anterior vertebral wedging. Schmorl, however, theorized that congenital weakness in the vertebral cartilaginous endplate led to continuous disc protrusion and subsequent sustained damage, ultimately culminating in growth cessation and posterior convex deformity. Additionally, based on family studies of Scheuermann's disease, it is considered that the disease follows an autosomal incomplete dominant inheritance pattern and exhibits a variety of phenotypes. Other etiological hypotheses include mechanical anomalies, vitamin A deficiency, strenuous physical labor, poliomyelitis, tumors, chondrodystrophy, excessive growth hormone secretion, prolonged sitting, osteochondrosis, adolescent osteoporosis, and extended periods of standing, among others.

12.3.7.2 Clinical Manifestations

Scheuermann's disease often manifests as kyphosis of the spine, which can occur in the thoracic vertebrae, thoracolumbar vertebrae, and lumbar vertebrae, with the thoracic region being the most common location. It may be accompanied by lumbar back pain, while neurological abnormalities are relatively infrequent. In current clinical practice, the quantitative diagnosis proposed by Sorensen in 1964 is widely used: at least three contiguous vertebrae must exhibit wedging deformities exceeding 5° each. Other criteria include thoracic kyphosis, narrow intervertebral space, irregular endplate, and at least one wedge-shaped vertebral body; two or more wedge-shaped vertebral bodies with a kyphosis angle greater than 45°; and characteristic imaging features like Schmorl nodules, irregular endplates, wedge-shaped vertebral bodies, and kyphosis (Figs. 12.27 and 12.28).

12.3.7.3 Classification

In addition to the typical occurrence of Scheuermann's disease in the thoracic or thoracolumbar vertebrae, there is also a variant known as lumbar Scheuermann's disease, sometimes referred to as Type II Scheuermann's disease. This type primarily affects male adolescents who engage in heavy exercise or individuals frequently subjected to heavy loads.

12.3.7.4 Treatment Principles

Non-surgical treatment options primarily involve follow-up observation, bracing, plaster casts, exercise, and physical therapy. For patients with mild deformities who have not yet reached skeletal maturity, regular examinations should be conducted every 6 months to monitor the progression of the deformity. Patients with a deformity degree of 55–70° and immature bones can be treated with plaster casts or braces. Adolescent patients with a deformity less than 60° should receive physical therapy or exercise therapy. Regular imaging checks are necessary until bone maturity is achieved.

The surgical indications for Scheuermann's disease are subject to ongoing debate. Generally, surgical intervention is considered for Scheuermann's disease in the following situations: severe and progressive thoracic kyphosis (>75–80°) in the absence of skeletal maturity; if the deformity continues to progress despite plaster or brace treatment; in cases of severe thoracolumbar kyphosis (>50–55°) accompanied by significant lower back pain and poor response to conservative measures; when there is neurological impairment due to the malformation; and when the physical appearance is deemed unacceptable by the surgeon, patient, or family members. Orthopedic surgery can be performed in stages or as a one-stage procedure involving anterior release, posterior internal fixation, and bone graft fusion. In cases of severe deformity, options may include posterior transpedicular osteotomy or vertebral column resection.

12.3.8 Spondylolisthesis

Spondylolisthesis refers to the forward displacement of the upper vertebral body in relation to the lower vertebral body.

12.3.8.1 Etiology

Due to the natural lumbar lordosis in the human spine, the sacral endplate assumes an inclined position. Normally, the bony structures posterior to the vertebral bodies, along with the posterior ligaments and intervertebral discs, work together to prevent anterior slippage of the sacral endplate's inclination. Among groups engaging in repetitive lumbar hyperextension and rotational movements, such as gymnasts, the increased occurrence of this condition suggests that mechanical stress plays a crucial role in its development. Ongoing research also suggests a connection between lumbar lordosis, imbalanced shearing forces, forced rotation, excessive flexion loads, and genetic factors in relation to spinal slippage.

12.3.8.2 Clinical Manifestations

The primary symptoms of this condition encompass pain experienced during activities, prolonged sitting, or standing. This pain can radiate toward the hips as well as the posterior and lateral aspects of the thighs. In instances of mild spondylolisthesis (where the displacement is less than 50% of the length of the affected vertebra), patients generally exhibit normal gait and posture. However, pain and muscle spasms may lead to reduced or even limited lumbar mobility. Conversely, individuals with severe spondylolisthesis (where the displacement exceeds 50% of the length of the displaced vertebra) may present with symptoms indicative of cauda equina compression, including muscle weakness, numbness, difficulties in walking, and potential issues with bowel movements. During a physical examination, localized tenderness may be identified at the site of slippage, and a sensation resembling a "step-off" may be observed between the spinous processes at the level of the slippage (Fig. 12.29).

A standing anteroposterior X-ray of the lumbar spine provides insight into the sequence of lumbar vertebrae and the extent of slippage. In cases of isthmic spondylolisthesis, oblique radiographs on both sides may reveal the characteristic "dog collar sign." Additionally, sagittal CT reconstruction proves valuable in identifying congen-

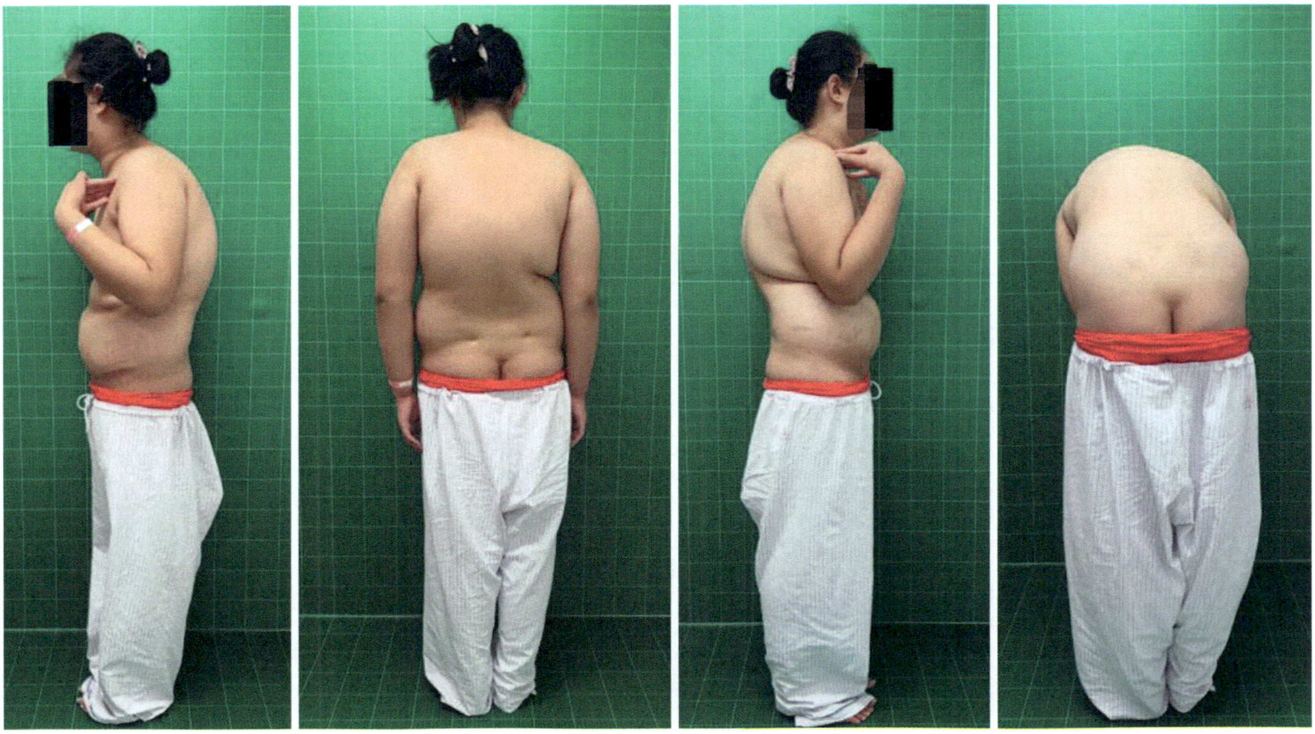

Fig. 12.27 General picture of Scheuermann's disease with kyphosis

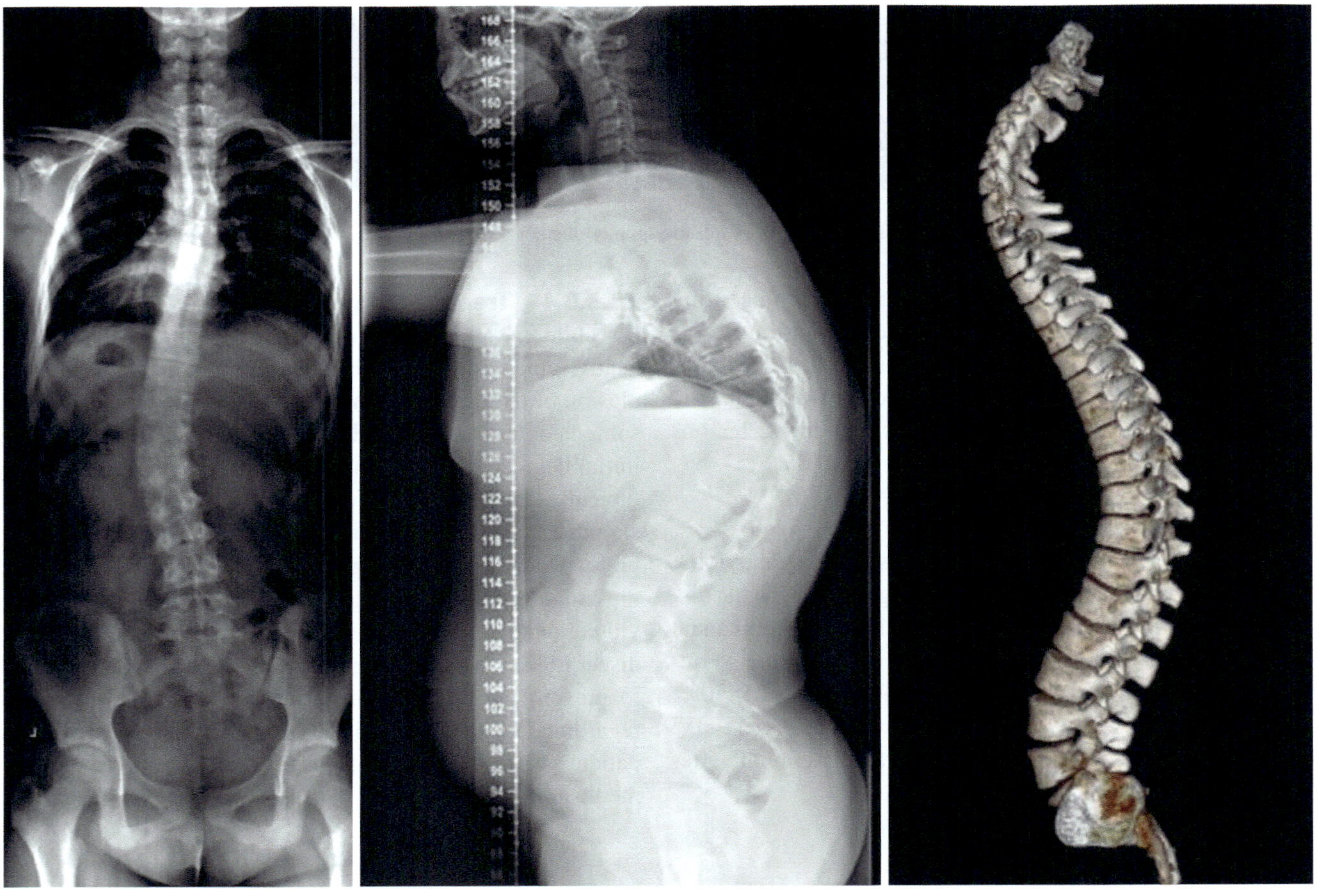

Fig. 12.28 Imaging examination of a patient with Scheuermann's disease and kyphosis shows wedge-shaped changes of the vertebral body

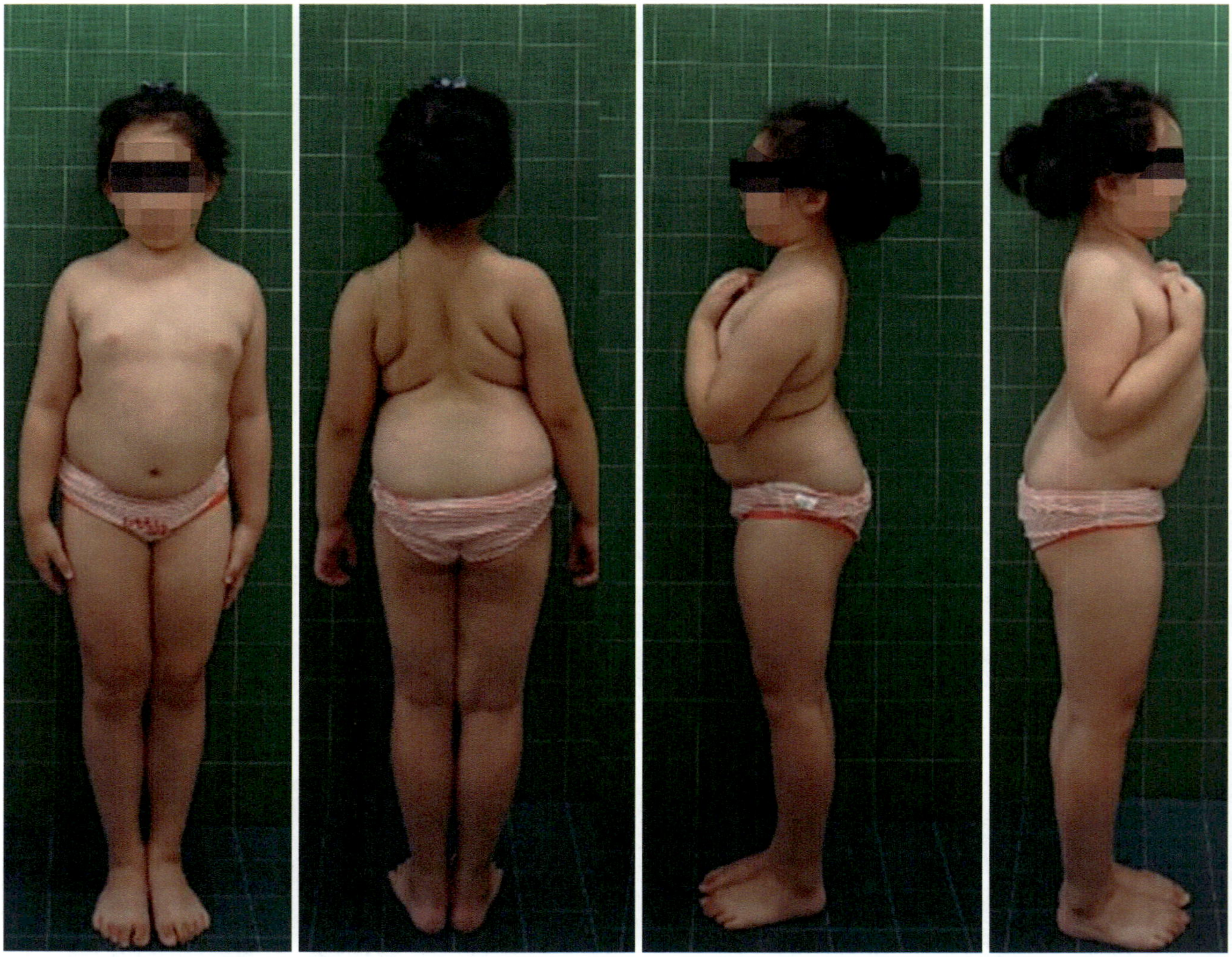

Fig. 12.29 Patient, a 6-year-old female, was diagnosed with dysplastic spondylolisthesis

ital developmental anomalies. For individuals presenting with neurological symptoms, an MRI examination is crucial to assess potential neural compression. SPECT imaging can be employed to differentiate between chronic isthmic spondylolisthesis and more recent active lesions (Fig. 12.30).

12.3.8.3 Classification

The Meyerding classification categorizes spinal spondylolisthesis into five grades based on the degree of forward displacement of the cranial vertebra in relation to the caudal vertebra: Grade I: anterior displacement of the cranial vertebra by 0–25%; Grade II: forward displacement of 25–50%; Grade III: 50–75% forward displacement; Grade IV: 75–100% forward displacement; and Grade V: cranial vertebra prolapse.

12.3.8.4 Treatment Principles

For children in the pre-pubertal or pubertal growth phase, it is advisable to conduct periodic examinations until the conclusion of the rapid growth period. The frequency of lumbar spine lateral radiography should be determined based on the initial degree of slippage and the child's age, with intervals typically set at every 6–12 months. In cases of mild vertebral slippage, non-surgical treatment measures, such as reducing physical activity and strengthening the abdominal and dorsal musculature, are the primary treatment modalities. For individuals with severe slippage, regardless of the presence of discernible symptoms, surgical intervention is recommended to prevent the progression of the condition. The decision regarding surgery should be made by considering the patient's individual circumstances and the expertise of the medical professional.

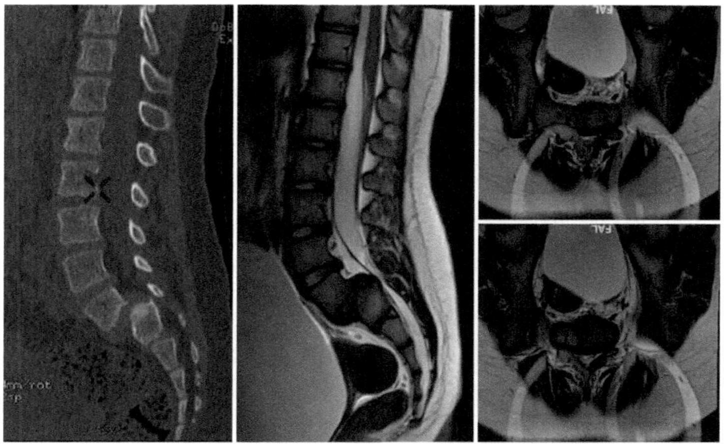

Fig. 12.30 Patient is a 6-year-old female diagnosed with dysplastic spondylolisthesis

12.4 Spinal Cord Malformation

12.4.1 Syringomyelia

Syringomyelia is a chronic and progressive disease of the spinal cord, distinguished by the formation of cystic within the spinal cord.

12.4.1.1 Etiology

At present, the cause and exact pathogenesis of syringomyelia are still unclear, and there are different hypotheses for different types.

12.4.1.2 Clinical Manifestations

As cyst-like changes develop within the spinal cord, they gradually expand outward, exerting pressure and causing damage to the nerve tissue of the spinal cord. This process leads to a progressive weakening of limb strength, along with stiffness in the back, shoulders, arms, and legs. Additionally, chronic pain, headaches, loss of temperature sensation, and impaired bladder and sphincter function may occur. While the condition typically progresses slowly, acute symptoms can also arise from factors like coughing or increased stress (Fig. 12.31).

MRI is of great value in the diagnosis of syringomyelia and can be used as a basis for classification (Fig. 12.32).

12.4.1.3 Classification

Based on MRI findings, syringomyelia can be categorized into three types: Type I, characterized by communicating syringomyelia; Type II, presenting as non-communicating syringomyelia; and Type III, which is characterized by atrophic syringomyelia.

12.4.1.4 Treatment Principles

When asymptomatic syringomyelia is incidentally discovered, there is currently no unanimous consensus on the necessity of surgical intervention. However, in cases where symptoms do arise, early surgical intervention is typically recommended.

12.4.2 Split Cord Malformation

Split cord malformation (SCM) is a congenital developmental anomaly affecting the spinal cord. It is used to describe the presence of bifid spinal cords resulting from various underlying causes, and this terminology is predominantly employed by most scholars.

12.4.2.1 Etiology

The pathogenesis of split cord malformation has not yet been fully elucidated. Several embryologically related hypotheses have been proposed, including abnormalities in the neural tube, presence of a double spinal cord, and anomalies in the neurogenic intestinal tube, among others.

12.4.2.2 Clinical Manifestations

Lesions associated with split cord malformation are primarily found in the lower thoracic and lumbar segments. In the majority of cases, there is an additional related disorder causing tethering of the spinal cord. These may include thickening of the conus medullaris, protrusion of the spinal cord or meninges, low-lying spinal cord, dermal sinus, subdural arachnoid cyst, or conus medullaris lipoma. The clinical presentations of nerve injury vary between children and adults with split cord malformation. In children, one may observe an unsteady gait, swaying, weakness in both lower limbs, scoliosis, and distinct skin changes around the waist and back. In contrast, adults often experience pain and prolonged weakness in the affected limb as their primary symptoms (Fig. 12.33).

CT, CTM, and MRI are of great value for diagnosis, and MRI is the preferred examination method (Fig. 12.34).

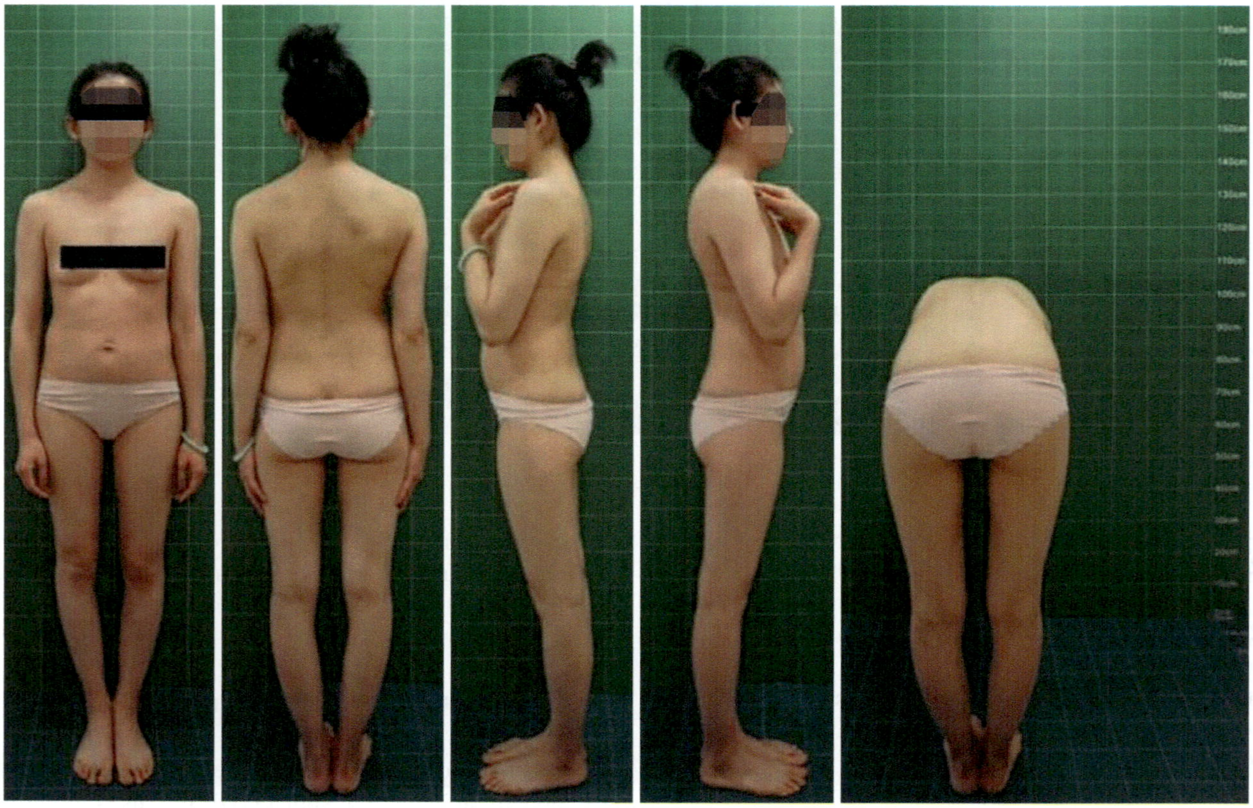

Fig. 12.31 Patient, female, 30 years old, diagnosed with syringomyelia

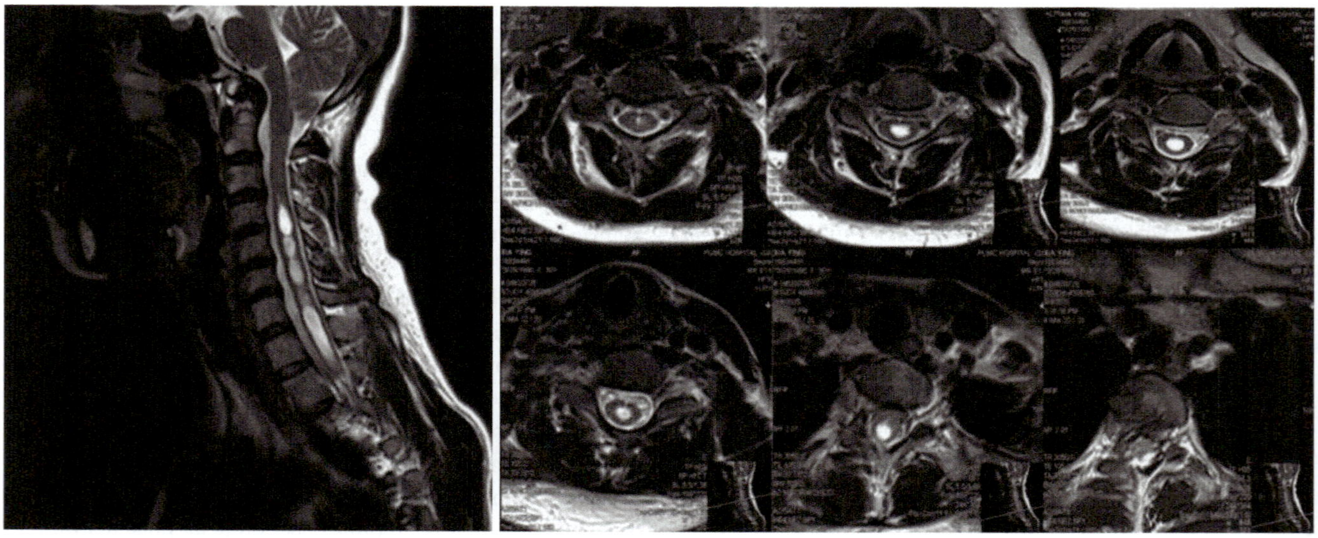

Fig. 12.32 A 30-year-old female patient was diagnosed with syringomyelia, and syringomyelia was seen on cervical MRI

12.4.2.3 Classification

According to Pang's classification, it can be categorized into three types. Type I: Both hemi-spinal cords have their individual dura mater sheaths, separated in between by an osseous or cartilaginous septum. Type II: Both hemi-spinal cords share a common dura mater sheath but are partitioned by a fibrous septum. Type III, Complex type: Spinal cord longitudinal cleft deformities occur in two or more locations within the same patient, combining different types of spinal cord longitudinal clefts.

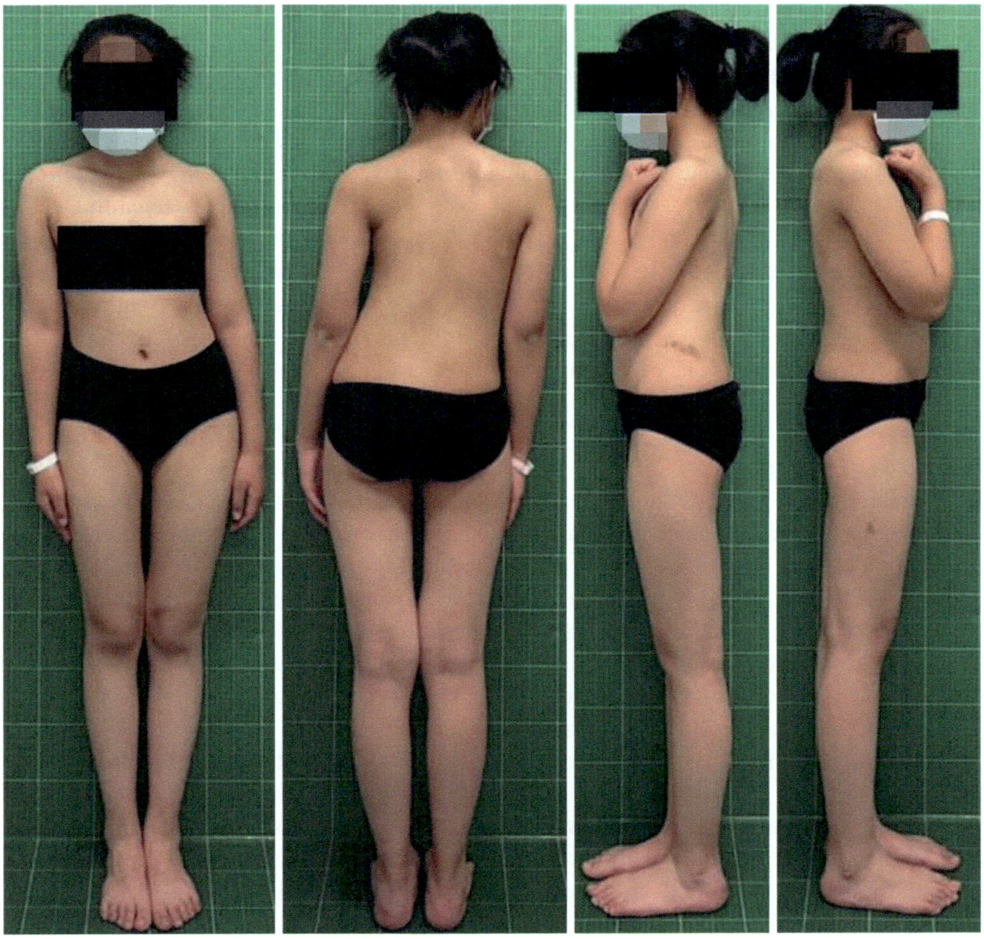

Fig. 12.33 Patient, a 14-year-old female, was diagnosed with scoliosis and split cord malformation

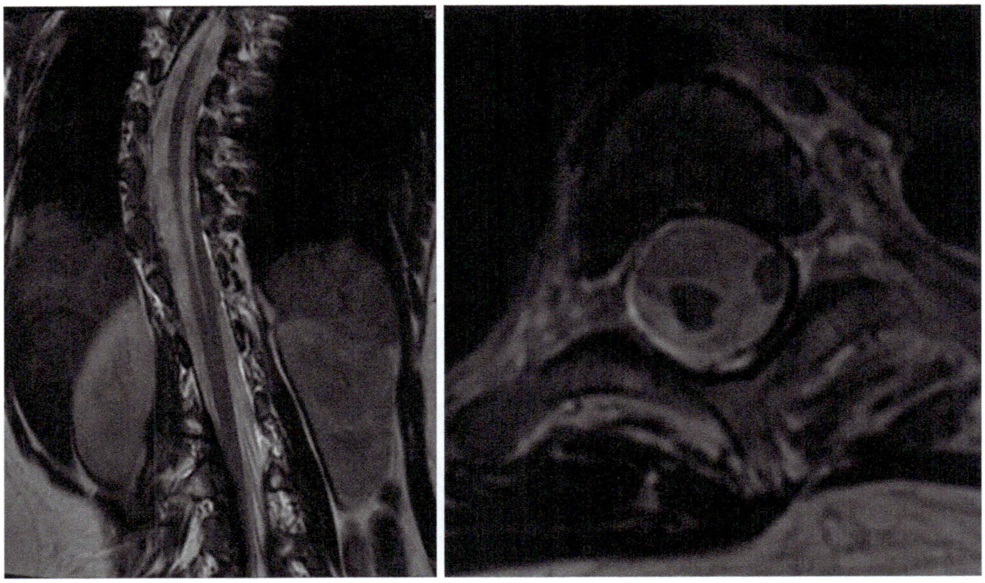

Fig. 12.34 A 14-year-old female patient was diagnosed with scoliosis combined with split cord malformation, and the split cord was seen on MRI

12.4.2.4 Treatment Principles

Surgical intervention is presently the only effective method. However, it should be noted that surgery does not reverse existing neurological impairments. Its primary aim is to prevent further deterioration of preexisting neural dysfunction and the development of new symptomatic manifestations.

12.4.3 Myelomeningocele

Myelomeningocele (MMC) is a congenital malformation of nervous system, which is one of the important causes of neonatal disability and death.

12.4.3.1 Etiology

Myelomeningocele primarily arises from neural tube defects during embryonic development, typically occurring between weeks 18 and 21 of gestation when the neural tube undergoes closure and folding. While there are various proposed pathogenic hypotheses, both environmental and genetic factors are recognized by most international scholars as contributing to its multifactorial etiology. The central emphasis, however, lies in understanding the intricate interplay between genetics and the environment.

12.4.3.2 Clinical Manifestations

The primary clinical feature is the presence of a localized cystic lesion along the infant's midline back at birth. This is often accompanied by excessive hair on the surrounding skin at the base of the cyst. The protrusion of the spinal cord and meninges in the lumbosacral region leads to a tethered spinal cord, a result of neuronal ischemia and hypoxia caused by the tension on the spinal cord and nerves due to the growth in age and stature. Consequently, this results in more prevalent and severe neurological impairment symptoms compared to cervical and thoracic spinal lesions. These symptoms include urinary and fecal incontinence, sensory and motor disturbances in the lower extremities and perineum, muscle atrophy, uneven length of lower limbs, scoliosis, and varus and valgus deformities (Fig. 12.35).

MRI is the preferred examination method (Fig. 12.36).

12.4.3.3 Treatment Principles

Researchers worldwide advocate for a multidisciplinary and comprehensive approach to intervention. This involves meticulous procedures such as exploratory vertebral canal expansion, neurolysis of the spinal cord and spinal nerves, and mending of the dura mater. However, there is considerable debate regarding the optimal timing for surgery. The prevailing consensus among the majority of experts leans toward early intervention. It is widely believed that performing the surgery at a younger age tends to yield more favorable postoperative outcomes.

12.4.4 Tethered Cord Syndrome

Tethered Cord Syndrome (TCS) is an abnormality, either congenital or acquired, affecting the spine, spinal canal, and spinal cord. This condition arises from variations, shortening, thickening, and tension of the terminal filament. These factors lead to the traction of the low-lying spinal cord cone, resulting in a series of syndromes characterized by neurological dysfunction.

12.4.4.1 Etiology

Spinal cord tethering can arise from various causes. Congenital factors are the most prevalent and may include abnormalities in terminal filament development, leading to shortening, thickening, and tension. Other factors may involve spinal deformities, incomplete closure of the spinal canal, split cord malformation, as well as the presence of teratomas and lipomas within the spinal canal, collectively known as primary tethering of the spinal cord. Acquired factors are predominantly due to adhesions between the spinal cord and dura mater or the formation of scar tissue in the surgical area following procedures like myelomeningocele repair or other intraspinal surgeries. These are referred to as secondary spinal cord tethering.

12.4.4.2 Clinical Manifestations

Due to variations in etiology, pathological changes, and the extent of traction in tethered cord syndrome, the onset and

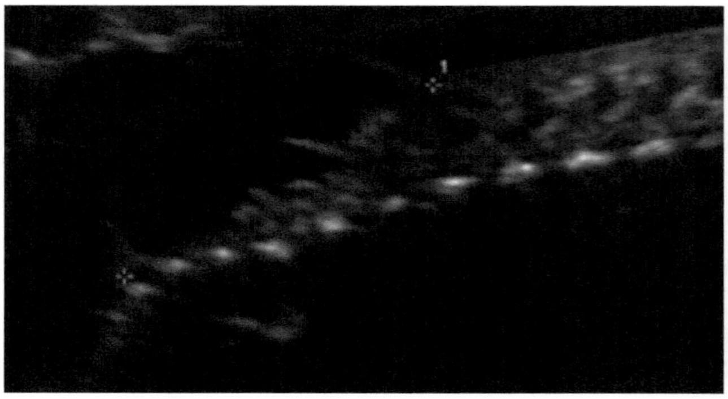

Fig. 12.35 Ultrasound image of myelomeningocele. (Reproduced with permission from [3])

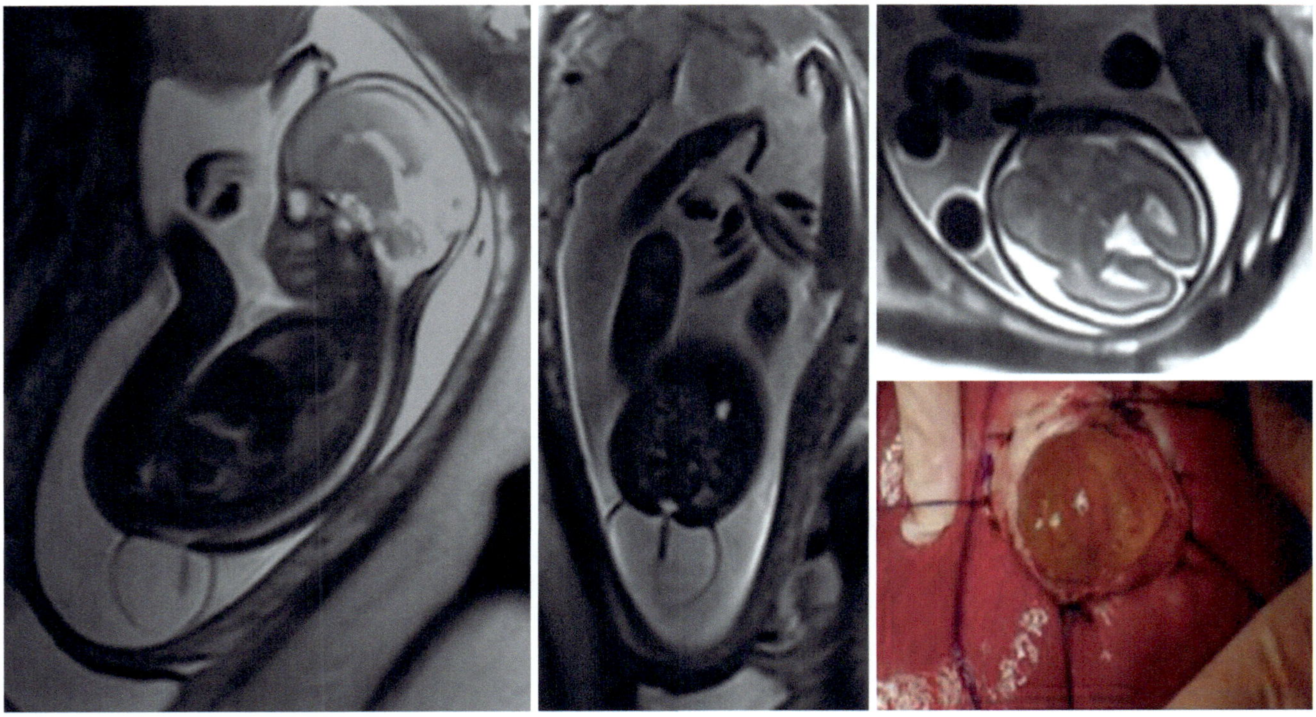

Fig. 12.36 MRI T2WI image and intraoperative photos of myelomeningocele. (Reproduced with permission from [3])

severity of neurological symptoms can greatly differ. The primary clinical manifestations include:

1. Lumbosacral median skin irregularities, such as soft tissue masses, tufts, skin recessions, or areas of pigmented bruising. However, it is important to note that approximately half of the patients may present with normal skin in this area.
2. Lower limb deformities, along with sensory and motor impairments. This encompasses conditions like lower limb shortening, muscular atrophy, muscle weakness, or even paralysis. Other indications may include abnormalities like foot malformation (such as clubfoot), saddle area discomfort, and reduced sensitivity in the foot's skin.
3. Impaired sphincter muscle function, involving issues like an enlarged urinary bladder, dribbling urinary incontinence, spastic neurogenic bladder, stress urinary incontinence, and potential enuresis. Fecal incontinence may also be observed.

X-ray examinations frequently reveal the presence of deformities. CT scans can provide valuable insights into the potential coexistence of osseous clefts in the spinal cord and excessive fatty thickening of the conus medullaris in cases of tethered spinal cord syndrome. Moreover, MRI scans not only help identify the presence or absence of spinal cord lesions, but also elucidate the relationship between the lowest position of the conus medullaris and the direction and morphology of the terminal filament and other tissues within the spinal canal (Figs. 12.37 and 12.38).

12.4.4.3 Classification

It can be divided into primary type and secondary type.

12.4.4.4 Treatment Principles

The spinal cord untethering is the main method for the treatment of TCS.

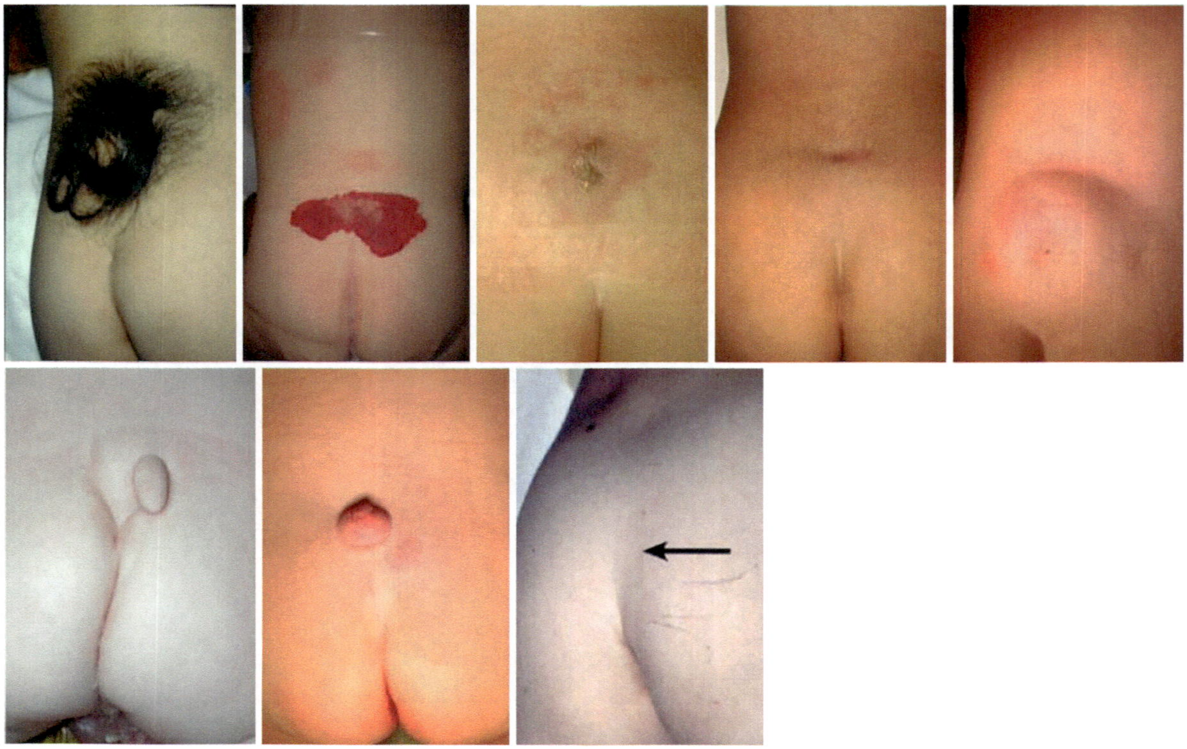

Fig. 12.37 General picture of a patient with tethered cord syndrome, showing tufts, soft tissue masses, and sunken skin. (Reproduced with permission from [4])

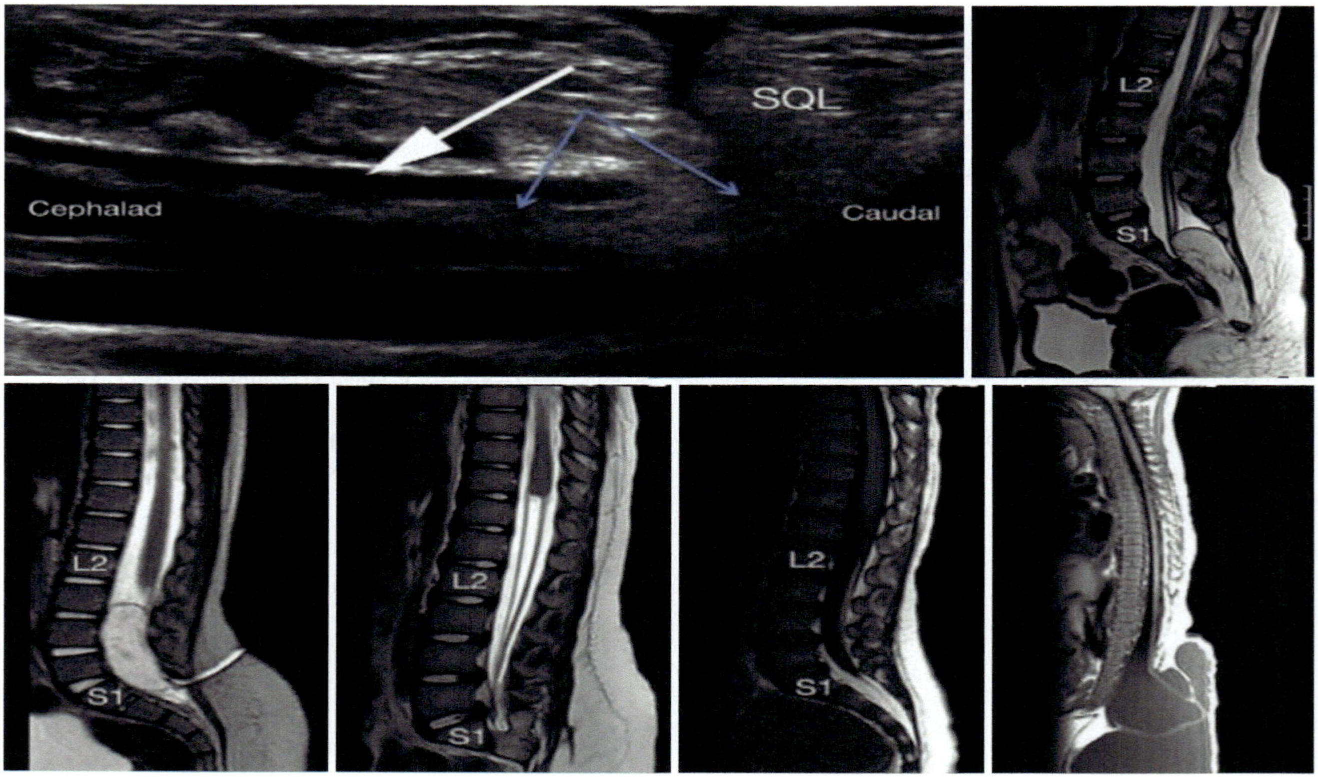

Fig. 12.38 Ultrasound and MRI of patients with tethered cord syndrome showed that the conus medullaris was pulled down. (Reproduced with permission from [4])

12.5 Congenital Cervical Hyperextension Deformity

Professor Qin's team successfully diagnosed and treated a case of congenital cervical hyperextension deformity, a condition classified as cervical developmental deformity. Given the absence of documented reports in the existing literature, this case is introduced as a novel pathological condition.

12.5.1 Etiology

The etiology is unknown.

12.5.2 Clinical Manifestations

Since birth, a 22-year-old male has displayed a noticeable posterior inclination of the head, coupled with reduced anterior neck flexion compared to typical infants. As he matured, this cervical malformation, marked by a progressively pronounced retroflexion of the neck, became increasingly severe, eventually reaching a relatively fixed state in adulthood. Due to this extreme retroflexion, he faces difficulty in perceiving the ground beneath his feet, significantly impacting his appearance, mobility, daily activities, as well as his educational and professional endeavors.

Physical Examination: The cervical region displays an extreme hyperextension, with the occiput primarily positioned against the posterior cervical area, causing the face to be directed upwards, making it difficult to see the ground ahead. As a result, walking requires careful attention. There is minimal rotational movement in the neck, and when passively manipulated, slight flexion is observed in the posterior neck. However, voluntary flexion is not achievable. Evaluation of the pectoralis major muscle reveals an absence of contraction. The soft tissues in the cervical-thoracic region demonstrate stiffness. The patient has no familial medical history, and there are no evident anomalies in other areas of the body (Fig. 12.39).

The lateral cervical spine X-ray illustrates a retroflexion angle of 77° at the cervical vertebra, accompanied by a noticeable gap between the atlas and axis vertebrae's articulation. No spacing is observed among the spinous processes of the other cervical vertebrae, confirming the retroflexed fixation in the cervical vertebrae below the axis during the developmental process (Fig. 12.39).

12.5.3 Treatment Principles

Following orthopedic principles, Professor Qin employed a specialized head-neck-chest push-pull orthosis. This apparatus exerted a continuous push-pull force, centered on the occipital bone. After 34 days of application, the cervical vertebra with reverse flexion exhibited a correction of 30°.

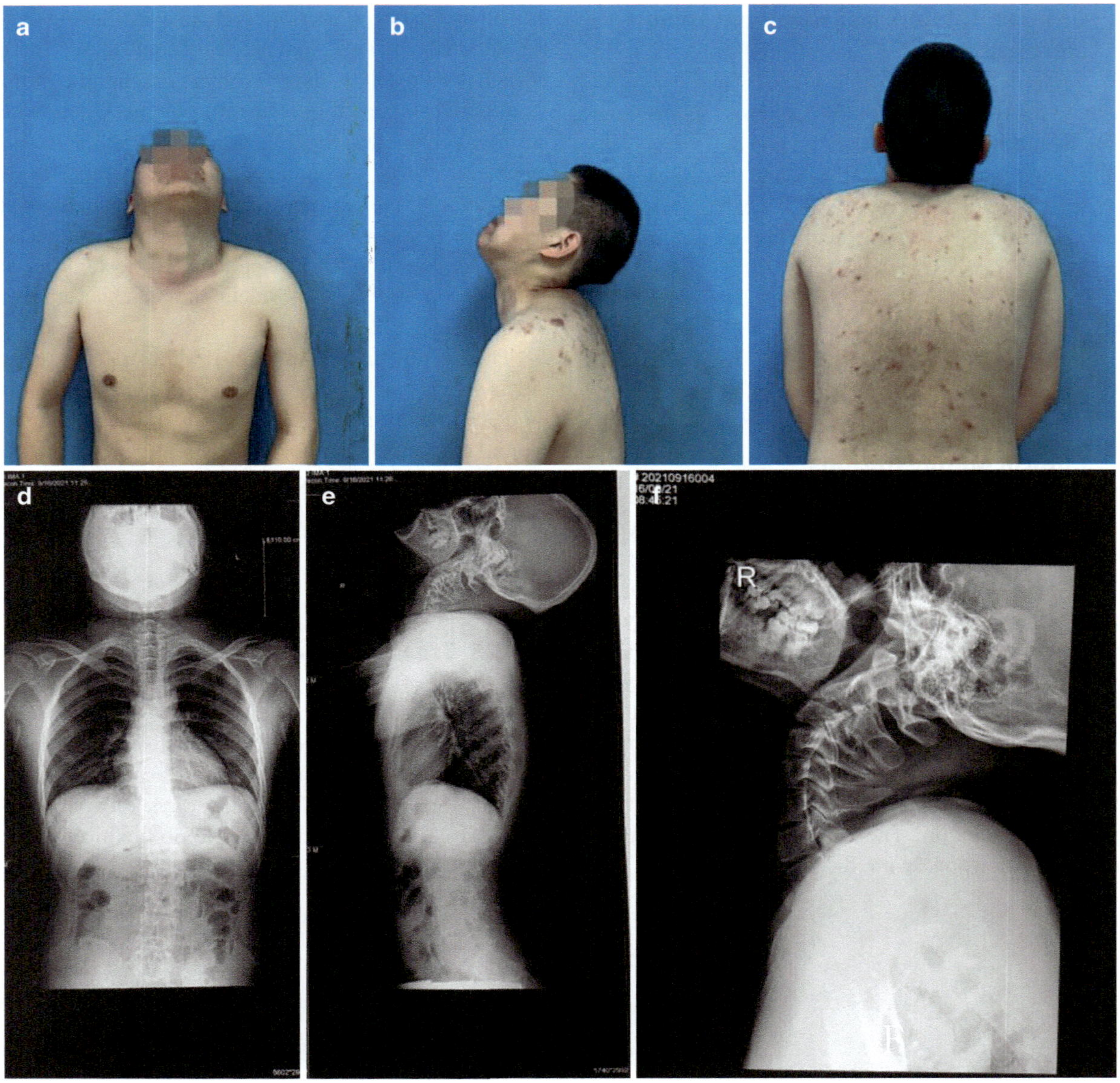

Fig. 12.39 Congenital cervical hyperextension deformity. (**a**) Cervical hyperextension can be seen from the front view of cervical spine; (**b**) lateral view of neck; (**c**) posterior view of neck; (**d**) anteroposterior radiograph of full spine; (**e**) lateral radiograph of full spine; (**f**) lateral radiograph of cervical spine

12.6 Ankylosing Spondylitis with Severe Kyphosis (Folding) Deformity

12.6.1 Etiology

Ankylosing spondylitis (AS) is a chronic, non-specific inflammatory disease that primarily affects the bones and ligaments. It typically initiates in the sacroiliac joint and progressively involves the spine, ligaments, and intervertebral joints, ultimately leading to spinal ankylosis.

As AS progresses, individuals may experience not only pain in the sacroiliac joint and lower back, but also the development of progressive kyphosis in the thoracolumbar spine. In advanced cases, severe and rigid thoracolumbar kyphosis (with a Cobb angle exceeding 100°) can lead to sagittal imbalance of the spine. This results in noticeable appearance deformities and difficulty in maintaining direct eye contact. These conditions significantly impact various aspects of daily life, including lying flat, walking, standing, and sitting. In rare instances, the spine, pelvis, lower limbs may become folded together, potentially compressing thoracic and abdominal organs. This can have implications for heart, lung, and digestive functions.

12.6.2 Clinical Manifestation

Patients typically exhibit marked kyphosis in the thoracolumbar segment, along with a folding of the trunk and lower limbs. This can lead to a posture where the head is positioned between the knees, and there may be restricted mobility in the entire spine as well as in major joints like the hips, knees, and shoulders. It is important to note that these manifestations may not necessarily be associated with neurological impairment.

On physical examination, the patient presents with a slender physique, normal skin color, and no evident signs of cafe-au-lait spots, abnormal hair growth, or pigmentation irregularities. The normal physiological curvature of the spine is notably absent, with a pronounced kyphosis evident in the thoracolumbar region, resulting in a severe arched back deformity. The trunk and lower limbs exhibit significant folding, with the chest and abdomen closely approaching the bilateral thighs, and the head buried between the knees. There are no signs of redness, swelling, tenderness, or percussion pain in any of the joints. The patient displays a marked restriction in total spinal mobility as well as limited abduction and lifting activities of the shoulders. There is bilateral hip flexion ankylosis deformity, accompanied by restricted movement. Both knees present with a flexion deformity, limiting extension activities. Sensation and muscle strength in the limbs are within normal range, muscle tension is typical, and tendon reflexes are as expected. No pathological signs are elicited during examination. The patient's height measures 66 cm, and the lengths of the lower limbs are equal (Fig. 12.40).

12.6.3 Treatment Principles

Treatment Goals: Attain a flat alignment of the shoulders, back, and hips, normalize blood gas levels, and enhance lung function (Fig. 12.41).

Surgery decision-making: multidisciplinary cooperation; Staged correction.

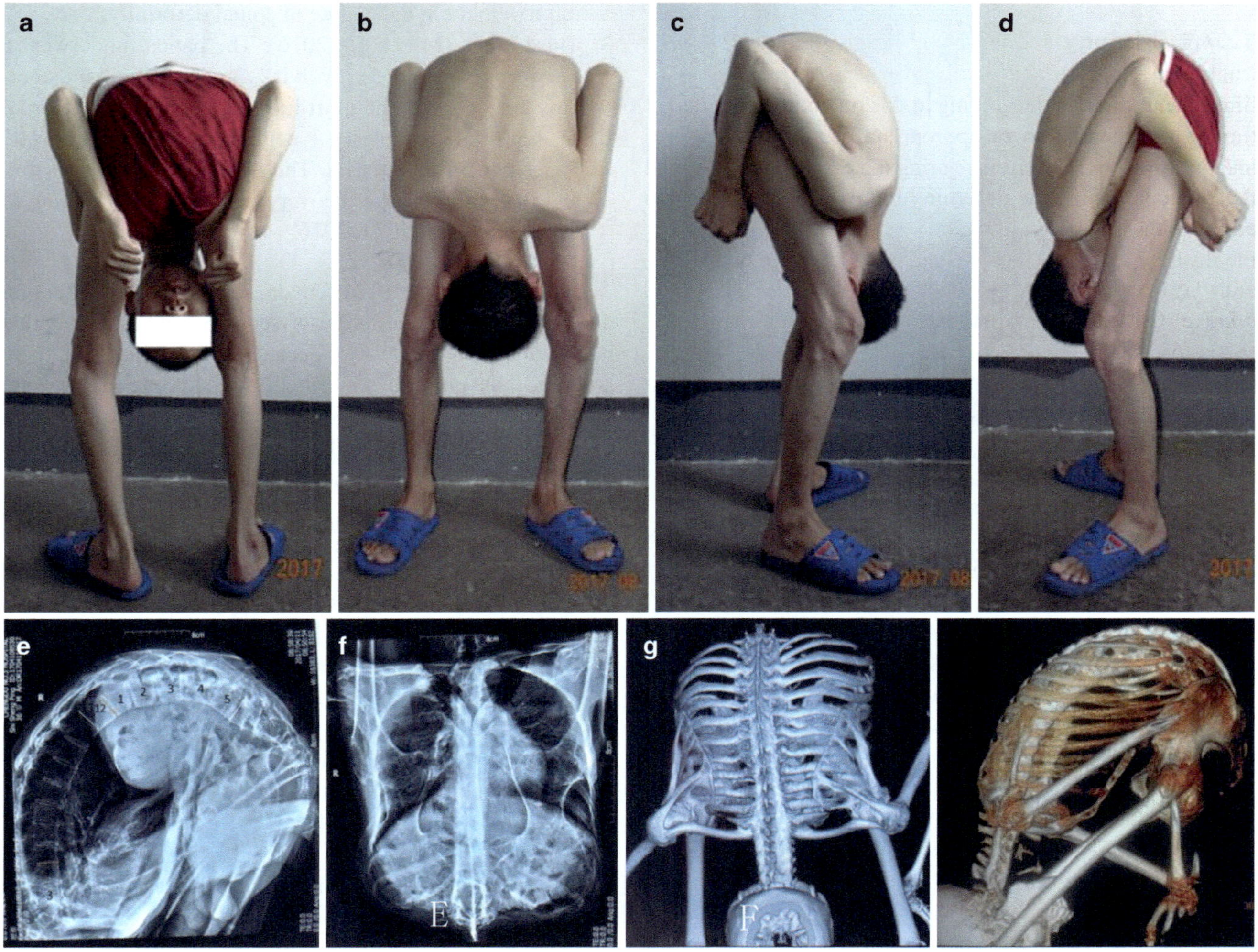

Fig. 12.40 Ankylosing spondylitis with very severe kyphosis (pre operation). (**a**) View from the back of standing position; (**b**) front view of standing position; (**c**, **d**) lateral view of standing position; (**e**) full-length anteroposterior and lateral view of spine; (**f**, **g**) full-length three-dimensional reconstruction of spine

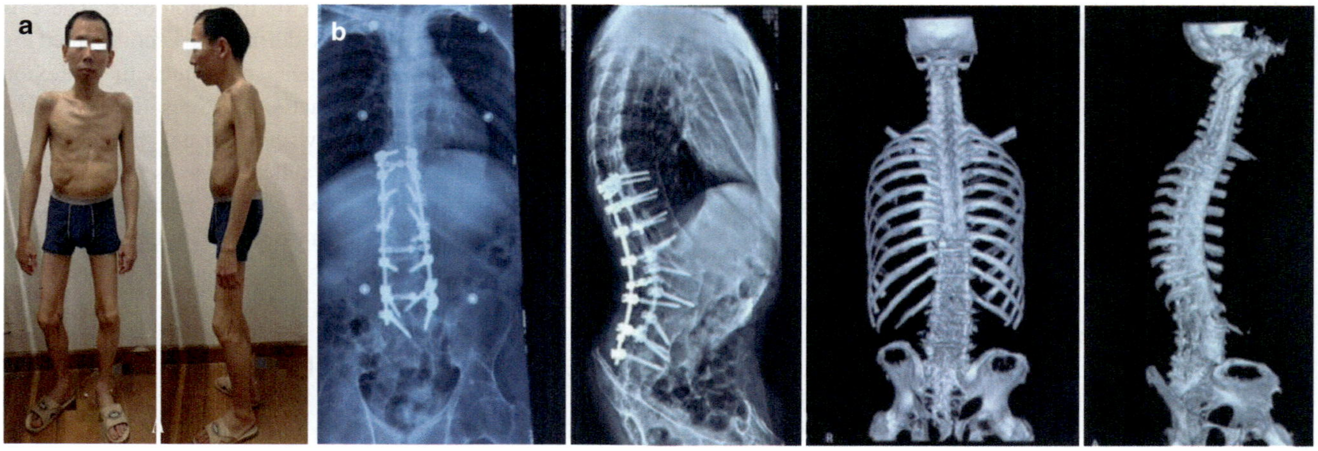

Fig. 12.41 Postoperative situation. (**a**) Postoperative frontal and lateral standing view photographs of the full body. (**b**) Postoperative full-length anteroposterior and lateral X-ray images, along with three-dimensional reconstruction of the spine

12.7 Extremely Severe Scoliosis Kyphosis

12.7.1 Etiology

The primary factor contributing to this outcome is the lack of timely implementation of appropriate preventive measures and orthopedic interventions during the early stages of spinal deformity, allowing the deformity to progress naturally into adulthood.

12.7.2 Clinical Manifestation

Case 1 involved a 27-year-old female who had been experiencing unevenness in her back for over 23 years. The diagnosis indicated:

1. Extremely severe scoliosis and kyphosis.
2. Thoracic deformity.
3. Severe impairment of lung function (Fig. 12.42).

Treatment goal: flat alignment of the shoulders, back, and hips, normalize blood gas levels.

Surgery decision-making: multidisciplinary cooperation; Staged orthopedics.

A staged Treatment approach was implemented for this case:

1. First Stage (November 6, 2014): One-stage cephalopelvic ring traction was initiated. Continuous traction, along with intermittent adjustments in height, led to significant improvements in the patient's spinal deformity and lung function.
2. Second Stage (October 16, 2015): Given the severity of the spinal deformity, a "posterior spinal release" procedure was performed under general anesthesia. Following the release operation, the patient continued cephalopelvic ring traction with height adjustments, leading to further improvement in the degree of spinal deformity.
3. Third Stage (March 16, 2016): The patient underwent a three-stage procedure involving "posterior spinal osteotomy correction, bone graft fusion, pedicle screw internal fixation + thoracoplasty + cephalopelvic ring removal" under general anesthesia. The operation was successful, and the postoperative recovery was favorable, leading to discharge on April 24, 2016.

Patient 2, a 21-year-old female, sought medical attention due to a long-standing issue of scoliosis and kyphosis that had been noted for over two decades. On examination, there are noticeable physical abnormalities, including a lateral and posterior bulge in the chest and back regions, along with unequal and elevated shoulders. Importantly, there is no indication of neurological impairment (Fig. 12.43).

Following admission, a thorough examination revealed the following conditions:

1. Extremely severe scoliosis and kyphosis.
2. Thoracic deformity.
3. Absence of ribs (with clear separation).
4. Wedge-shaped vertebrae from T6 to T8.
5. Impaired lung function.
6. Sacral vertebral spina bifida, not visible.
7. Enlargement of the left atrium.
8. Presence of thyroid nodules.

The treatment plan was implemented in stages as follows:

1. One-stage cephalopelvic ring traction on March 28, 2019. Continuous traction and periodic adjustments in height led to significant improvements in the patient's spinal deformity and lung function.

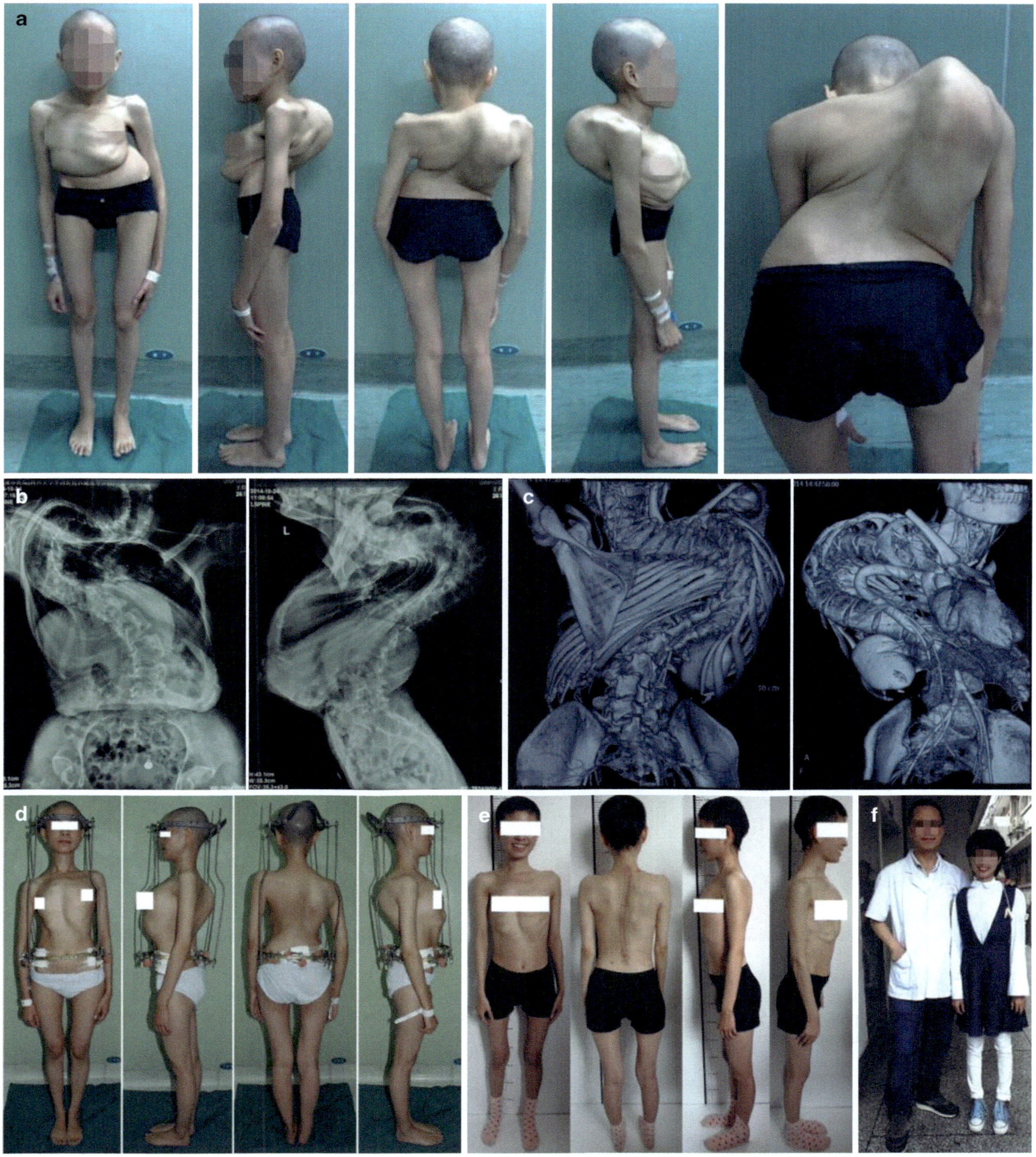

Fig. 12.42 (**a**) A full-length view from the front, back, and side while in a standing position: Both eyes appear level, with the right shoulder slightly higher than the left. There is a noticeable rightward curvature in the chest spine, accompanied by severe kyphosis. The left iliac spine is slightly elevated compared to the right. Movement in the thoracolumbar spine is significantly restricted. (**b**, **c**) Full-length anteroposterior and lateral X-ray images along with a three-dimensional reconstruction of the spine: These images reveal severe scoliosis and kyphosis of the spine. (**d**) A general photo taken after the application of external fixation and traction using the cephalopelvic ring. (**e**) Postoperative images show that the patient has achieved the desired correction and stabilization. The outcome is satisfactory. (**f**) A photograph of the patient with the surgical team after the operation, displaying good physical and mental well-being

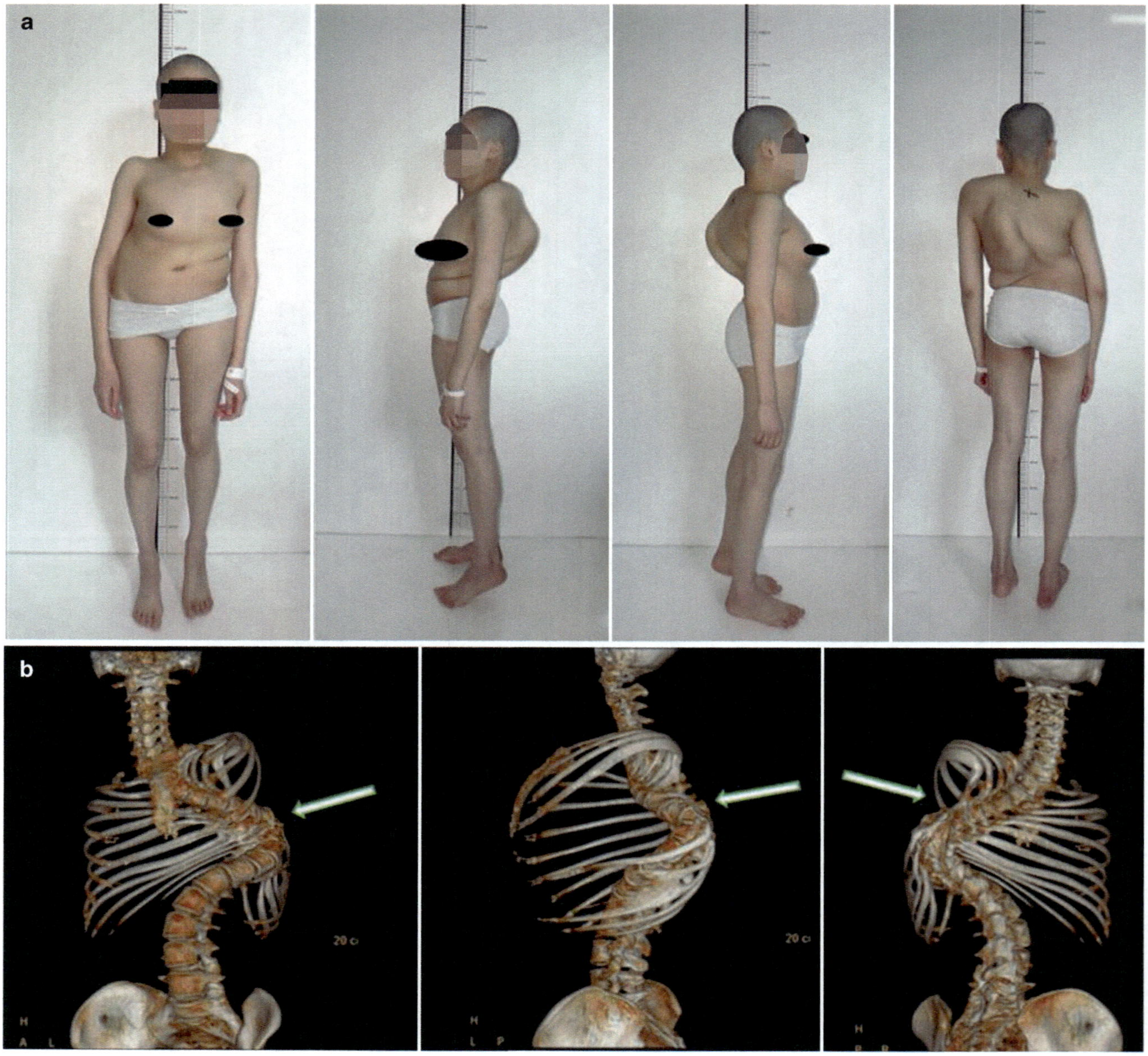

Fig. 12.43 (**a**) Standing front, back, and lateral photos of the patient at admission. (**b**) Preoperative three-dimensional reconstruction of the full-length spine. (**c**) Approximately 5 months after cephalopelvic ring traction, there was a notable improvement in the degree of scoliosis and kyphosis. (**d**) The postoperative photo of the patient shows substantial progress toward the goal of flat alignment of the shoulders, back, and hips, normalize blood gas levels, achieving a satisfactory outcome

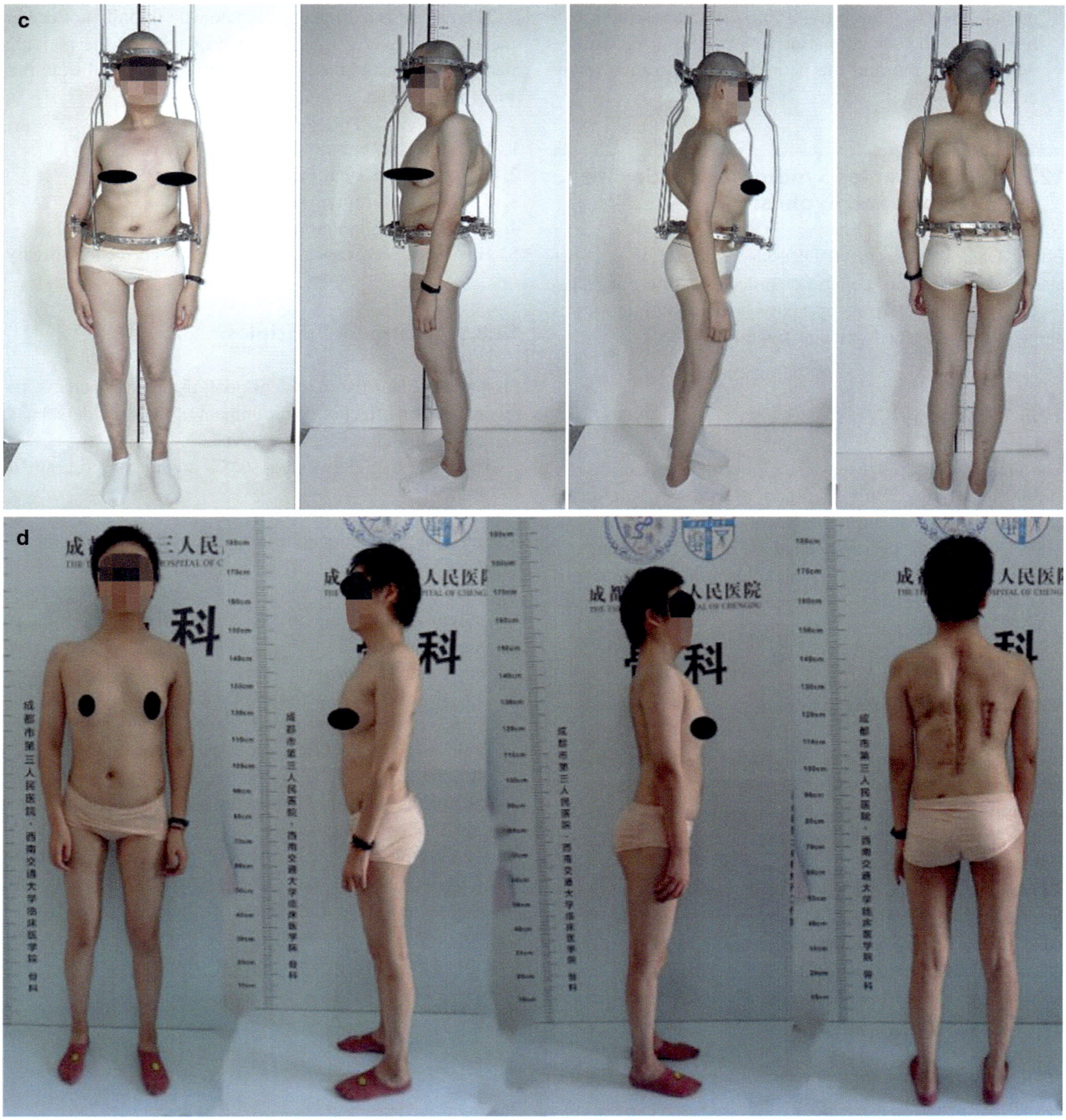

Fig. 12.43 (continued)

2. On August 2, 2019, the second stage involved a "posterior spinal release + concave thoracoplasty" procedure under general anesthesia. Following the release operation, cephalopelvic ring traction was maintained with further adjustments in height. This resulted in additional improvement of the patient's spinal deformity, along with expansion of the concave side of the thoracic cavity.
3. Despite notable progress, the patient's spinal deformity remained severe. Thus, on November 25, 2019, the third "posterior spinal release" was conducted under general anesthesia. Following the operation, cephalopelvic ring traction was resumed.
4. The final stage of the treatment plan took place on June 4, 2020, under general anesthesia. This encompassed "posterior spine correction, bone grafting, fusion, and

pedicle screw fixation + thoracic reconstruction + removal of the cephalopelvic ring." All four procedures were successful, and the patient's postoperative recovery was favorable.

12.8 Ehlers-Danlos Syndrome with Severe Scoliosis and Kyphosis

Ehlers-Danlos syndrome (EDS), also referred to as hyperelastic skin, is a rare genetic disorder affecting connective tissue. It is characterized by laxity in both skin and joints, along with heightened vascular fragility.

12.8.1 Etiology

The incidence of this disease is approximately 1 in 4000 to 10,000 individuals. Both men and women can be affected, although it tends to be more prevalent in males. There is often a family history associated with this condition, with most cases being inherited in an autosomal dominant manner, although in a few instances it may involve recessive inheritance of sex chromosomes.

12.8.2 Clinical Manifestation

Ehlers-Danlos syndrome often involves the skeletal muscle system, presenting as a triad of joint pain, swelling, joint instability, and spinal deformity. Based on clinical manifestations, pathological findings, and genetic diagnosis, Ehlers-Danlos syndrome can be classified into 13 types. These include the classic type, characterized by abnormally increased skin elasticity, as well as the vascular type, scoliosis type, joint laxity type, and skin fragility type, among others. It is worth noting that scoliosis is relatively uncommon, accounting for only 1% of all types (Fig. 12.44).

The patient is a 29-year-old male who initially noticed an uneven back over 26 years ago. Considering the patient's medical history and the findings from the physical examination, the diagnosis includes.

1. Extremely severe scoliosis and kyphosis.
2. Ehlers-Danlos syndrome.
3. Thoracic deformity.
4. Impaired lung function (extremely severe).
5. History of pectus excavatum deformity correction surgery.

12.8.3 Treatment Principles

First of all, clear the treatment goal, in order to achieve the reconstruction effect of flat alignment of the shoulders, back, and hips, normalize blood gas levels.

The patient underwent a staged treatment program as follows:

1. One-stage cephalopelvic ring traction on September 6, 2015.
2. After continuous cephalopelvic ring traction with intermittent adjustments to the traction height, significant improvement was observed in the patient's spinal deformity and lung function.
3. On June 1st, 2016, the second stage involved a "posterior spinal release" performed under general anesthesia. Following the release operation, the patient continued with cephalopelvic ring traction and adjustments to the traction height. This led to further improvement in the degree of spinal deformity.
4. On February 15 and April 7, 2017, the patient underwent two separate stages of "posterior spinal osteotomy, orthopedic bone graft fusion, pedicle screw fixation + thoracoplasty + cephalopelvic ring removal" under general anesthesia. The postoperative recovery was satisfactory.

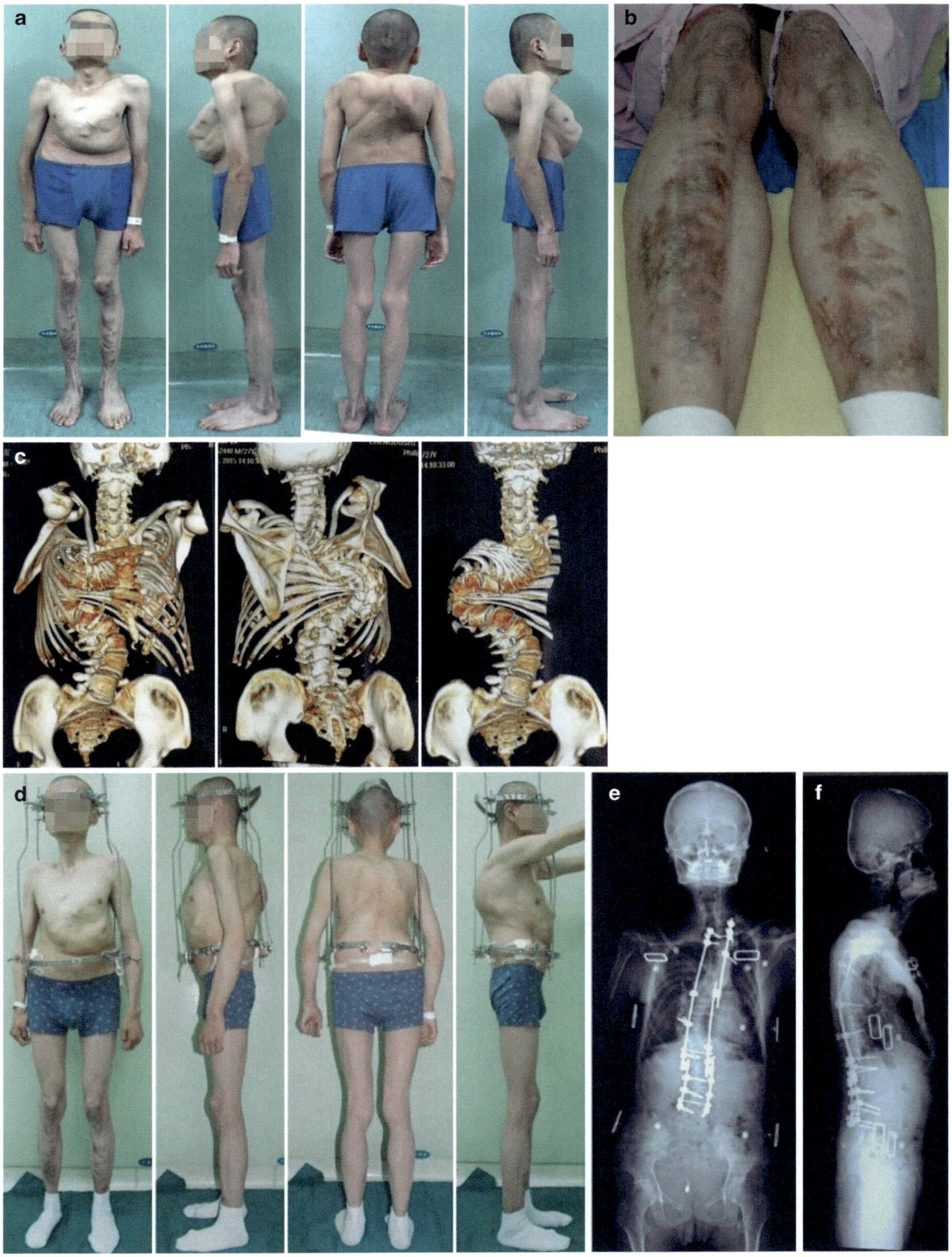

Fig. 12.44 (**a**) The patient with Erdang syndrome and severe spinal deformity. It shows the patient's full-body appearance while in a standing position at admission. (**b**) Subcutaneous pigmentation formed due to previous subcutaneous hemorrhage caused by increased vascular fragility. Notably, there are evident skin folds at the knee joint owing to skin laxity. (**c**) Full-length anteroposterior and lateral three-dimensional reconstruction of the spine. (**d**) The patient exhibiting significant improvement after cephalopelvic ring traction compared to their condition at admission. (**e**) After orthopedic surgery, a review of the whole spine through anteroposterior and lateral radiographs reveals a restoration of the patient's sagittal and coronal balance. (**f**) The patient successfully resumed normal social life after surgery

References

1. Antoniolli LP, Milman LM, Bonamigo RR. Dermoscopy of the iris: identification of Lisch nodules and contribution to the diagnosis of Neurofibromatosis type 1. An Bras Dermatol. 2021;96(4):487–9.
2. Cimino PJ, Gutmann DH. Neurofibromatosis type 1. Handb Clin Neurol. 2018;148:799–811.
3. Cavalheiro S, da Costa MDS, Moron AF, Leonard J. Comparison of prenatal and postnatal management of patients with myelomeningocele. Neurosurg Clin N Am. 2017;28(3):439–48.
4. Tuite GF, Thompson DNP, Austin PF, Bauer SB. Evaluation and management of tethered cord syndrome in occult spinal dysraphism: recommendations from the international children's continence society. Neurourol Urodyn. 2018;37(3):890–903.

13 Congenital Upper Limb and Hand Deformities Associate with Genetic Abnormalities

Wen Tian, Wenyao Zhong, and Sihe Qin

13.1 Congenital Upper Limb Deformity

13.1.1 Congenital High Scapula

Congenital high scapula, also known as Sprengel deformity, or congenital upward displacement of the scapula (congenital elevation of the scapula), is a deformity of the shoulder girdle. It is characterized by abnormal descent, position, and anatomical changes of the scapula. The scapula is in a higher position, the shoulder joint of the affected side is higher than that of the healthy side, the upper arm of the affected limb is limited, and the deformities of ribs, neck, and thoracic vertebrae can be combined at the same time. In 1891, Sprengel reported four cases and discussed the etiology, so the disease was also called Sprengel malformation. In addition to the high position of the scapula on the affected side, congenital high scapula is also characterized by limited abduction and elevation of the upper limb.

13.1.1.1 Etiology

The cause is unknown and may be related to the following factors: (1) genetic factors; (2) excessive intrauterine pressure caused by excessive amniotic fluid volume; (3) muscular tissue defect or abnormal joint between scapula and vertebral body. In the early embryonic stage, especially in the stage of cervical spine and upper limb bud development and scapular descent, the scapula fails to complete the descent process for various reasons and descends to the normal position, resulting in high scapula.

W. Tian
Beijing Jishuitan Hospital, Beijing, China

W. Zhong
Department of Hand Surgery, Beijing Jishuitan Hospital, Beijing, China

S. Qin (✉)
Department of Orthopaedics, Rehabilitation Hospital of the National Research Center for Rehabilitation Technical Aids, Beijing, China

13.1.1.2 Clinical Manifestation

It should be found that the affected shoulder is heightened after the child is 1 year old (Fig. 13.1a). "High" refers to the relationship between the scapula and the thorax, showing the shape of shrugging the shoulder and short neck. The abduction and lifting function of the shoulder joint is obviously limited (Fig. 13.1b). The muscles of the scapular girdle of the affected limb are not developed. Older patients may be combined with spinal and thoracic deformities. The scapula is small and the lower corner is raised. The upper and lower diameters become shorter and the transverse diameters become wider. The limitation of abduction and elevation of the shoulder joint is related to the position and developmental deformity of the scapula.

X-ray findings showed that the scapula of the affected side was small, the lower corner was elevated, the upper limit could exceed the height of the thorax, the width between the axillary edge of the scapula and the spinal edge (transverse diameter) increased, the lower corner turned to the axilla, the medial upper edge turned to the spine, the scapula, and the spine were connected by bone bridges, and other thoracic, cervical, and rib deformities could be seen (Fig. 13.1c).

13.1.1.3 Treatment Principle

If the deformity is not serious and the dysfunction is not significant, some passive and active upper limb activities can be done, such as abduction, elevation, depression and adduction, stretching and traction of shortened muscles, to improve and enhance shoulder abduction and elevation function. Children with severe deformity and obvious dysfunction can be treated by surgery.

13.1.2 Congenital Macrodactyly

Congenital macrodactyly refers to congenital limb overgrowth disorders caused by different causes, including macrodactyly (lipodystrophic macrodactyly), congenital muscular hypertrophy syndrome, congenital muscular

S. Qin et al. (eds.), *Atlas of Limb Deformity*, https://doi.org/10.1007/978-981-97-0999-1_13

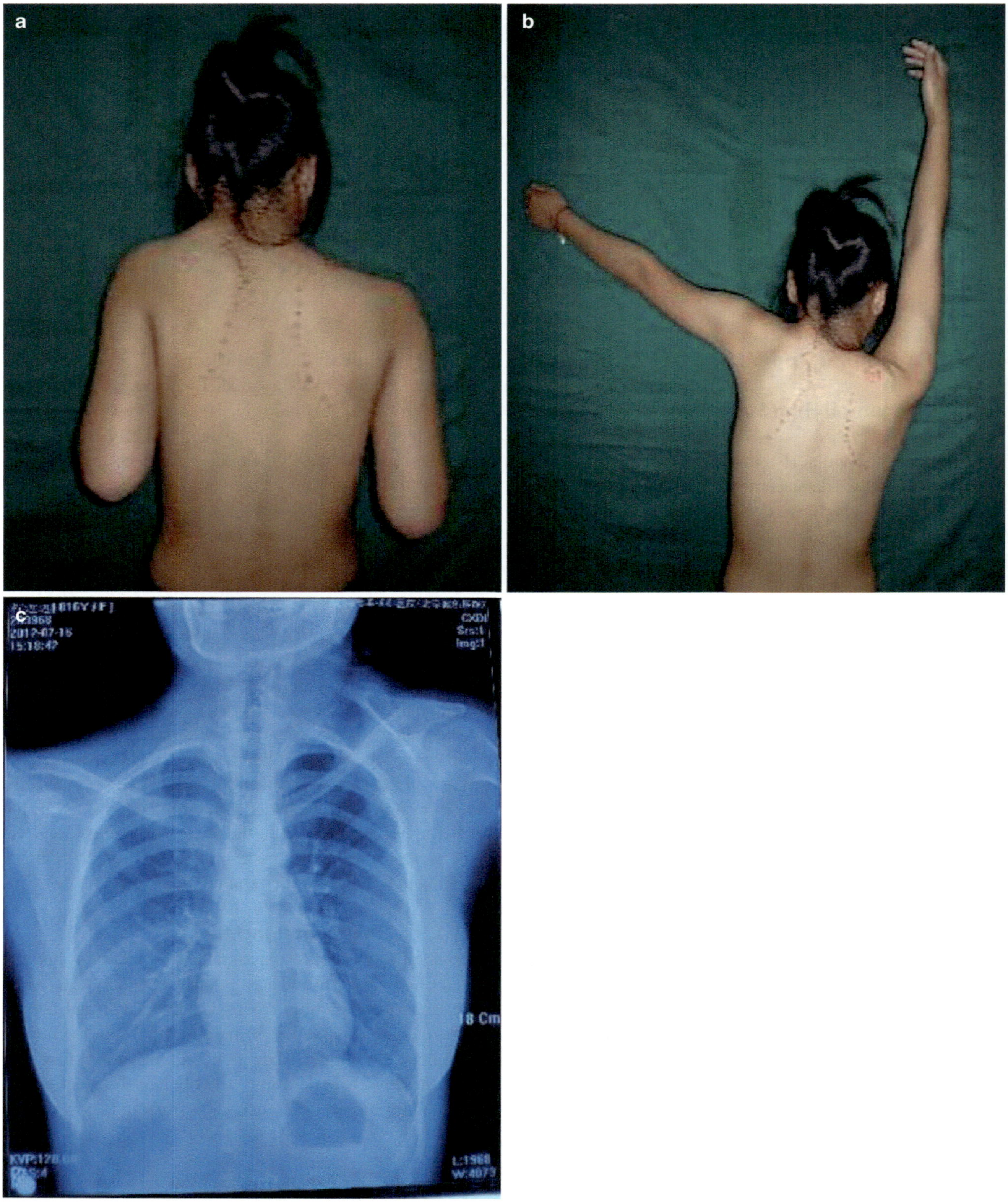

Fig. 13.1 (**a**) Affected shoulder heightening. (**b**) Limitation of abduction and elevation of shoulder joint. (**c**) X-ray shows elevation of left scapula

hypertrophy syndrome, Neurofibromatosis, proteus syndrome, and congenital tumor disorders. Macrodactyly with severe deformity can significantly affect the appearance and function of hands and limbs and cause great psychological pressure to patients and their families.

13.1.2.1 Etiology

At present, it is considered that true macrodactyly (lipodystrophic macrodactyly) and myogenic hypertrophy syndrome belong to PIK3CA-related overgrowth diseases (PROS), which are the results of chimeric mutations of PIK3CA gene in somatic cells. Congenital macrodactyly associated with other genetic mutations include neurofibromatosis type 1 (NF1 mutations) and Poseidon syndrome (AKT1 mutations).

13.1.2.2 Clinical Manifestations and Classification

There are many causes of macrodactyly, but from the point of view of morphological manifestations and surgical treatment, it can be classified according to the type of hypertrophic tissue (Figs. 13.2, 13.3, 13.4, 13.5, 13.6, 13.7, 13.8, 13.9, 13.10, 13.11, 13.12, 13.13, 13.14 and 13.15): (1) adipose tissue hyperplasia type, (2) nerve adipose tissue infiltration type, (3) muscle tissue type, (4) vascular tissue type, (5) osteoarticular hypertrophy type, (6) tumor tissue type, and (7) other types. In fact, limb hypertrophy seen clinically is often caused by simultaneous hyperplasia of multiple tissues. The etiological classification of most macrodactyly (limbs) still needs a lot of research work to confirm, except that some of them can be found to have a clear etiology.

13.1.2.3 Treatment Principle

It is necessary to choose the surgical method according to different clinical manifestations, but the operation can only improve the appearance and function of the affected hand to a certain extent, and with the growth and development of the child, the deformity may require multiple operations. For those with poor function and poor appearance, amputation of fingers/toes/limbs can be considered.

13.1.3 Congenital Deformity of Split Hand

Split hand, also known as cleft hand, is a malformation caused by the formation of the central longitudinal row of the hand. Typical cleft hand deformity is characterized by a deep "V" shaped cleft in the center of the hand, which can involve both hands and feet, combined with severe deformities of the forearm or leg. Atypical split hand is actually a special type of syndactyly of brachydactyly, which is not discussed in this section.

13.1.3.1 Etiology

Congenital split hands can be hereditary and sporadic; it may be solitary or part of the clinical phenotype of other malformations or syndromes, such as Carpenter syndrome, ectrodactyly syndrome, etc. At present, according to the underlying genetic mechanism, the split hand/foot deformity can be divided into seven subtypes, corresponding to different pathogenic mutations, involving genes such as DLX5, TP63, WNT10B, and so on.

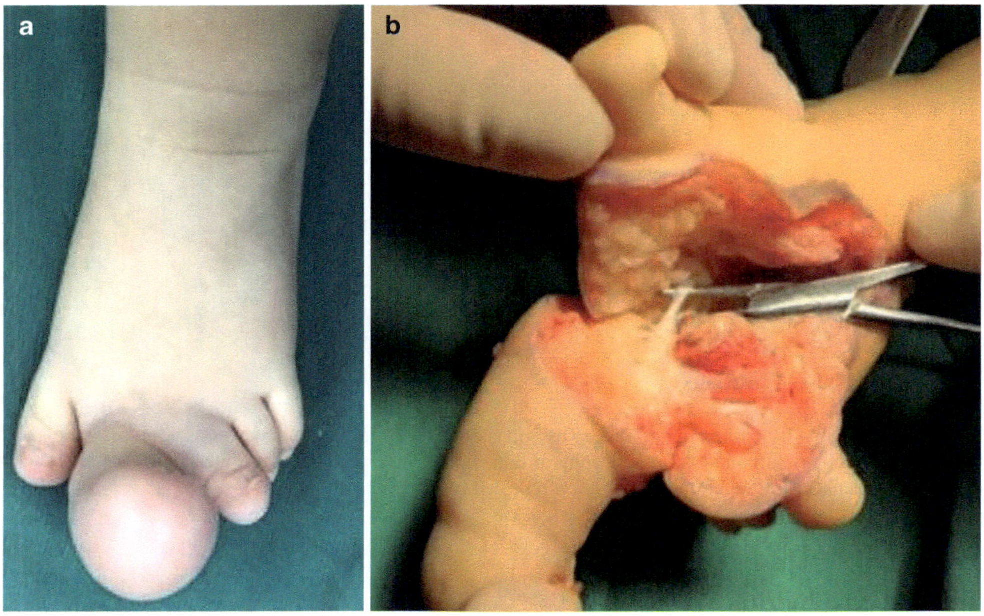

Fig. 13.2 (**a**) The first to third toes of the left foot are macrodactyly, especially the second toe is severely hypertrophy. (**b**) Surgical exploration shows a large amount of adipose tissue hyperplasia, but the digital nerves are basically normal

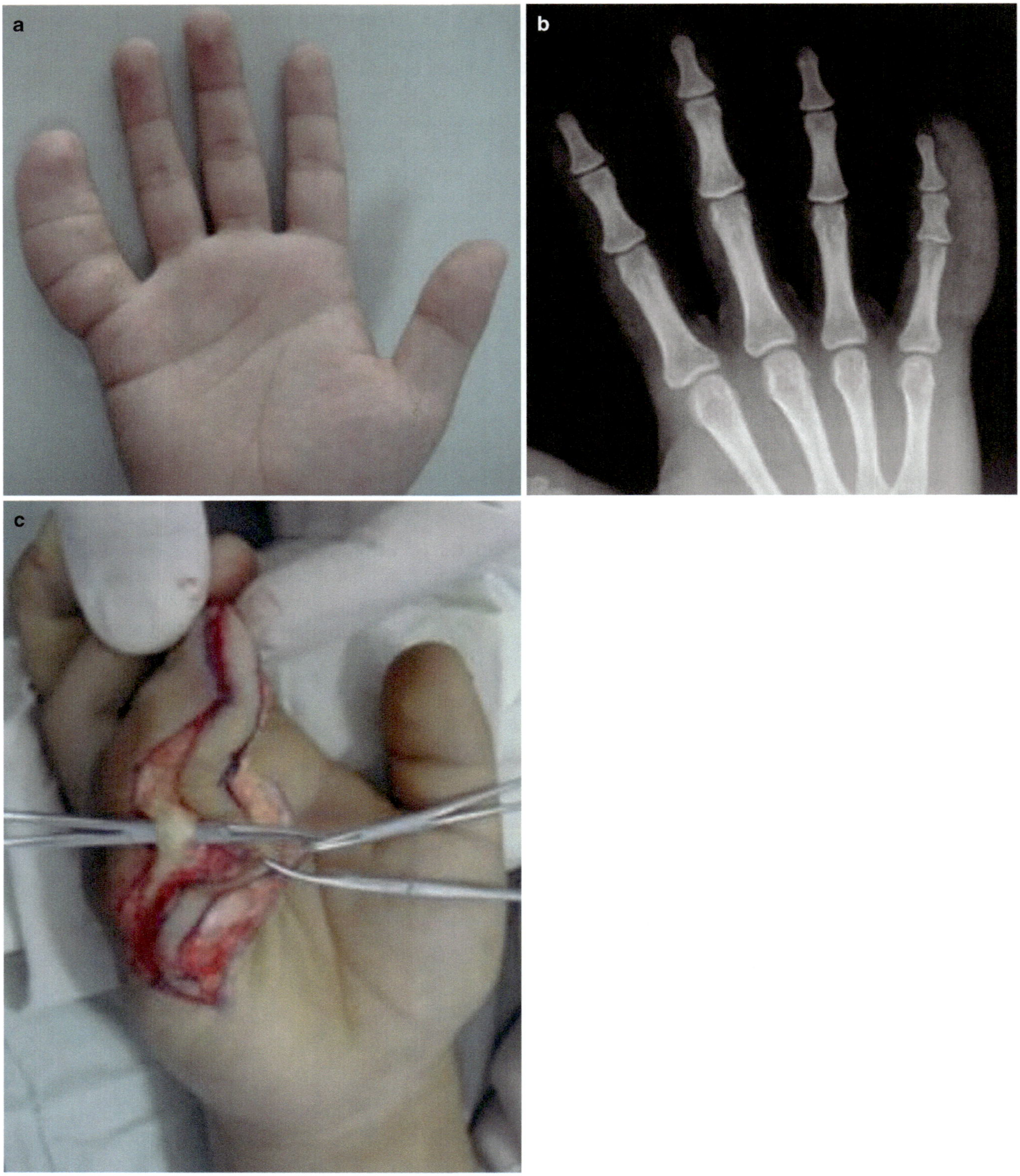

Fig. 13.3 (**a**) Right little finger giant finger. (**b**) Soft tissue shadow can be seen on the X-ray film, and no hypertrophy of bone and joint structure can be seen. (**c**) Intraoperative exploration revealed overgrowth of subcutaneous adipose tissue and fatty infiltration and thickening of the ulnar proper digital nerves

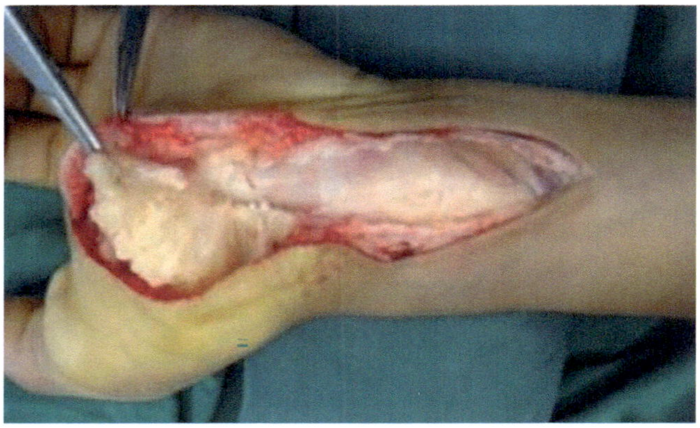

Fig. 13.4 The left thumb, index macrodactyly and index had been amputated, and the second surgical exploration showed extensive infiltration of adipose tissue in the median nerve and excessive hyperplasia of subcutaneous adipose tissue in the thenar

13.1.3.2 Clinical Manifestations and Classification

The typical split hand is characterized by a deep fissure in the center of the hand. The hands are usually asymmetrical. The fingers on both sides of the deep fissure are often thickened, deviated or rotated toward the center, and may be accompanied by syndactyly, polydactyly, phalangeal fusion, hyperplastic transverse bone (cross bone), flexion deformity, Delta bone, etc. (Fig. 13.16).

Manske and Halikis divided the deformity into five types according to the need of surgery (1995), which is the most commonly used classification in clinic at present. Type I: normal thumb (Fig. 13.17). Type II: stenosis of the thumb, which can be further divided into type IIA (Fig. 13.18): mild stenosis of the thumb, and type IIB: severe stenosis of the thumb (Fig. 13.19). Type III: syndactyly of the thumb, syn-

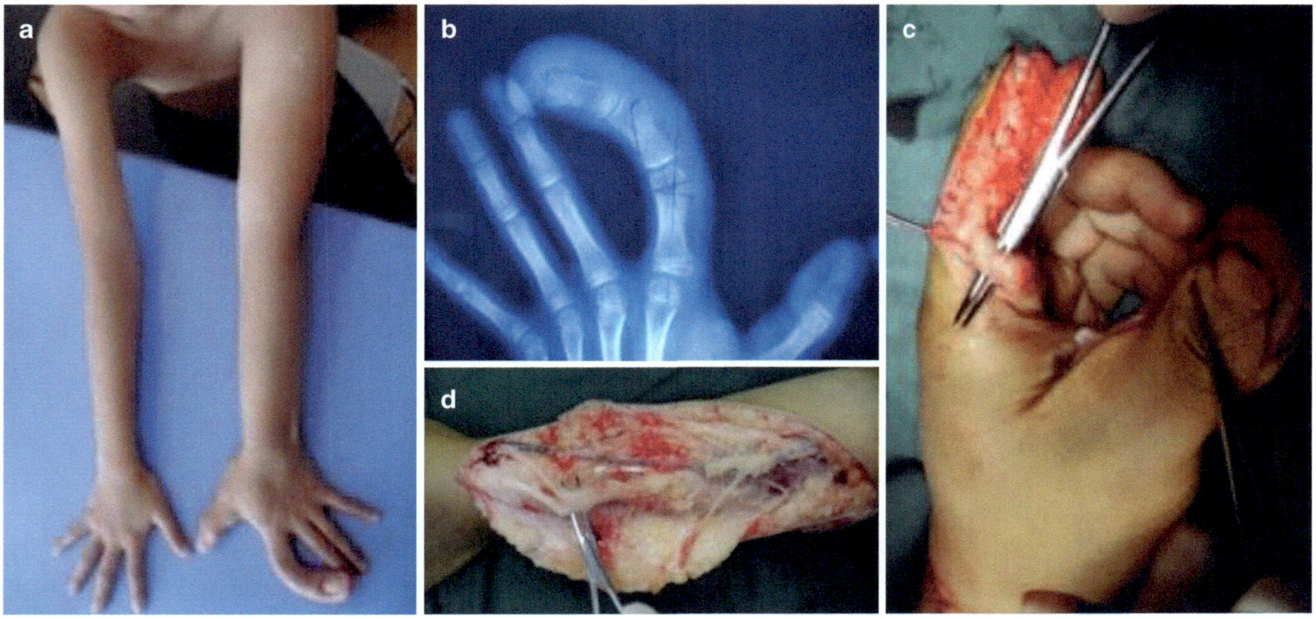

Fig. 13.5 (**a**) Giant left upper limb with fingers spreading to thumb and index finger. (**b**) Radiography showing hypertrophy of the phalanx of the index finger and deviation of the interphalangeal joint. (**c**) Intraoperative exploration shows fatty infiltration of finger nerves in addition to excessive proliferation of local adipose tissue. (**d**) Local fatty infiltration of the sensory branch of the radial nerve in the forearm

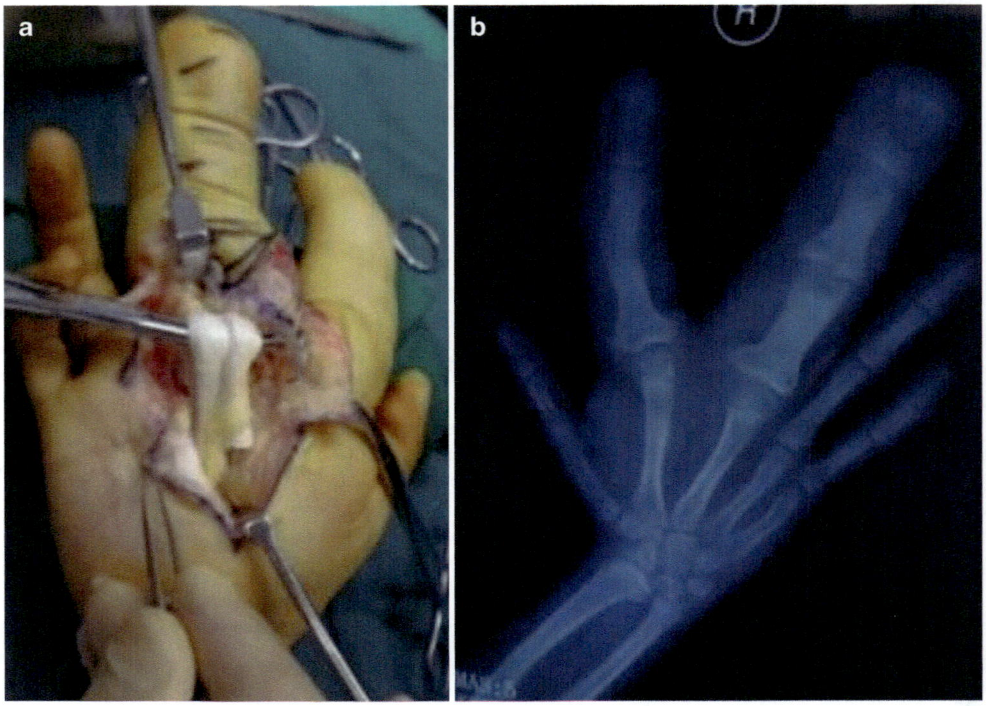

Fig. 13.6 (**a**) The right hand shows macrodactyly of the middle finger. Surgical exploration reveals excessive proliferation of subcutaneous adipose tissue and thickening of the flexor tendon of the finger. (**b**) X-ray film shows that the metacarpal and phalangeal bones are bulky, especially the phalanges are obviously bulky and deformed

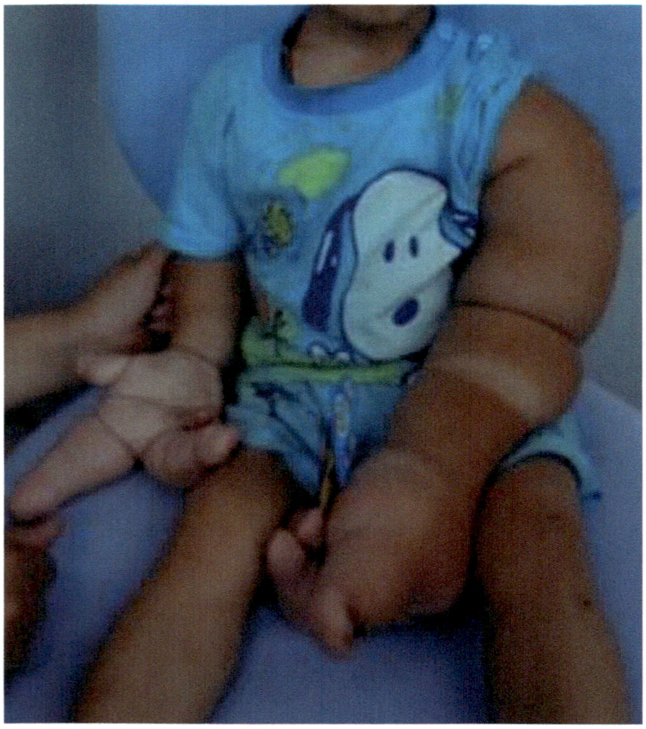

Fig. 13.7 The hypertrophic tissue spread to the chest, which seriously affected the function and appearance of the child's limbs. The etiology of this case is still unclear

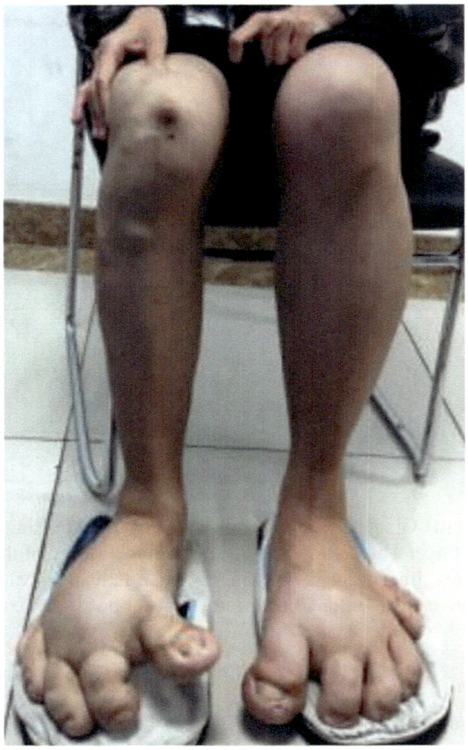

Fig. 13.8 A case of Klippel-Trenaunay syndrome with macrodactyly and bilateral vascular malformations of the lower extremities

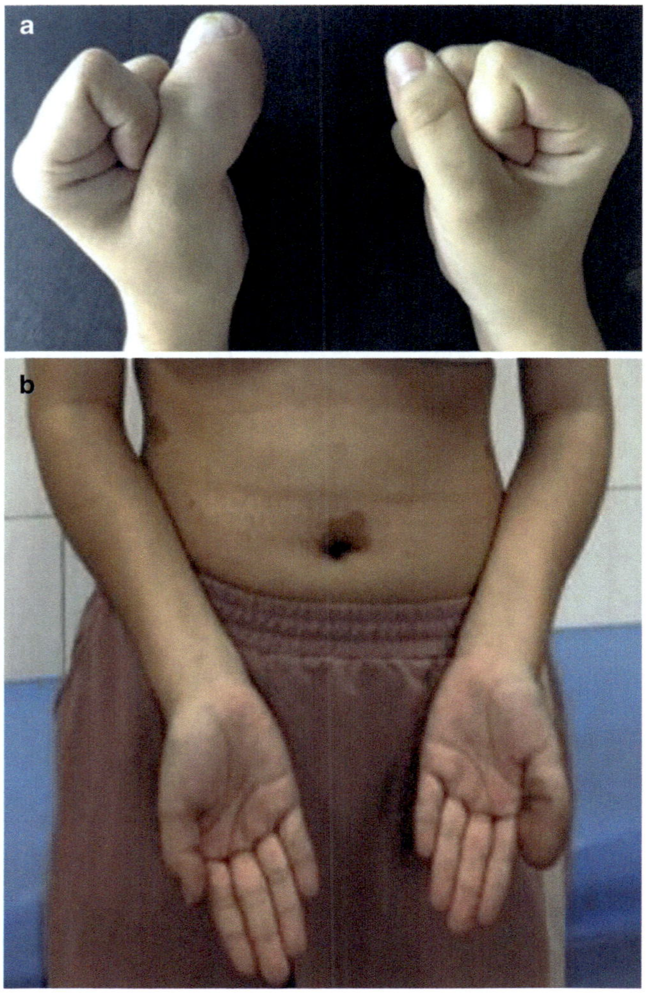

Fig. 13.9 (**a**) Hypertrophy of the left thumb with pigmentation. (**b**) The cafe-au-lait spots and pigmented freckles on the trunk and abdomen. This is neurofibromatosis type 1 (NF1)

dactyly of the axis of the thumb and index finger, and disappearance of the thumb (Fig. 13.20). Type IV: fusion of the thumb and finger, the development of the axis of the index finger is inhibited, and the thumb and finger are partially fused (Fig. 13.21). Type V: The thumb is absent, the development of the thumb is inhibited, the ulnar row still exists, and the thumb is absent (Fig. 13.22).

13.1.3.3 Treatment Principle

The purpose of the operation includes eliminating the deep fissure of the hand to improve the appearance, improving the first web stenosis and flexion deformity of the fingers, and improving the rotation deformity of the fingers. Surgical treatment of the cracked hand usually improves the appearance more significantly and may sacrifice part of the hand function, so if the child is older and the function of the cracked hand is still good, surgical treatment cannot be recommended.

13.1.4 Congenital Joint Contracture Involving the Hand

Congenital joint contracture of the hand is a kind of congenital disease characterized by ankylosis and limitation of movement of the finger and wrist joints, mostly manifested as flexion contracture, involving multiple joints can be called multiple joint contracture. Clinically, the more common disease types include single flexion deformity, thumb deformity, congenital multiple joint contracture, distal joint contracture, and so on. Some children with congenital central or peripheral nervous system abnormalities may also have joint contracture.

13.1.4.1 Etiology

At present, more than 300 congenital diseases can be manifested as hand joint contracture, with a variety of causes, including genetic and environmental factors. Environmental factors include fetal crowding and compression, such as multiple births or oligohydramnios caused by renal hypoplasia and early persistent amniotic fluid leakage, which directly lead to fetal joint movement limitation.

At present, the etiology of congenital multiple joint contracture is not clear, which may be caused by congenital neurogenic or myogenic lesions, and no heredity has been found. Distal joint contracture is a group of multiple joint contractures associated with genetic mutations, which is hereditary.

13.1.4.2 Clinical Manifestation

The clinical manifestations of hand joint contracture are usually related to the structure involved and the course of contracture, including skin, subcutaneous tissue, joint capsule ligament, tendon, muscle, bone joint, and neurovascular bundle. The degree of contracture deformity may be further aggravated with the growth and development of patients with long course of disease and without intervention.

1. Flexion deformity often involves bilateral little fingers, showing flexion contracture of the proximal interphalangeal joint (Fig. 13.23).
2. Thumb deformity (Fig. 13.24) can be divided into three types according to anatomical characteristics and severity of deformity. Type I is the lightest.

   It is characterized by dysplasia or absence of the extensor pollicis brevis, and there is usually no significant limitation in the movement of the interphalangeal and carpometacarpal joints of the thumb. Type II is characterized by limited movement of the metacarpophalangeal and carpometacarpal joints of the thumb, but not of the interphalangeal joints. Type III, on the basis of type II, also has limited movement of interphalangeal joints.

   The passive extension of the metacarpophalangeal joint and the abduction of the thumb were limited, and the

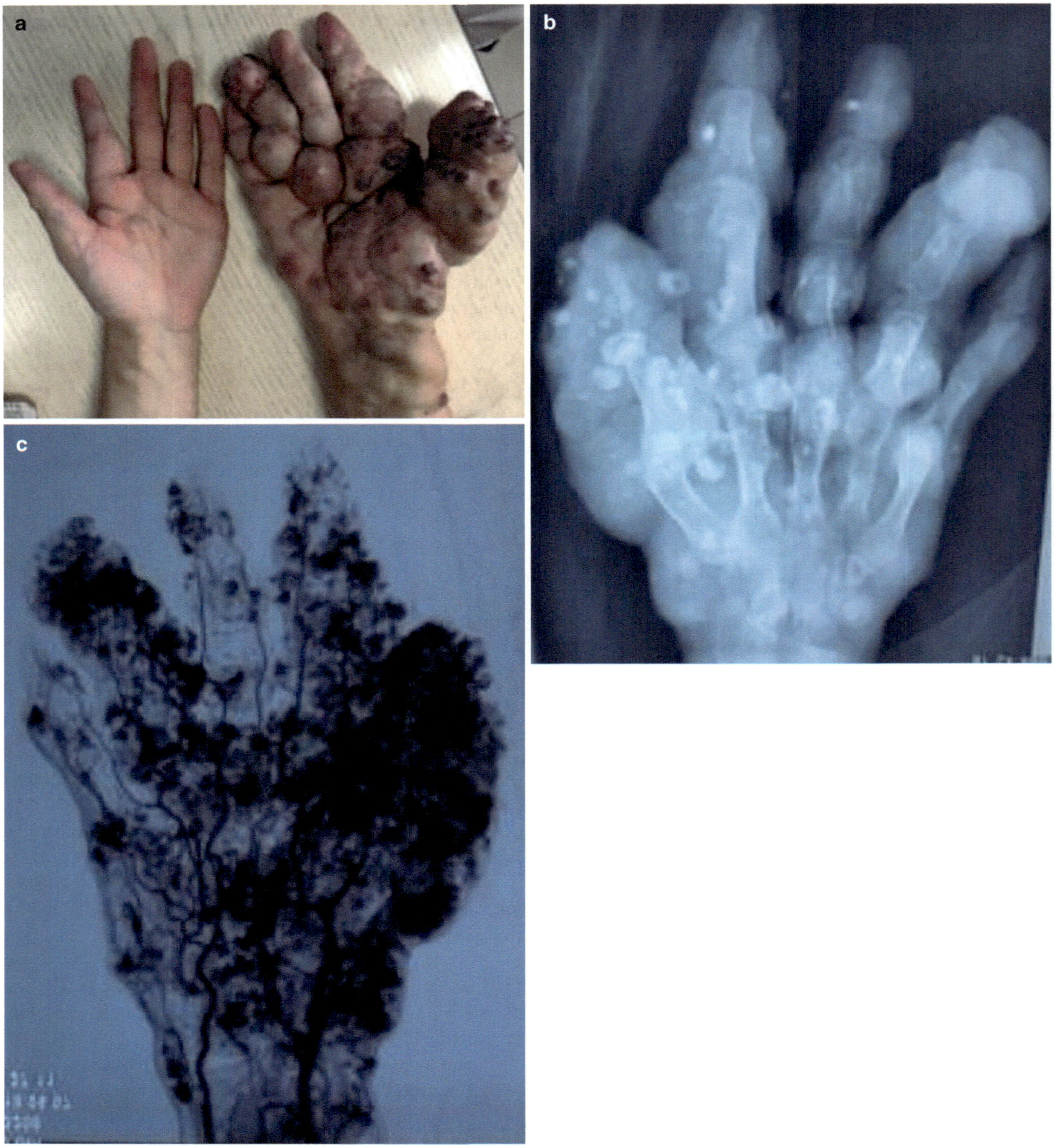

Fig. 13.10 (**a**) Extensive vascular lesions and hypertrophy in the right hand and mild lesions in the left hand. (**b**) X-ray shows multiple enchondromas and phleboliths in the metacarpal and phalangeal bones. (**c**) Angiography of (**c**) shows a diffuse venous malformation. This is Maffucci's syndrome

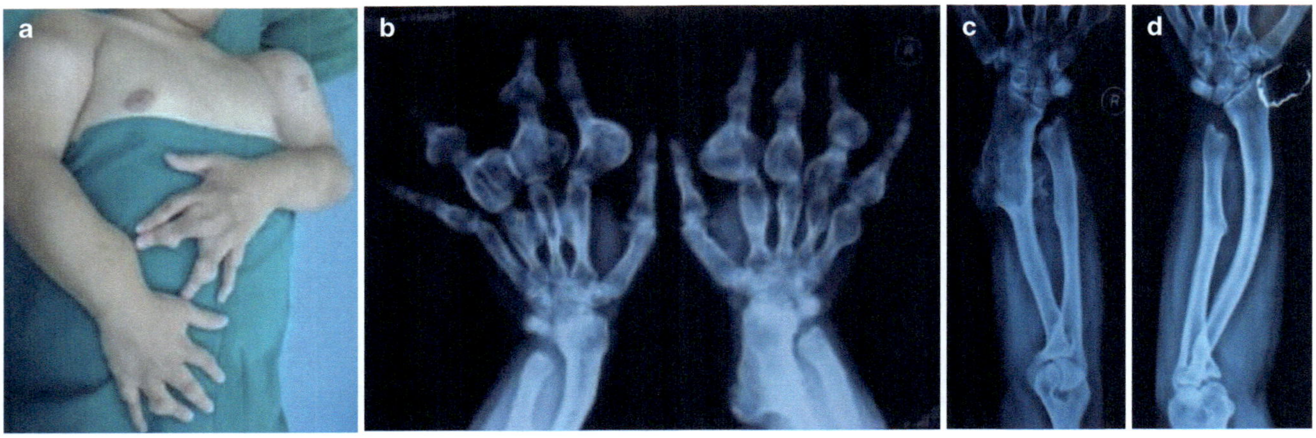

Fig. 13.11 (**a**) Bilateral hypertrophy of the upper limbs in varying degrees, with multiple localized masses bulging. (**b**) Radiographs show multiple enchondromas in the radius and ulna of both hands. (**c**) X-ray film of right forearm. (**d**) Radiography of left forearm. The tumor also extends to the upper arm. This is Ollier's disease (multiple enchondromatosis)

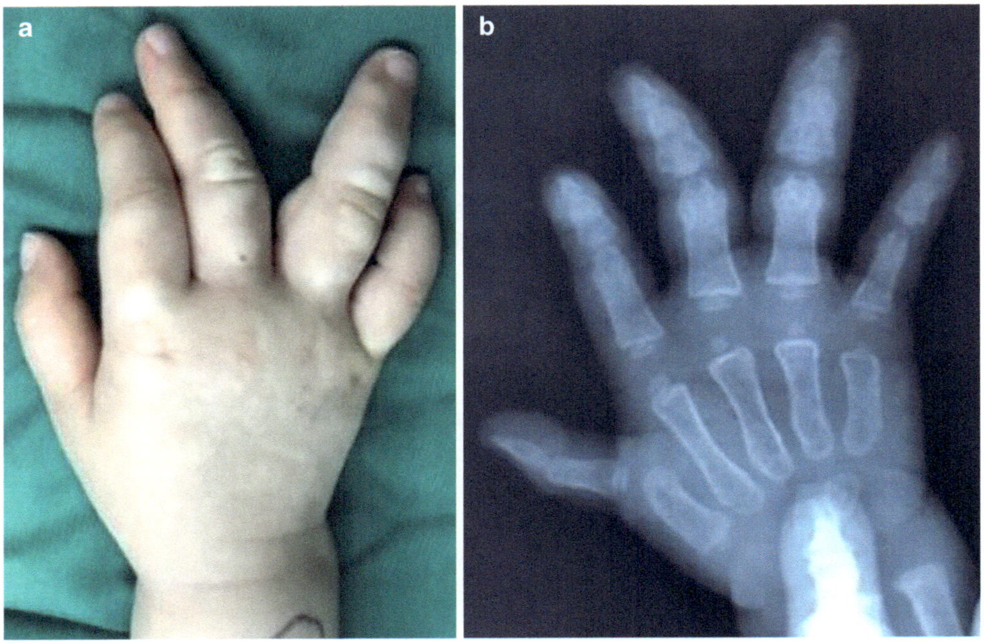

Fig. 13.12 (**a**) Sulcus and gyrus lesions are seen in the right macrodactyly, index finger to ring finger, and dorsum of hand. (**b**) X-ray film shows phalangeal hypertrophy and deformation. This case is Proteus syndrome (Poseidon syndrome)

passive extension of the interphalangeal joint was not significantly limited, which was type II.

3. Children with multiple joint contractures usually have thin limbs, insufficient muscle capacity and abnormal skin lines. A classic case of multiple joint contractures.

   Shoulder collapse, internal rotation and adduction of shoulder joint, extension contracture of elbow joint, pronation of forearm, flexion contracture of wrist joint and finger joint, adduction of thumb, and joint contracture of lower limbs (Figs. 13.25, 13.26, 13.27 and 13.28).

Some syndromic multiple joint contractures, such as Freeman-Sheldon syndrome, Beals syndrome, Poland syndrome, etc., may be accompanied by facial and other organ system abnormalities in addition to the manifestations of limb joint contractures (Figs. 13.29, 13.30, 13.31 and 13.32).

13.1.4.3 Treatment Principle

Early intervention after birth, including traction and massage of joints, orthopedic braces, plaster series, etc., usually improves joint contracture. Surgical treatment can be per-

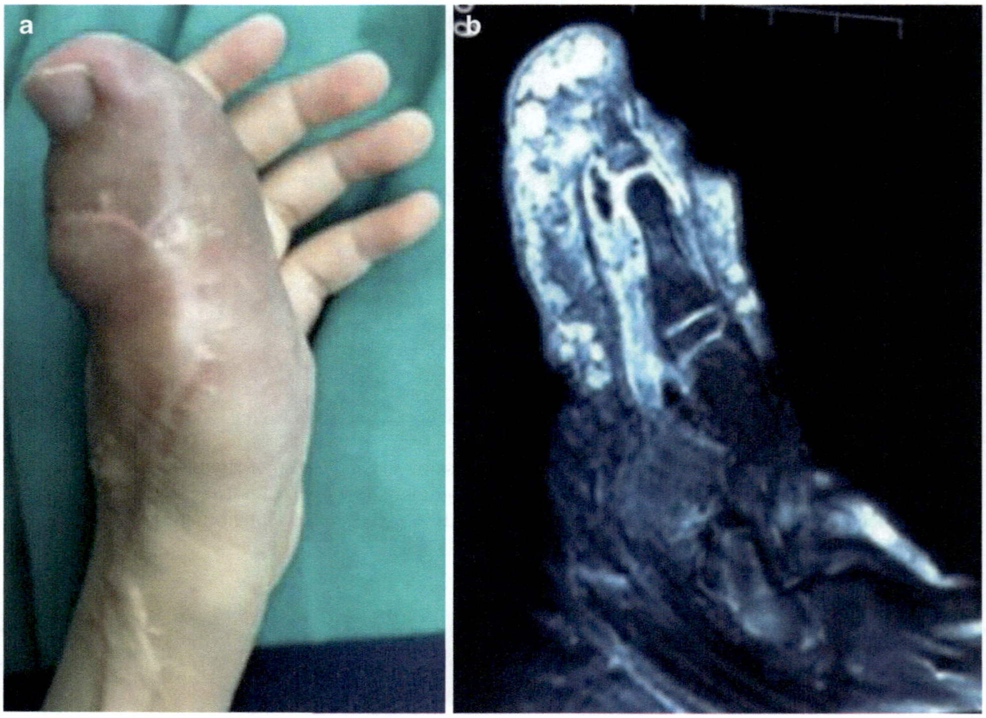

Fig. 13.13 (**a**) Left thumb hypertrophy with purple skin color. (**b**) MRI shows a large amount of blood flow signals. This case was confirmed to be hemangioma by pathological examination

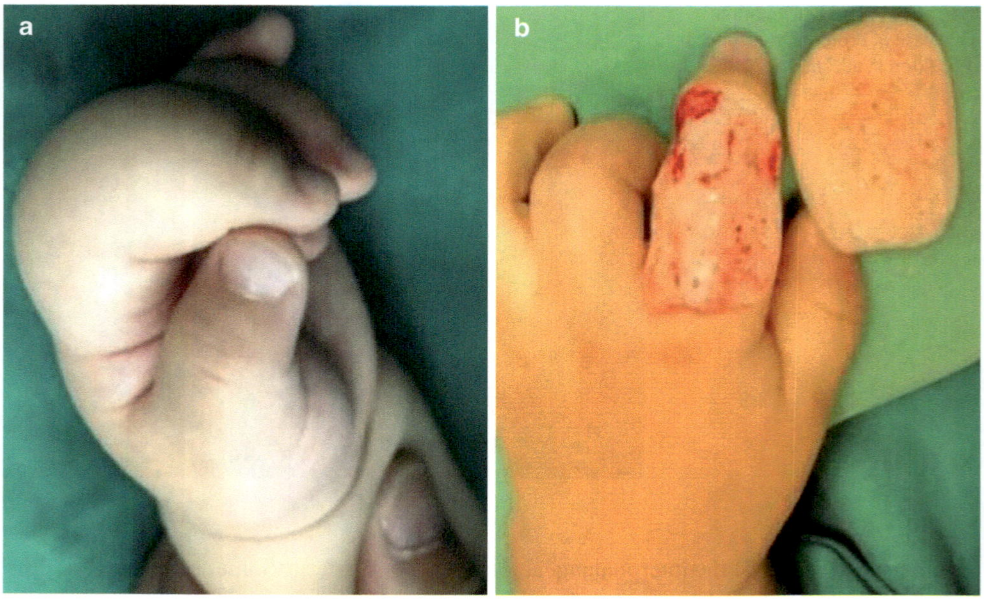

Fig. 13.14 (**a**) Hypertrophy of the left index finger with marked dorsal hypertrophy. (**b**) The hypertrophic tissue on the dorsum of the finger was resected. Dense adipose tissue and lymphatic structures were found. At the same time, yellowish transparent fluid was found flowing out of the lymphatic vessels. This case is an angiolymphoma

formed according to the specific deformity, including skin and soft tissue release and skin grafting, joint capsule release, tendon lengthening or displacement, osteotomy, and correction of bone and joint. For the surgical treatment of the hand, the grasping function should be carefully evaluated before the operation to avoid damaging the original limb function.

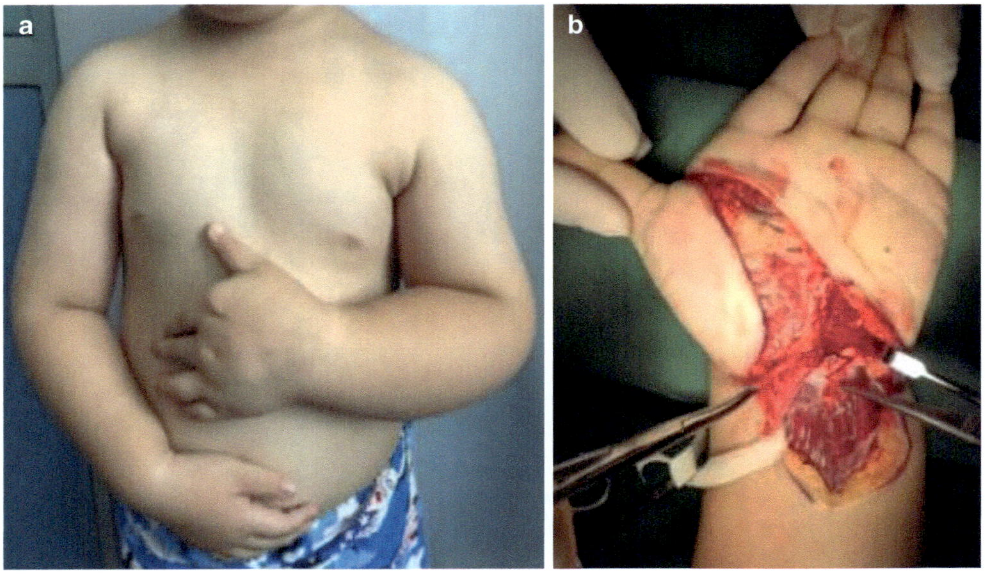

Fig. 13.15 (**a**) Hypertrophy of left upper limb and severe deformity of hand. (**b**) Surgical exploration reveals a large amount of hyperplastic muscle tissue. This is a case of muscular hypertrophy syndrome

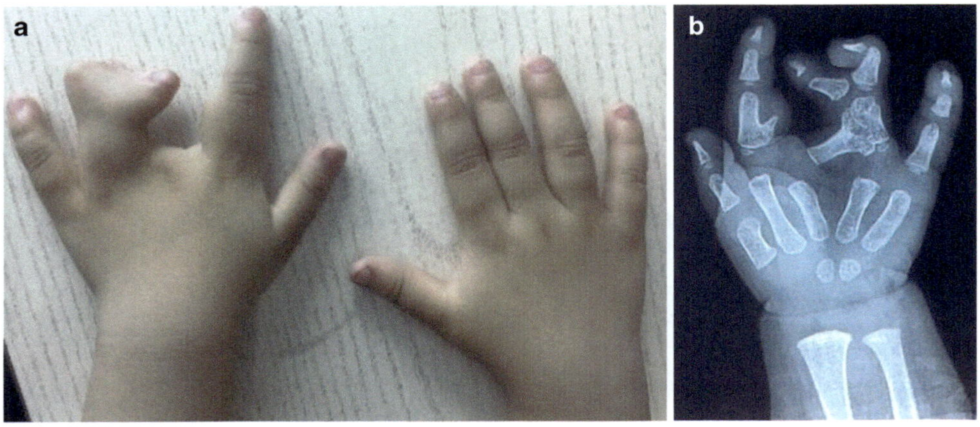

Fig. 13.16 (**a**) A deformity of the cleft hand of the right hand, except for the central fissure of the hand. (**b**) X-ray shows bony syndactyly and transverse phalanx

Fig. 13.17 Right hand split hand type I: normal thumb

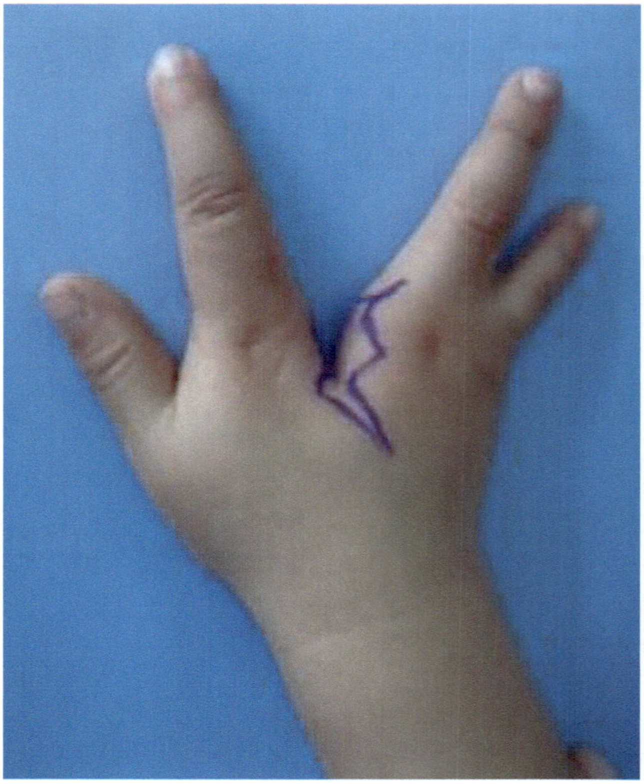

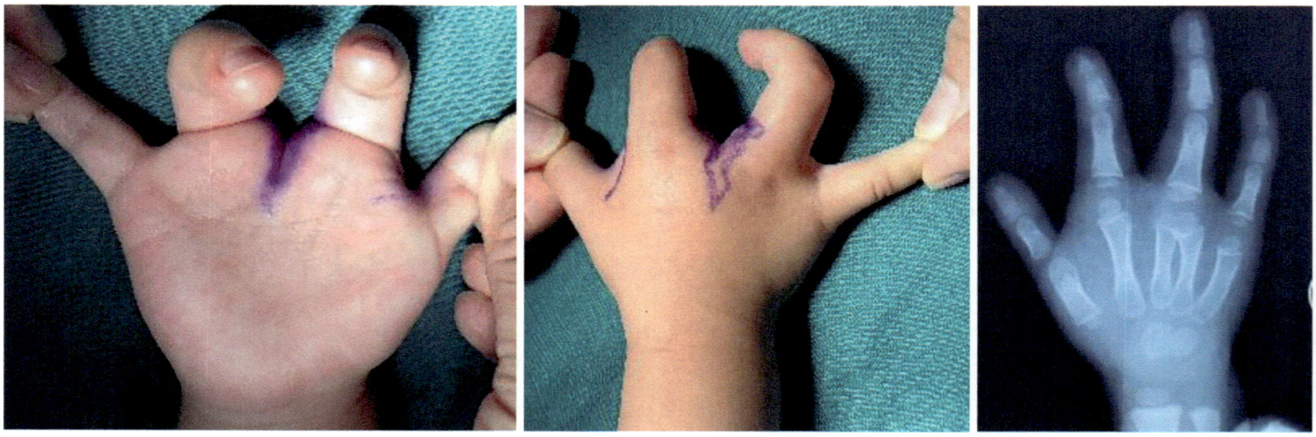

Fig. 13.18 Right hand split hand type IIA: slight stenosis of the thumb

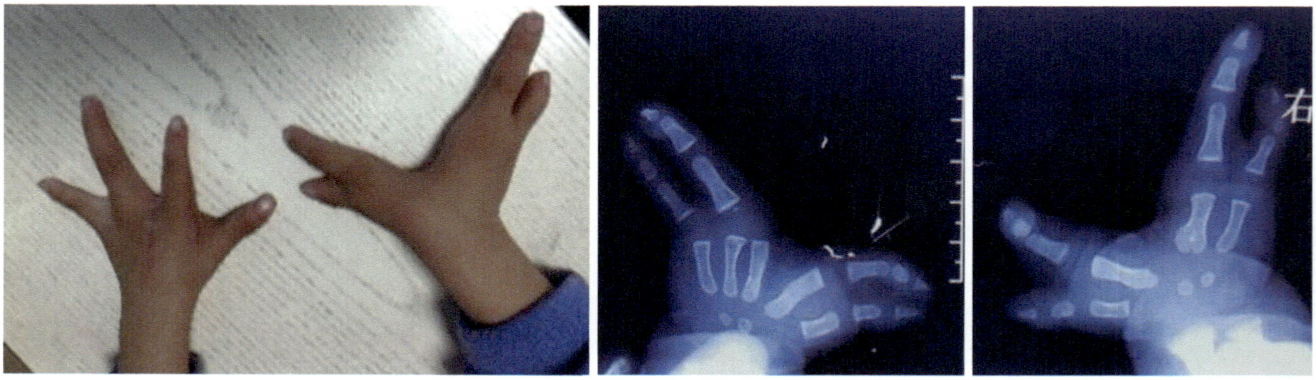

Fig. 13.19 Both hands were split, the right hand was type IIB: severe stenosis of the thumb, the left hand was type III: syndactyly of the thumb and the left hand. After the operation, the X-ray showed syndactyly of the thumb and the left hand before the operation

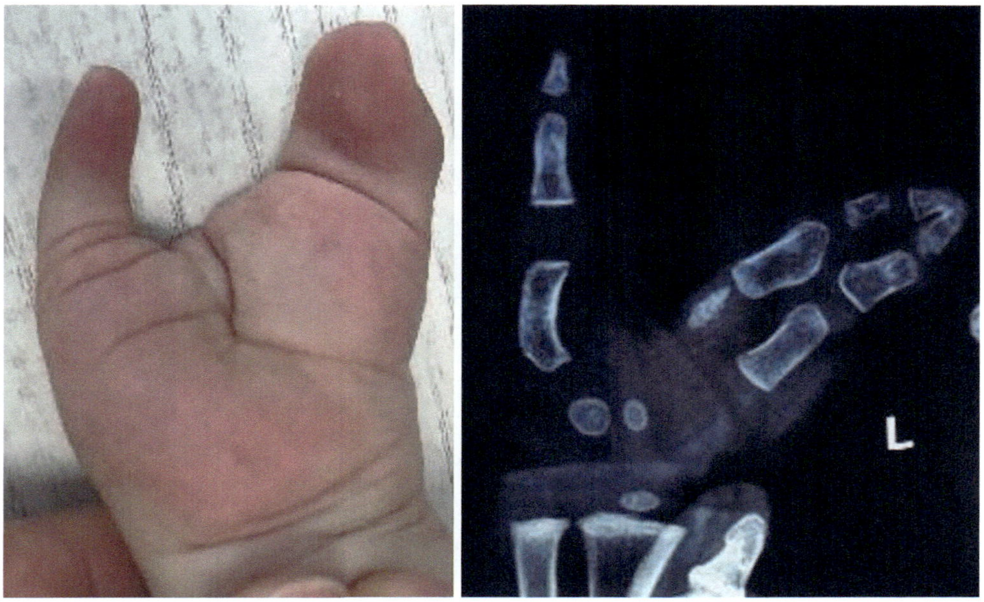

Fig. 13.20 Left split hand type III: thumb fusion type, combined with radial phalangeal syndactyly

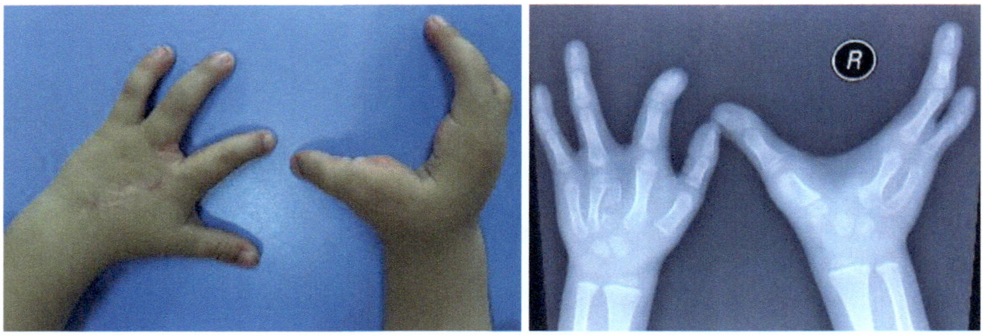

Fig. 13.21 The left hand is the normal type of thumb web (already operated), and the right hand is the type IV: the fusion type of thumb web

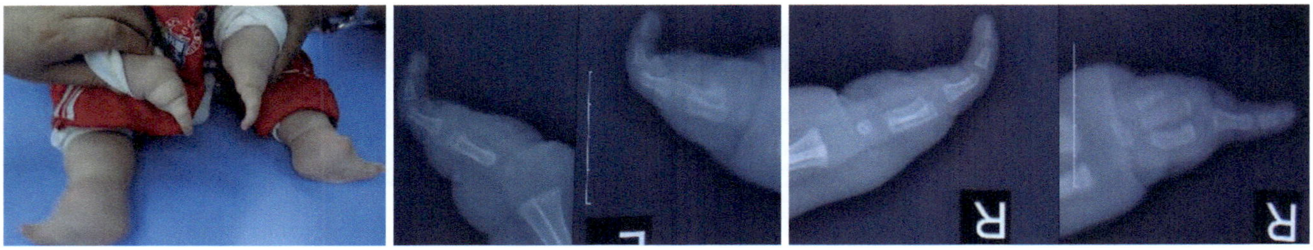

Fig. 13.22 Both hands are V-shaped: the thumb is absent and the little finger is still present

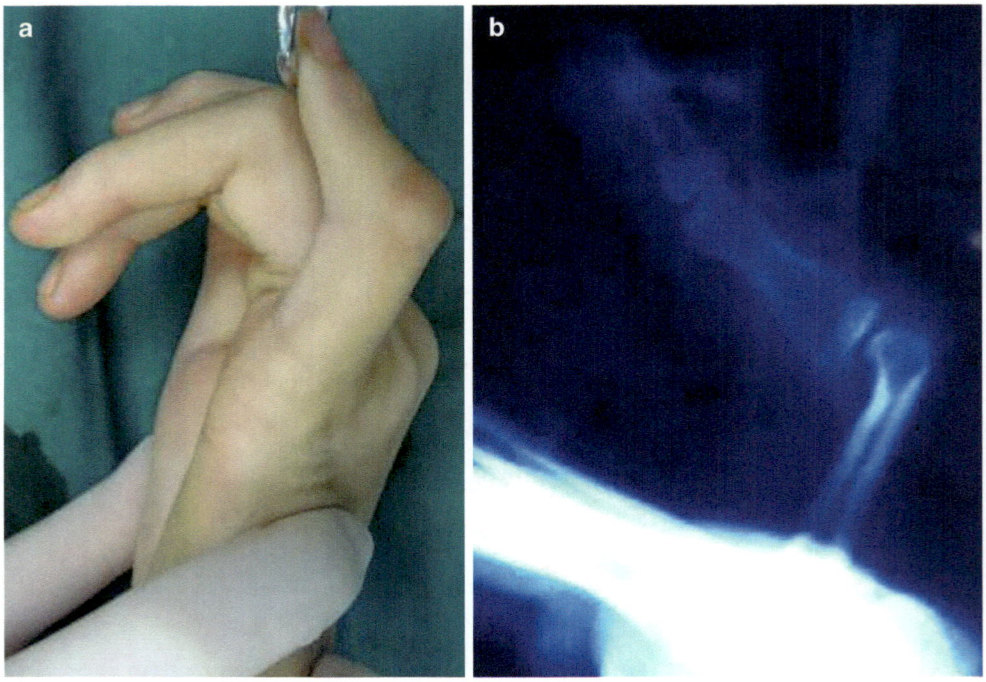

Fig. 13.23 (**a**) A flexion deformity of the left little finger with flexion contracture of the proximal interphalangeal joint. (**b**) X-ray film shows that the proximal phalanx is abnormal in shape, and the middle phalanx has a tendency of volar dislocation

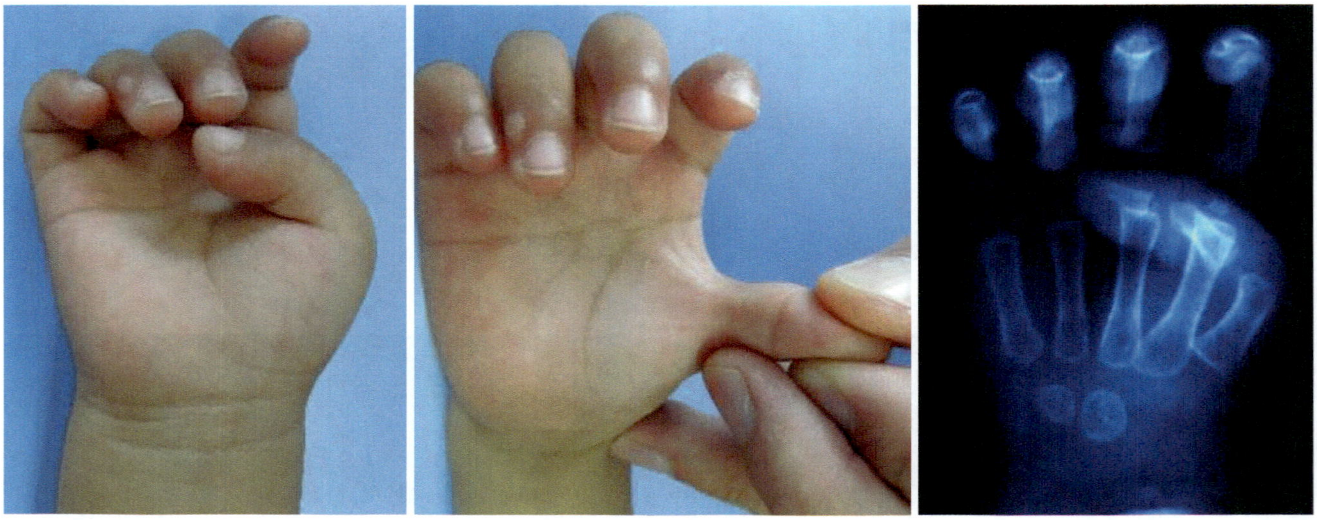

Fig. 13.24 Thumb deformity. Flexion of the metacarpophalangeal joint of the thumb can be seen at rest, suggesting dysplasia or absence of the extensor pollicis brevis

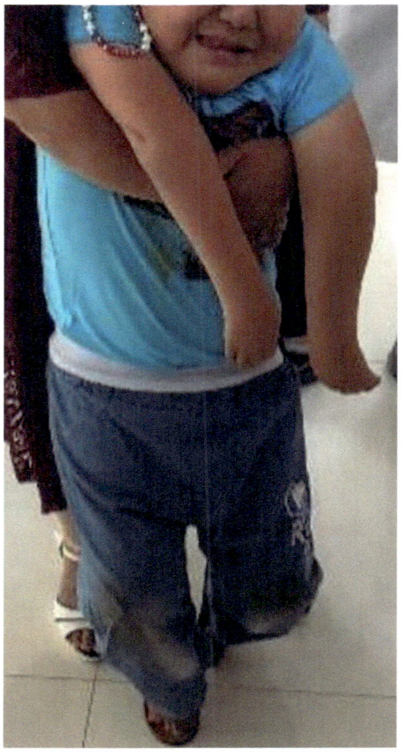

Fig. 13.25 The typical upper limb manifestations of multiple joint contracture include shoulder joint internal rotation and adduction, elbow joint extension contracture, forearm pronation, wrist joint flexion contracture, and lower limb joint contracture

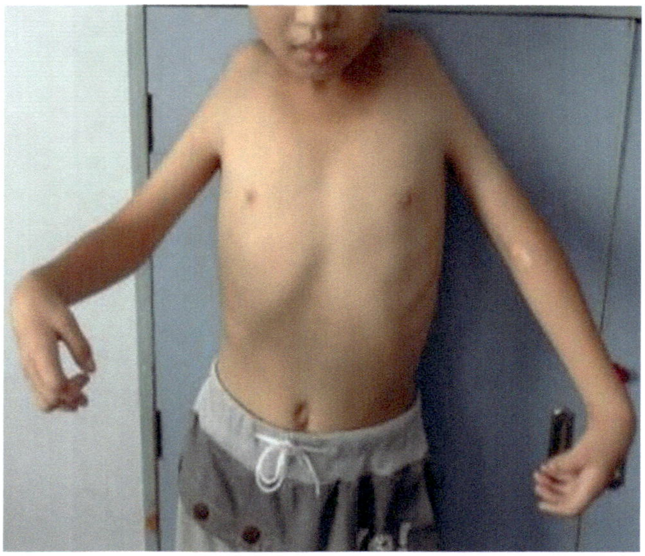

Fig. 13.27 Bilateral multi-joint contracture of upper limbs, including shoulder joint contracture

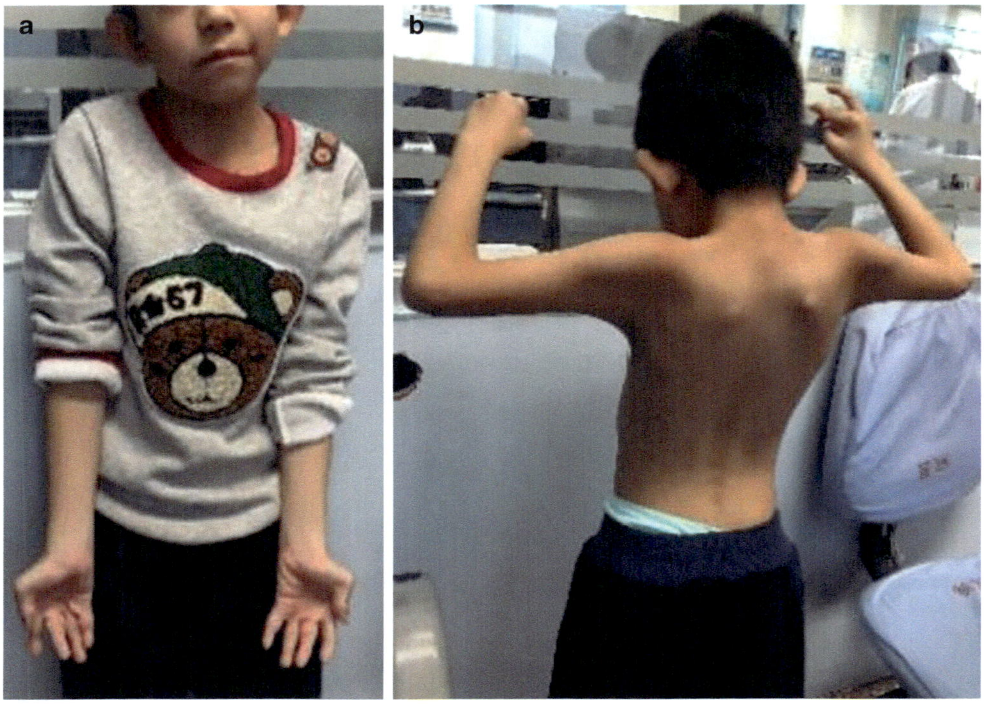

Fig. 13.26 (**a**) Bilateral flexion contracture of finger joints with adduction of thumb. (**b**) Decreased latissimus dorsi muscle volume

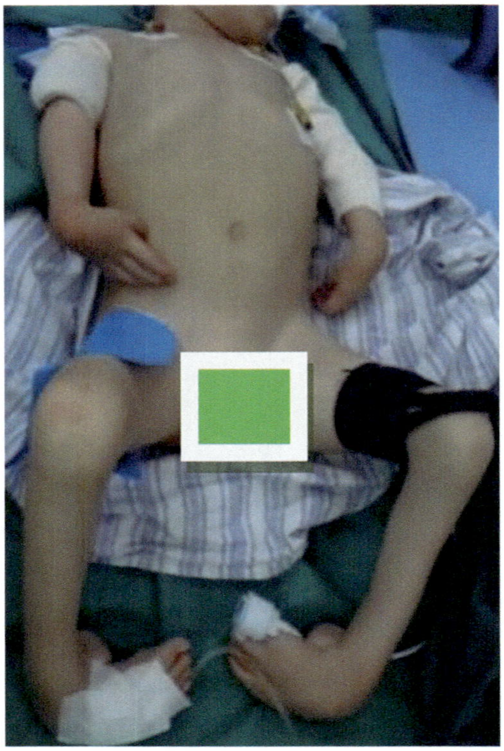

Fig. 13.28 Multiple joint contractures of bilateral upper and lower extremities

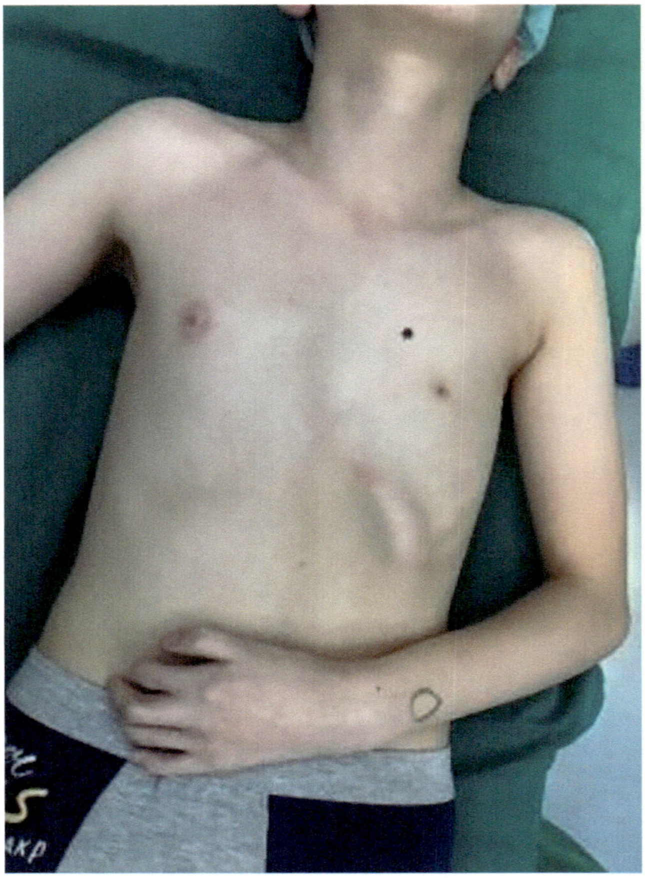

Fig. 13.30 Upper extremity joint contracture with chest wall deformity

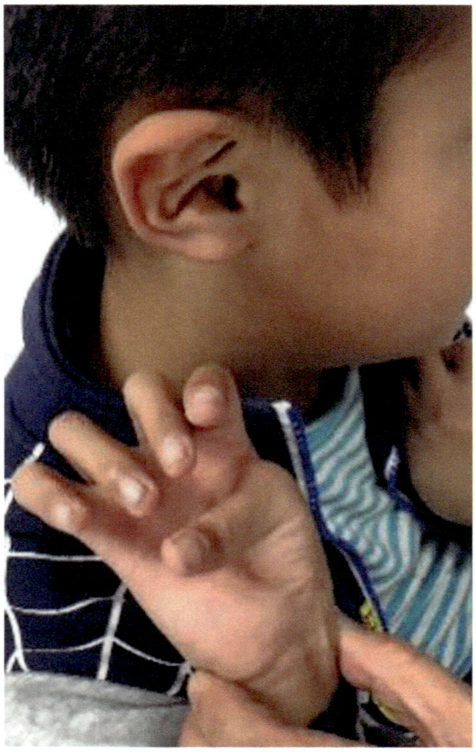

Fig. 13.29 Hand deformities include spider-finger deformity, flexion finger deformity, and thumb deformity, combined with ear deformity

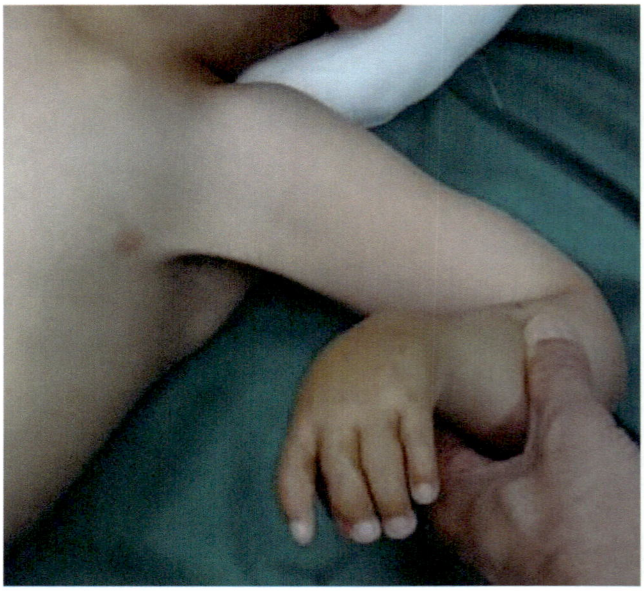

Fig. 13.31 A case of joint contracture of left upper extremity with pectoral muscle dysplasia and axillary web was diagnosed as Poland's syndrome

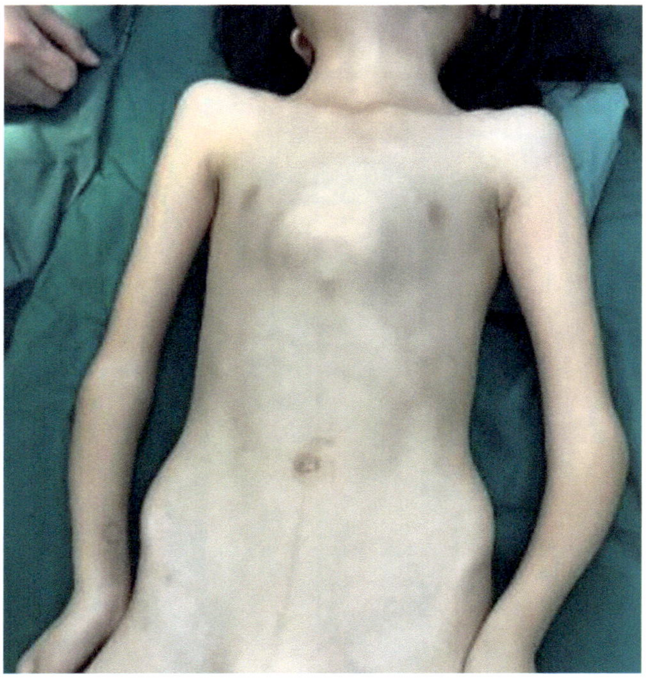

Fig. 13.32 Bilateral upper limb joint contracture with "chicken breast"

13.2 Congenital Syndactyly and Polydactyly

13.2.1 Congenital Syndactyly

Syndactyly is a pathological condition in which the tissue structure of two or more fingers is not physiologically connected, and it is one of the most common congenital hand deformities.

13.2.1.1 Etiology

At the fourth week of embryo, the finger contour began to appear at the end of the limb bud of the upper limb, and the finger differentiation was completed at the eighth week. Apoptosis, degradation of extracellular matrix, and differentiation of interdigital tissue are the basis for the formation of normal interdigital space from the end of the finger to the proximal web. Different reasons lead to the occurrence and abnormal development of the above processes, which may induce syndactyly, such as gene mutation, chromosome variation, and other genetic factors. Chemical drugs, viral infection, ionizing radiation, abnormal intrauterine environment, maternal diseases, and other non-genetic factors.

13.2.1.2 Clinical Manifestations and Classification

Syndactyly can be divided into complete syndactyly (Fig. 13.33), incomplete syndactyly (Fig. 13.34), soft tissue syndactyly (Fig. 13.35), and bony syndactyly (Fig. 13.36).

Syndactyly may occur alone, and may also occur in other hand deformities, such as syndactyly of split hand, syndactyly of multiple fingers, syndactyly of longitudinal dysplasia, syndactyly of ectrodactyly, and syndactyly of macrosomia (Figs. 13.37, 13.38, 13.39, 13.40 and 13.41). It can also occur in some malformation syndromes, such as Apert syndrome, Poland syndrome, band syndrome, multiple joint contractures and fingers (Figs. 13.42, 13.43, 13.44 and 13.45).

13.2.1.3 Treatment Principle

The conventional treatment principles of syndactyly include: (1) syndactyly of thumb, index finger, ring and little finger should be treated preferentially. (2) Bilateral syndactyly of the same finger is recommended to be treated by stages. Related combined malformations should be treated in the same period or by stages according to relevant principles.

13.2.2 Congenital Polydactyly

Polydactyly is the most common congenital malformation of the hand and upper limbs, which can be divided into radial polydactyly, ulnar polydactyly, and central polydactyly. The incidence of radial polydactyly was the highest among the three.

13.2.2.1 Etiology

Most polydactyly is sporadic and non-syndromic, which may be the result of both endogenous and exogenous factors. It is usually unilateral. Familial polydactyly is mostly bilateral. Mutations in genes such as GLI3 and ZRS/SHH can lead to polydactyly.

Polydactyly can also occur in some syndromic malformations, such as Holt-Oram syndrome, Fanconi anemia, Rubinstein-Taybi syndrome, Meckel syndrome, oro-facio-digital syndrome type 1, etc.

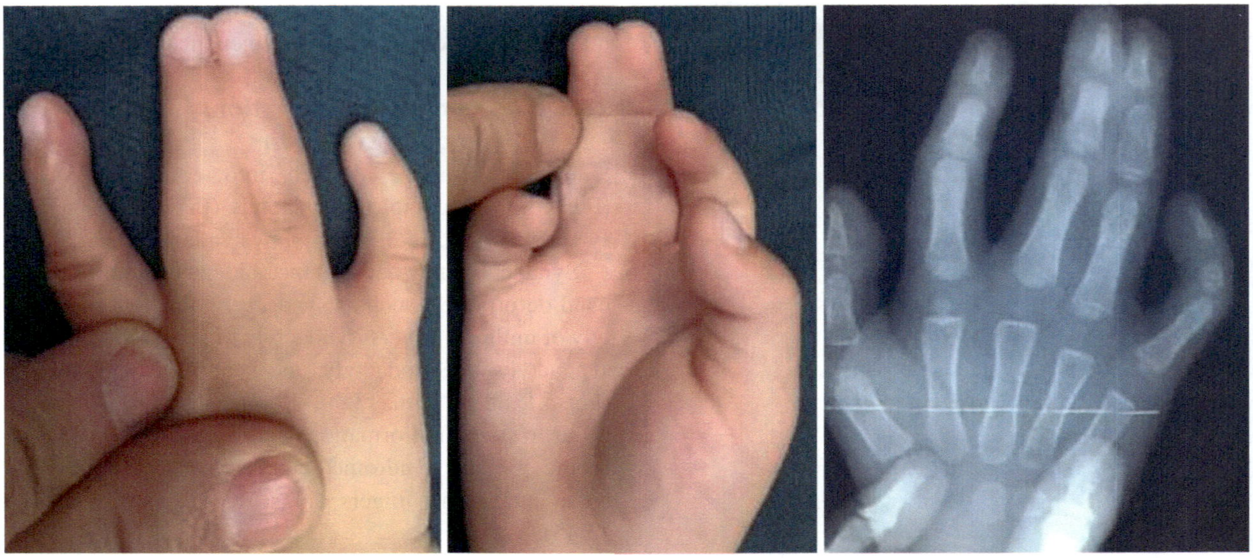

Fig. 13.33 Complete syndactyly

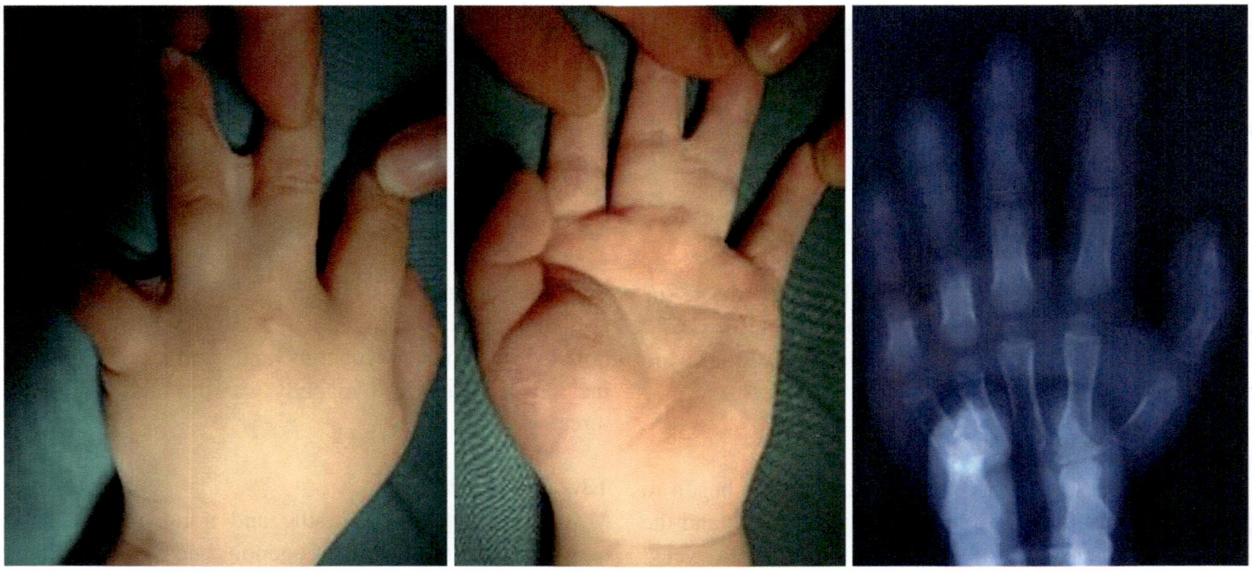

Fig. 13.34 Incomplete syndactyly

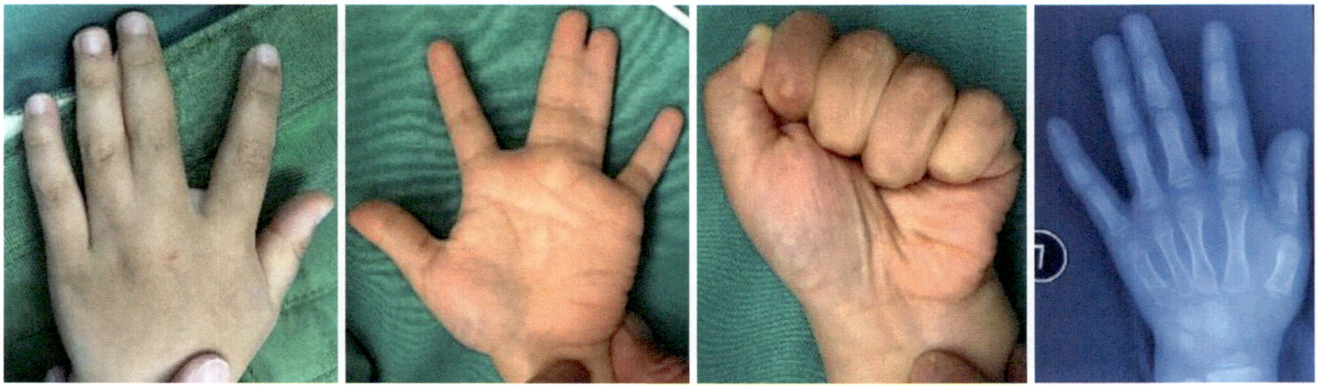

Fig. 13.35 Soft tissue syndactyly

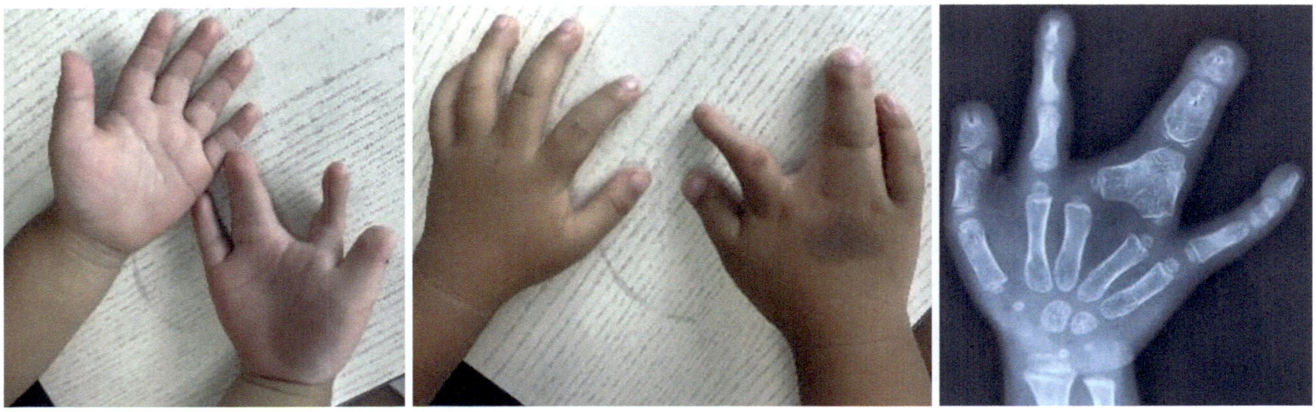

Fig. 13.36 Skeletal syndactyly of the middle ring finger of the right hand. Combined with ipsilateral polypthalmos

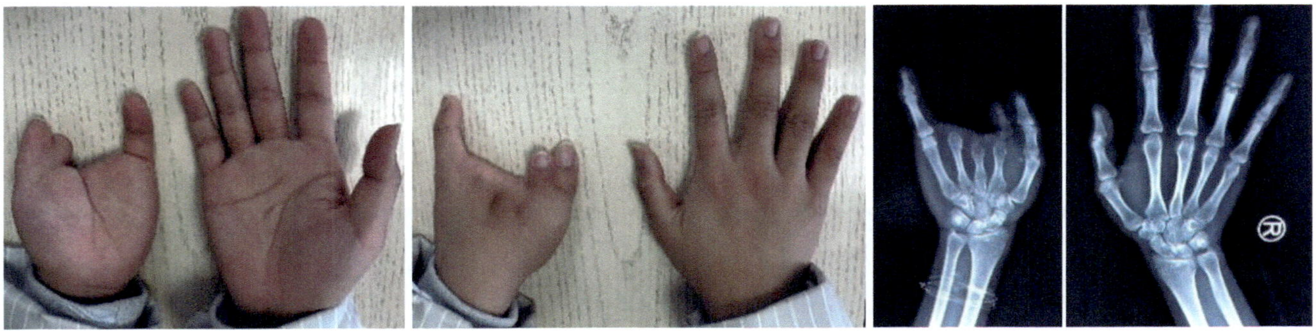

Fig. 13.37 Poland syndrome, left brachydactyly, and syndactyly

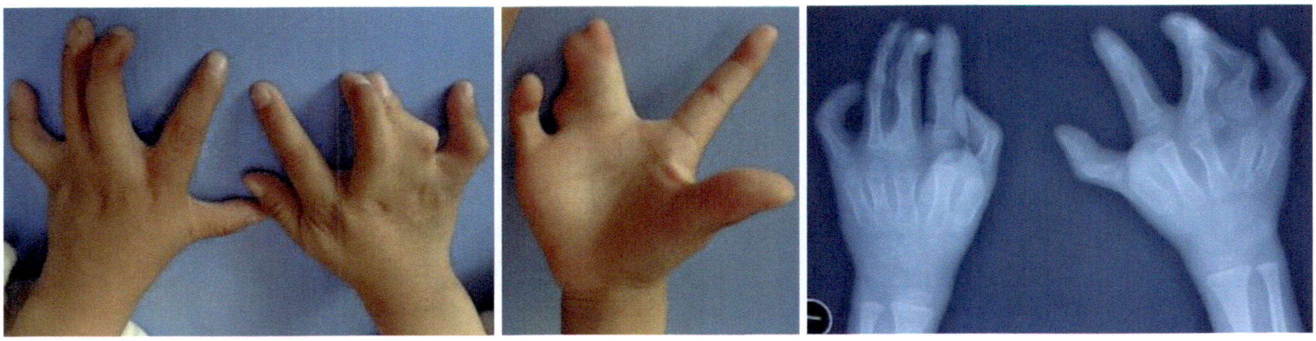

Fig. 13.38 The right hand is the central row of multi-fingered syndactyly

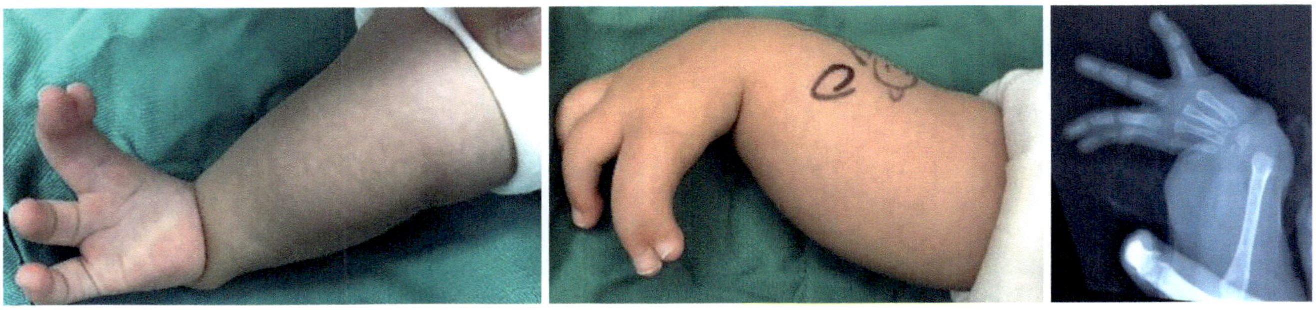

Fig. 13.39 Dysplasia of interhemispheric fissure with syndactyly and the absence of thumb

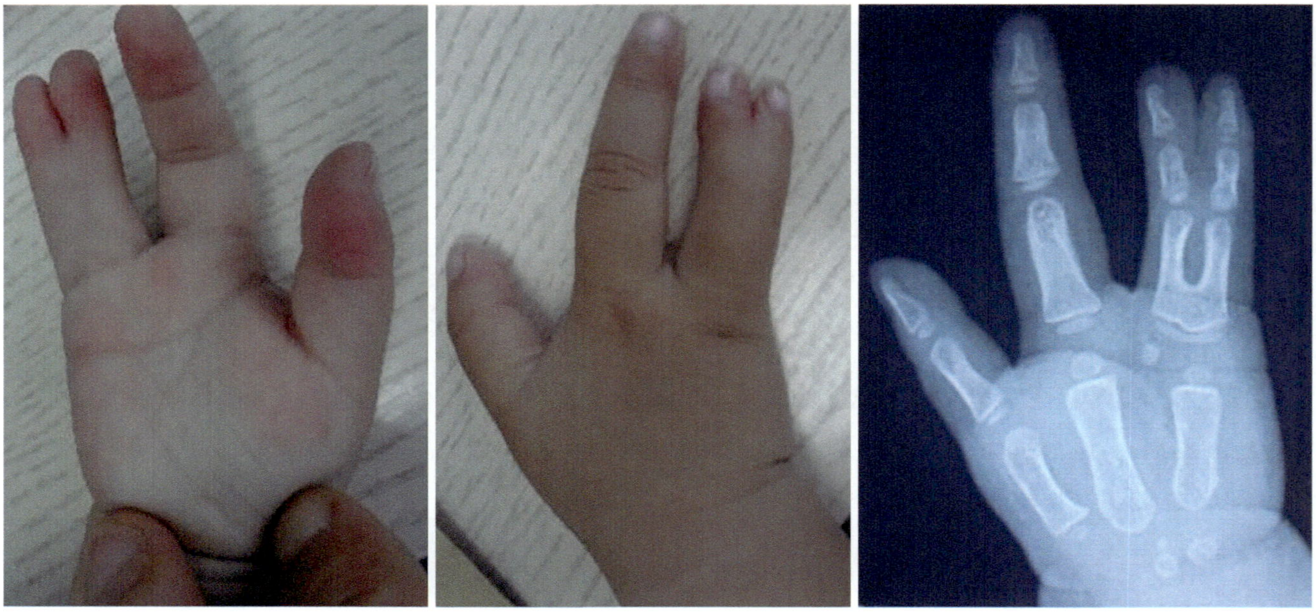

Fig. 13.40 Ectrodactyly with bony syndactyly

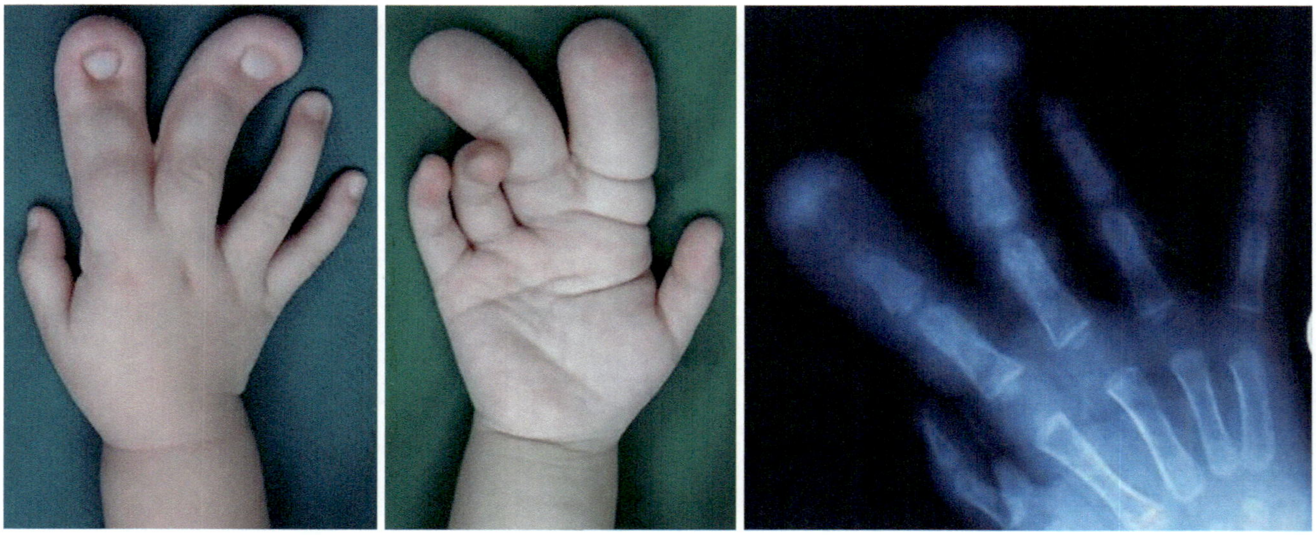

Fig. 13.41 Macrodactyly and syndactyly

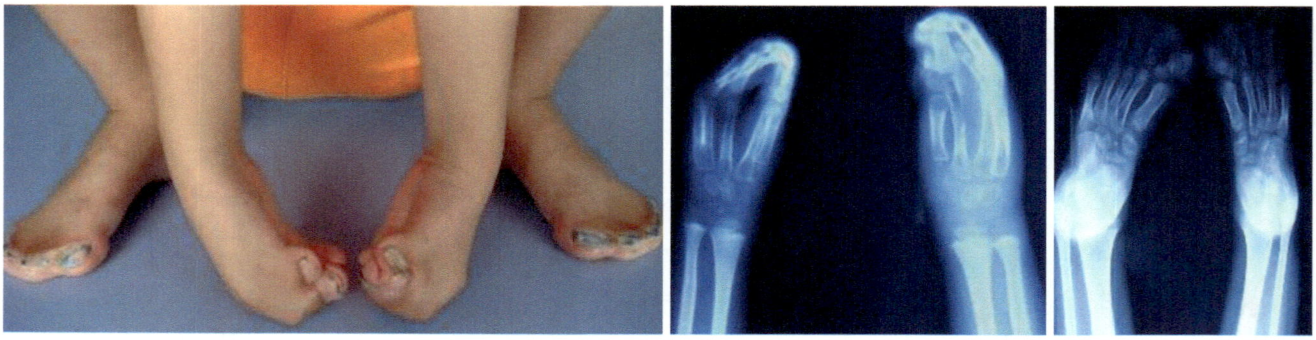

Fig. 13.42 Apert syndrome syndactyly and syndactyly

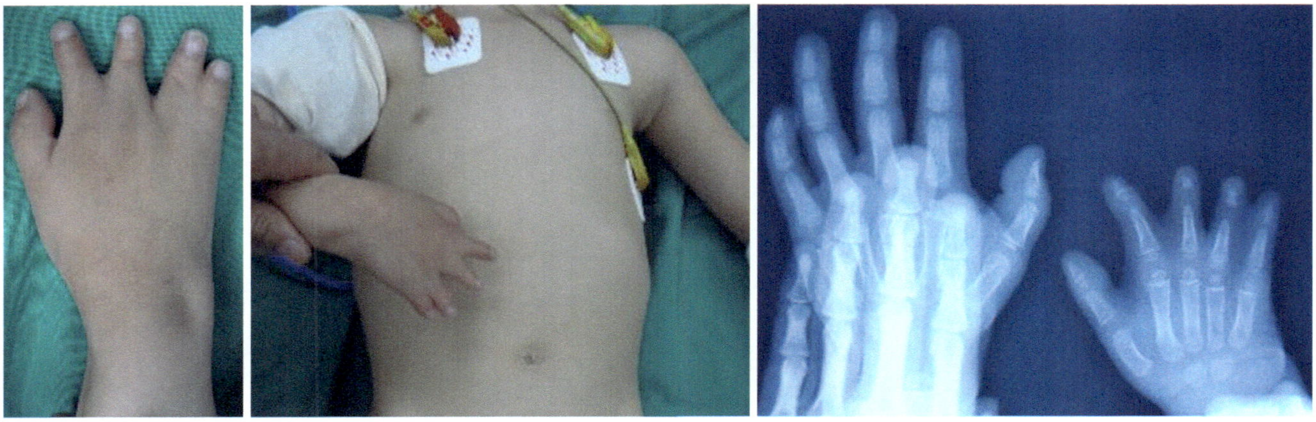

Fig. 13.43 Poland syndrome brachysyndactyly with ipsilateral chest wall and pectoral muscle dysplasia

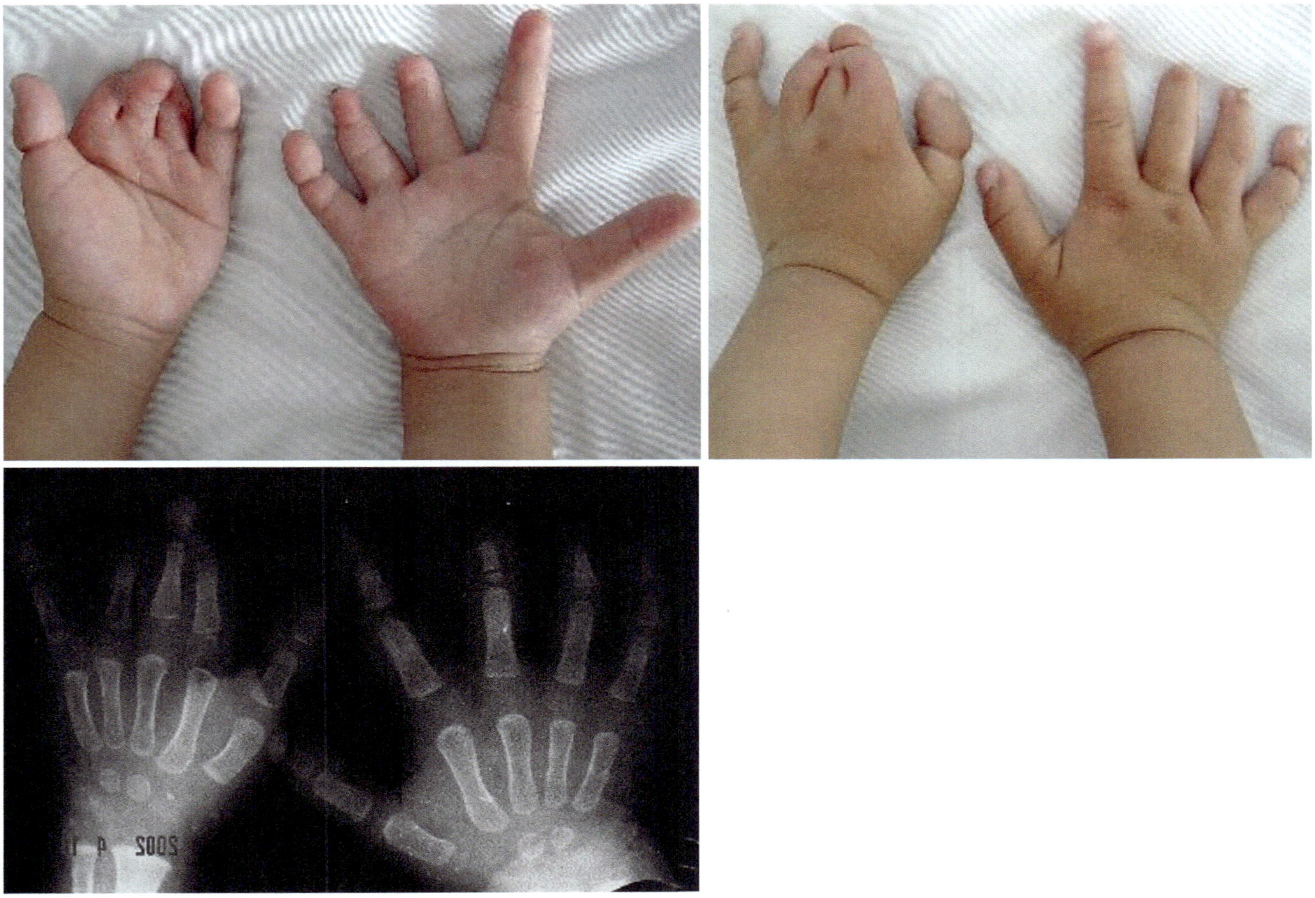

Fig. 13.44 Band syndrome syndactyly

13.2.2.2 Classification and Treatment Principle

1. Radial polydactyly occurs in polydactyly on the radial side of the hand. Polydactyly or double thumb deformity is the most common (Figs. 13.46, 13.47 and 13.48). Polydactyly with three or even four deformed thumbs is also present (Figs. 13.49 and 13.50). Wassel classification divides double thumb deformities into seven types, mainly based on the level of thumb repetition, which has been commonly used for radial polydactyly.

Treatment principles: The floating thumb can be simply resected, but most of the radial polydactyly need to make full use of all the structures of the polydactyly to

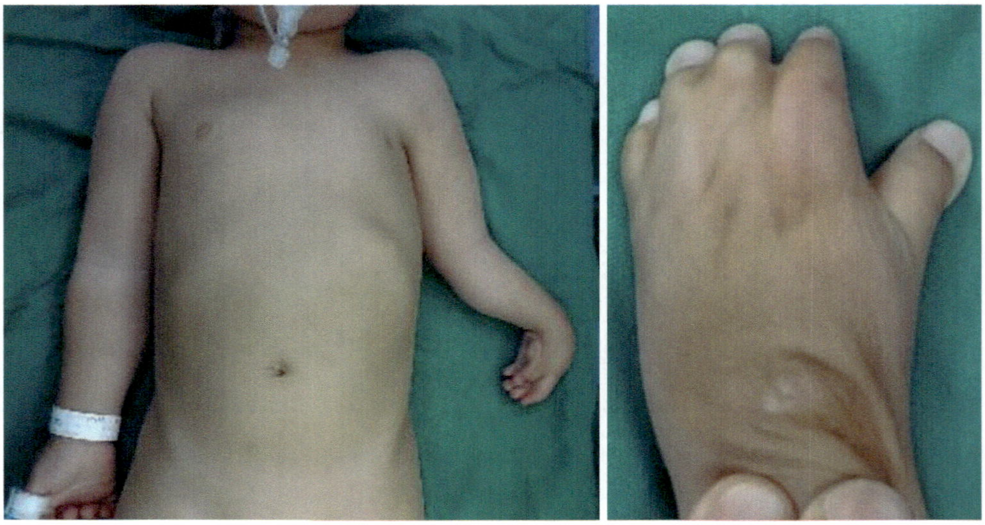

Fig. 13.45 Poland syndrome with multiple joint contractures of the left upper extremity and syndactyly of the left brachydactyly

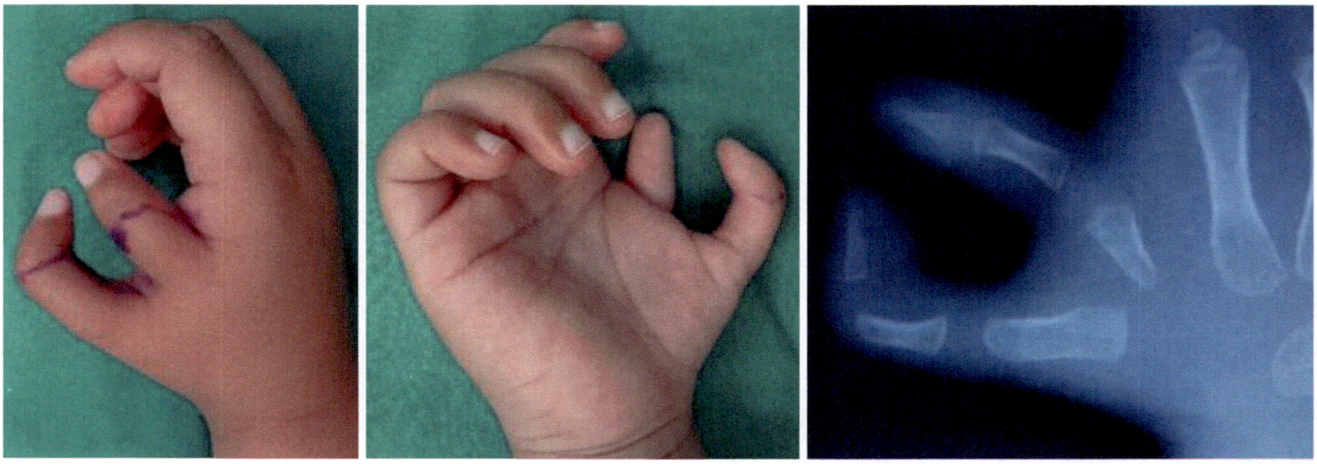

Fig. 13.46 Wassel type VI polydactyly

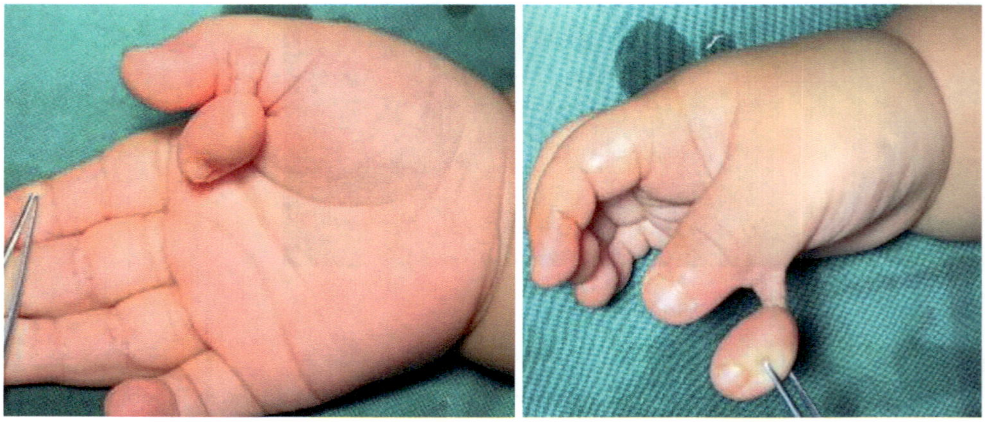

Fig. 13.47 The right thumb has a floating polydactyly, and the supernumerary thumb is connected with the main thumb by a small soft tissue pedicle

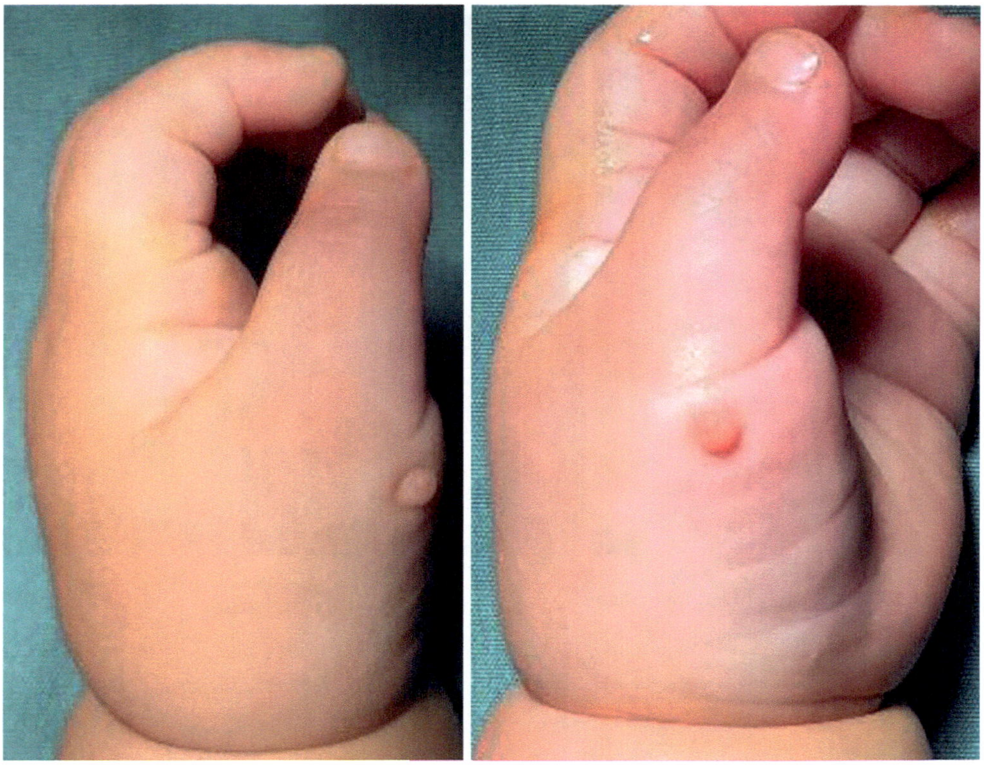

Fig. 13.48 Polydactyly of left thumb

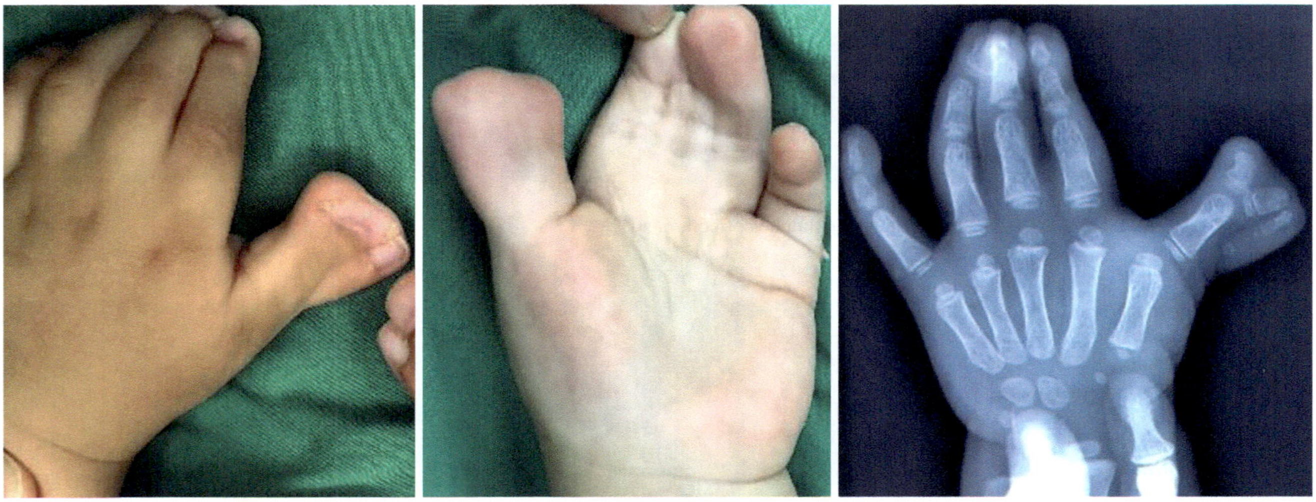

Fig. 13.49 Polydactyly of left three thumbs

reconstruct a thumb with satisfactory appearance and function as far as possible, that is, polydactyly resection and reconstruction. Other special procedures include Bilhaut-Cloquet and on-top plasty.

2. Ulnar Polydactyly Polydactyly occurring on the ulnar side of the hand (Figs. 13.51, 13.52 and 13.53) may be associated with polydactyly of the toes. Although polydactyly repetition level can be used to describe its morphological manifestations, it is often divided into soft tissue type and osteoarticular type in clinical practice.

   The principle of treatment is basically the same as that of radial polydactyly, but most ulnar polydactyly is simple in anatomy and relatively uncomplicated in treatment.
3. Central polydactyly is rare and is often associated with syndactyly and severe osteoarticular deformities (Figs. 13.54, 13.55 and 13.56).

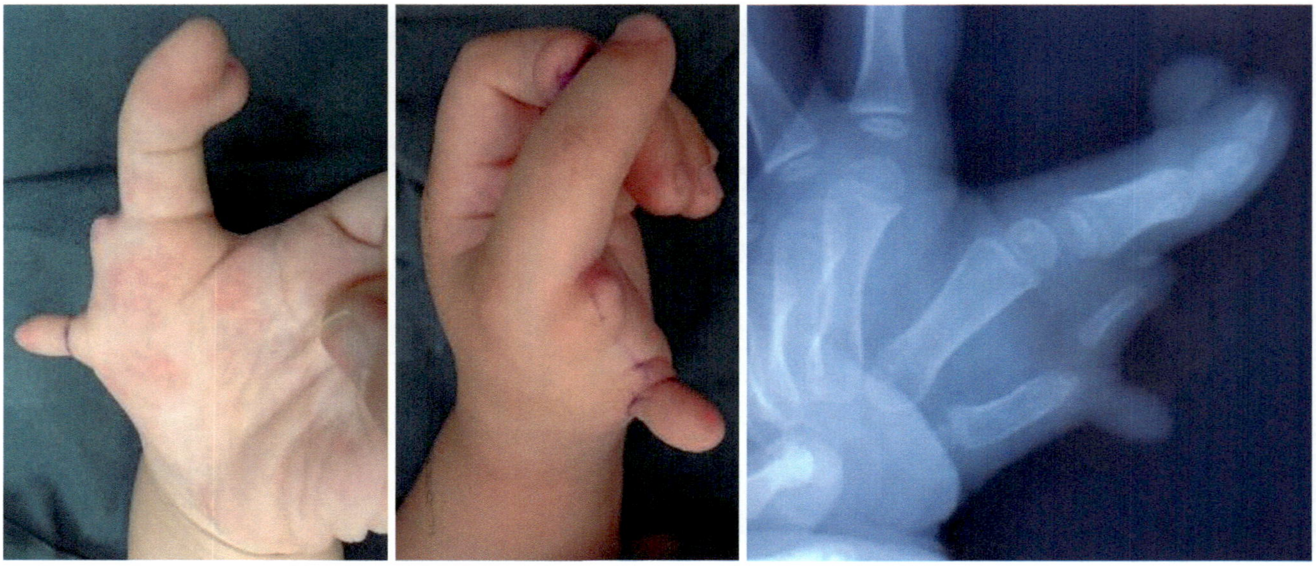

Fig. 13.50 Polydactyly of left four thumbs

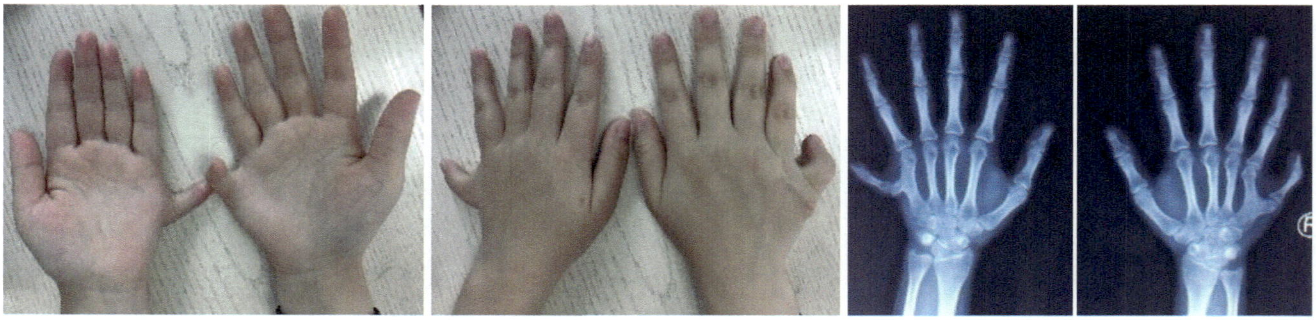

Fig. 13.51 Horizontal ulnar polydactyly of metacarpal bones of both hands

Fig. 13.52 Polydactyly on the horizontal ulnar side of the proximal phalanx of the right hand, with severe bone and joint deformity

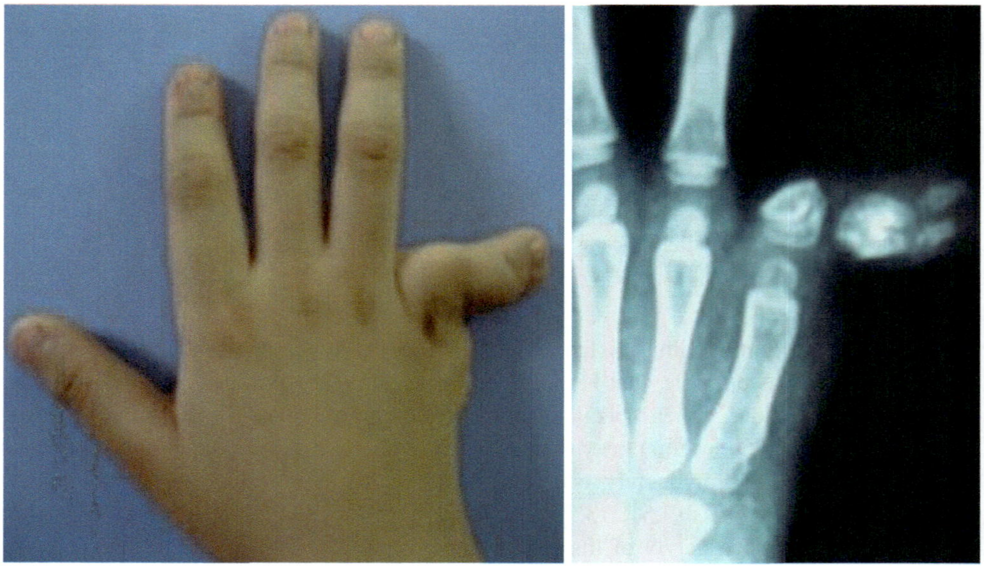

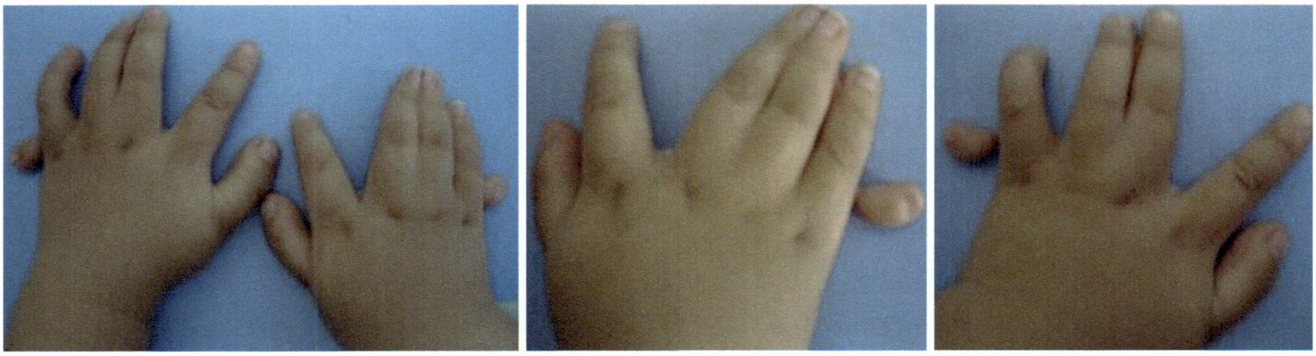

Fig. 13.53 Floating ulnar polydactyly of both hands combined with syndactyly of other fingers

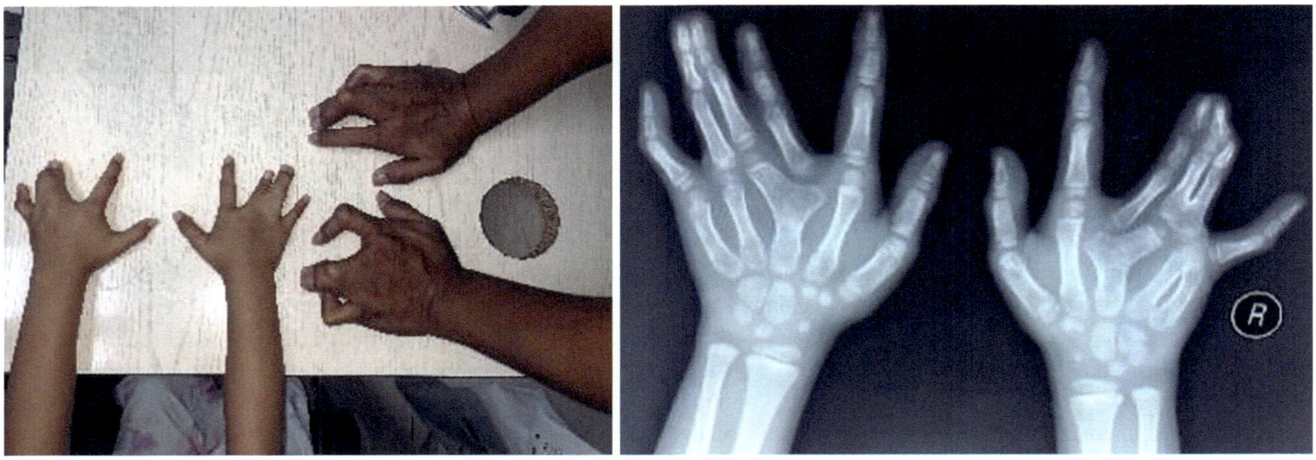

Fig. 13.54 Central polysyndactyly of both hands with positive family history

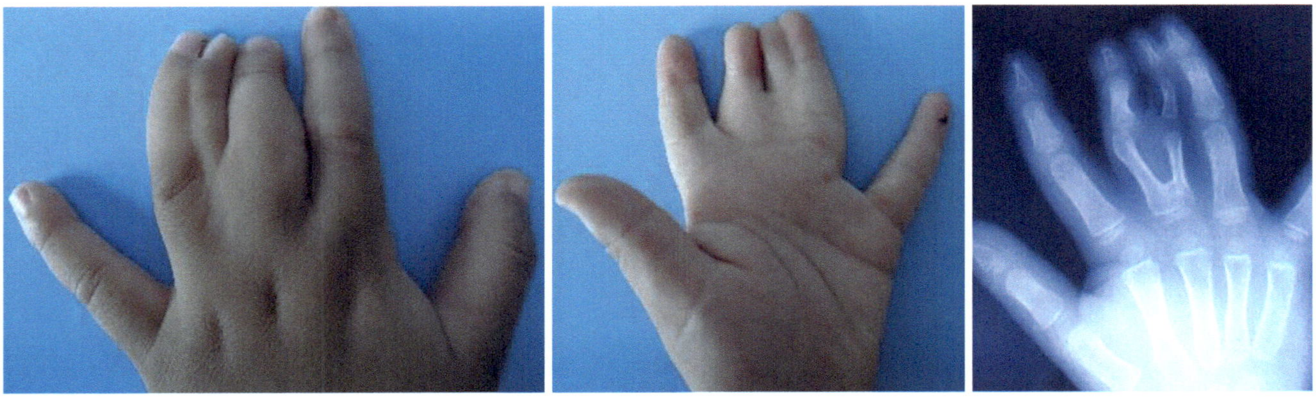

Fig. 13.55 Central polysyndactyly of left hand

Treatment principle: Most of the central polydactyly have complex morphology, complex pathological anatomy mechanism, and often combined with bony syndactyly. It is necessary to evaluate the hand function of patients before operation, and carefully select the operation to avoid further limitation of function after operation.

13.2.3 Mirror Hand

13.2.3.1 Etiology

The mirror hand, a rare congenital deformity of the hand, is named after another finger with fingers and incomplete metacarpals on the radial side of the thumb, which looks like the

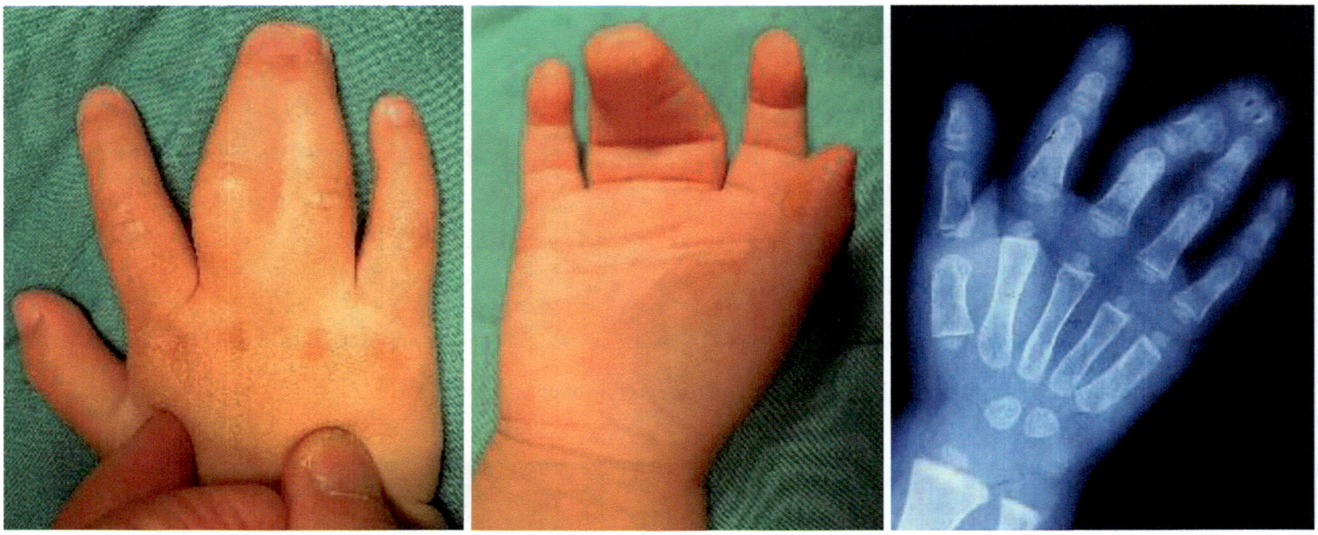

Fig. 13.56 Central polysyndactyly of right hand

shadow of the hand in the mirror. The etiology is unknown, which may be related to heredity, the key stage of embryonic hand development in the early stage of pregnancy, and the influence of internal and external harmful factors on the embryo.

13.2.3.2 Clinical Manifestations

It is characterized by polydactyly without thumb, symmetrical twin development and distribution on both sides of the fingers, generally seven fingers, but lacking the shape and structure of the thumb. The patient's hand can only be flexed and extended, and there is no palm function. X-ray examination showed that the structure development of seven fingers, metacarpals, and wrist joints was basically normal, but the thumb-like structure was absent (Fig. 13.57).

According to the principle of mirror hand reconstruction, preoperative evaluation was performed to determine how to resect the multiple fingers and metacarpals on the radial side, shorten one of the metacarpals, change the angle to the opposite palm state and fix it, and if necessary, skin plasty was performed.

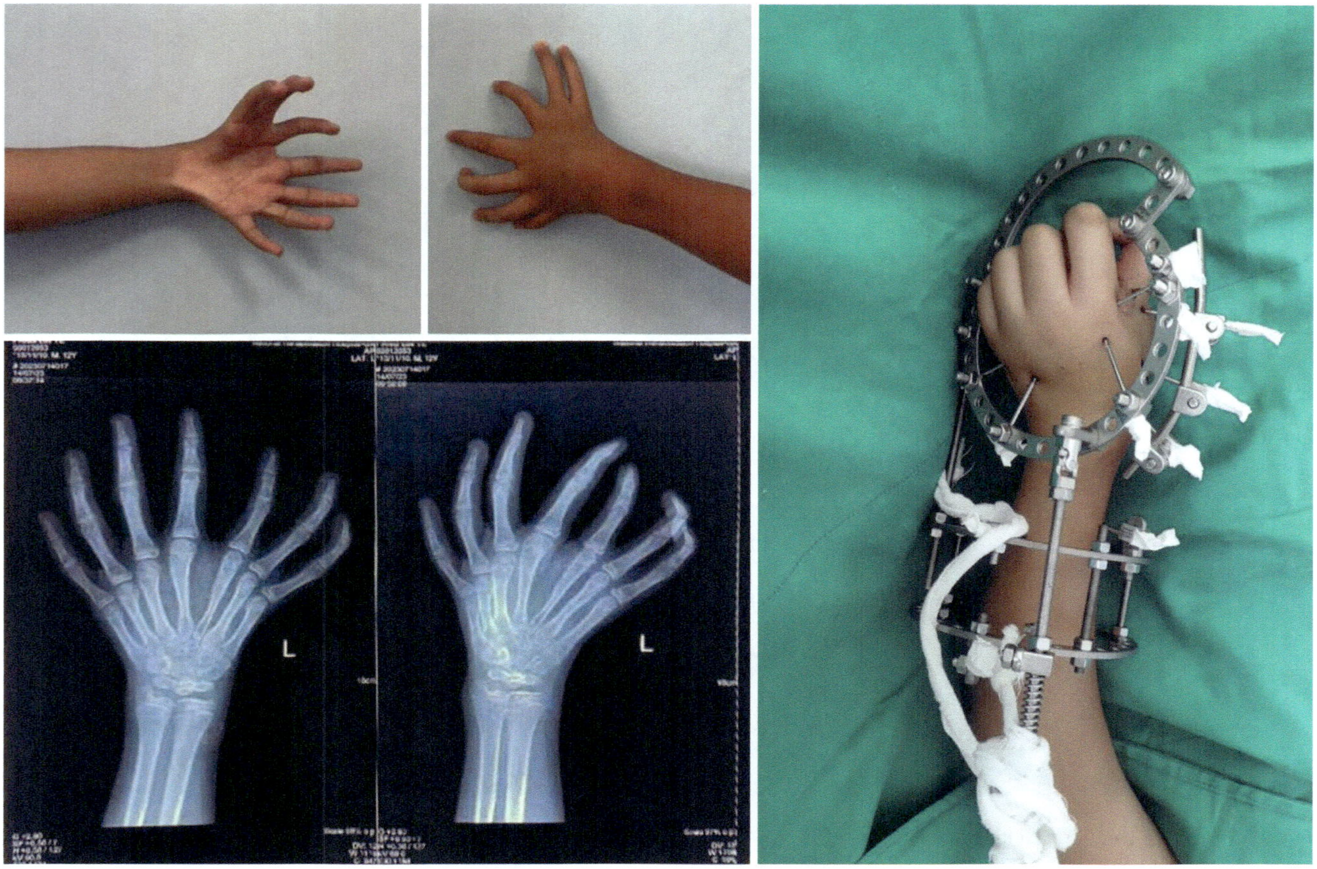

Fig. 13.57 Male, 12 years old. Left mirror image of hand shape and X-ray features before operation. Two fingers and metacarpals were resected, and one finger was fixed with a needle after reconstruction of the opposite palm shape

13.3 Congenital Radial and Ulnar Longitudinal Dysplasia with Joint Fusion

13.3.1 Radial Longitudinal Dysplasia

Radial longitudinal dysplasia is a series of deformities caused by the formation of the radial row of the hand and upper limbs, which can also be called radial dysplasia, radial crutch hand, and so on. It mainly involves the radius, radial carpus and thumb, showing dysplasia or even absence of bone joints and soft tissues to varying degrees, and can be combined with abnormalities of other parts of the limbs or organ systems, such as scoliosis, cardiovascular system defects, digestive system defects, hematopoietic system dysfunction, etc.

13.3.1.1 Etiology

Potential causes of radial longitudinal dysplasia include intrauterine compression, vascular insufficiency, trauma, maternal drug exposure, and genetic mutations, which can be one of the phenotypes of a congenital syndrome.

13.3.1.2 Clinical Manifestations and Classification

Bayne classification is commonly used to classify radial longitudinal dysplasia into four types: type I: the radius is slightly shortened relative to the ulna, but the anatomical shape is still normal (Fig. 13.58); type II: the basic shape of the radius is present, but significantly short (Fig. 13.59); type III: the radius is partially absent (Fig. 13.60); Type IV (Fig. 13.61): Complete absence of the radius: the most severe and common type.

Thumb dysplasia is often associated and is discussed separately in view of its functional importance.

13.3.1.3 Treatment Principle

The disease requires systematic and continuous treatment, treatment and correction should be started from the discovery of deformities, and non-surgical methods and surgical

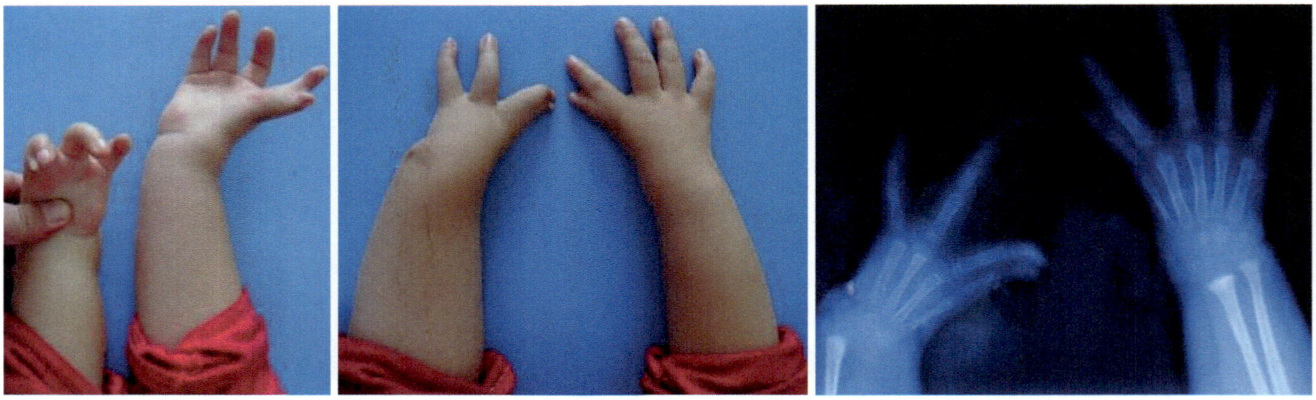

Fig. 13.58 Bilateral radial longitudinal dysplasia. The right side is Bayne I type

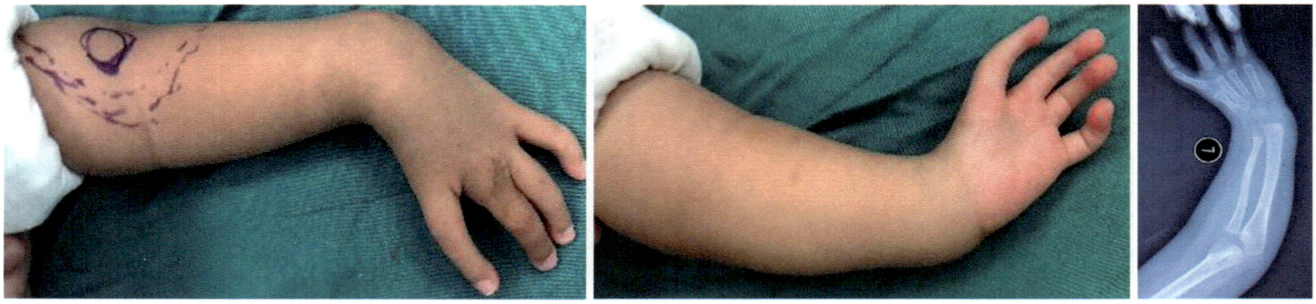

Fig. 13.59 Bayne type II radial longitudinal dysplasia

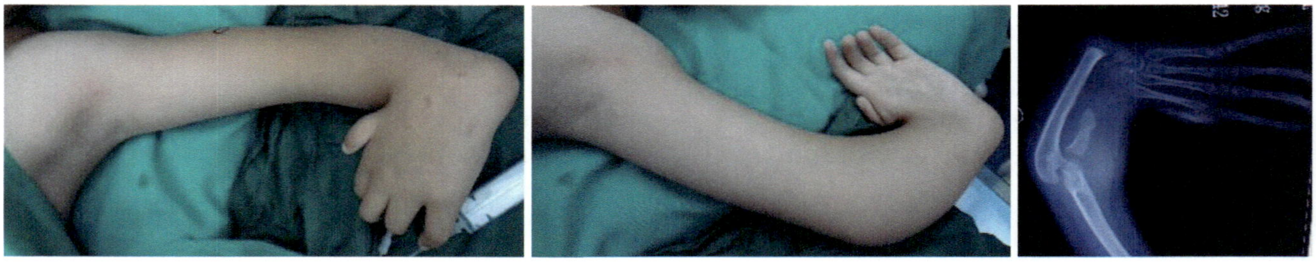

Fig. 13.60 Bayne type III radial longitudinal dysplasia

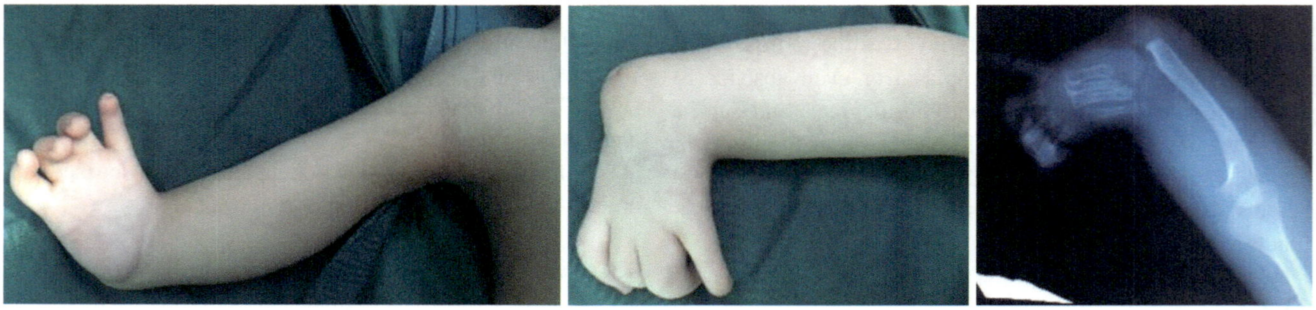

Fig. 13.61 Bayne type IV radial longitudinal dysplasia

treatment should be coordinated. However, for those who are older, miss the opportunity of early intervention, and whose hand function can meet the needs of daily life, they cannot be treated by surgery.

13.3.2 Thumb Dysplasia

Thumb hypoplasia is a part of radial longitudinal dysplasia, and the severity of the deformity can range from a slight reduction in thumb size to complete absence.

13.3.2.1 Etiology

It is basically the same as the dysplasia of the radial inter-hemispheric fissure.

13.3.2.2 Clinical Manifestation

The modified Blauth classification is often used clinically: type I: the thumb is smaller than the contralateral side, the thenar muscle is slightly hypoplastic, but the thumb function is basically normal (Fig. 13.62). Type II: Thumb is significantly developed and small, mainly manifested as dysplasia of internal structures of the thumb, such as metacarpophalangeal joint capsule ligament, thenar muscle, etc. (Fig. 13.63). Type III: In addition to type II manifestations, the first carpometacarpal joint dysplasia and external muscle abnormalities were present. It can be further divided into IIIA (Fig. 13.64): carpometacarpal joint is present; IIIB (Fig. 13.65): carpometacarpal joint is absent. IV: floating thumb (Fig. 13.66). The thumb of the V: is completely absent (Fig. 13.67).

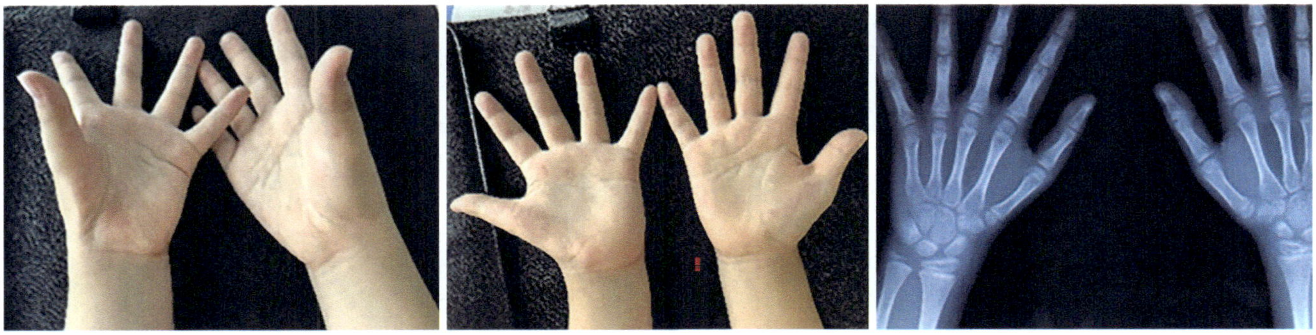

Fig. 13.62 Modified Blauth I thumb dysplasia in the left hand

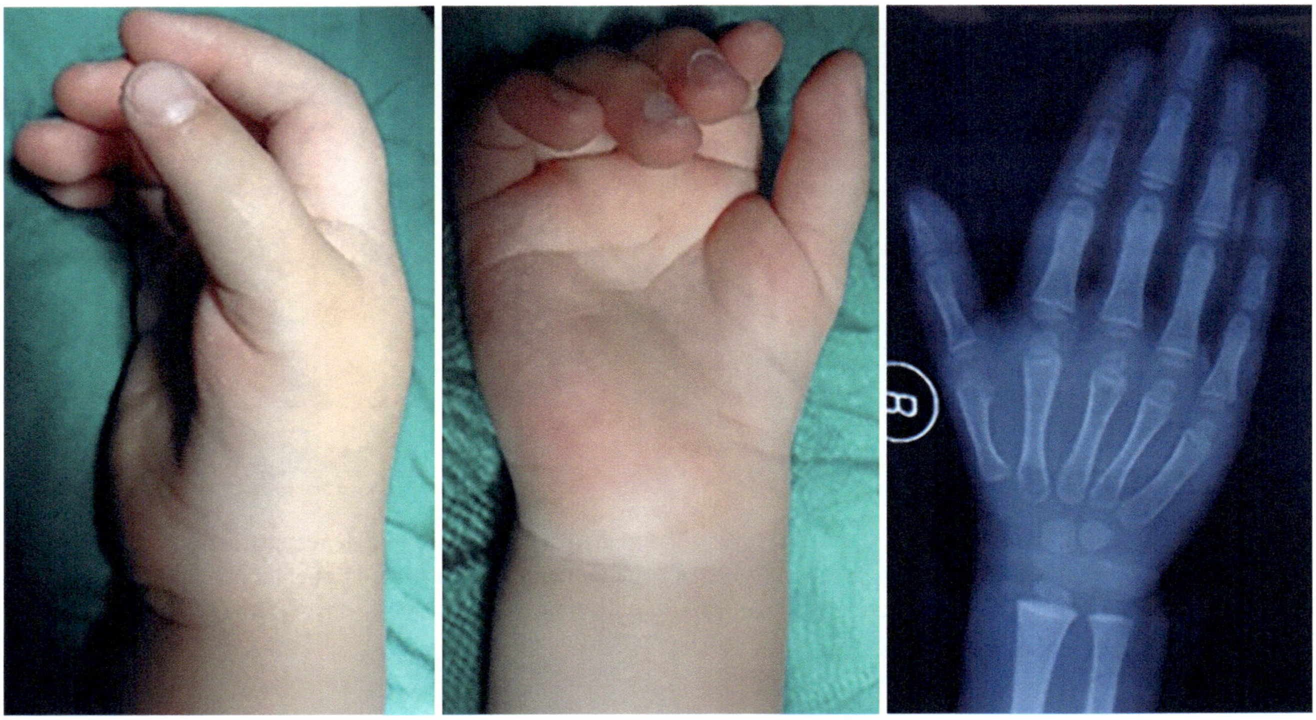

Fig. 13.63 Modified Blauth II thumb dysplasia

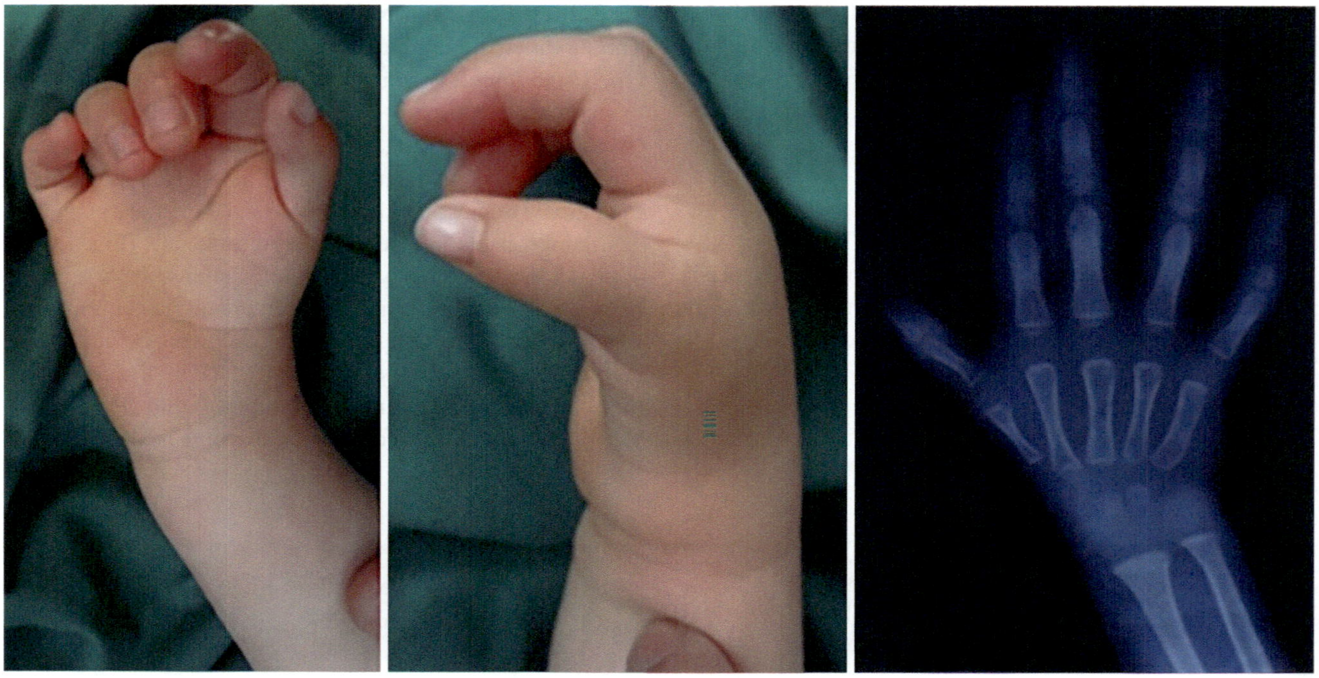

Fig. 13.64 Modified Blauth type IIIA thumb dysplasia

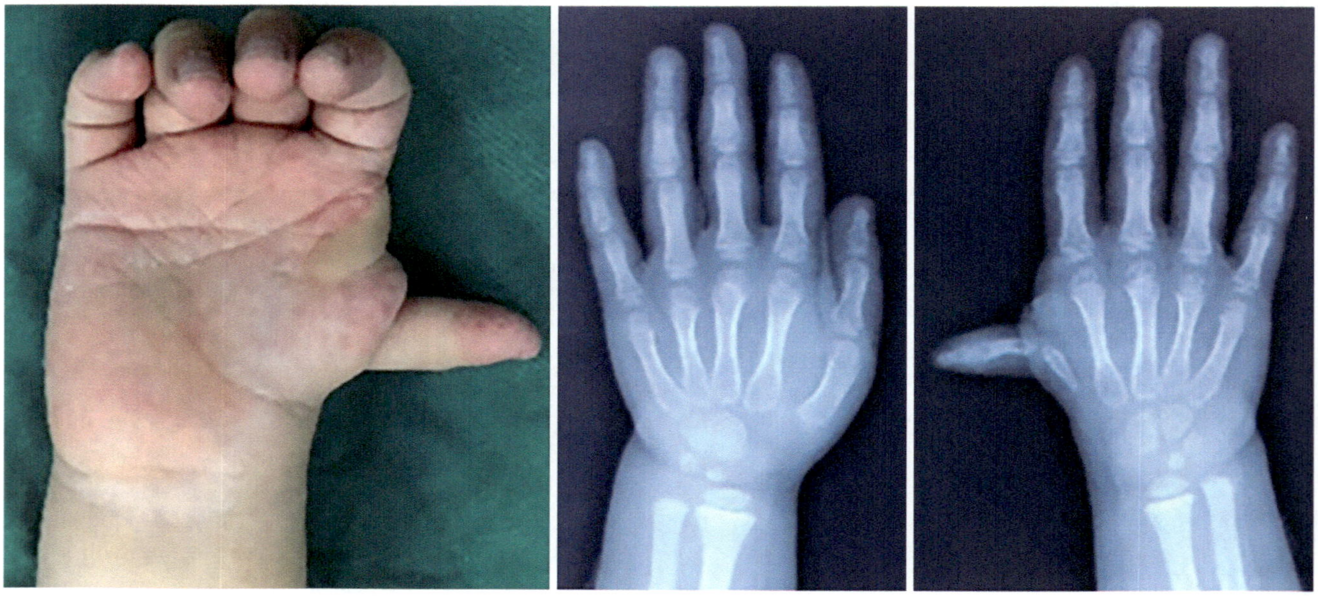

Fig. 13.65 Modified Blauth type IIIB thumb dysplasia in the right hand

13.3.2.3 Treatment Principle

According to the clinical classification, type II and type IIIA can be treated with various thumb function reconstruction operations, while type IIIB, type IV, and type V can be treated with various thumb reconstruction operations and index thumb reconstruction operations, and the timing and indications of various operations should be strictly controlled.

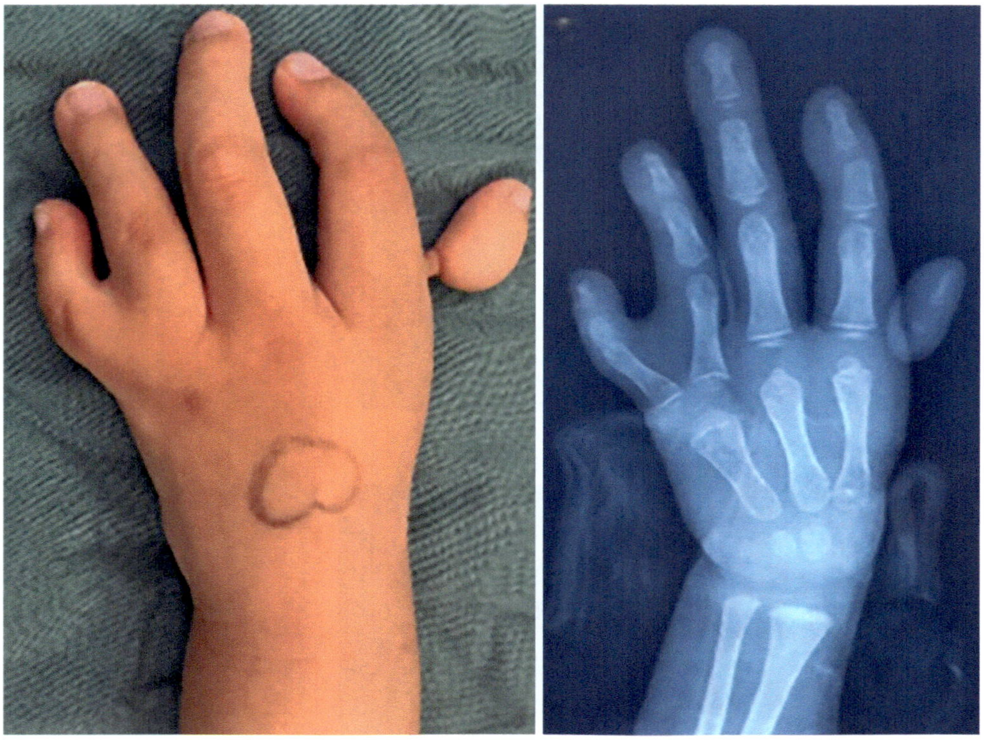

Fig. 13.66 Modified Blauth type IV thumb dysplasia

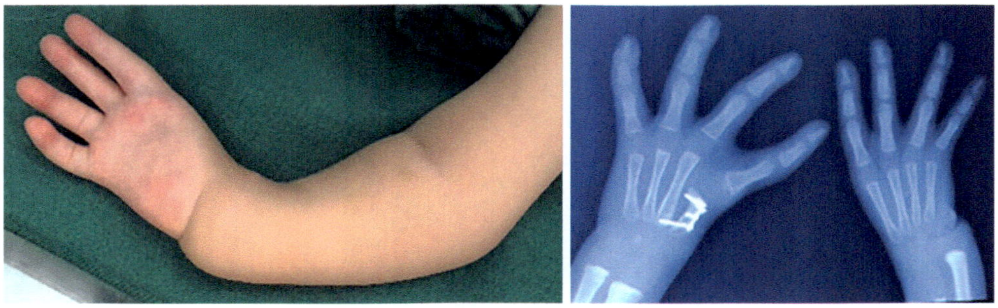

Fig. 13.67 The right hand was modified Blauth V thumb dysplasia with complete absence of the thumb

13.3.3 Ulnar Longitudinal Dysplasia

Ulnar longitudinal dysplasi, also known as ulnar crutch-hand deformity, includes a series of deformities caused by the formation of the ulnar row of the upper limb.

13.3.3.1 Etiology

The etiology of ulnar longitudinal dysplasia is unknown, and it is currently considered to be a sporadic, non-genetic disorder, but there are reports of positive family history. The disease may be associated with other musculoskeletal disorders, such as focal proximal femoral defects, fibular defects, fibular deformities, and scoliosis.

13.3.3.2 Clinical Manifestation

The typical manifestations are shortening of the forearm, bowing to the dorsal side of the radius, deviation of the hand and wrist to the ulnar side, and other deformities of the hand and upper limbs, such as syndactyly, ectrodactyly, thumb dysplasia, etc.

According to the degree of ulnar dysplasia, it can be divided into five types. Type I: slight shortening of ulna with complete shape (Fig. 13.68); Type II: small ulna with more than 2 cm shortening (Fig. 13.69); Type III: partial absence of ulna (Fig. 13.70); Type IV: complete absence of ulna (Fig. 13.71); Type V: combined with brachioradial fusion or radioulnar fusion (Fig. 13.72).

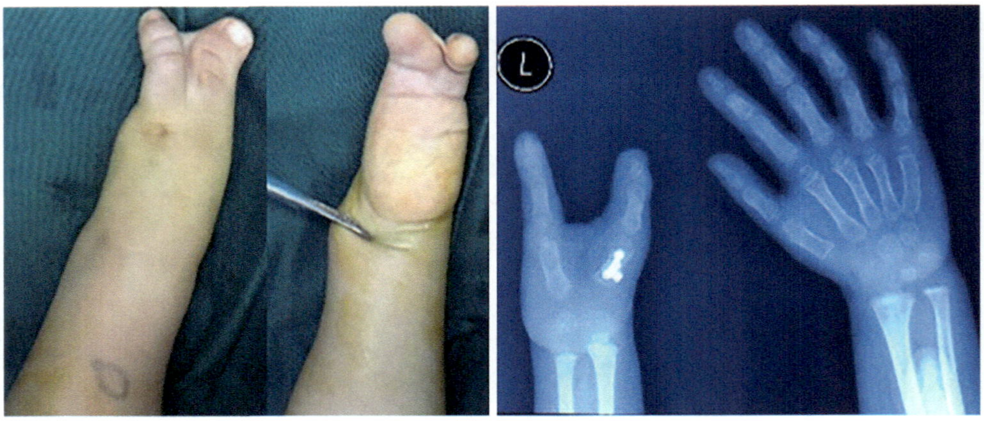

Fig. 13.68 Left ulnar longitudinal dysplasia type I: the ulna is slightly shortened and the shape is still intact. X-ray showed that the finger was separated and the first metacarpal bone was osteotomized

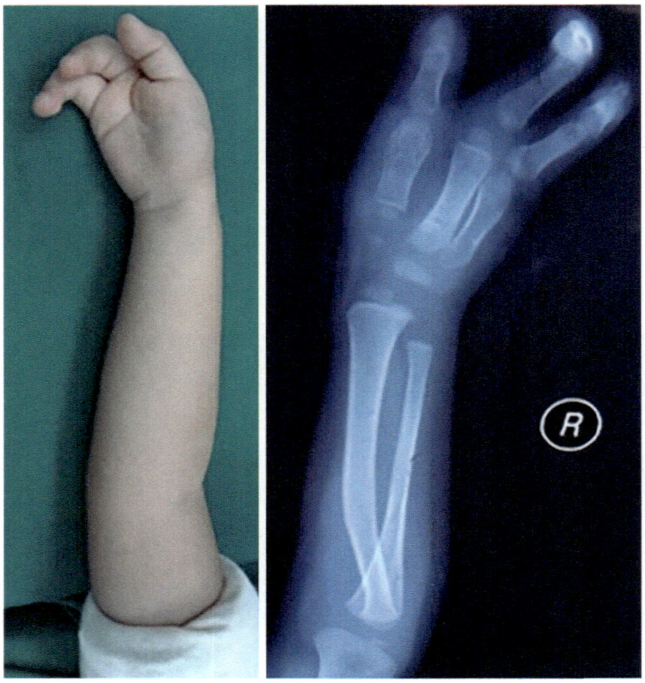

Fig. 13.69 Right ulnar longitudinal dysplasia type II: the ulna is small and shortened by more than 2 cm

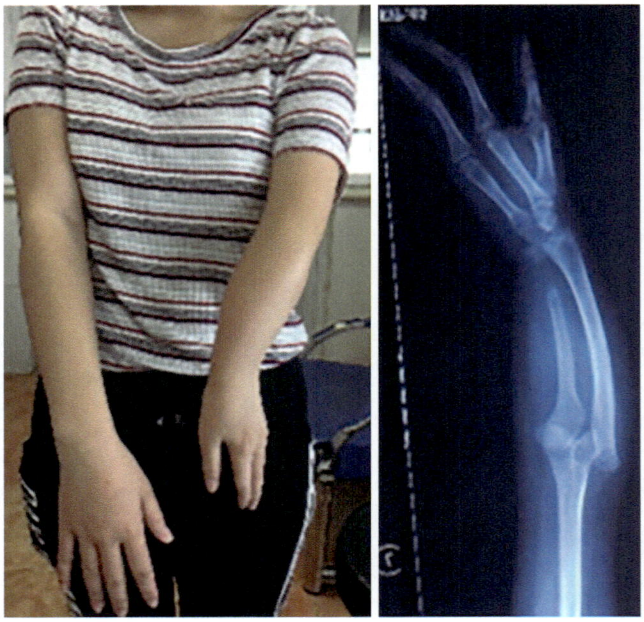

Fig. 13.70 Left ulnar longitudinal dysplasia type III: partial absence of the ulna with visible dislocation of the radial head

13.3.3.3 Treatment Principle

The disease can involve the elbow joint, ulna and radius, wrist joint, and hand deformities with impaired function, and the treatment should be considered comprehensively to improve hand function.

13.3.4 Madelung Deformity

Madelung deformity, mainly involving the wrist and forearm, is a rare upper limb deformity, which is a common type of wrist deformity caused by distal radius dysplasia. The radiographic features include volar and ulnar deviation of the distal radius, and the change of the proximal carpal bone of the proximal row of the wrist joint from a curved arch to a pointed shape. Madelung deformity with the presence of Vickers ligament, which can be called true Madelung deformity, accounts for about 90% of cases.

13.3.4.1 Etiology

The direct cause is the dysplasia of the ulnar and palmar epiphyses of the distal radius, which may be related to trauma, osteochondral dysplasia, dystrophic dysplasia, genetic factors, and so on. Syndromic Madelung deformities mainly include Leri-Weill dyschondrosteosis (LWD) and Turner syndrome (TS), both of which are related to SHOX gene (short homeobox containing gene).

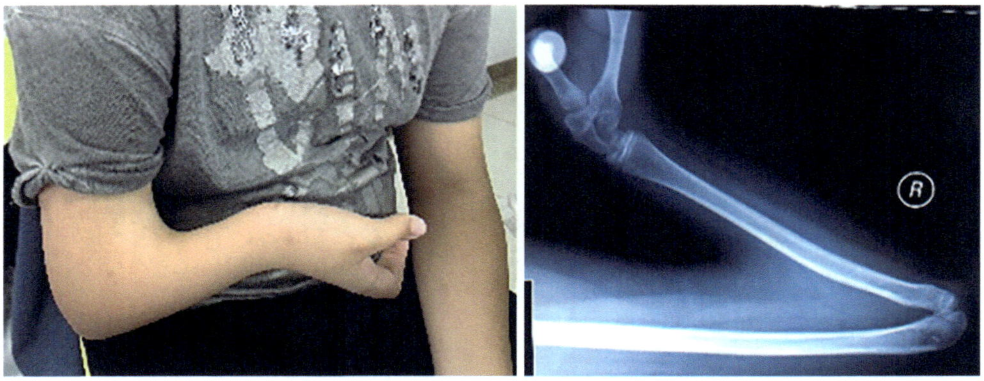

Fig. 13.71 Right ulnar longitudinal dysplasia type IV: complete absence of the ulna

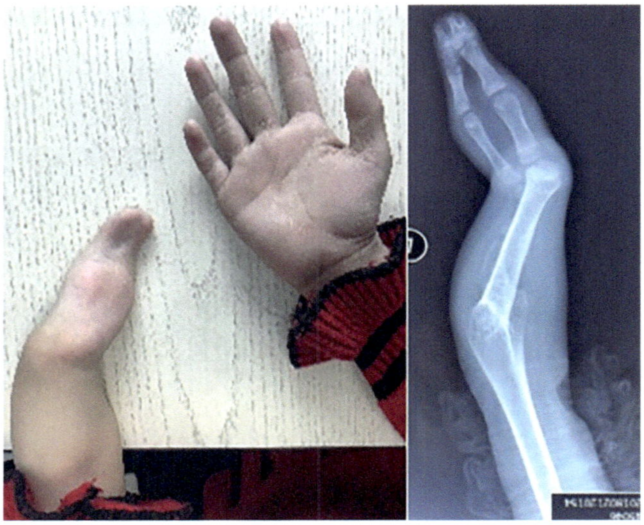

Fig. 13.72 Left ulnar longitudinal dysplasia V: combined with brachioradial fusion

13.3.4.2 Clinical Manifestation

This kind of malformation can occur in both men and women, but it is more common in women, and it can occur unilaterally or bilaterally. Clinical manifestations include distal ulna protrusion dorsally and distally to the radius. Wrist joint movement was limited, especially in dorsiflexion and ulnar deviation, while wrist flexion increased. When the deformity is severe or the course of disease is long, the wrist is painful, weak, and unstable.

Typical radiographic findings include (Figs. 13.73, 13.74, 13.75 and 13.76): volar and ulnar flexion of the distal radius, increased inclination of the distal radial articular surface, inverted triangular arrangement of the carpal bones, proximal volar displacement of the lunate, significant positive ulnar variation, and dorsal dislocation of the ulnar head. Bone and joint degeneration and spontaneous rupture of tendons may occur in the elderly. Madelung deformity can be evaluated on radiographs, and there are 3 thresholds to assist in diagnosis: ulnar deviation angle ≥30°, lunate subsidence ≥4–5 mm, and volar carpal displacement ≥15 mm on standard anteroposterior wrist radiographs.

13.3.4.3 Treatment Principle

Asymptomatic patients can be treated conservatively, and early deformity with pain can be treated by wearing orthopedic braces and adjusting activity patterns.

The main surgical indications for Madelung deformity include wrist deformity, recurrent and persistent pain, and limited mobility. At present, there is no unified standard for the surgical treatment of this disease.

For patients with skeletal immaturity, indications for surgery include: (1) no pain, but progressive deformity and unsatisfactory appearance; (2) Symptomatic deformity. Vickers ligament release and distal radial epiphyseal release are recommended as early as possible to prevent further deterioration of the disease if the child has great growth potential and obvious deformity progression, and distal ulnar epiphyseal block is necessary.

For patients with skeletal maturity, surgical treatments include radial osteotomy alone, ulnar osteotomy alone, combined radioulnar osteotomy, DRUJ plasty (Sauv Sauvé-Kapandji procedure), DRUJ arthroplasty, arthrodesis, and selective wrist denervation.

13.3.5 Congenital Radioulnar Arthrodesis

Radioulnar synostosis refers to the different forms of fusion of the radius and ulna, which is characterized by limited rotation of the forearm and fixation at a certain angle. Most of them were proximal fusion of radius and ulna, and distal fusion was rare, which could be combined with bony fusion of elbow joint.

13.3.5.1 Etiology

The disease is caused by ossification without separation between ulna and radius cartilage during embryonic development or by filling mesodermal tissue between ulna and

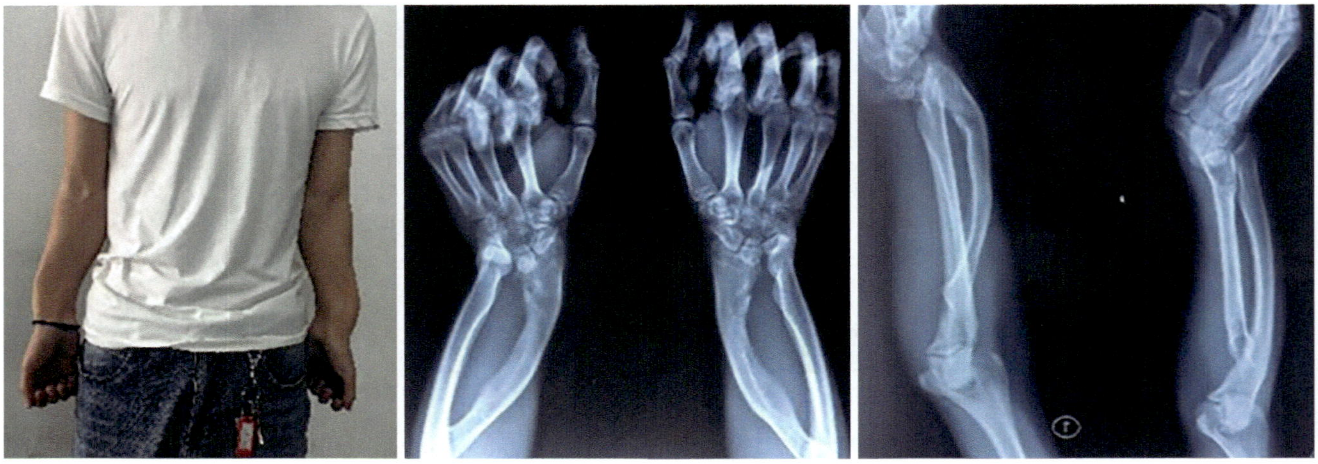

Fig. 13.73 Young male, bilateral Madelung deformity, with typical gross appearance and radiographic appearance

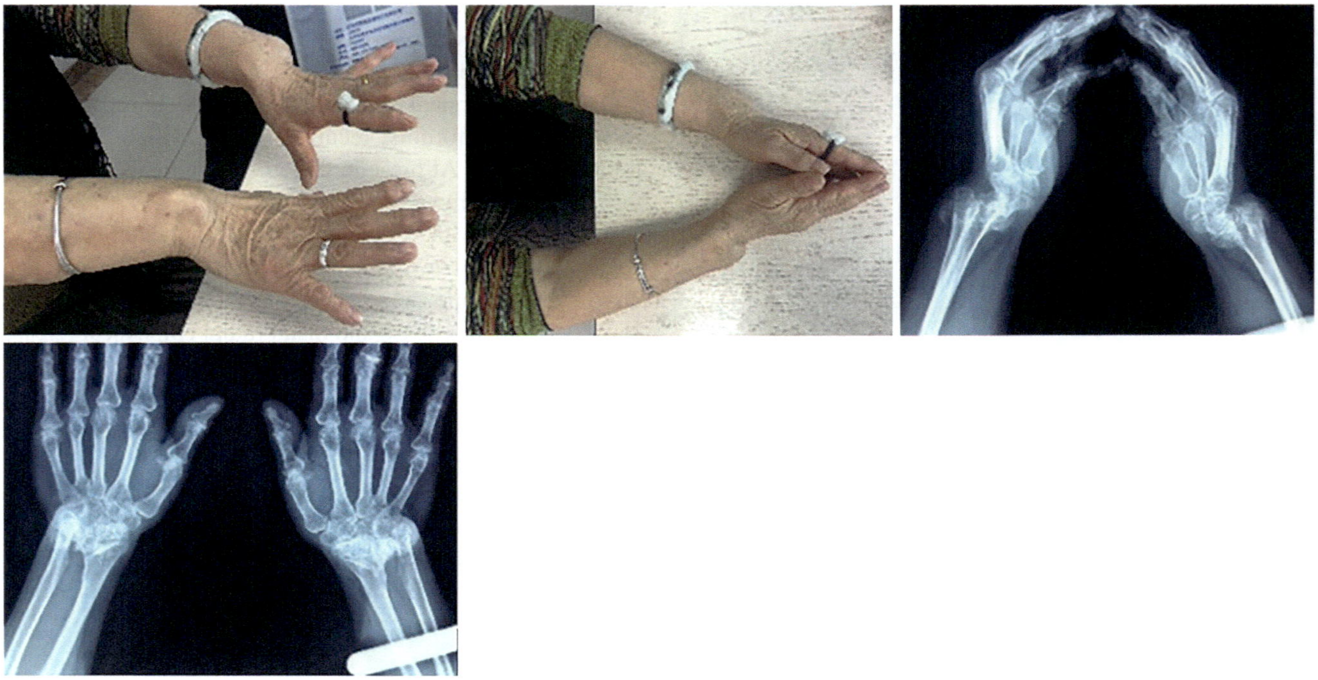

Fig. 13.74 Elderly female, bilateral Madelung deformity, in addition to typical gross appearance and X-ray findings, has degenerative arthritis of bone and joint

radius. Some cases have family history, and most of them are autosomal dominant inheritance. The disease can also be seen in Poland syndrome, Holt-Oram syndrome, Cornelia de Lange syndrome, and other congenital diseases.

13.3.5.2 Clinical Manifestation

The clinical manifestation is that the forearm rotation is limited, and most of them are fixed in the pronation position of the forearm. The degree of limitation of forearm function depends on the fixed position of forearm rotation and whether it is bilateral involvement. The movement of shoulder joint and wrist joint compensates part of the forearm rotation function.

At present, the disease is divided into four types according to imaging findings (Figs. 13.77, 13.78, 13.79, 13.80, 13.81 and 13.82). Type I: no bony symphysis was found on the X-ray film, and the radial head was reduced, but the overall shape was normal. Type II: osseous symphysis can be seen, and other structures are basically normal (Fig. 13.77). Type III: osseous symphysis with radial head hypoplasia and

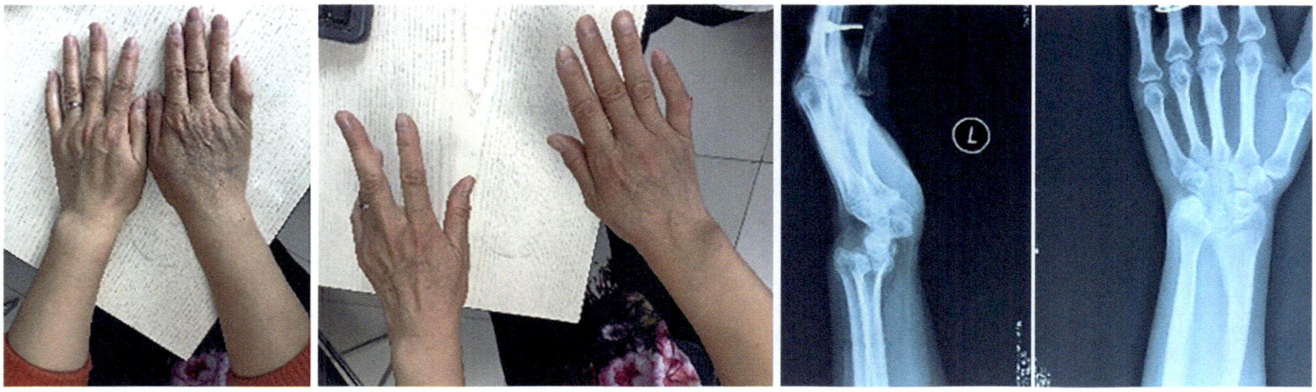

Fig. 13.75 This is an elderly female with left Madelung deformity. In gross appearance, the active extension of the ring and little finger is limited, suggesting spontaneous rupture of the tendon

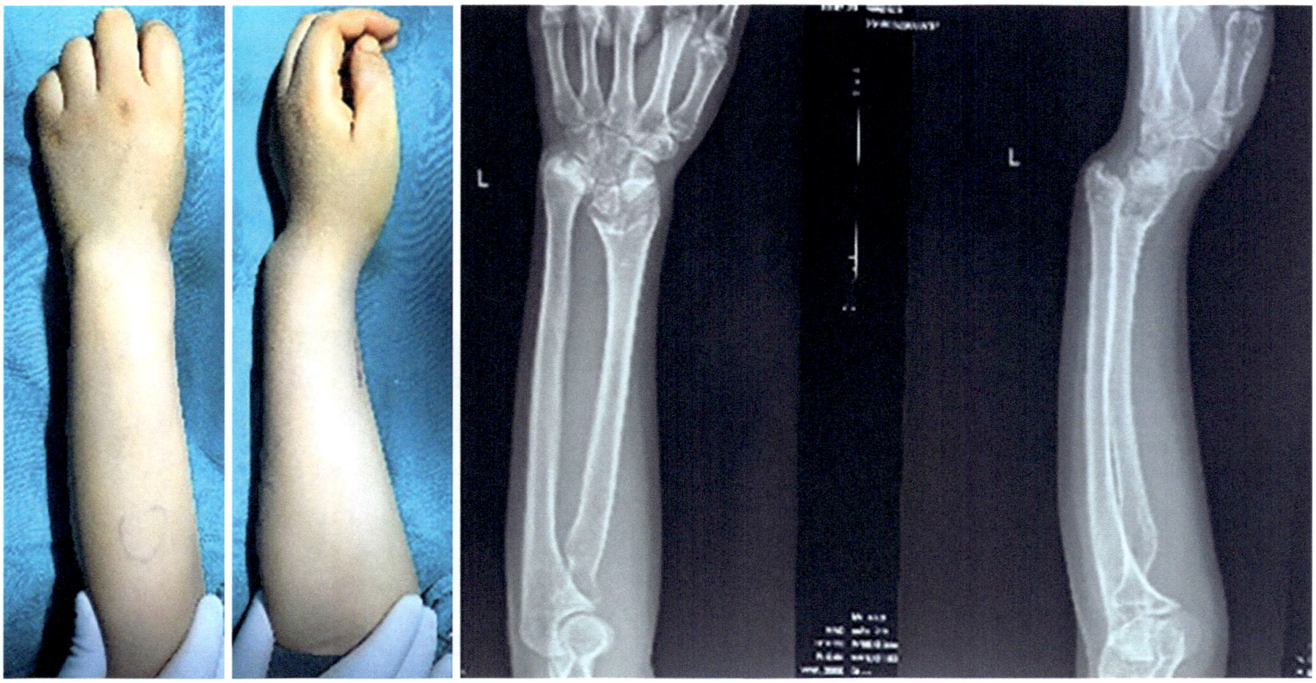

Fig. 13.76 Adolescent female, 14 years old, left Madelung deformity, proximal radius dysplasia

posterior dislocation of the radial head can be seen (Fig. 13.78). Type IV: short bony symphysis with anteriorly dislocated mushroom-shaped radial head (Fig. 13.79). There is no specific classification for more types of ulnar and radial fusion (Figs. 13.80 and 13.81).

13.3.5.3 Treatment Principle

The optimal treatment of congenital ulnar and radial fusion is still uncertain, which usually depends on the location and degree of fusion, the degree of functional limitation and bilateral involvement. If the disease occurs on one side or on both sides, but the fixed position of rotation is close to the neutral position, conservative treatment can be considered.

13.3.6 Congenital Elbow Fusion

Congenital elbow fusion (Elbow Synostosis) is very rare and may occur alone, but it is often associated with other malformations or is the manifestation of a syndrome.

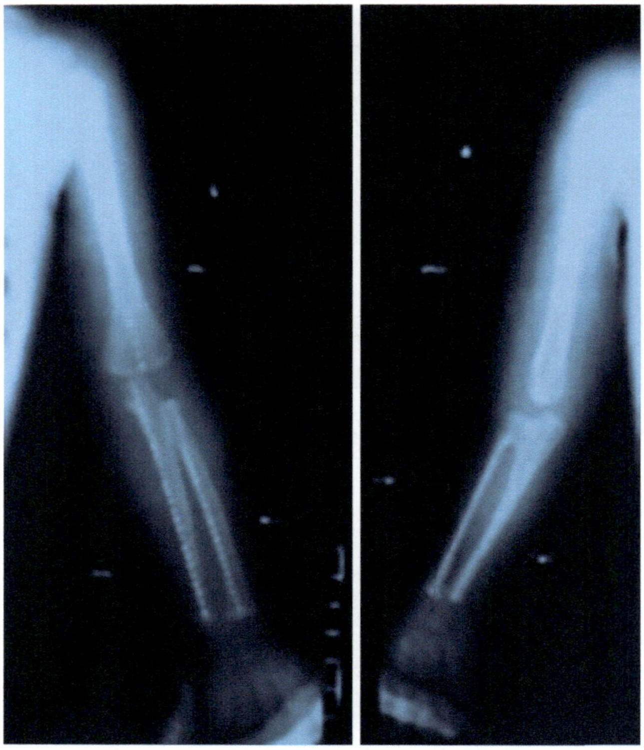

Fig. 13.77 Bilateral type II ulnar and radial fusion

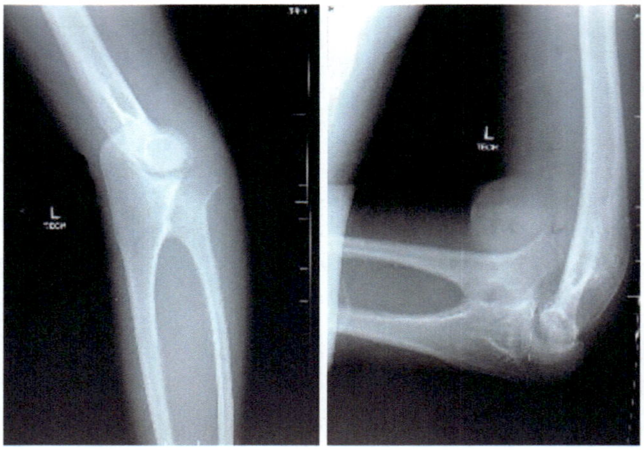

Fig. 13.79 Left type IV ulnoradial fusion with anteriorly dislocated mushroom-shaped radial head

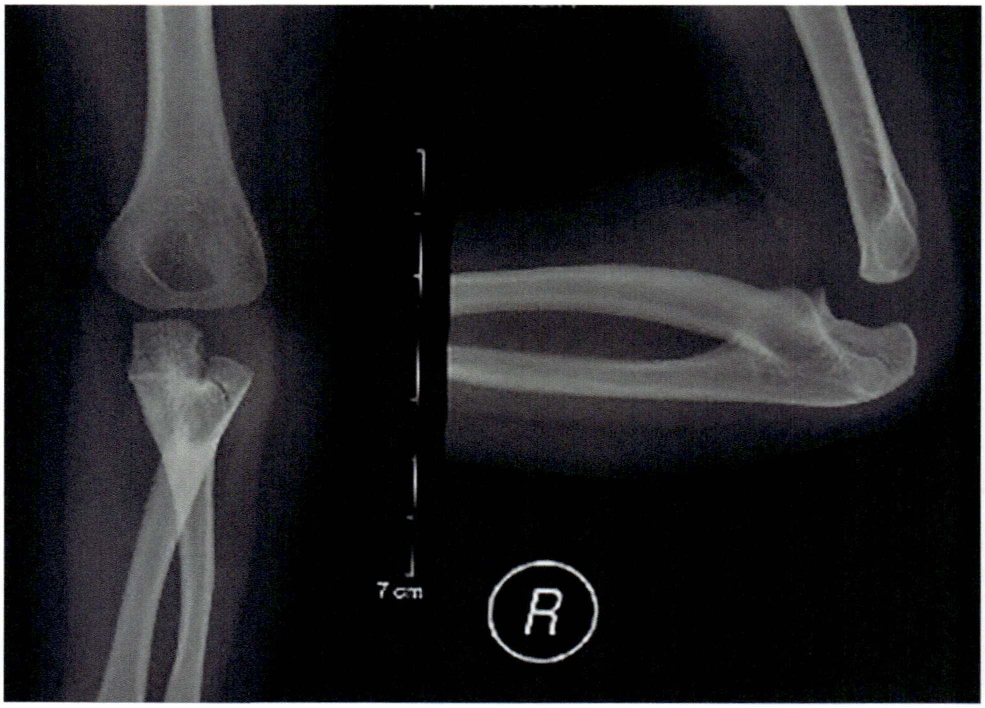

Fig. 13.78 Type III ulnoradial fusion on the right. In addition to the osseous symphysis, radial head hypoplasia and posterior dislocation of the radial head are also seen

13.3.6.1 Etiology

The pathogenesis is not clear. Dysplasia of the ulnar interhemispheric fissure, Apert syndrome, Herrmann's multiple fusion syndrome, and some chromosomal abnormalities may present with congenital elbow fusion.

13.3.6.2 Clinical Manifestation

Elbow fusions that occur alone often involve one limb, while syndromic elbow fusions often involve both limbs.

According to the fusion, it can be divided into humeral-radial-ulnar fusion (Fig. 13.82), humeral-radial fusion

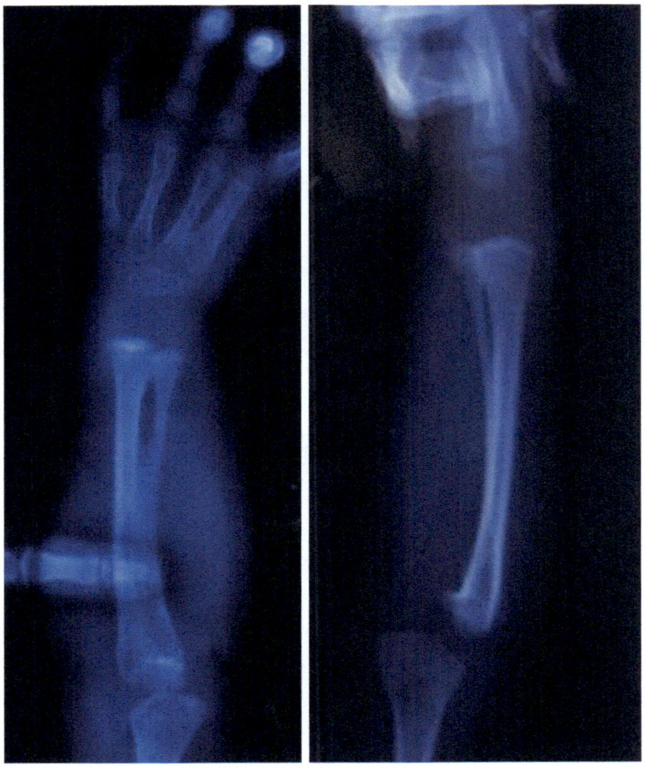

Fig. 13.80 Special type of ulna and radius fusion, distal and proximal fusion separately

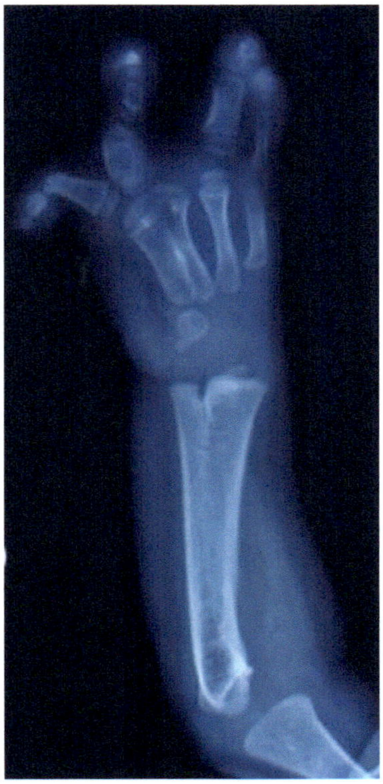

Fig. 13.81 Special type of ulna and radius fusion, almost complete fusion

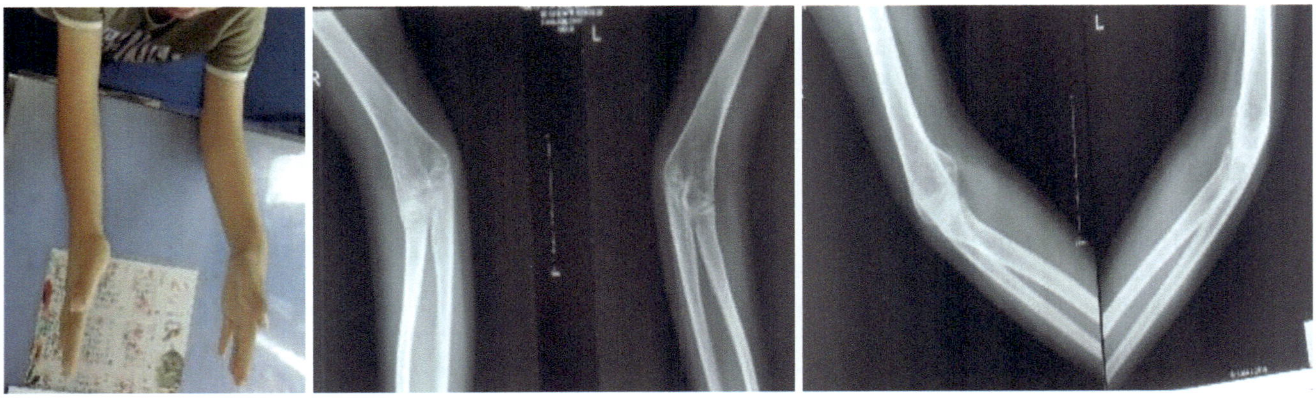

Fig. 13.82 Fusion of left brachial-radial-ulnar joint

(Fig. 13.83), and humeral-ulnar fusion, which can be combined with proximal ulnar and radial fusion. The clinical manifestations are elbow joint deformity with active and passive range of motion deficiency, forearm shortness, and hand deformity, which may be combined with other organ system abnormalities. In infancy, arthrodesis may be cartilaginous and not visible on radiographs. With the increase of age and the gradual ossification of cartilage, the elbow joint fusion can be shown on the X-ray film.

13.3.6.3 Treatment Principle

The prognosis of this deformity is poor, and the treatment is mainly to improve limb function, which can achieve basic daily use. If only the appearance is considered, orthopedic surgery can be performed to correct the forearm bending deformity, and the elbow flexion angle and forearm length can be increased appropriately.

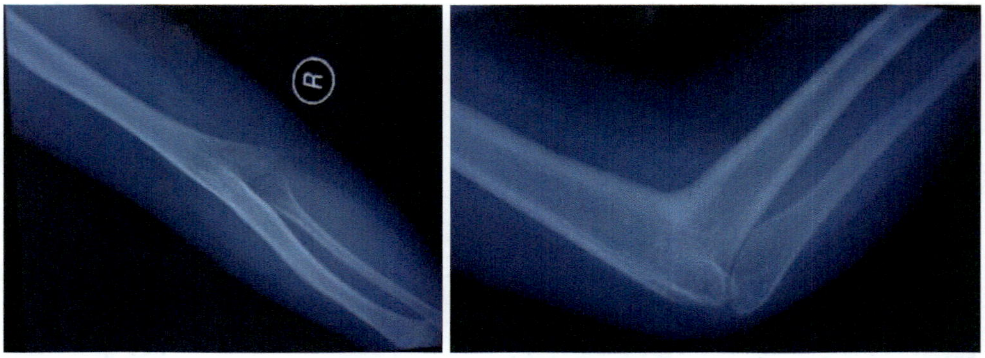

Fig. 13.83 Fusion of right humeroradial joint

13.4 Hand Deformity Syndromic

13.4.1 Apert Syndrome

Apert syndrome is a rare congenital syndrome involving the hand, foot, craniofacial, and other important internal organs, with characteristic morphological features of hand, foot, and craniofacial deformities.

13.4.1.1 Etiology

More than 80% of the cases are caused by mutations in the FGFR2 gene, which is located at 10q25-q26.

13.4.1.2 Clinical Manifestation

It mainly includes the following aspects. Cranial deformities: Facial deformities: midface dysplasia, exophthalmos; Limb deformities: Bilateral symmetric complex syndactyly with wide deviation of the thumb (hallux) (Figs. 13.84, 13.85, 13.86 and 13.87). It may also be associated with cleft palate (Fig. 13.88), scoliosis, heart disease, etc.

13.4.1.3 Treatment Principle

The standard of treatment for hand and foot deformities is to separate syndactyly and restore the basic grasping, grasping and pinching functions of the hand, and priority should be given to the treatment of syndactyly of thumb and index finger. For foot deformities, if patients can complete basic walking, running, and other functions, they can communicate with their parents without surgical treatment.

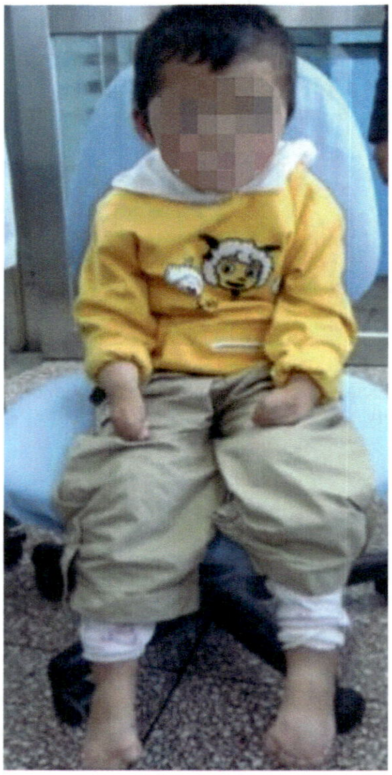

Fig. 13.84 Facial deformity and syndactyly of hands, feet, and fingers characteristic of Apert syndrome

13.4.2 Poland Syndrome

Poland syndrome is a group of congenital upper limb malformation sequence combination with the main clinical manifestations of unilateral pectoral muscle absence or dysplasia, short upper limb, especially the hand, brachydactyly or brachysyndactyly.

13.4.2.1 Etiology

At present, it is generally accepted that at the sixth or seventh week of gestation, abnormal changes in mesodermal differentiation lead to the distortion of subclavian artery development, resulting in dysplasia of one side of subclavian artery or its branches, internal thoracic artery, etc., resulting in chest wall and hand deformities. Poland syndrome is considered to be a non-hereditary disease, and some patients have a clear history of abnormal pregnancy (referring to the history of viral infection, antibiotic use, threatened abortion or trauma in early pregnancy).

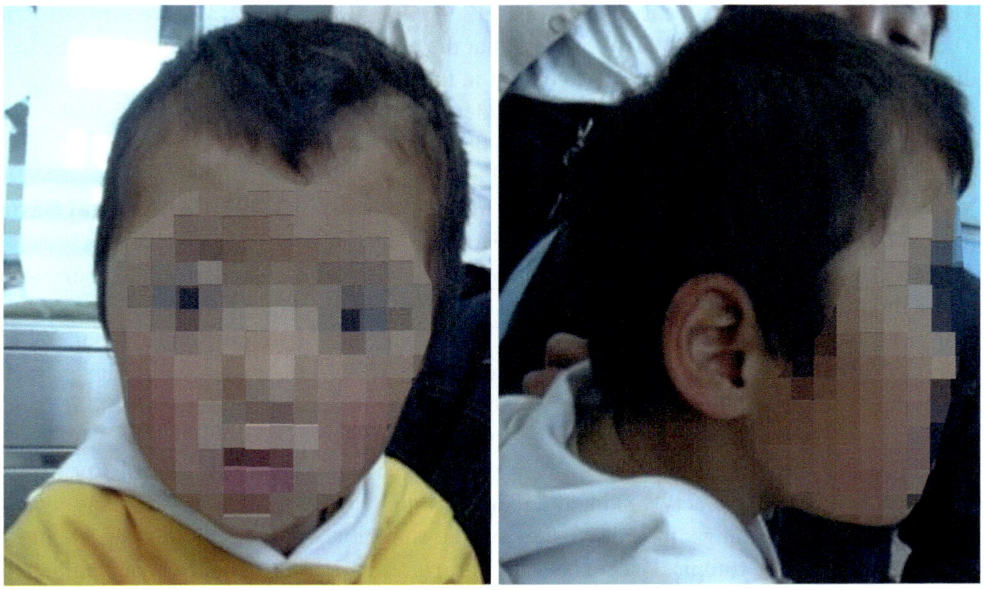

Fig. 13.85 Characteristic facial features of Apert syndrome: cranial malformation, midface dysplasia, exophthalmos, etc.

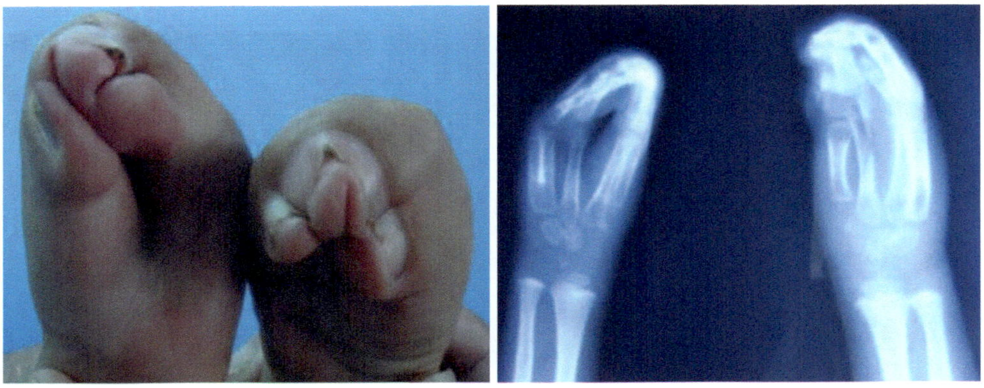

Fig. 13.86 Symmetric complex syndactyly of both hands

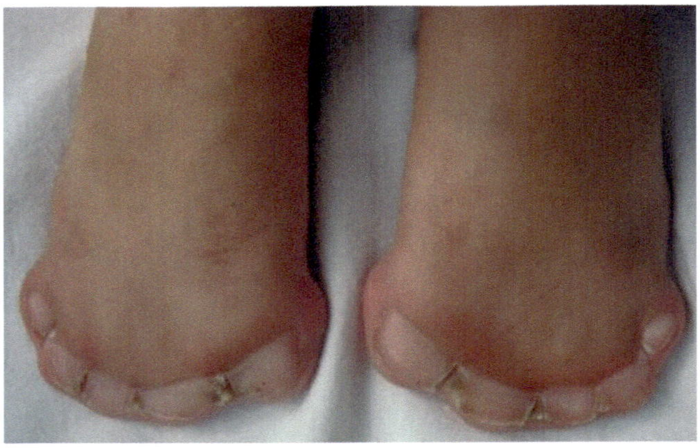

Fig. 13.87 Bilateral symmetrical syndactyly with wide and deviated toes

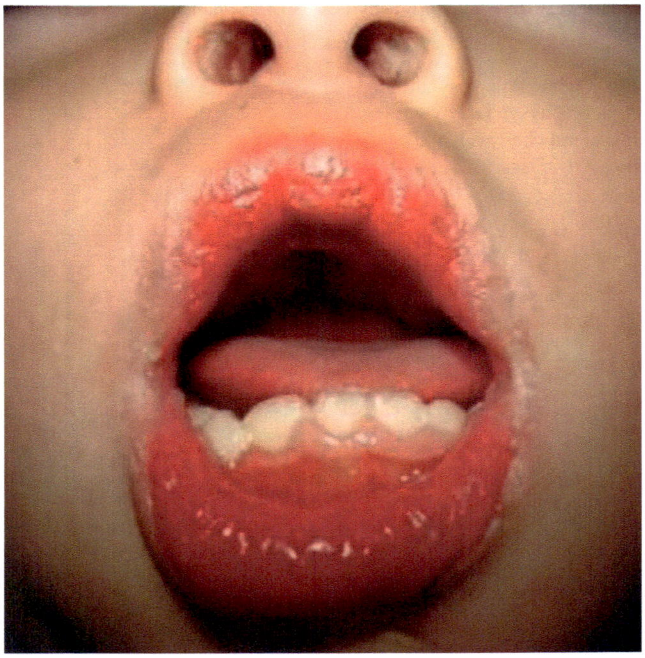

Fig. 13.88 Apert syndrome with cleft palate

13.4.2.2 Clinical Manifestation

The main clinicopathological features were that the affected upper limbs were heavy at both ends and light in the middle, that is, the deformities around the chest, shoulder girdle, and hand were serious, while the deformities of the upper arm and forearm were relatively light. The typical clinical manifestations are the absence or dysplasia of the ipsilateral pectoral muscle, the small, ectopic or absence of the nipple compared with the contralateral development, the short upper limbs and hands, the short fingers, and the syndactyly (Fig. 13.89). All patients had unilateral onset. Some patients were accompanied by chest wall dysplasia, such as thoracic flattening, local bulge, bilateral asymmetry, scapular dysplasia, latissimus dorsi dysplasia, axillary deformity, and band deformity. All the syndactyly fingers were partial or complete syndactyly of polydactyly skin, and there was no bony syndactyly. Rare findings include fusion of the superior radioulnar joint, heterotopic viscera, joint contracture, and banding (Figs. 13.90, 13.91, 13.92 and 13.93).

13.4.2.3 Treatment Principle

Hand deformities can be treated according to the severity of deformities to improve hand function to the greatest extent. The separation of syndactyly of brachydactyly is valuable.

13.4.3 Congenital Band Syndrome

Congenital band syndrome (Constriction band syndrome) is a rare congenital disease that mainly affects the extremities. Its clinical manifestations vary greatly, and the band around the extremities is its characteristic manifestation, which can also be called amniotic band, constrictive band, and so on.

13.4.3.1 Etiology

The etiology of band syndrome is unknown, and there are three main theories about its pathogenesis. (1) The endogenous theory that banding syndrome is the result of focal defects within the embryo. (2) Exogenous theory. Early

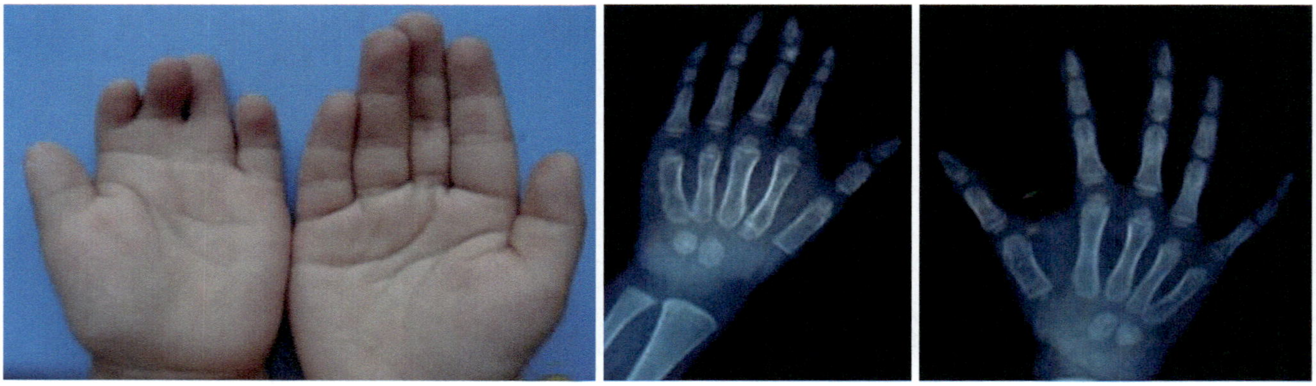

Fig. 13.89 Syndactyly brachydactyly of left hand

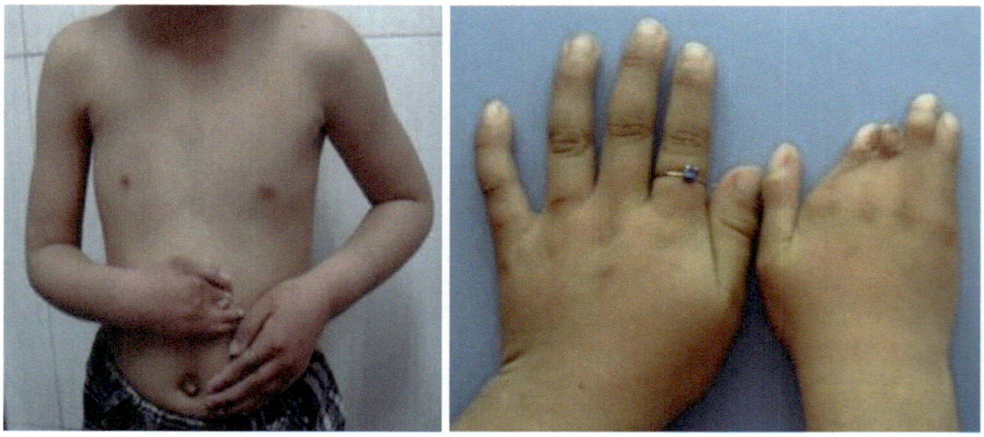

Fig. 13.90 Poland syndrome, right brachysyndactyly with ipsilateral chest wall and breast dysplasia

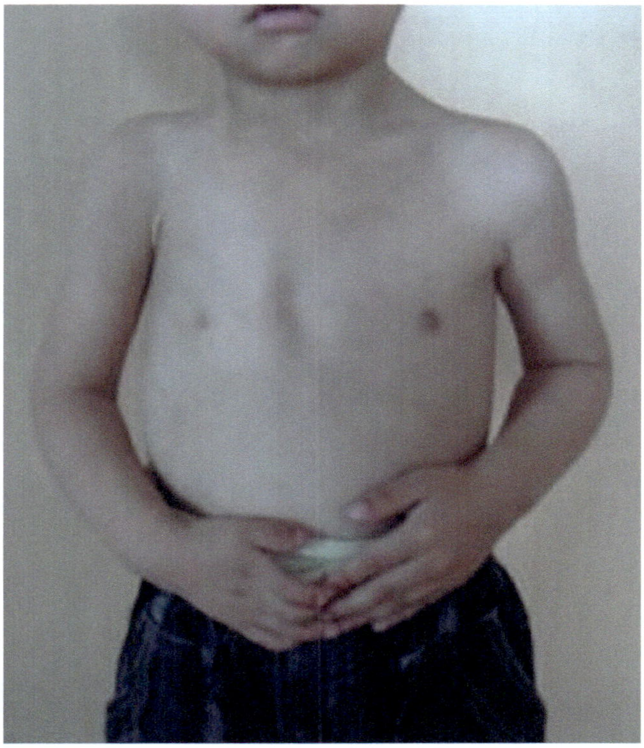

Fig. 13.91 Poland's syndrome, depression of right thorax

rupture of the amniotic membrane causes the mesodermal bands to wrap around the limb, resulting in typical limb deformities. (3) Theory of intrauterine injury and extrauterine injury. At present, there are many evidences supporting the exogenous theory. The disease is caused by the abnormal intrauterine environment during pregnancy, and its influencing factors are very complex.

13.4.3.2 Clinical Manifestation

Typical clinical features include finger (toe, limb) banding (Fig. 13.94), intrauterine amputation (Fig. 13.95), syndactyly and short fingers (Fig. 13.96), which are often associated with lower limb deformities (Fig. 13.97). In addition to the limb bands, the characteristic syndactyly of the bands is another feature of the disease, and its morphological features are far more complex than known (Figs. 13.98, 13.99 and 13.100).

13.4.3.3 Treatment Principle

If there is lymphedema at the distal end of the band, poor venous return or even blood supply disorders, surgery should be performed as soon as possible. Hand deformity should be operated according to the morphological characteristics of the deformity, and attention should be paid to protecting the blood supply of the fingertip, if necessary, the operation should be staged.

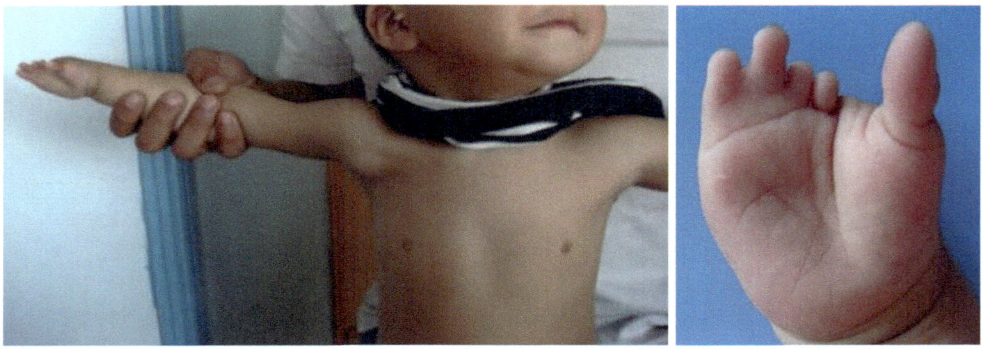

Fig. 13.92 Poland syndrome brachysyndactyly with hand band (right thumb)

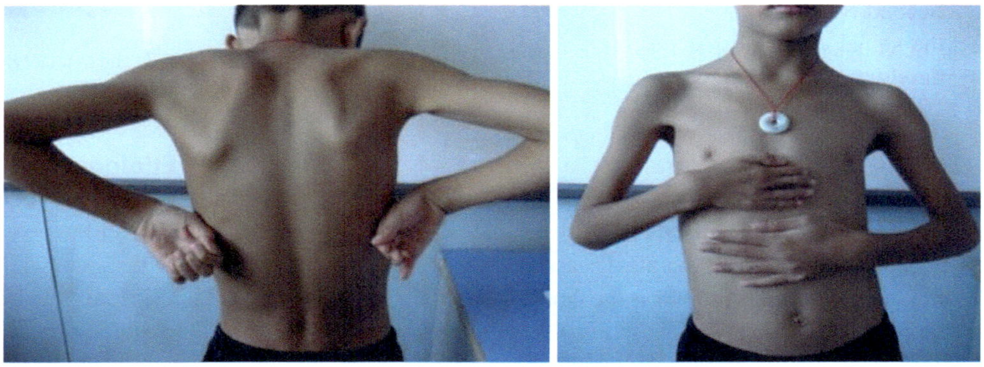

Fig. 13.93 Poland syndrome with latissimus dorsi and scapular dysplasia (right)

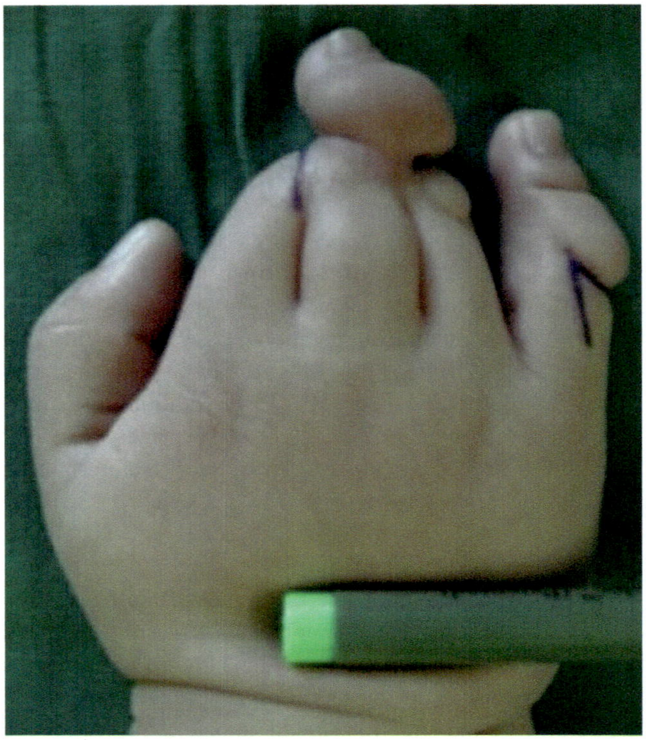

Fig. 13.94 Right finger strap, combined fingertips and fingers

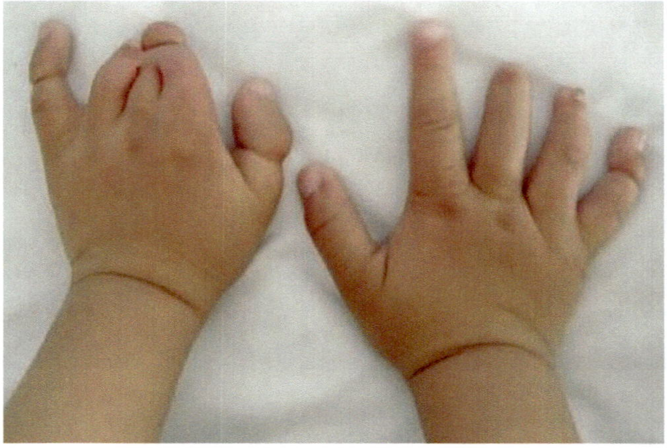

Fig. 13.95 Finger bands of both hands, combined with skin bridge syndactyly of the left hand

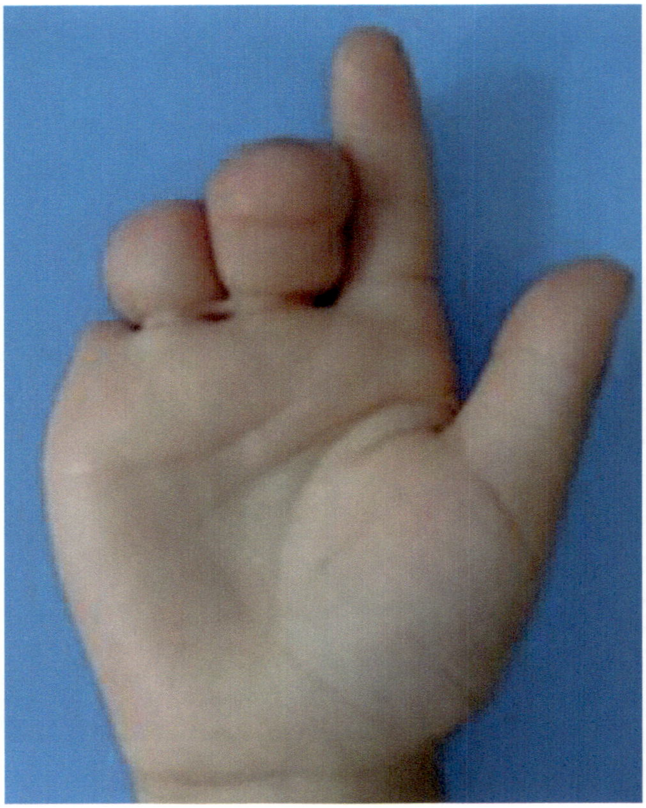

Fig. 13.96 In this case, in addition to the band, intrauterine amputation and skin bridge syndactyly can be seen

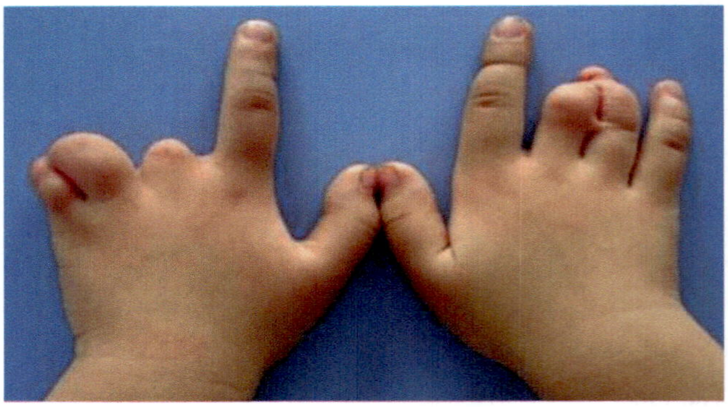

Fig. 13.97 Bands and syndactyly of fingers of both hands

13.4.4 Proteus Syndrome

Proteus syndrome was first described by Cohen in 1979. Wiedemann listed it as a separate disease in 1983 and named it "Proteus syndrome." Proteus is the God of the sea in Greek mythology, unpredictable. The clinical phenotypes of this syndrome are quite different, and no clinical cases with identical morphological characteristics have been found, so it is also called "deformed syndrome."

13.4.4.1 Etiology

The disease is rare and is believed to be caused by mutations in the somatic AKT1 gene.

13.4.4.2 Clinical Manifestation

Hand and foot deformities are often characterized by irregular enlargement of the hands and feet, and sulcus and gyrus changes in the skin of the palms and soles are sometimes characteristic of the disease (Figs. 13.101, 13.102 and

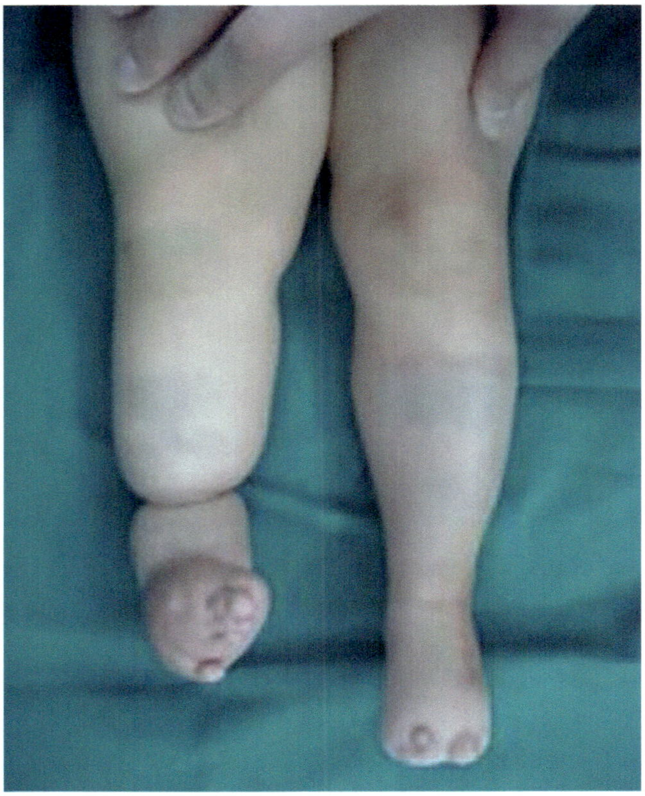

Fig. 13.98 Lap band syndrome with right clubfoot and toe deformity

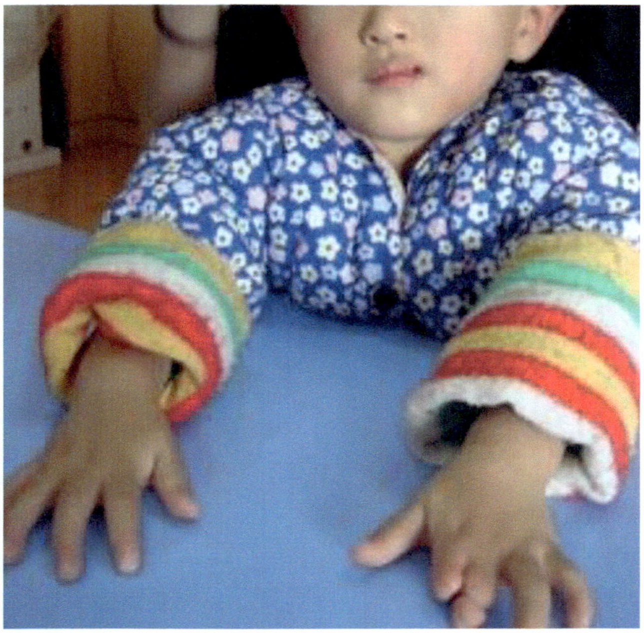

Fig. 13.100 Hair band syndrome with facial abnormality

Fig. 13.99 Bimanual girdle combined with cutaneous tube-like neoplasm on limbs and back

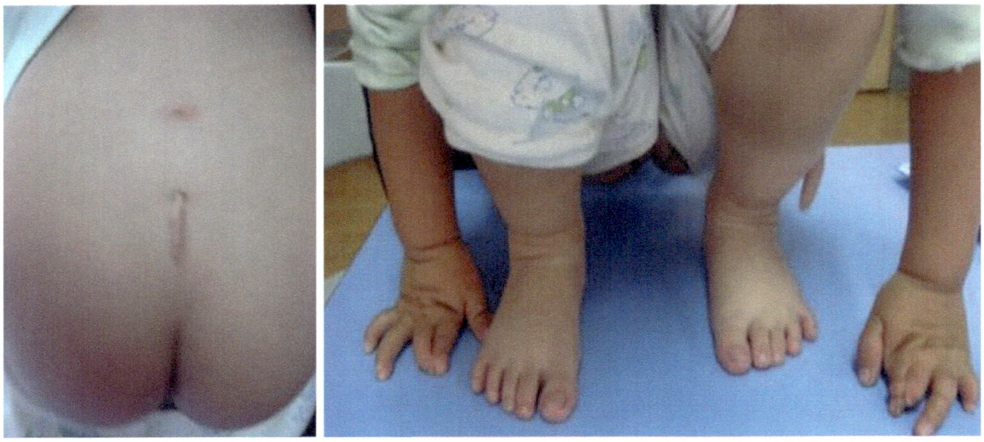

13.103). Intraoperative exploration revealed that the overgrown tissue was a cartilage-like lesion (Fig. 13.104), which restricted the flexion of the fingers, resulting in severe limitation of grasping and pinching, and could also be combined with a variety of other tissue or organ disorders (Fig. 13.105).

13.4.4.3 Treatment Principle

In order to improve the appearance and function of the main, if necessary, cut the finger.

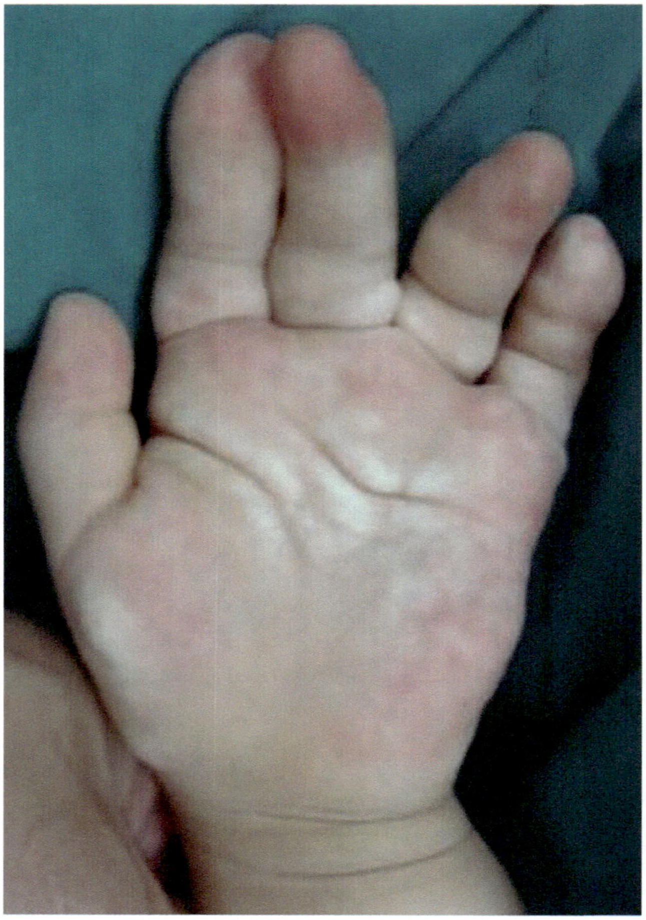

Fig. 13.101 Sulcus and gyrus like changes in the skin of left palm

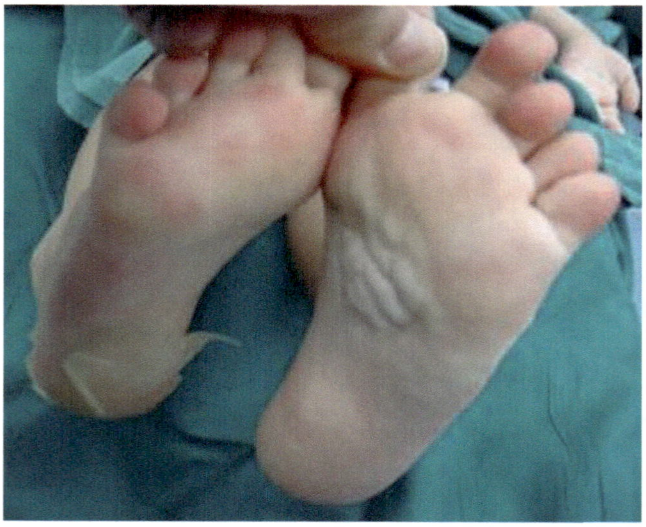

Fig. 13.102 Sulcus and gyrus changes of left plantar skin

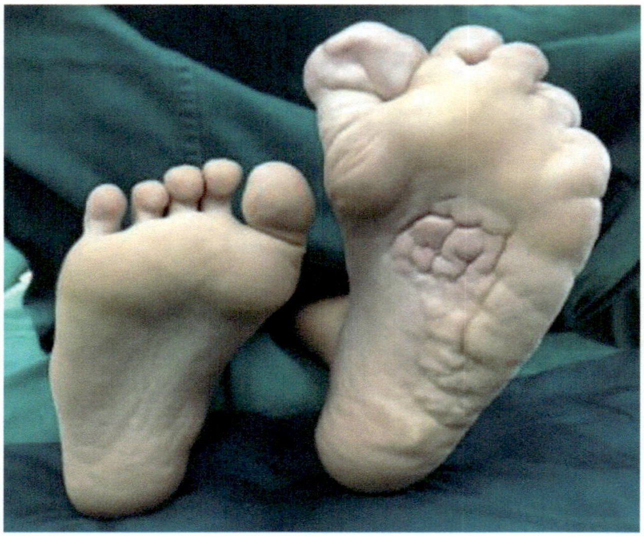

Fig. 13.103 Hypertrophy of the left foot, multiple masses in the toes, and sulcus and gyrus changes in the plantar skin

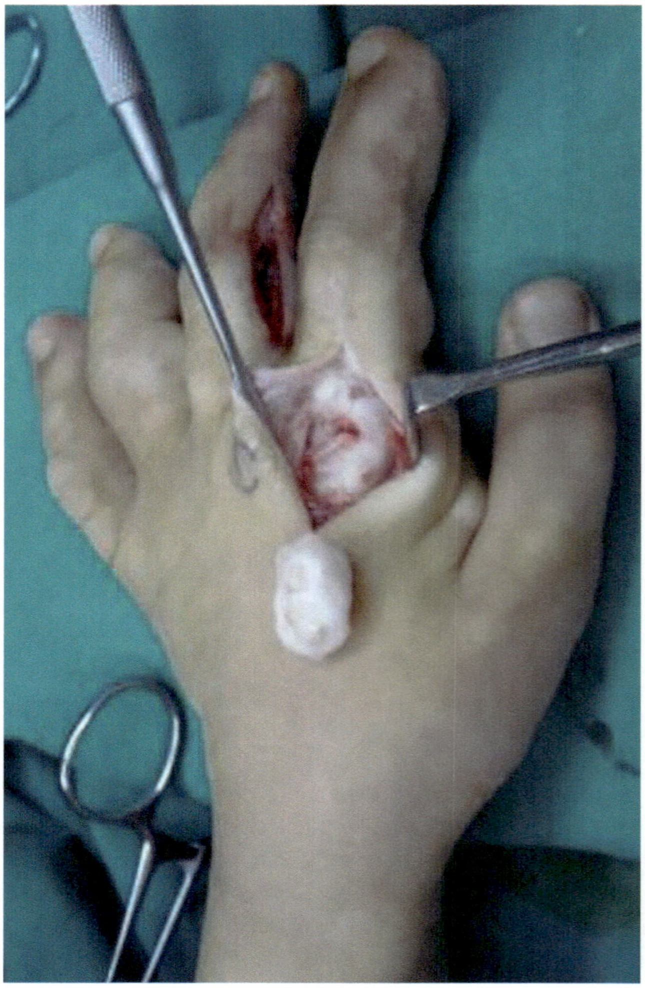

Fig. 13.104 Intraoperative exploration showed that the overgrowth tissue was a cartilage-like mass

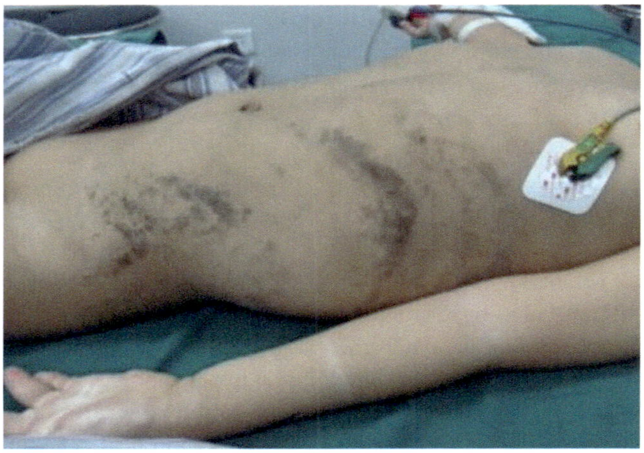

Fig. 13.105 Patients may have abnormal pigmentation of the skin

13.4.5 Freeman-Sheldon Syndrome or Whistling Face Syndrome

Freeman-Sheldon syndrome is also called "Whistling face syndrome" in English literature, because it is characterized by multiple joint contractures as the main limb manifestation, combined with facial abnormalities, such as small mouth and pouting lips, similar to the state of flute player when playing the flute.

13.4.5.1 Etiology

A type of distal joint contracture often associated with mutations in the MYH3 gene.

13.4.5.2 Clinical Manifestation

Morphological abnormalities mainly involve the face (Fig. 13.106), hands, and feet and are also accompanied by

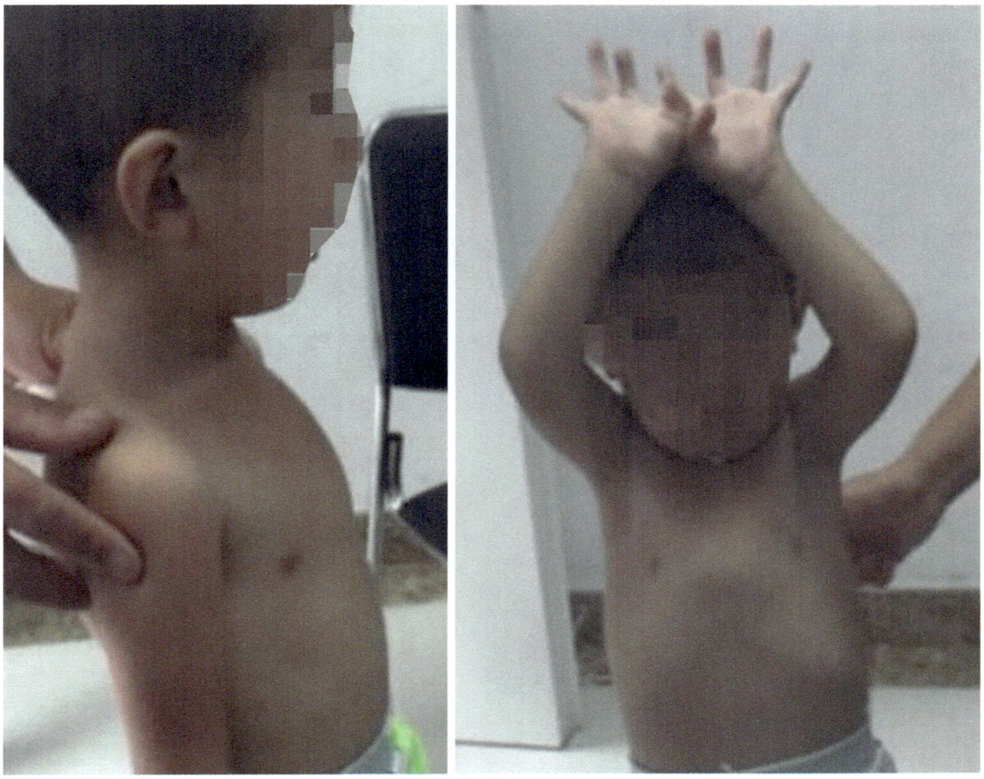

Fig. 13.106 Pied Piper Facial Syndrome Special face, hand deformities are finger joint contracture and thumb deformity

wide neck (Fig. 13.107), short deformity, facial stiffness, short stature, etc., but flexion contracture of hand joints and facial dysplasia are common deformities. In addition to joint contracture, hand deformities are often accompanied by blowing hand deformities (Fig. 13.108).

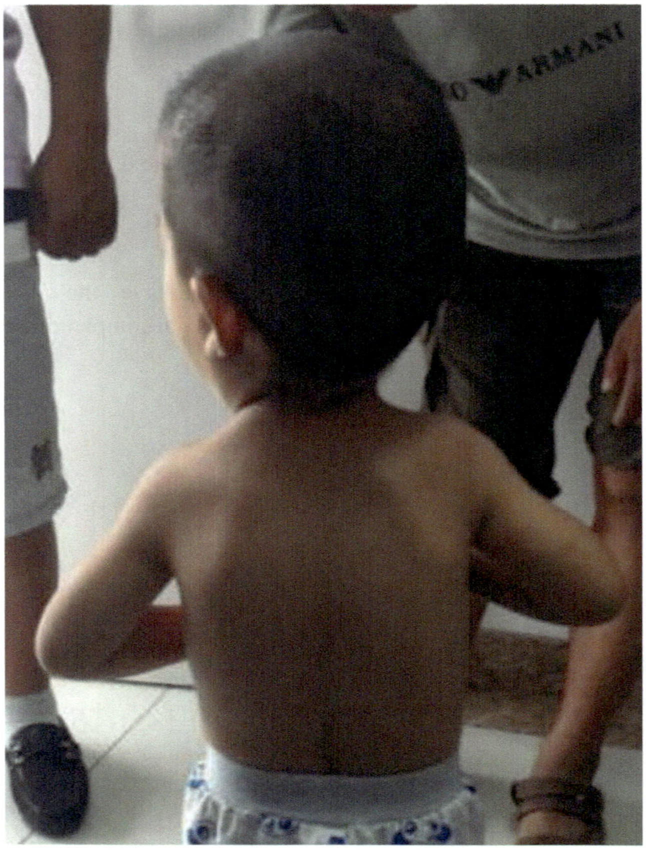

Fig. 13.107 Wide neck, short neck deformity

13.4.5.3 Treatment Principle

The treatment principle of hand deformity is the same as that of congenital joint contracture, and there is no special treatment for facial deformity.

13.4.6 Myogenic Limb Hypertrophy Syndrome

Congenital myogenic limb hypertrophy syndrome (congenital muscular hypertrophy syndrome), formerly known as accessory muscle syndrome, vagus muscle syndrome, congenital unilateral upper limb muscle hypertrophy, and so on, is an overgrowth disease. The authors propose the term "congenital myogenic limb hypertrophy syndrome" for this malformation.

13.4.6.1 Etiology

At present, the disease belongs to PIK3CA-associated overgrowth disease (PROS), which is the result of PIK3CA gene chimeric mutation in somatic cells.

13.4.6.2 Clinical Manifestation

Most of them involve unilateral upper limbs or lower limbs, but the involvement of bilateral limbs and trunk can also be seen. The clinical manifestations are hypertrophy of the involved limbs and abnormal muscle volume (Figs. 13.109, 13.110, 13.111 and 13.112). The main reason is the excessive proliferation of limb muscles (Fig. 13.113).

Upper extremity involvement has little effect on shoulder and elbow function, while hand function is usually more severely affected, with severe grasping, grasping, and pinching dysfunction (Fig. 13.114). Lower limb involvement can lead to unequal length of limbs, foot hypertrophy, affecting walking, and wearing shoes.

Fig. 13.108 Hands deformity

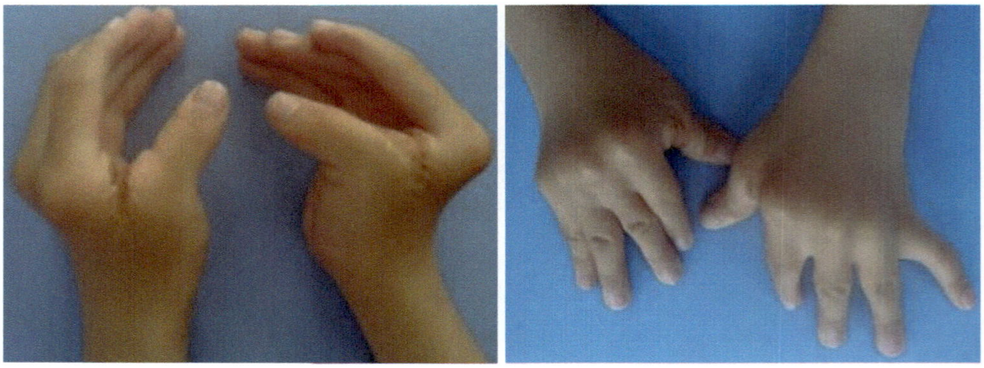

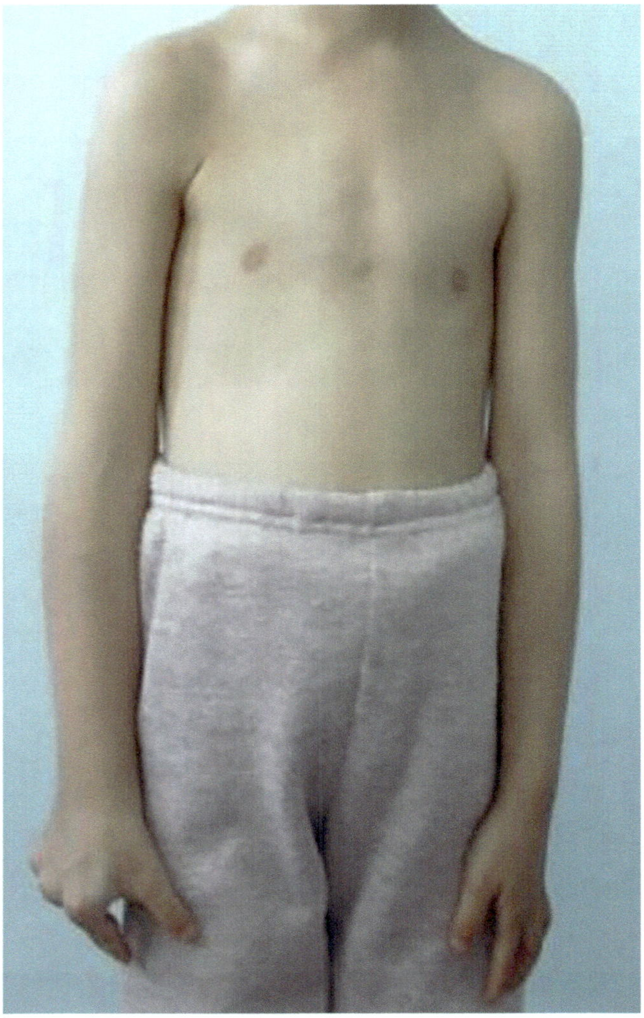

Fig. 13.109 Overall hypertrophy of the right upper limb

13.4.6.3 Treatment Principle

At present, there is no unified treatment principle. Hypertrophic variant muscle can be surgically resected to some extent to improve the shape and function of the affected hand and foot, but complete resection is almost impossible.

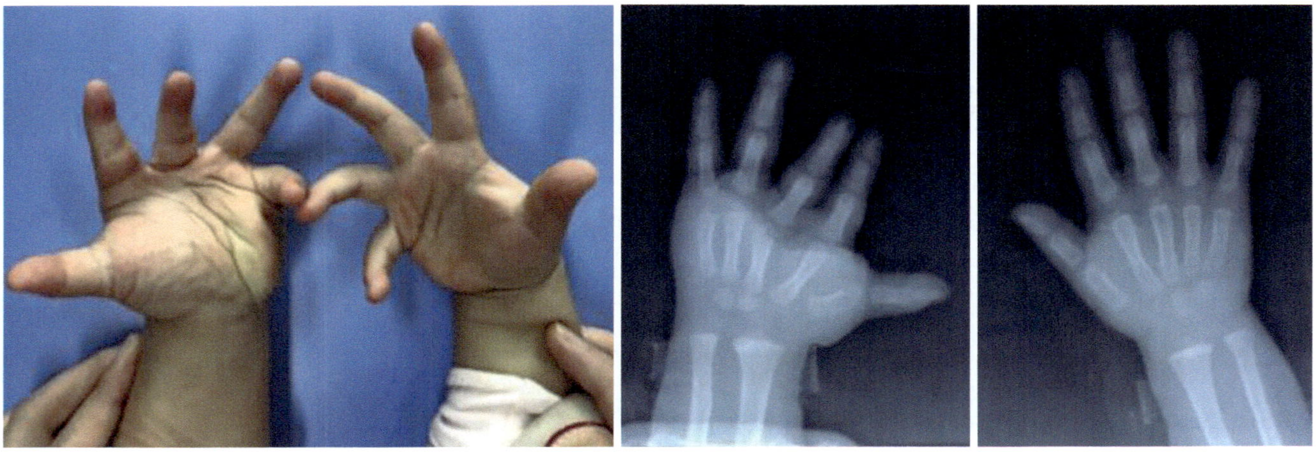

Fig. 13.110 Increased muscle volume in the left hand, hypertrophy of the palm, marked by the thenar and hypothenar, and excessive abduction of the thumb. Radiographs showed various degrees of deformity of the bones and joints

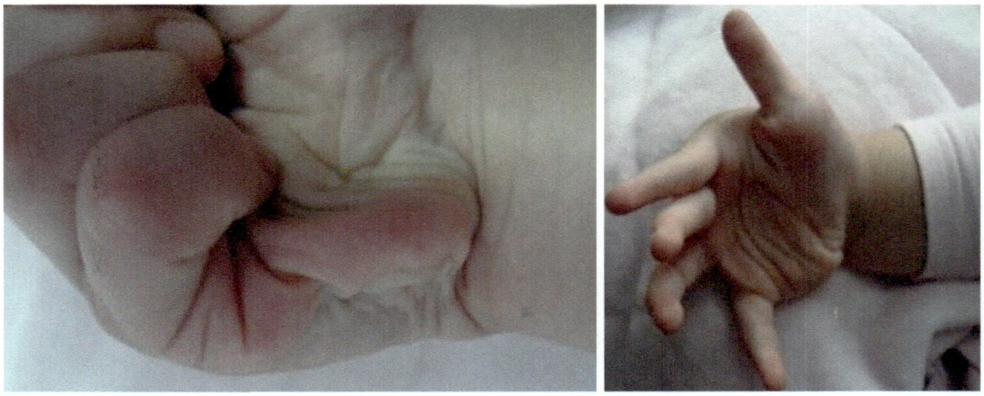

Fig. 13.111 Characteristic dermatoglyphics and palmprint caused by abnormal skin and muscle

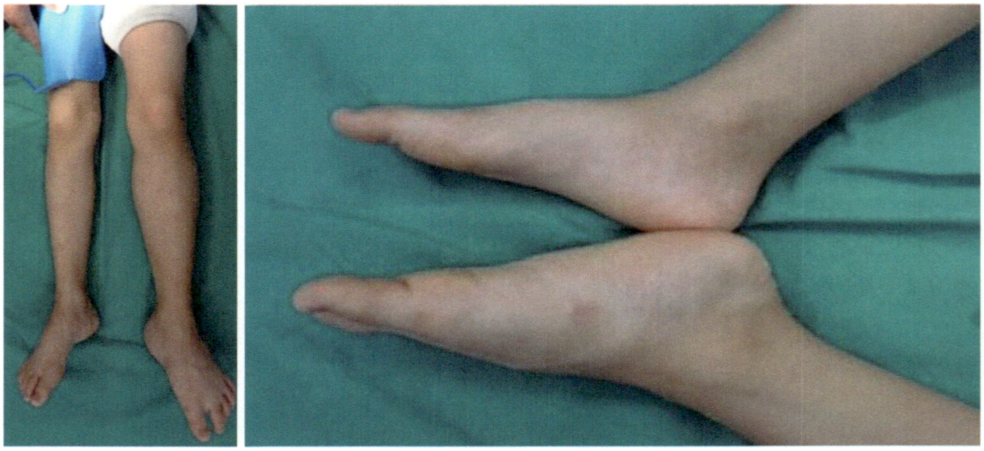

Fig. 13.112 Increased muscle volume in the left lower extremity

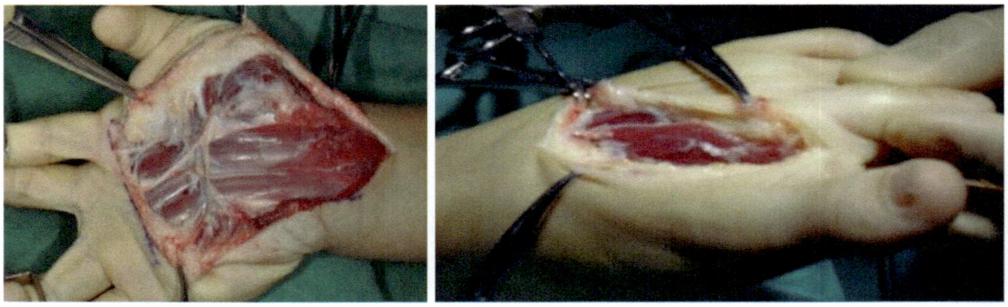

Fig. 13.113 In this patient, a large amount of hypertrophic muscle tissue was found during the operation. The left picture shows the right hand, and the right picture shows the left foot. This picture shows different patients

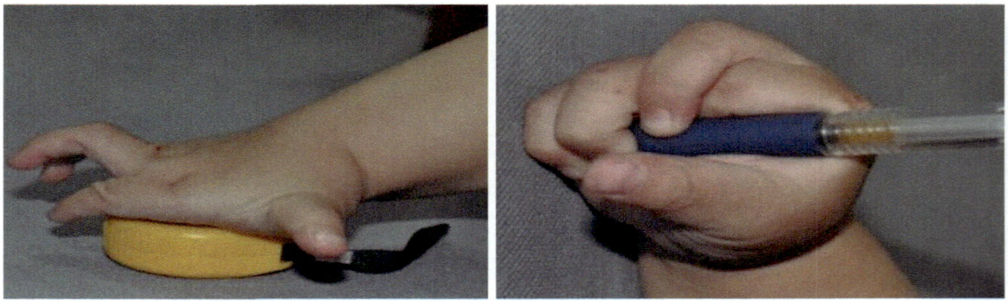

Fig. 13.114 Hand deformities caused by myogenic hypertrophy have a significant impact on hand function

13.5 Other Congenital Diseases

13.5.1 Multiple Osteochondroma Limb (Upper Limb) Deformity

The disease is also known as hereditary multiple osteochondroma (HME), diaphyseal continuity disease, multiple exostoses, etc. It is a rare autosomal dominant genetic disease, which often occurs in the epiphysis of long tubular bones, but also in short tubular bones and flat bones.

13.5.1.1 Etiology

Most of them are related to mutations of EXT gene (EXT1, EXT2 or EXT3).

13.5.1.2 Clinical Manifestation

The lower extremities are more common in the distal femur and proximal and distal tibia and fibula (Fig. 13.115), and the upper extremities are more common in the distal ulna and radius (Fig. 13.116), scapula, and short tubular bones.

The forearm is involved in 30–60% of patients. In addition to multiple bony protuberances, the affected bones may also have secondary deformities or dysfunction, such as forearm shortening and bending, ulnar deviation of wrist joint, dislocation of radial head, deviation of finger joint,

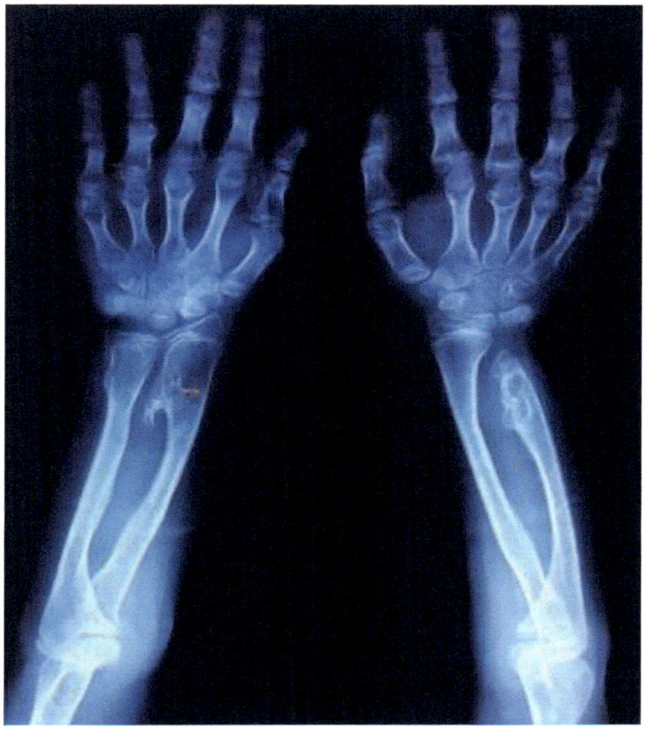

Fig. 13.116 Radiographic findings of multiple osteochondromas in the forearm

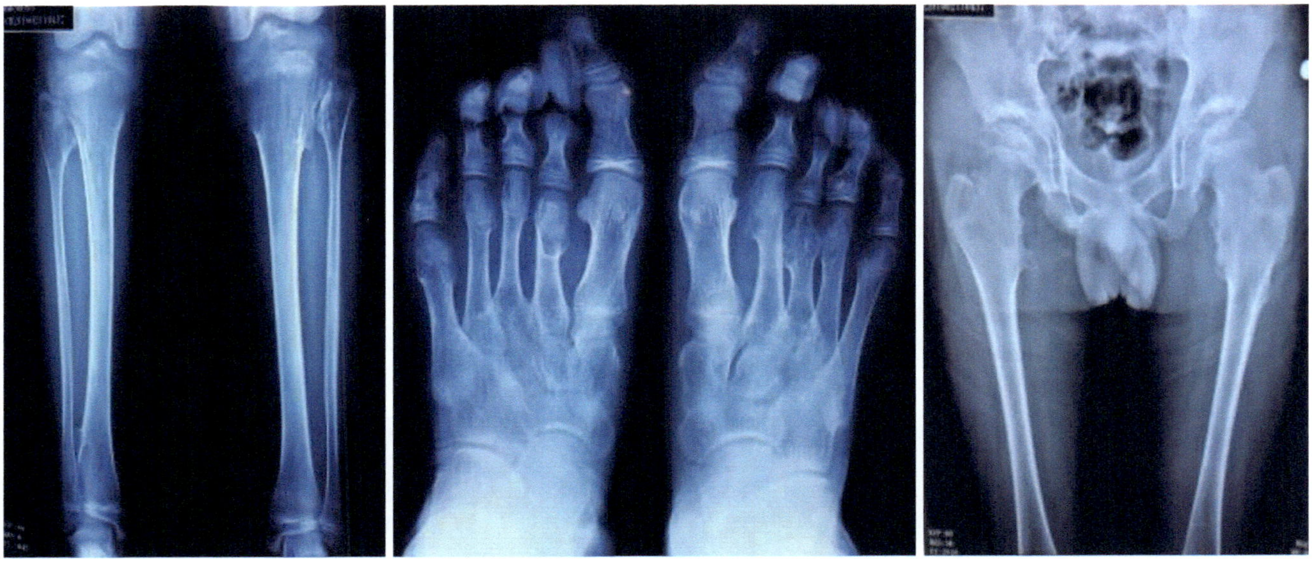

Fig. 13.115 Radiographic findings of multiple osteochondromas in the lower extremities

rotation of forearm or limitation of flexion and extension of finger, wrist and elbow joints (Fig. 13.117). Bone lesions can compress or irritate adjacent nerves, blood vessels, or tendons, producing corresponding symptoms. Malignant transformation may occur in this disease.

13.5.1.3 Treatment Principle

When bone lesions affect the function and appearance of upper limbs, or produce compression symptoms, tumor resection is feasible. Some developmental malformations require more complex bone and joint reconstruction.

13.5.2 Multiple Enchondromatosis Limb (Upper Limb) Deformity

Multiple enchondromatosis, also known as Ollier disease when combined with bone and joint deformities, is a rare disease that often occurs in children. The disease can be diagnosed if there are more than three parts of the whole body with enchondroma.

13.5.2.1 Etiology

The pathogenesis and genetic background are still unclear, which may be related to heterozygous mutation of isocitrate dehydrogenase (IDH) gene.

13.5.2.2 Clinical Manifestation

It can occur in both long and short bones of the body. For the upper limbs, the short bone of the hand is the predilection site, showing multiple phalangeal or metacarpal bone masses (Figs. 13.118 and 13.119), and the short tubular bone of the foot is also the predilection site (Fig. 13.120). The functional impact is related to the extent of the lesion, and the involved bone is prone to pathological fracture. Bone lesions have a certain probability of malignant transformation (Fig. 13.121).

On the X-ray film, the lesions can be divided into four types: internal expansion growth (Fig. 13.122), central

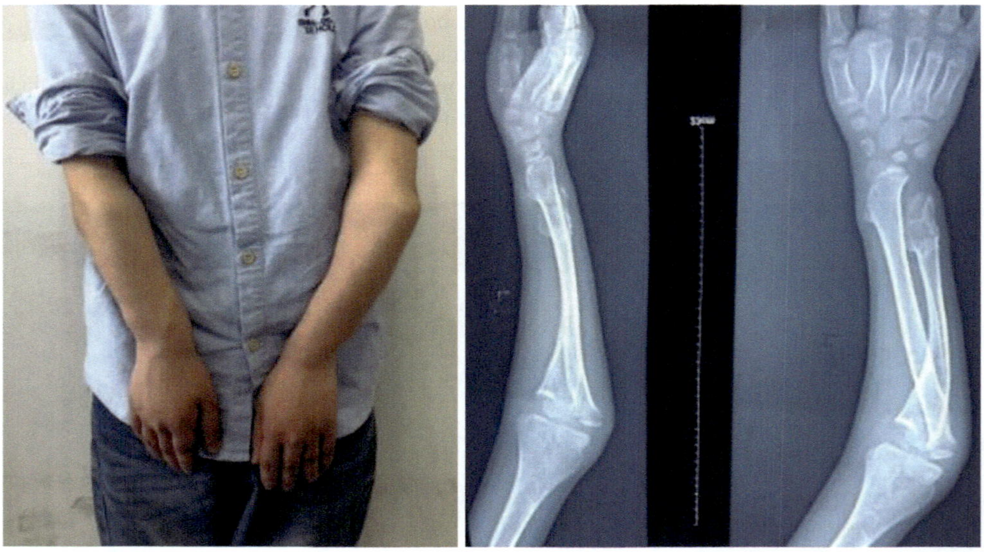

Fig. 13.117 Patient with multiple osteochondromas, multiple bone lesions in the left upper limb, dislocation of the radial head

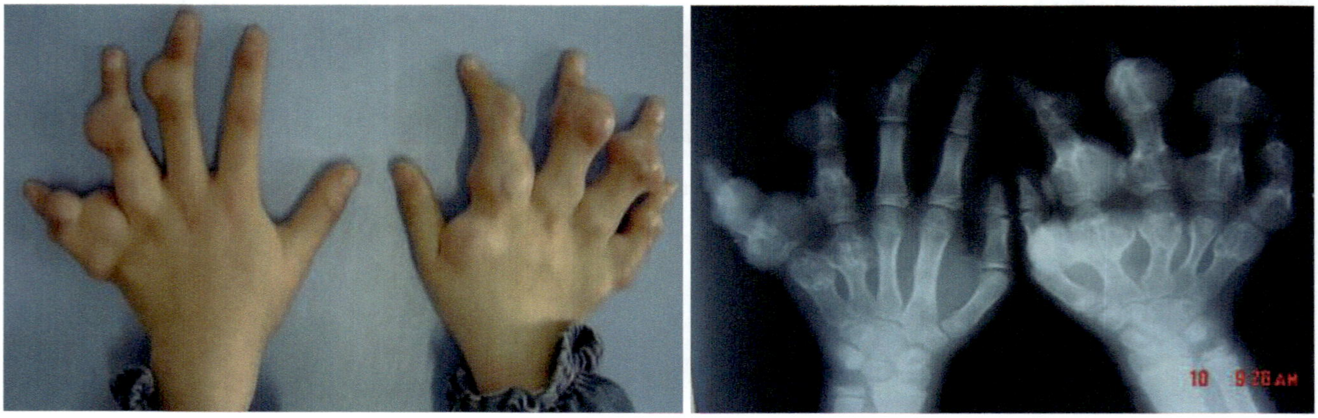

Fig. 13.118 Multiple phalangeal and metacarpal masses on both hands

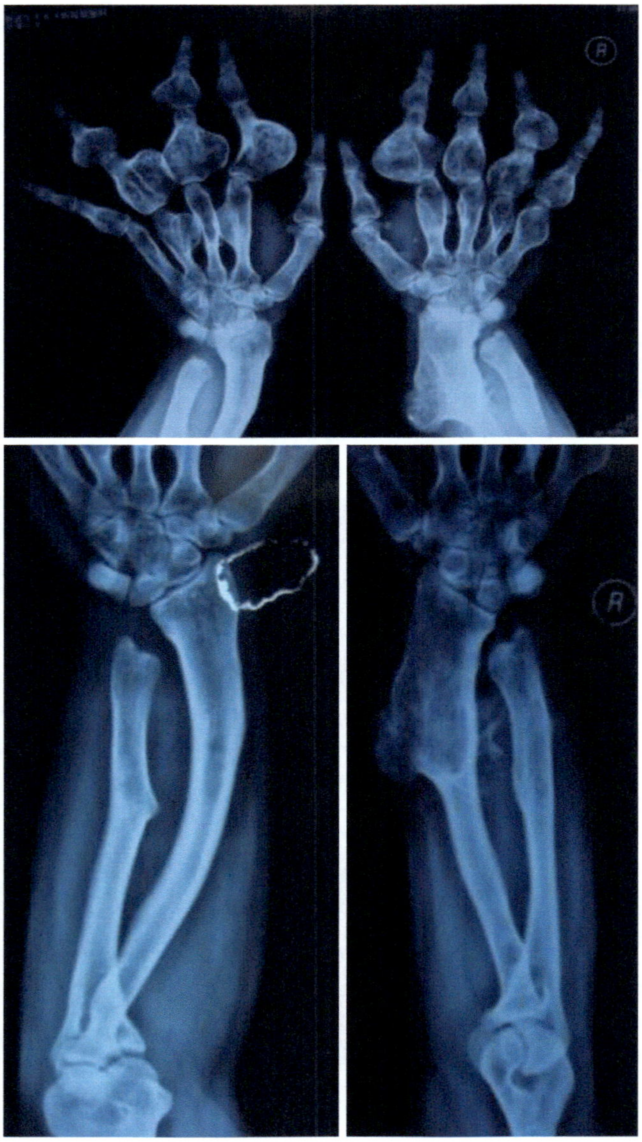

Fig. 13.119 In addition to multiple phalangeal and metacarpal bone lesions in both hands, the forearm also has secondary deformities due to bone lesions

expansion growth (Fig. 13.123), eccentric expansion growth (Fig. 13.124), and mixed expansion growth (Fig. 13.125).

13.5.2.3 Treatment Principle

For children, if the hand lesion grows faster or affects the function and appearance when it is found, it can be treated by early surgery, which can be treated by curettage of enchondroma combined with cortical osteoplasty. Most adult patients need to be filled with bone graft after curettage.

Developmental deformities caused by forearm lesions, such as shortening and bending, should be considered for bone and joint reconstruction in the later stage.

If the bone lesions become malignant, amputation of limbs/fingers should be considered, and medical oncology intervention should be carried out after operation.

13.5.3 Limb (Upper Limb) Deformity Caused by Neurofibromatosis

Neurofibromatosis (NF) is a group of autosomal dominant genetic diseases, mainly involving the nervous system, with bone, skin, and other organ system abnormalities.

13.5.3.1 Etiology

Neurofibromatosis is an autosomal dominant genetic disorder caused by mutations in the NFUNK1 neurofibromatosis UNK2 gene. It is divided into two types in clinic and genetics: neurofibromatosis type 1 UNK3 neurofibromatosis type 1, NF 1 UNK1, neurofibromatosis type 2 UNK2, NF 2 UNK3, and Schwannoma to sis UNK4 UNK5. Neurofibromatosis type 1 is the most common cause of upper limb deformities. (2) Clinical manifestations of neurofibromatosis type 1.

Clinical manifestations of neurofibromatosis type 1 (Figs. 13.126, 13.127, 13.128, 13.129, 13.130 and 13.131): (1) cafe-au-lait spots (2) multiple neurofibromas (3) neurological symptoms: most patients have no special discomfort. A small number of patients have mental decline, memory impairment, seizures, limb weakness, numbness, etc. (4) Skeletal damage: a small number of patients have abnormal skeletal development at birth, such as pseudarthrosis, scoliosis, lordosis and kyphosis deformity, skull asymmetry, defect or depression, or compression of bone during tumor growth, resulting in different skeletal abnormalities (5) Visceral damage. Splanchnic neurofibromas can cause compression symptoms.

13.5.3.2 Treatment Principle

Neurofibroma mass or overgrowth in the limbs can be treated surgically.

The pseudarthrosis can be treated by periosteal excision, fibrous tissue excision, reduction, bone grafting and Ilizarov external fixation. Proximal osteotomy and lengthening can be performed at the same time if there is bone defect.

13.5.4 Shortening of Upper Limbs and Hands Caused by Achondroplasia

Achondroplasia (ACH), including pseudoachondroplasia, is a physical retardation or disorder (dwarfism) caused by insufficient secretion of growth hormone due to various reasons.

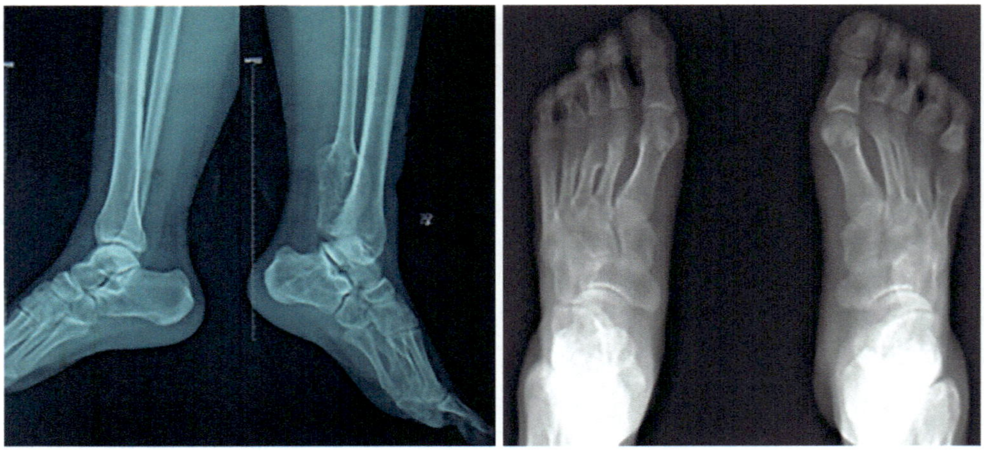

Fig. 13.120 X-ray manifestation of multiple enchondromatosis in both lower limb

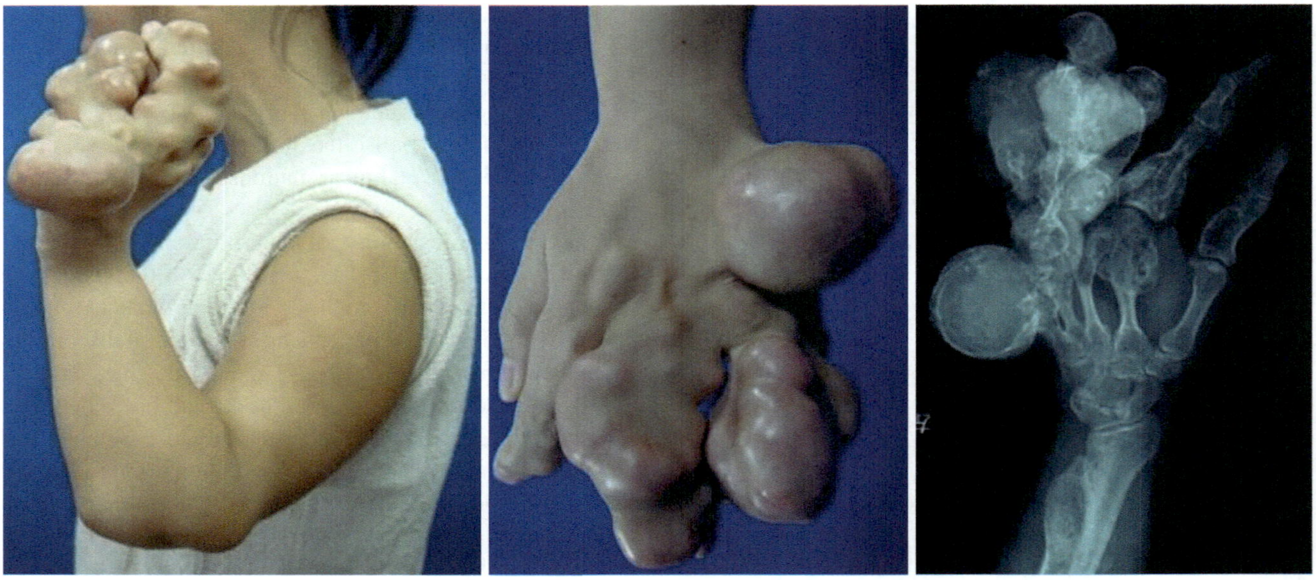

Fig. 13.121 Malignant change of multiple enchondromas in the left hand

13.5.4.1 Etiology

It can be divided into primary type and secondary type. The etiology of primary type is unknown. It is mostly caused by congenital hypoplasia or genetic diseases. It may be autosomal recessive inheritance. It is familial. It is mainly caused by growth hormone deficiency alone. Boys are more common than girls. The ratio of male to female is about (2–4): 10. Secondary diseases can be secondary to hypothalamic-pituitary diseases, such as tumors, infections, craniocerebral trauma, surgery or radiotherapy, which directly damage the pituitary, or damage the hypothalamus, or interrupt the pituitary portal vein system. Hypothalamic-pituitary tumors are an important cause of secondary pituitary dwarfism.

13.5.4.2 Clinical Manifestation

Because of the weak growth ability of cartilage, the longitudinal growth retardation of bone path, the formation of severe dwarfism, family heredity, not endocrine. The clinical features are as follows: (1) the length of trunk bones is often normal, while the limbs are obviously short, and the lower body is significantly shorter than the upper body; (2) lordosis of the spine, the abdomen forward, the buttocks backward, and the fingers short and thick; (3) normal intelligence development; (4) sexual organs are normal and have reproductive capacity.

Achondroplasia with upper limb shortening is shown in Fig. 13.132.

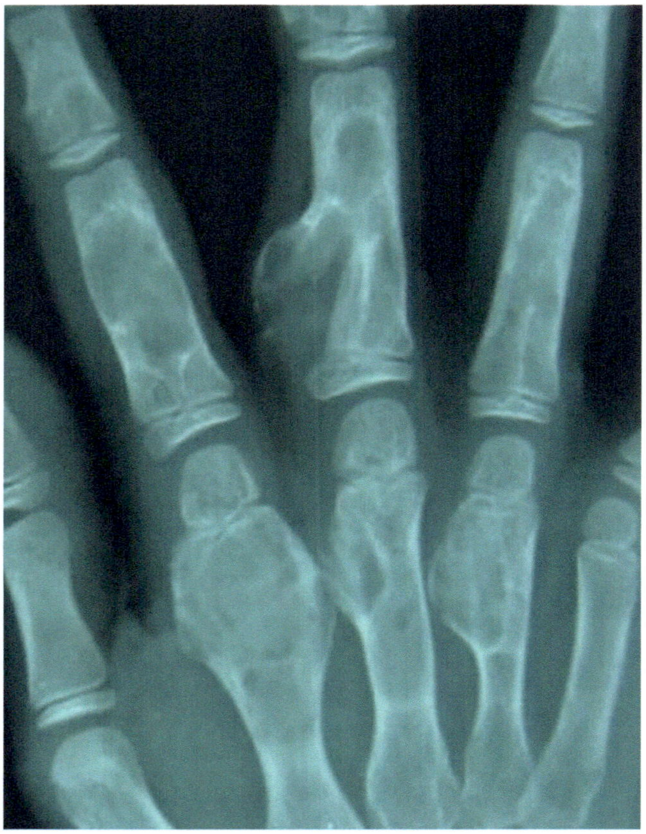

Fig. 13.122 Enchondroma in the proximal phalanx of the ring finger

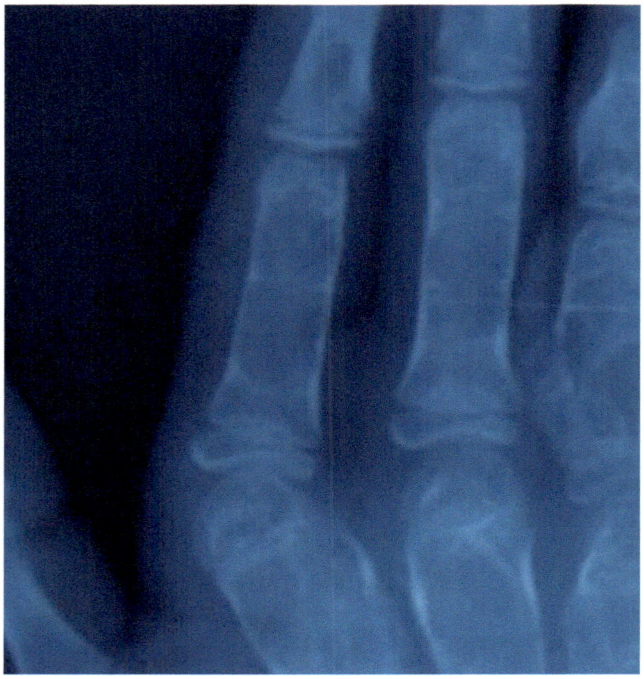

Fig. 13.123 Central expansive growth enchondroma of proximal phalanx of index and middle finger

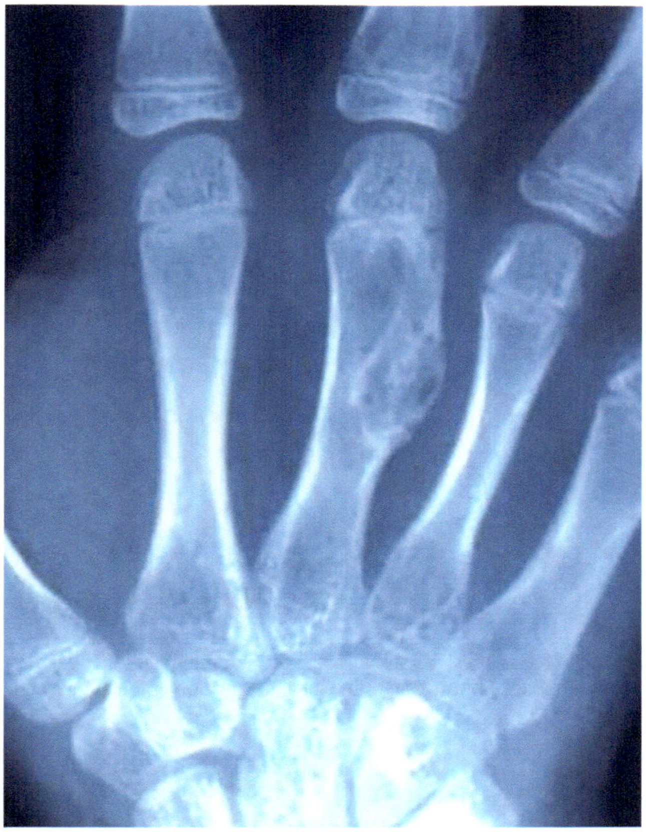

Fig. 13.124 Eccentric expansive growth enchondroma of the third metacarpal bone

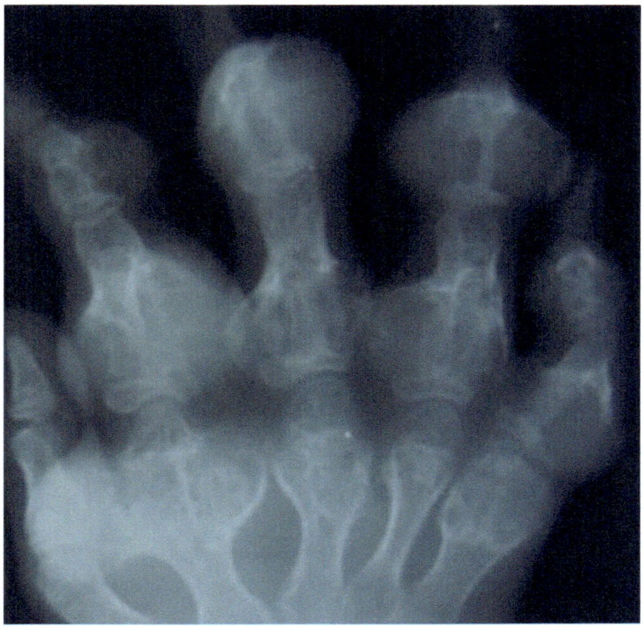

Fig. 13.125 Mixed expanding and growing enchondroma

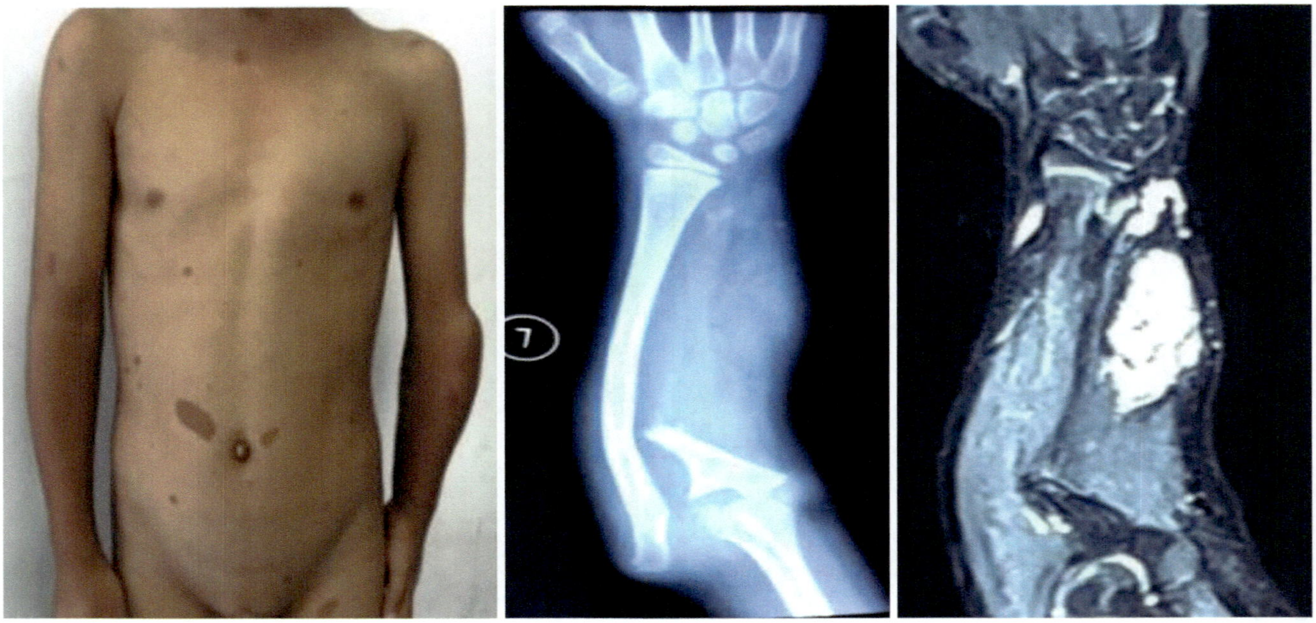

Fig. 13.126 Extensive cafe-au-lait spots and pigmented freckles were scattered on the limbs and trunk. The left forearm was deformed. X-ray showed massive destruction of the ulna, dislocation of the humeroradial joint, and curvature of the radius. MRI showed soft tissue mass shadows

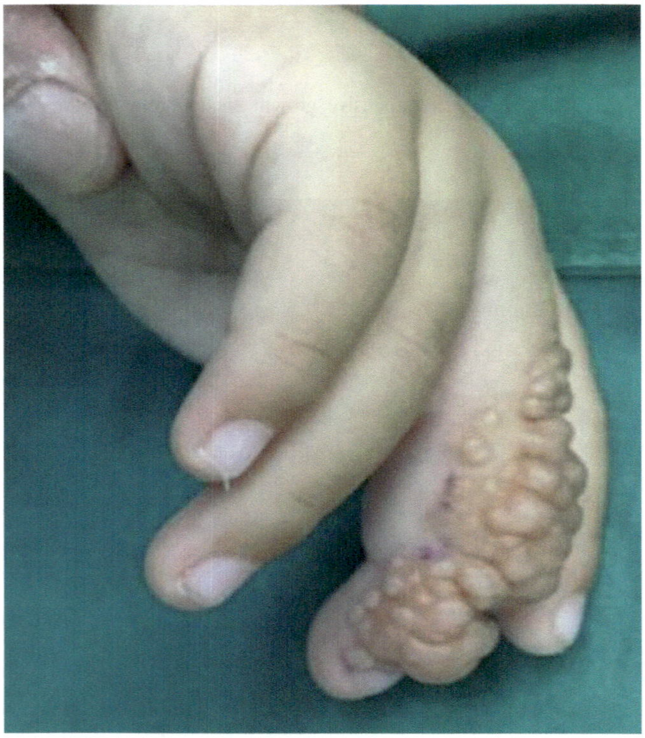

Fig. 13.127 Dense distribution of tumor-like skin lesions in the skin of the right hand (cutaneous type)

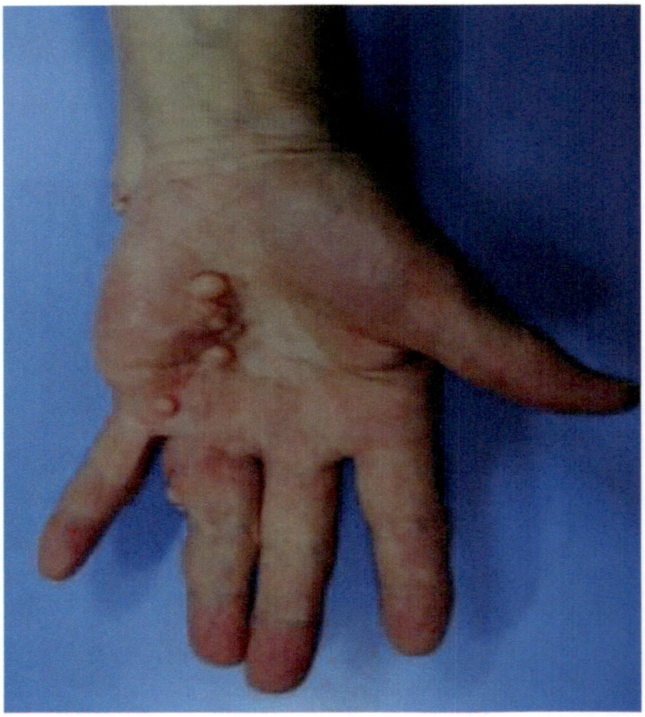

Fig. 13.128 Scattered skin tumors and subcutaneous masses on the left hand (mixed skin and subcutaneous nodules)

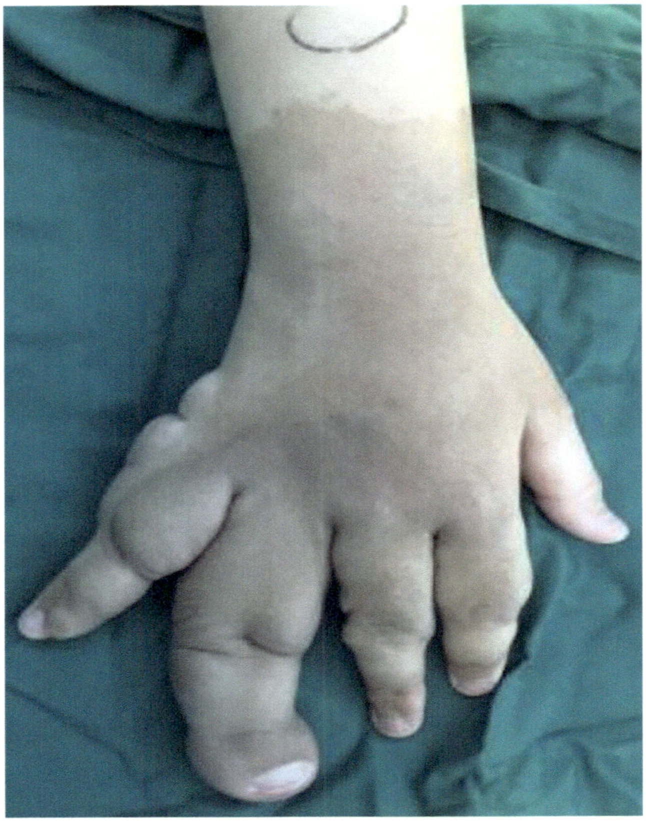

Fig. 13.129 Hypertrophy of the fingers of the right hand with diffuse skin lesions with pigmentation (plexiform neurofibromatosis type)

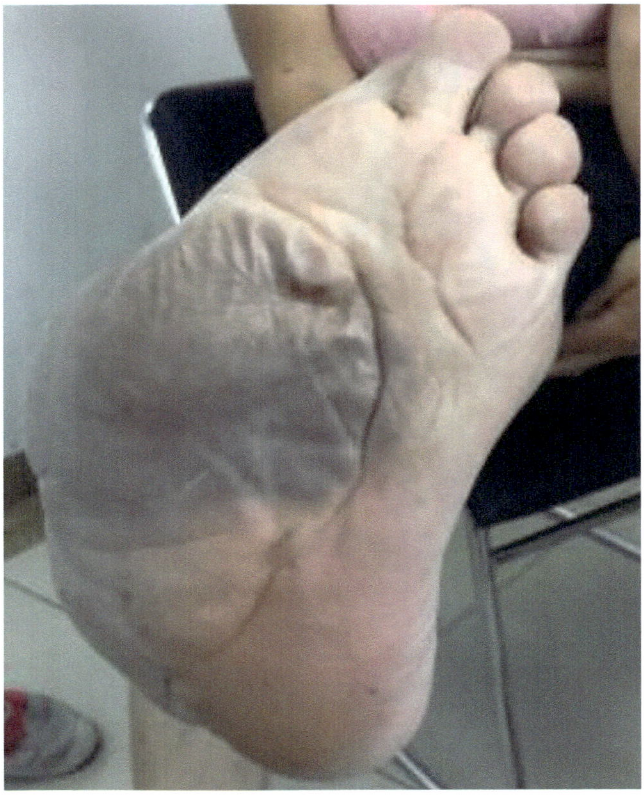

Fig. 13.130 Plexiform neurofibroma of left sole

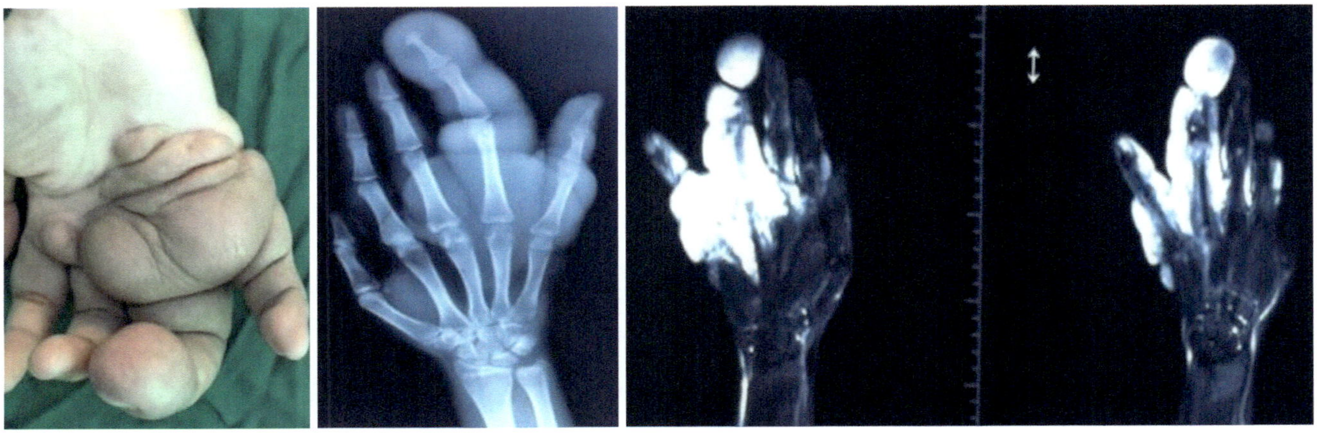

Fig. 13.131 Plexiform neurofibroma in the right hand. X-ray film showed obvious soft tissue shadow and bone atrophy in the fingers. MRI showed extensive and diffuse lesion invasion

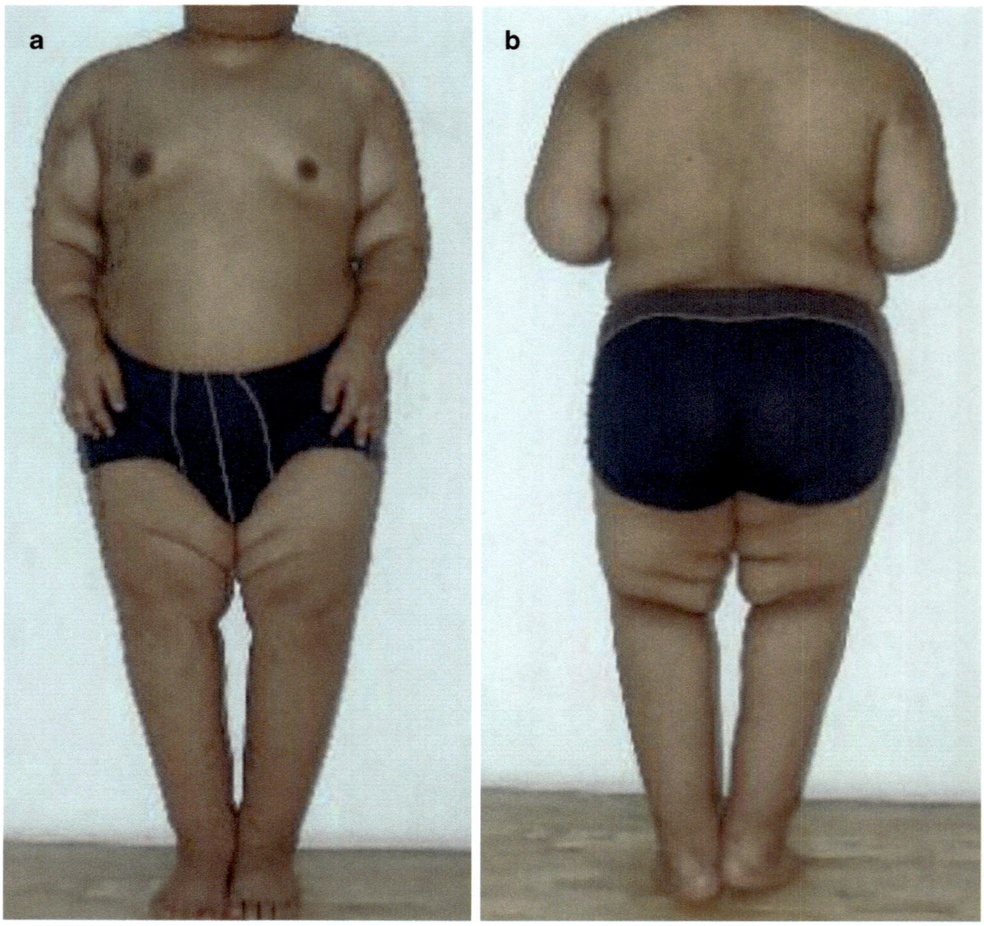

Fig. 13.132 (**a**) Frontal view. Shortening of upper limbs due to achondroplasia (both legs have been lengthened). (**b**) Back view

13.5.5 The Cause of the Disease Is Unknown. The Finger (Toe) Cartilage Dysplasia Is Short (Figs. 13.133 and 13.134)

Case 1 Fig. 13.133.

Case 2 Fig. 13.134.

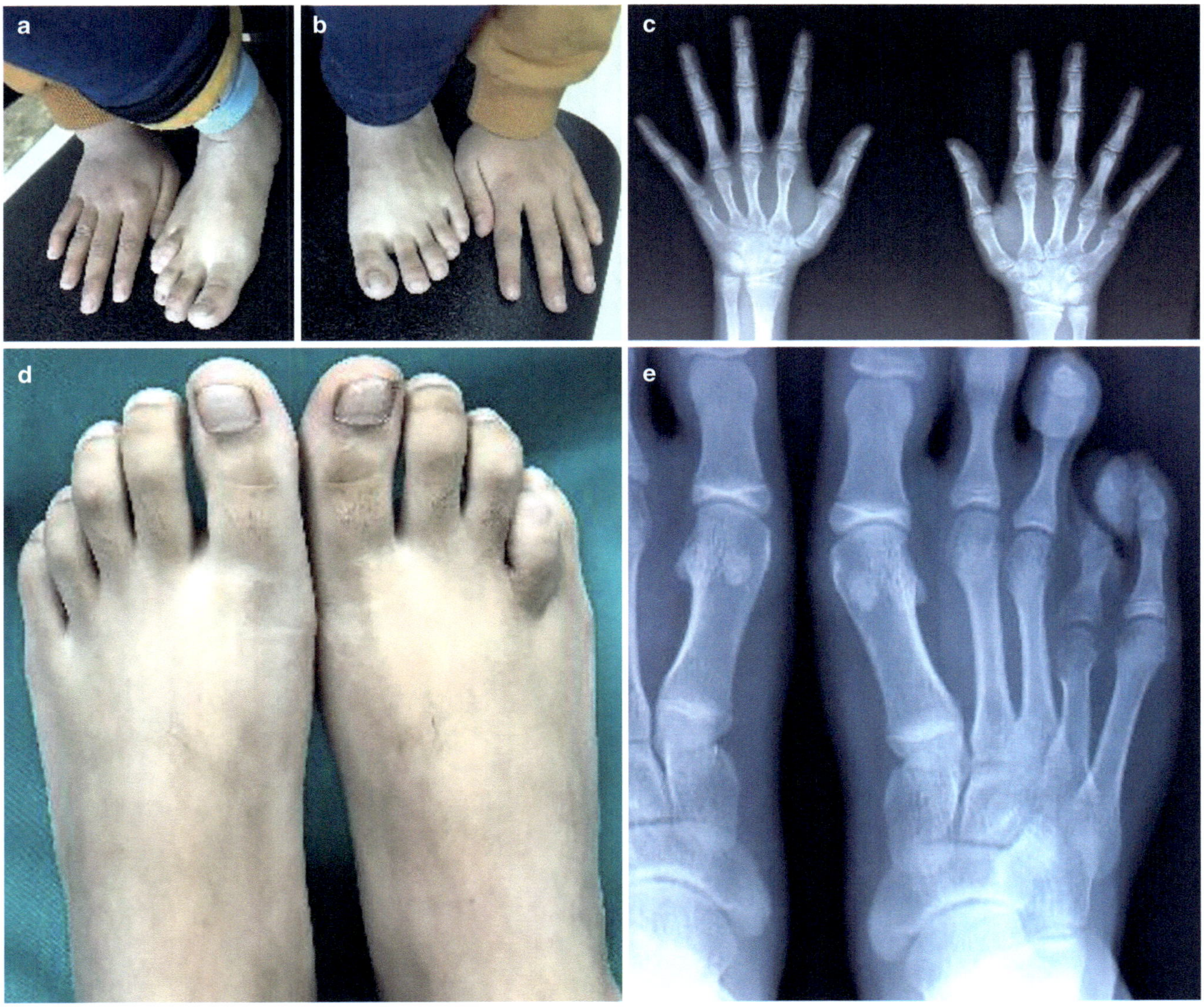

Fig. 13.133 (**a**, **b**) The little finger of both hands and the fourth toe of the right foot are short. (**c**) Radiographs of both hands show premature closure of the epiphyses of the fourth and fifth metacarpals with short bone length. (**d**) Short fourth toe of right foot. (**e**) X-ray of the right foot showing a short fourth metatarsal

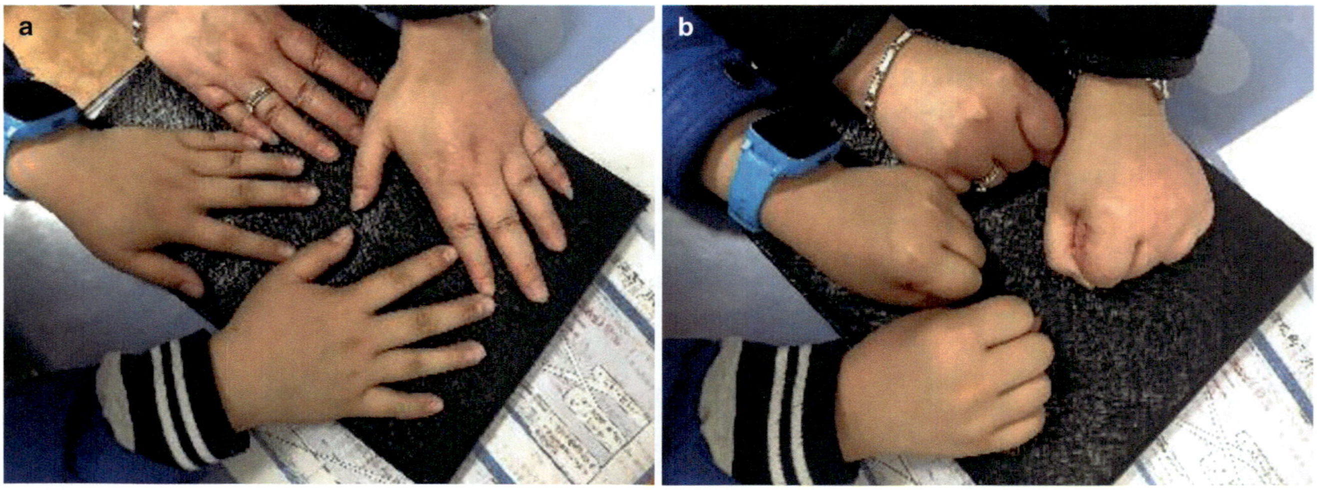

Fig. 13.134 (**a**) Both the child and the mother have short fingers (the mother's left hand ring, little finger and right little finger, and the son's left hand little finger and right-hand ring and little finger are short). (**b**) When the fingers are flexed to make a fist, the metacarpal bone of the short little finger can be seen to "sink"

14 Acquired Upper Limb–Hand Deformity

Sihe Qin, Wen Tian, and Wenyao Zhong

14.1 Central Neurogenic Upper Limb, Hand Deformity

14.1.1 Upper Limb Deformity of Cerebral Palsy

Cerebral palsy involving the upper limbs alone is rare, more common in hemiplegia or double paralysis.

14.1.1.1 Etiology

Cerebral palsy can be caused by brain injury caused by premature delivery, neonatal asphyxia, neonatal low weight, neonatal jaundice, hydrocephalus, and other reasons. Juvenile brain trauma is also a cause of cerebral palsy.

14.1.1.2 Clinical Manifestation

The most common deformities of cerebral palsy patients with upper limb involvement are shoulder joint adduction and internal rotation, elbow flexion and wrist drooping, forearm pronation deformity (Fig. 14.1), finger flexion and fist clenching, shoulder joint abduction, elbow joint extension, forearm supination, and wrist joint dorsiflexion. The severity of the above symptoms varied, with only increased muscle tension and mild motor function limitation in mild cases, which had little impact on function. In severe cases, severe fixed deformity and complete loss of upper limb function are formed.

Case: Fig. 14.2.

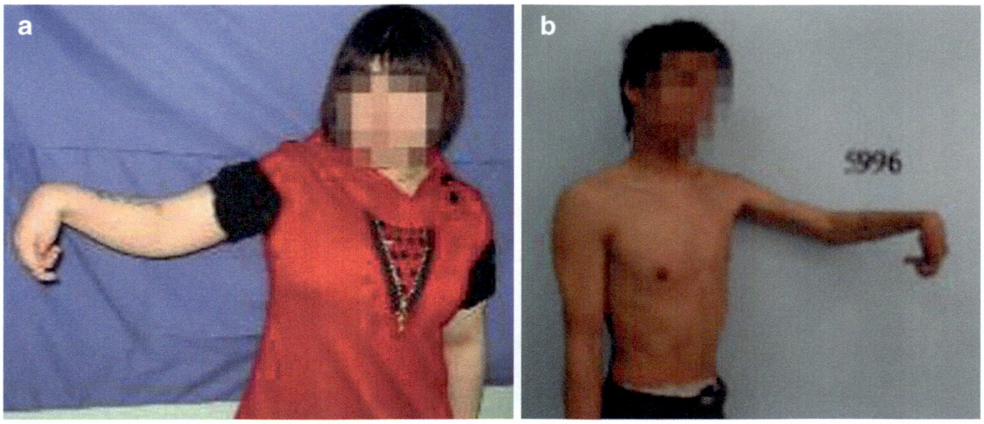

Fig. 14.1 Upper limb deformity of cerebral palsy. (**a**) Right upper limb deformity; (**b**) left upper limb deformity

S. Qin (✉)
Department of Orthopaedics, Rehabilitation Hospital of the National Research Center for Rehabilitation Technical Aids, Beijing, China

W. Tian
Beijing Jishuitan Hospital, Beijing, China

W. Zhong
Department of Hand Surgery, Beijing Jishuitan Hospital, Beijing, China

S. Qin et al. (eds.), *Atlas of Limb Deformity*, https://doi.org/10.1007/978-981-97-0999-1_14

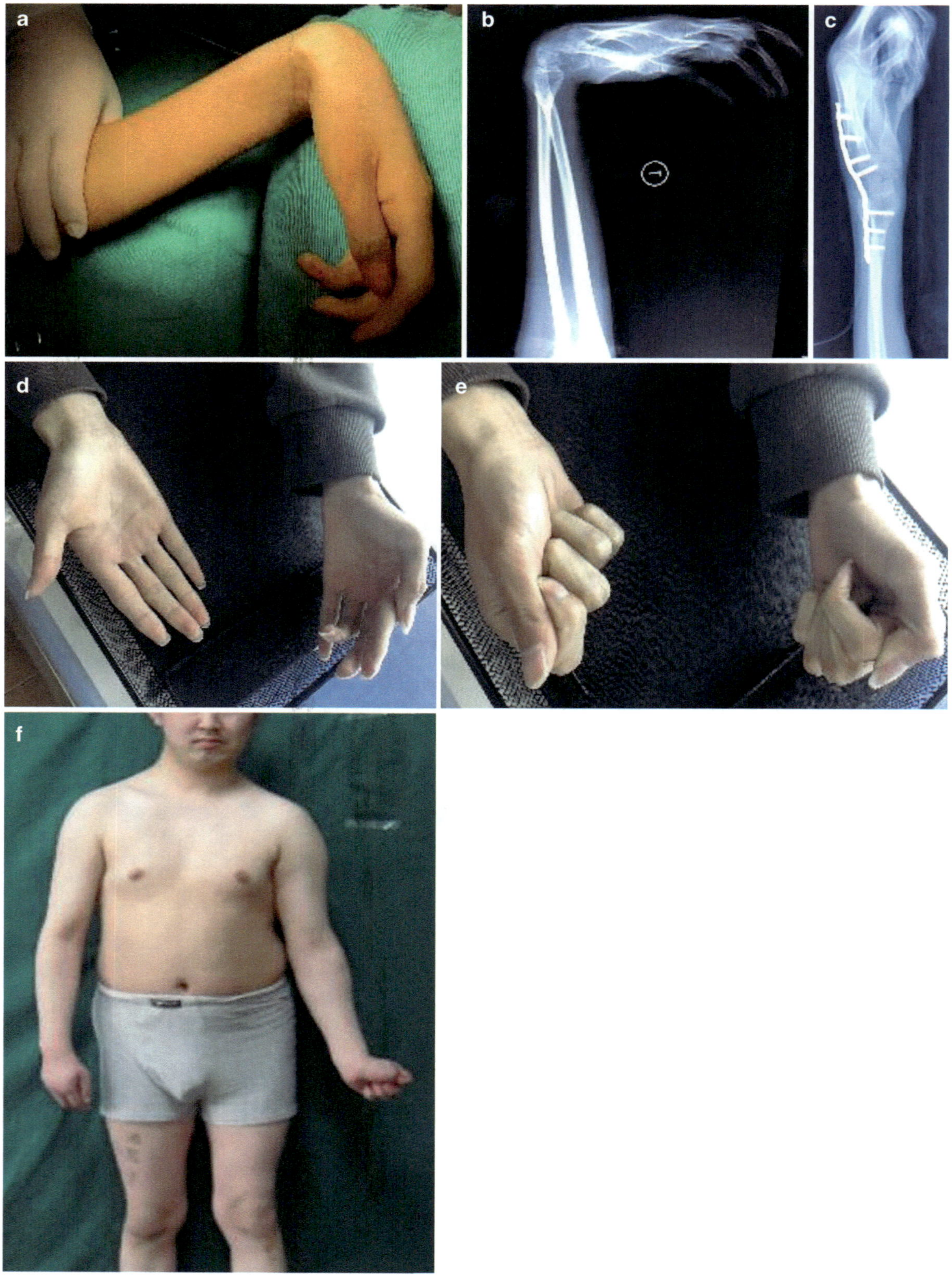

Fig. 14.2 (**a**) A 18-year-old patient suffered from cerebral palsy due to cerebral hypoxia after birth. With the growth, the flexion contracture of the left wrist joint was gradually aggravated. At present, the wrist joint was extremely flexion contracture, the active extension was severely limited, and the hand function could not be exerted. (**b**) X-ray film shows that the left wrist joint has been flexed for a long time, resulting in a deformity of carpal bone development, showing a "wedge" change. (**c**) Radiographs show the wrist was surgically fused in a neutral position. Wrist fusion is shown 1 year after surgery. (**d**) One year after wrist arthrodesis, the fingers of the affected hand are straightened and the fused wrist joint is stable. (**e**) Flexion of the affected hand 1 year after carpal fusion. (**f**) Left upper limb deformity of encephalitis sequela

14.1.1.3 Treatment Principle

(1) Selective constriction of muscular branches of peripheral nerves was performed to reduce muscle tension and spasm in patients with spasticity, no fixed deformity or mild deformity. (2) In case of fixed deformity, soft tissue release and tendon transfer should be performed to balance muscle strength, and wrist arthrodesis should be performed if necessary.

14.1.2 Upper Limb Deformity in Encephalitis and Stroke

14.1.2.1 Etiology

Brain injury caused by epidemic encephalitis B, epidemic cerebrospinal meningitis, cerebral thrombosis or cerebral hemorrhage, involving the upper limb motor center, can lead to spastic paralysis of the upper limb.

14.1.2.2 Clinical Manifestation

Similar to the sequelae of cerebral palsy, it is characterized by different degrees of shoulder adduction and internal rotation, elbow flexion, wrist drooping, forearm pronation deformity, and finger flexion deformity. Shoulder deformity is rare, while elbow, wrist, and hand deformity are common.

Sequelae of encephalitis (Fig. 14.2).

14.1.3 Stroke (Cerebrovascular Disease) Upper Limb Deformity (Fig. 14.3)

14.1.3.1 Treatment Principle

In the acute stage, rehabilitation treatment is the main method to restore the function to the greatest extent. In the sequela stage, surgical intervention can be used, and the treatment principles and methods can refer to the treatment of upper limb deformities of cerebral palsy.

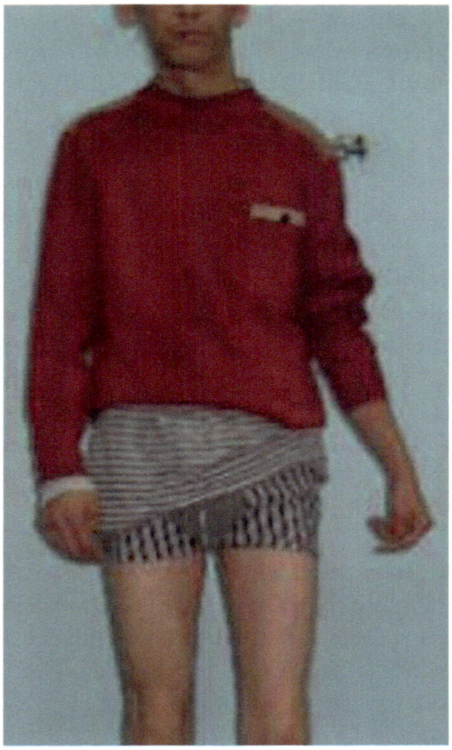

Fig. 14.3 Left upper limb deformity of cerebral hemorrhage sequela

14.2 Peripheral Neurogenic Upper Limb, Hand Deformity

14.2.1 Brachial Plexus Injury

14.2.1.1 Etiology

Brachial plexus injuries are mostly closed injuries, such as traffic accidents, violent traction, direct impact, and so on. There were occasional direct stab wounds and local vascular injuries. Local compression, such as cervical ribs, transverse process hypertrophy, tumors, or local soft tissue fiber cords, muscle hypertrophy, vascular variation, can cause brachial plexus injury. Obstetric brachial plexus injuries also occur.

14.2.1.2 Clinical Manifestation

The diagnosis of brachial plexus injury is relatively complex, which needs to be combined with clinical manifestations, electrophysiological examination, imaging examination, etc to determine whether the brachial plexus was injury, the level of injury, the nature of injury, etc. According to the anatomical structure, it can be divided into brachial plexus upper trunk, middle upper trunk, lower trunk injury, and total brachial plexus injury. Total brachial plexus root avulsion injury often leads to the loss or partial loss of motor and sensory function of the whole upper limb, and the treatment effect is still not very ideal.

14.2.1.3 Treatment Principle

Treatment is more complex, requiring a combination of various factors to develop a systematic and continuous treatment plan, including a strict rehabilitation plan. The results of treatment vary greatly with different injuries.

Case 1: Fig. 14.4.
Case 2: Fig. 14.5.
Case 3: Fig. 14.6.

14.2.2 Radial Nerve Injury

14.2.2.1 Etiology

Various traumas are common causes of radial nerve injury, such as cutting injury, direct stab injury or traction during fracture, direct stab injury at the fracture end or nerve entrapment at the fracture end. There are also cases of accidental injury caused by surgery. Radial nerve entrapment caused by various reasons is also a common cause.

14.2.2.2 Clinical Manifestation

After radial nerve injury, it mainly causes the loss or partial loss of wrist extension, finger extension and thumb extension, resulting in wrist drop, finger drop and thumb drop deformity, and the corresponding decrease or disappearance of skin sensation on the dorsal side of the thumb web and the radial side of the back of the hand. Clinical symptoms or signs may vary or form different combinations depending on the level of radial nerve injury.

14.2.2.3 Treatment Principle

The treatment of radial nerve injury depends on the specific injury situation, such as the nature of injury, the time of injury, the level of injury, age, general condition, and so on.

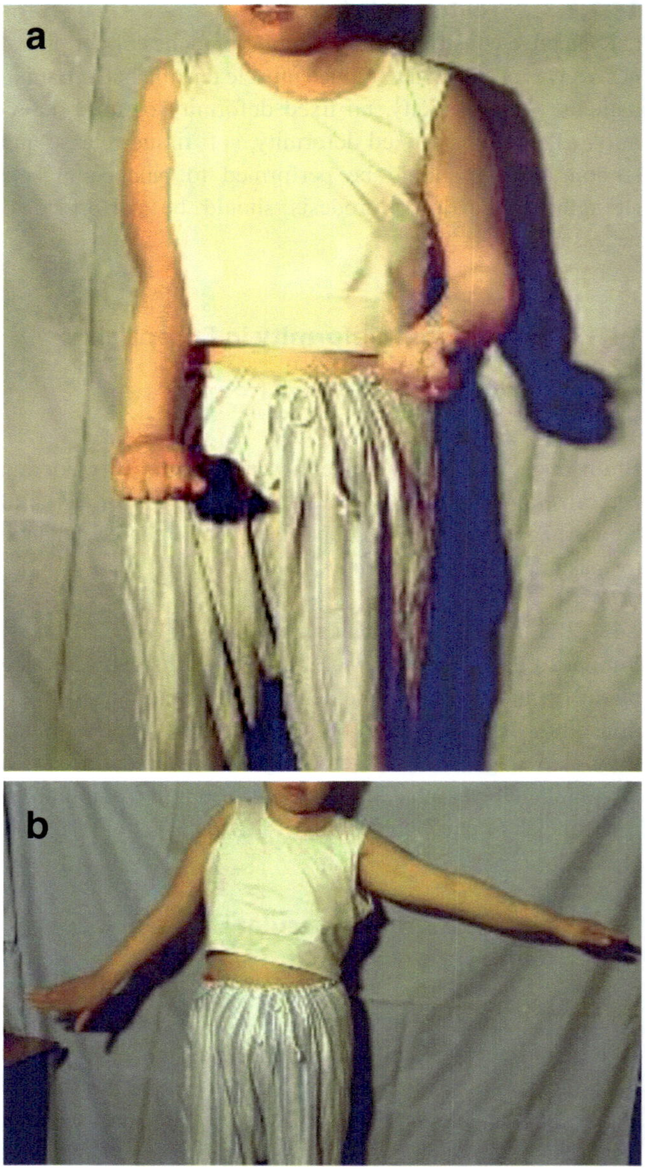

Fig. 14.4 (**a**) The patient is 22 years old. The upper trunk of the right brachial plexus nerve is not completely injured due to a traffic accident. The active abduction of the right shoulder joint and the flexion of the elbow joint are impaired. The skin sensation outside the shoulder joint is reduced. The elbow flexion function of the patient is limited. The function of the affected hand is basically normal. (**b**) Shows the limitation of abduction function of the right shoulder joint. This is an incomplete injury of the upper trunk of the brachial plexus

The commonly used methods are direct nerve suture, nerve release, nerve transplantation, and so on. For those who have poor recovery after repair or have been injured for a long time, functional reconstruction can be carried out by tendon transfer.

Case 1: Fig. 14.7.
Case 2: Fig. 14.8.

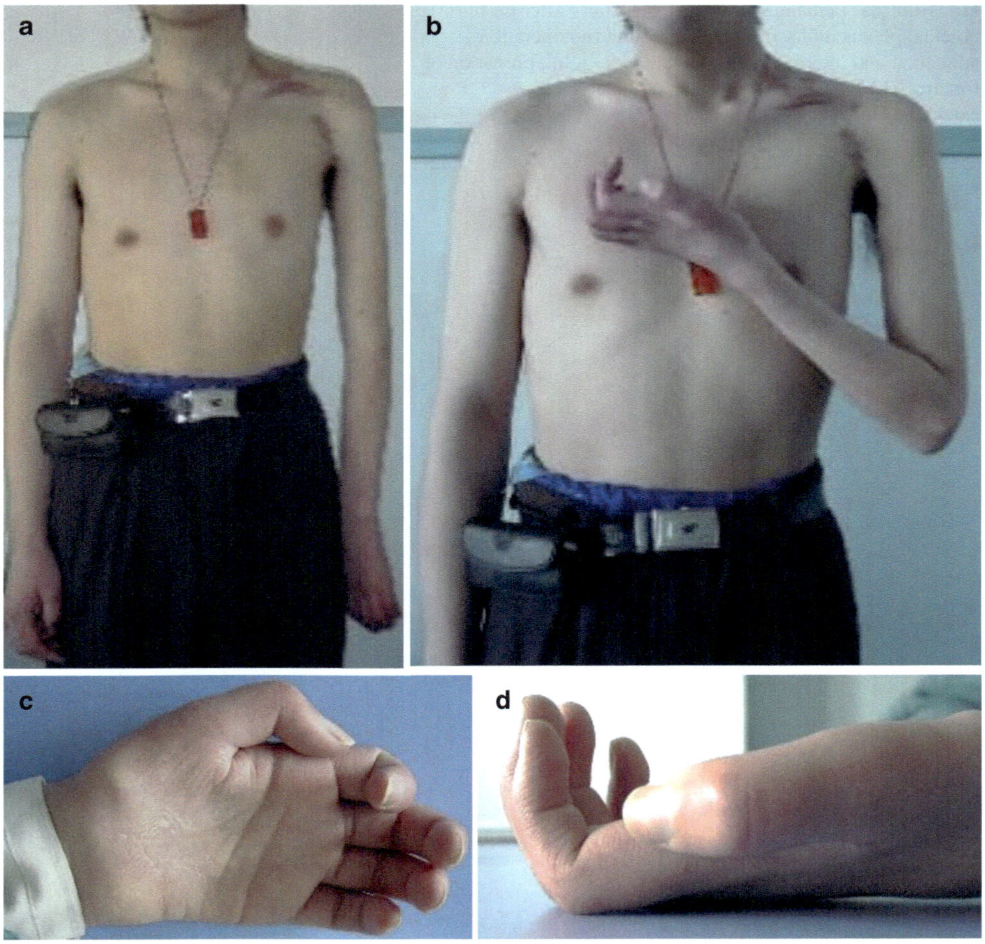

Fig. 14.5 (**a**) Male, 25 years old, with total brachial plexus root avulsion caused by traction injury of left upper limb, 1 year after nerve transfer. (**b**) Partial recovery of elbow flexion. (**c**) No recovery of hand function. (**d**) No recovery of hand function

14.2.3 Ulnar Nerve Injury

14.2.3.1 Etiology

There are many causes of ulnar nerve injury, most of which are various traumas. Ulnar nerve entrapment at the elbow is also a common cause. The causes of entrapment include elbow degeneration, cubitus valgus, fibrous scar tissue, mass, variant muscle, and so on.

14.2.3.2 Clinical Manifestation

Ulnar nerve injury often seriously affects the flexion function of the ring and little finger and the sensory function of the ulnar and little fingers of the ring finger, as well as the functions of division, syndactyly, and wrist flexion, and obvious atrophy of the hypothenar muscles and the first dorsal interosseous muscles can be seen. Claw hand deformity is an important clinical sign of ulnar nerve injury, and the severity of this sign varies with the level of injury. Tinel's sign and Froment's sign were positive. Sometimes the palmaris brevis reflex disappears. Ulnar nerve injury often seriously affects the fine hand movements of patients.

14.2.3.3 Treatment Principle

The treatment principle is basically the same as that of radial nerve injury.

Case 1: Fig. 14.9.

Case 2: Fig. 14.10.

Case 3: Fig. 14.11.

14.2.4 Median Nerve

14.2.4.1 Etiology

Trauma and wrist entrapment are the main causes of median nerve injury.

14.2.4.2 Clinical Manifestation

According to the different levels of injury, the corresponding clinical symptoms and signs may appear. Carpal tunnel syndrome is a common type of median nerve entrapment injury.

14.2.4.3 Treatment Principle

It is basically the same as radial nerve and ulnar nerve injury.

Case 1: Fig. 14.12.

Case 2: Fig. 14.13.

Fig. 14.6 (**a**) Female, 9 years old, deformity after obstetric brachial plexus injury of right upper limb (no operation), adduction and internal rotation of shoulder joint, pronation of forearm. (**b**) Weakness in shoulder abduction, elbow extension, and forearm supination

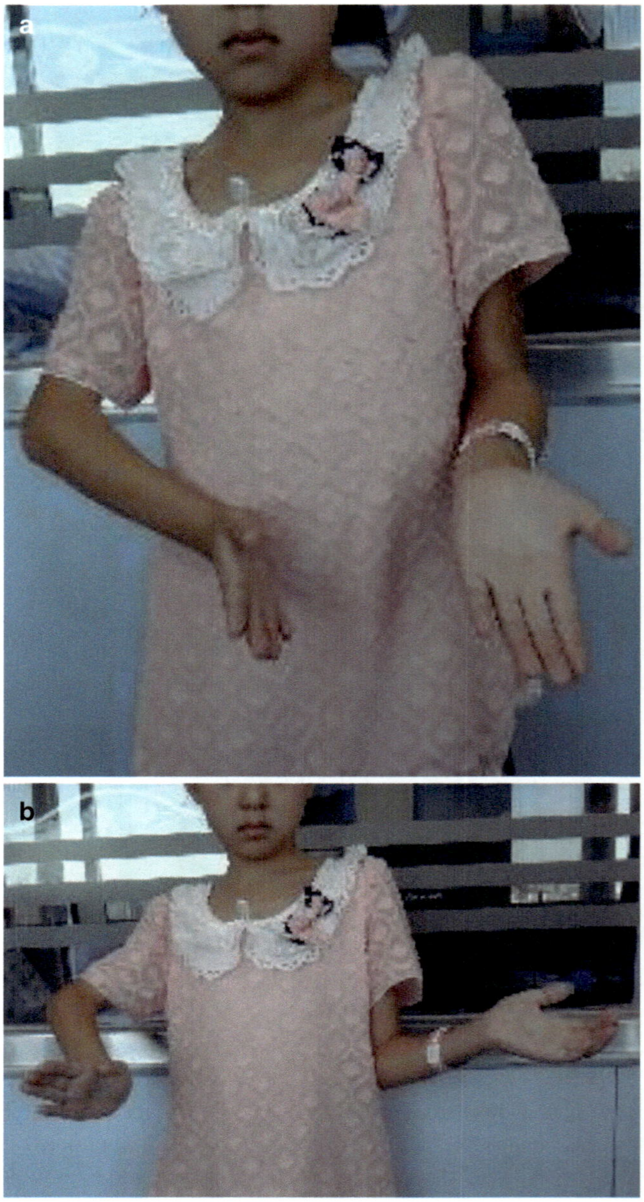

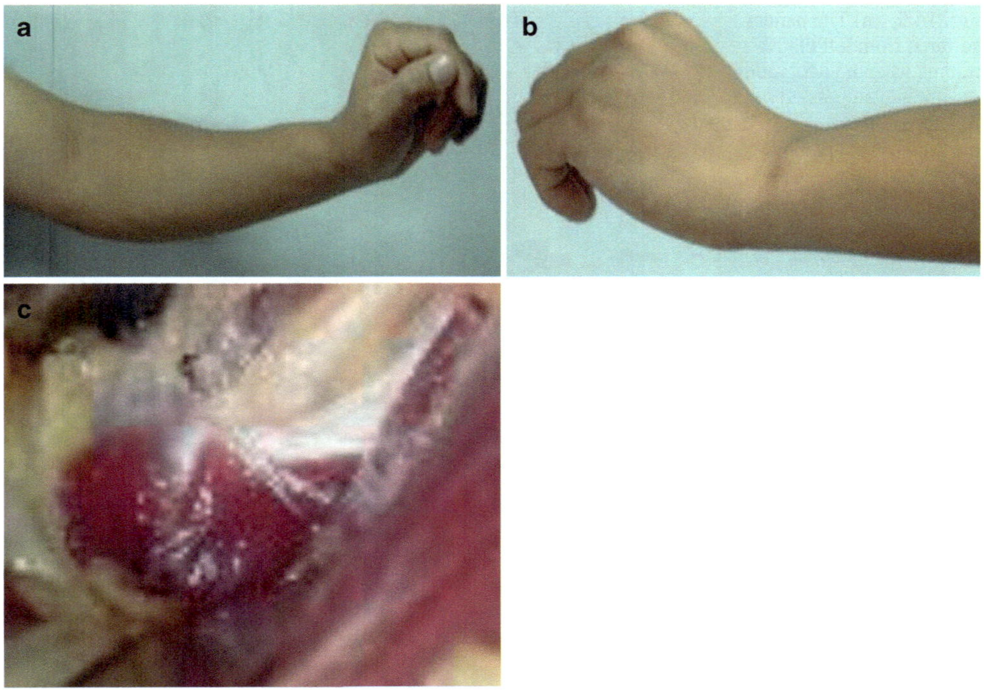

Fig. 14.7 (**a**) The patient has left finger extension and thumb extension dysfunction without obvious inducement, with normal wrist extension function and normal sensation on the dorsal side of the thumb web. (**b**) Shows normal wrist extension. This case is diagnosed as "radial nerve entrapment" (proximal forearm). (**c**) Surgical exploration revealed that the radial nerve and the dorsal interosseous nerve of the forearm were compressed at the entrance of the supinator muscle

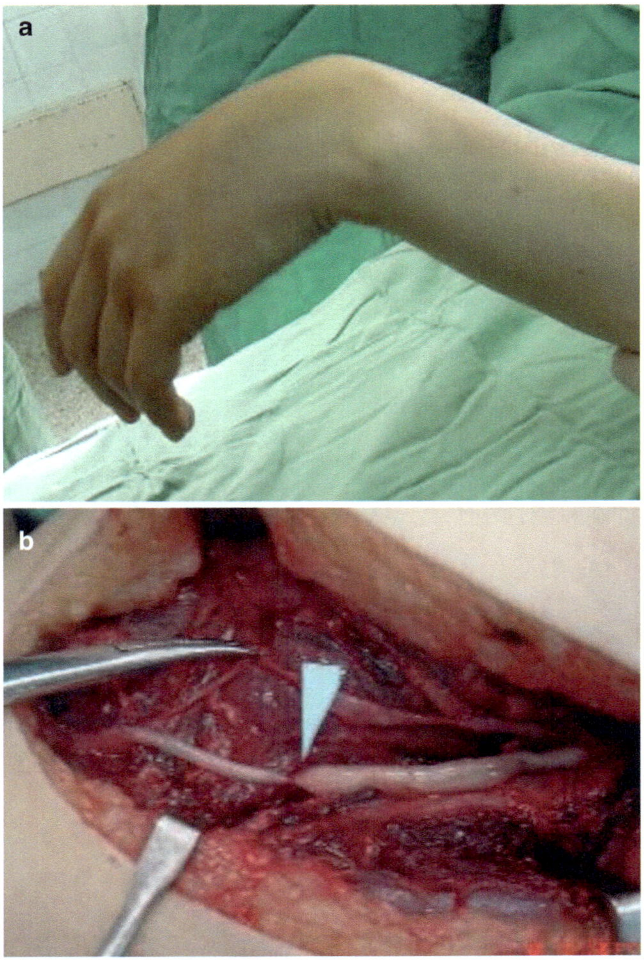

Fig. 14.8 (**a**) The patient was diagnosed as "radial nerve entrapment" (upper arm) due to left wrist drop, finger drop, and thumb drop without obvious inducement, loss of active wrist extension, finger extension and thumb extension, and obvious decrease of skin sensation on the dorsal side of the thumb web. (**b**) The surgical exploration found that the radial nerve trunk had an "hourglass" stenosis (indicated by the arrow) at the level of the middle and lower segments of the upper arm, and the nerve proximal to the stenosis was irregularly thickened and edematous

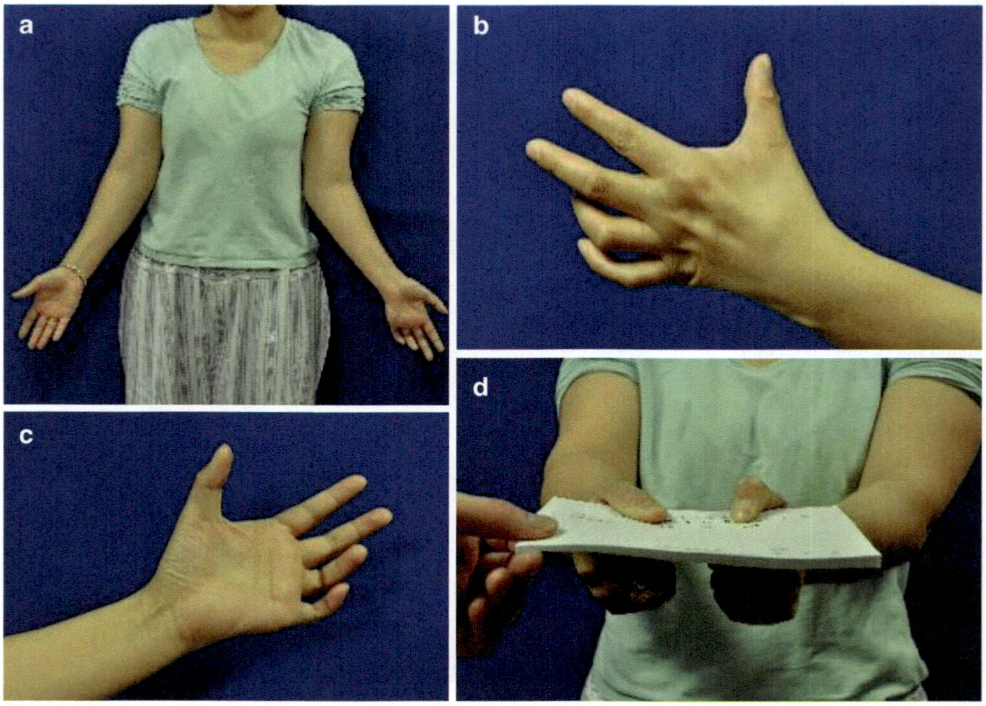

Fig. 14.9 (**a**) The patient suffered from left elbow trauma when he was young, resulting in supracondylar fracture of the humerus. With the growth, he gradually developed cubitus valgus deformity. At present, the ring little finger is numb and hypoesthesia, and the intrinsic muscles of the hand and the flexor muscles of the forearm are atrophied. (**b**) It shows marked atrophy of the first dorsal interosseous muscle with claw hand deformity. (**c**) It shows hypothenar muscle atrophy and claw hand deformity. (**d**) The Froment sign is positive. This is a case of ulnar nerve entrapment at the elbow caused by valgus deformity of the elbow

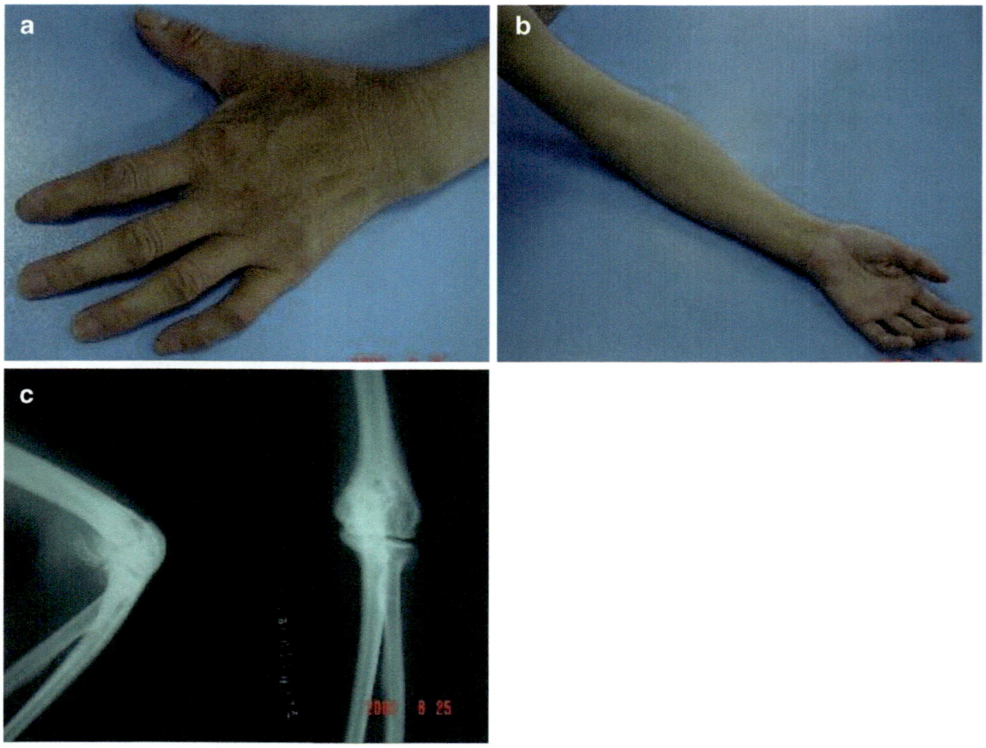

Fig. 14.10 (**a**) Patient A is an elderly female, who gradually developed hand intrinsic muscle atrophy, hypoesthesia of ring and little finger, hypodynamia, and mild claw hand deformity without inducement. (**b**) In addition to the intrinsic muscular atrophy of the hand, there is muscular atrophy of the flexor aspect of the forearm. (**c**) Radiographs show typical degenerative arthritic changes in the elbow joint. This is an example of ulnar nerve entrapment at the elbow caused by retirement arthritis (apophysis)

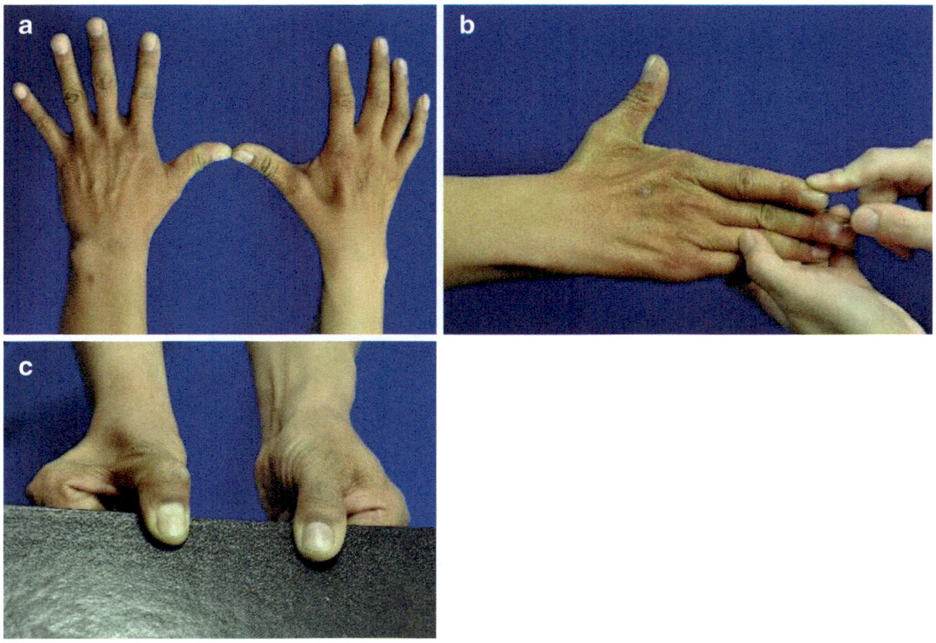

Fig. 14.11 (**a**) A patient is an adult male with progressive hypoesthesia of the ring and little finger of the right hand, atrophy of the intrinsic muscles of the hand, and claw hand deformity. The first dorsal interosseous and hypothenar muscles are atrophied, and claw hand deformity is shown. (**b**) Shows that the abduction function of the index finger is significantly reduced. (**c**) Shows a positive Froment sign (right). (**d**) Surgical exploration revealed that the right ulnar nerve was compressed and strangulated by local scar fibrous tissue in the ulnar nerve groove at the elbow

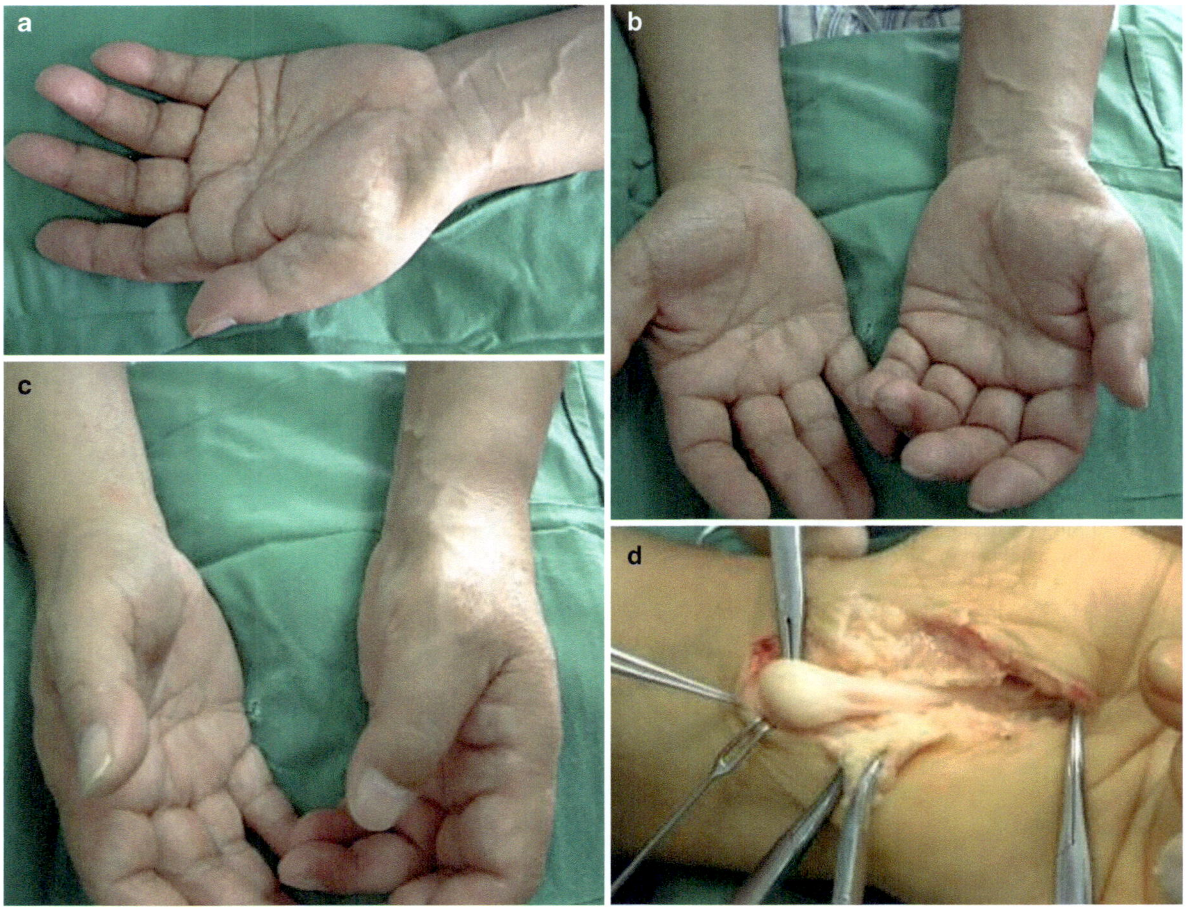

Fig. 14.12 (**a**) Patient A is an elderly female with numbness and hypoesthesia in the thumb, index finger, middle finger, and ring finger of the left hand, gradual atrophy of the thenar muscles, loss of abduction function of the thumb, positive Tinel sign of the median nerve on the palmar side of the wrist, and positive wrist flexion test. (**b**) Comparison of both hands. The left thenar muscles are obviously atrophied, and the thumb is adducted and supinated. (**c**) Flat left thenar muscle. (**d**) Surgical exploration revealed severe synovial hyperplasia in the left carpal tunnel and significant compression of the median nerve in the carpal tunnel

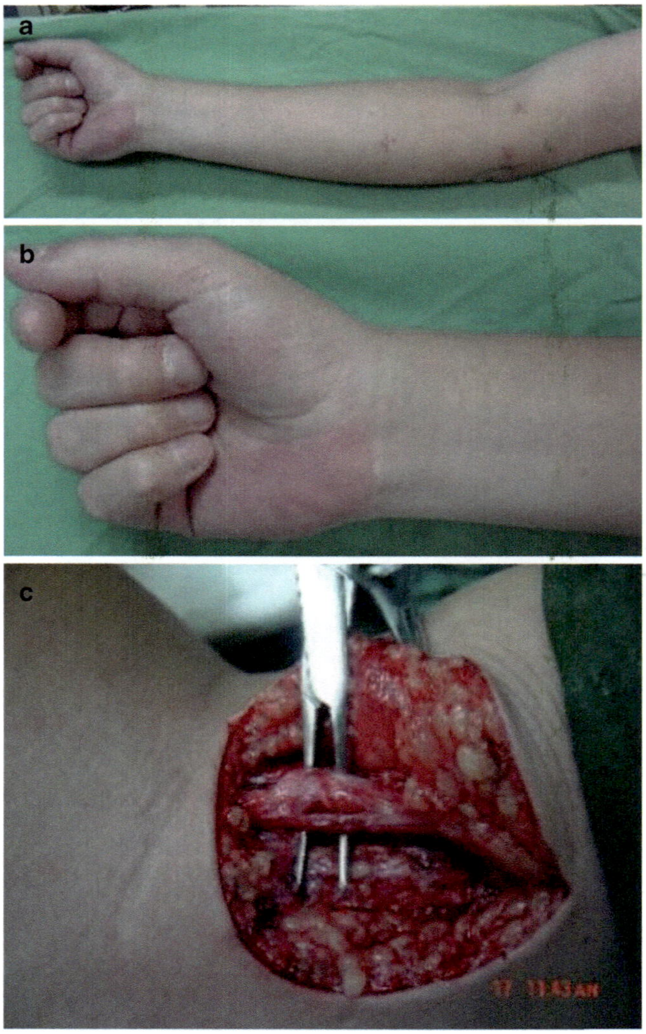

Fig. 14.13 (**a**) The right elbow joint was injured by multiple sharp instruments on the medial side. After the injury, the thumb, index, middle, and ring fingers were numb with hypoesthesia, the flexion function of the thumb and index fingers was impaired, and the abduction function of the thumb was partially impaired. (**b**) Shows normal flexion of the middle, ring, and little fingers and impaired flexion of the thumb and index fingers. (**c**) Surgical exploration revealed that the median nerve was broken at the proximal part of the elbow joint

14.3 Trauma and Infection Lead to Upper Limb, Hand Deformity

14.3.1 Ischemic Muscle Contracture of Forearm

Forearm ischemic muscle contracture, also known as VolkmAnns ischemic muscle contracture, is one of the serious complications that may occur after forearm trauma.

14.3.1.1 Etiology

It is common to have supracondylar fracture of the humerus or fracture of the forearm with poor reduction or without reduction. It can also be seen in vascular injury, severe soft tissue injury of the forearm, compression of the limbs after coma, too tight external dressing of the elbow or forearm, or too tight binding of external fixations (such as plaster, small splint, etc.).

14.3.1.2 Clinical Manifestation

Forearm muscle atrophy, forearm pronation deformity, wrist and finger flexion, thumb adduction, metacarpophalangeal joint hyperextension, claw hand, which cannot be corrected passively (Fig. 14.14).

Case 1: Fig. 14.14.
Case 2: Fig. 14.15.
Case 3: Fig. 14.16.

14.3.1.3 Treatment Principle

Surgical release of the contracted tendon and correction of claw finger deformity.

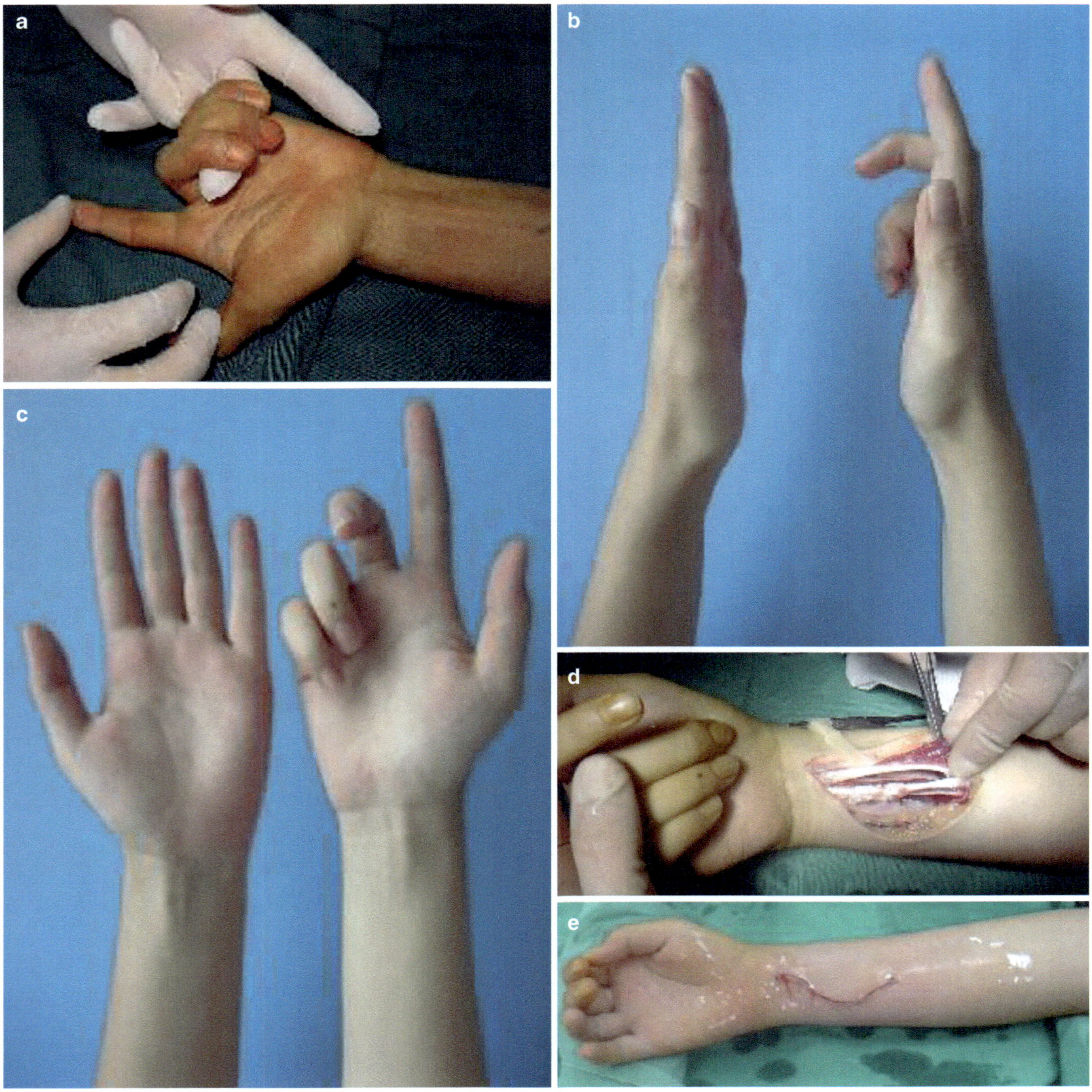

Fig. 14.14 (**a**) The patient was 12 years old, and the right forearm radial and ulnar fracture was externally fixed, resulting in "ischemic muscle contracture of the forearm," with flexion contracture of the index, middle, ring and little fingers, and relatively mild flexion contracture of the index finger. (**b**) Palmar view. (**c**) Left forearm VolkmAnns muscle contracture and limitation of passive extension of middle ring and little finger joint. (**d**) Transposition of the flexor digitorum superficialis muscle to the flexor digitorum profundus tendon of the middle and little fingers. (**e**) The flexion contracture of the fingers was significantly improved after (**d**) operation

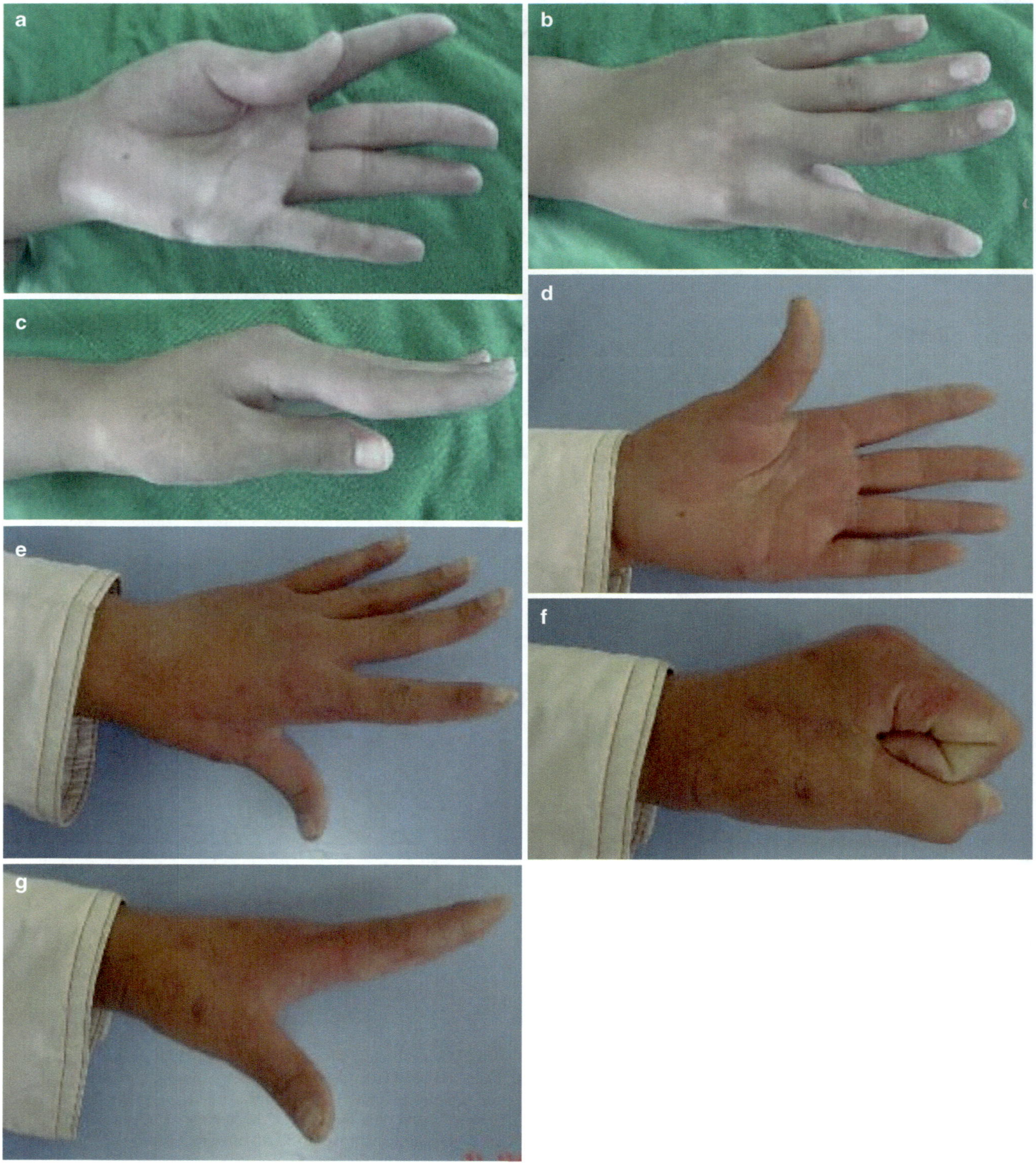

Fig. 14.15 (**a**) Female patient with "ischemic contracture of left intrinsic muscle" due to external cosmetic allergy, flexion of metacarpophalangeal joint of fingers, hyperextension of interphalangeal joint, and adduction of thumb. (**b**) Preoperative dorsal view. (**c**) Preoperative lateral view showing typical intrinsic myopositive sign. (**d**) Deformity improved significantly after endomuscular release. (**e**) Postoperative dorsal view. (**f**) The patient clenched his fist after surgery. (**g**) Postoperative finger straightening

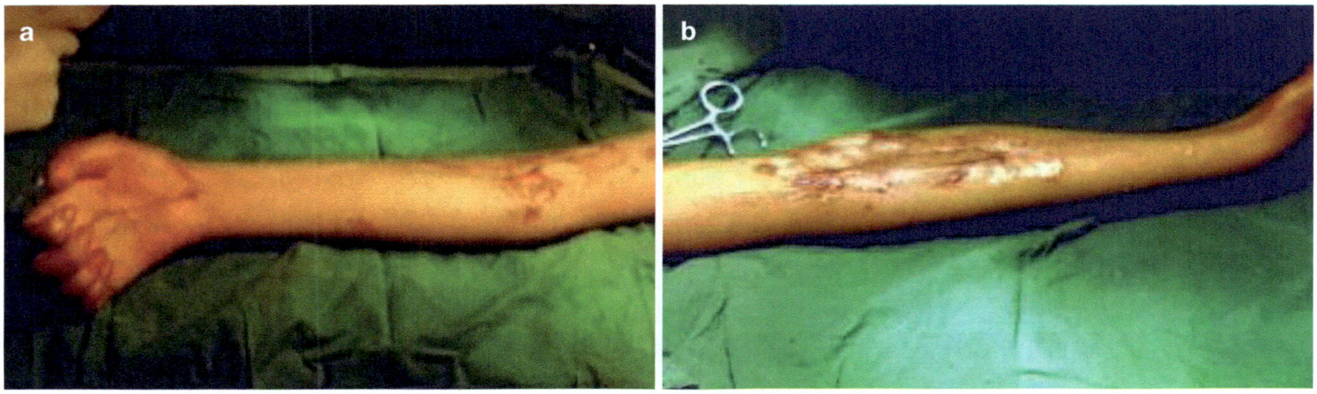

Fig. 14.16 (**a**) The patient suffered from "osteofascial compartment syndrome" in the right forearm after a traffic accident. He had undergone "forearm incision decompression." After the operation, there were still residual deformities, extensive scar tissue in the forearm, significantly reduced muscle volume, flat palm, disappearance of thenar and hypothenar protuberances, adduction and supination of the thumb, and flexion deformity of the wrist and fingers. (**b**) Extensive scar tissue in the forearm and flexion deformity of the wrist joint

14.4 Nonunion and Bone Defect of Upper Limb

14.4.1 Etiology

Severe trauma and osteomyelitis are the main causes of bone nonunion and bone defect in upper limbs.

14.4.2 Clinical Manifestation

History of severe trauma or bone infection, old scar, deformity, shortening, and/or abnormal movement of the upper arm or forearm. X-ray showed bone nonunion and/or bone defect.

Open fractures of the upper extremities caused by severe trauma can cause bone defects (Fig. 14.17 (1–3)); inappropriate treatment of closed or open fractures can cause nonunion (Fig. 14.17 (4, 5)).

14.4.3 Treatment Principle

Ilizarov femoral lengthening technique was used to repair the bone defect. The nonunion was cured and the hand function was improved by the optimized combination of local cleaning of nonunion, autogenous bone grafting and external fixation.

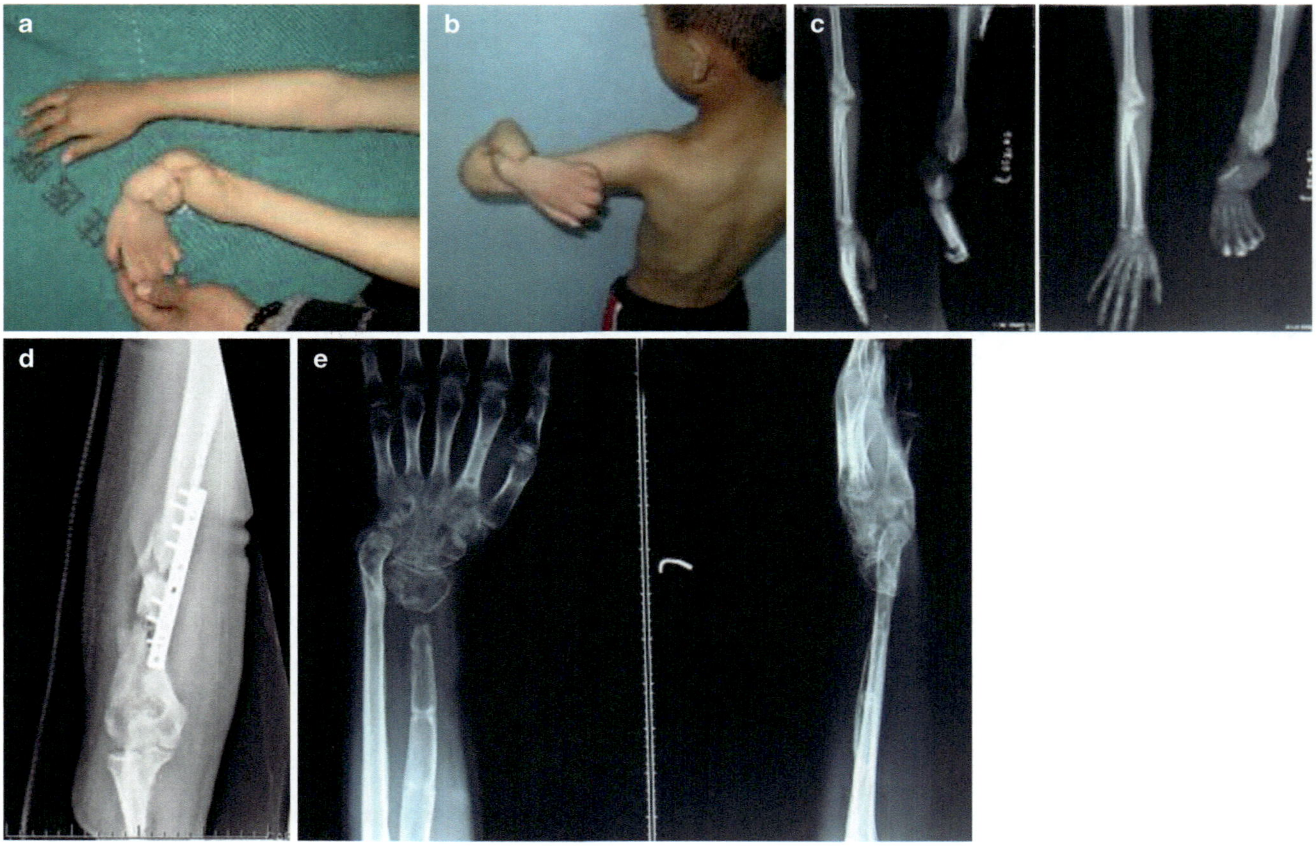

Fig. 14.17 (1–3) Infected bone defect of left forearm (1) Shortening of the left forearm; (2) No bony support of the forearm; (3) X-ray film. (4, 5) Postoperative nonunion of fracture. (4) Nonunion after internal fixation of humeral open comminuted fracture; (5) Nonunion and bone defect after open comminuted fracture of left radius

14.5 Joint Contracture Deformity of Upper Limb Caused by Burn or Trauma

14.5.1 Etiology

After the healing of the wound, the local scar contracture caused the deformity of the bone and joint. Trauma can also cause soft tissue injury on the flexor side of the joint, such as belt injury (treadmill, etc.), and scar healing after injury can also cause joint contracture.

14.5.2 Clinical Manifestation

Large area of burn and scald of skin or scar of trauma, contracture of the joint at the distal end of scar traction, elbow flexion deformity, dorsal wrist extension deformity, palmar scar flexion deformity, if the injury is deep, involving muscles or tendons, it will lead to more serious deformity and dysfunction.

Severe bone and joint deformity of upper limbs caused by scald (Fig. 14.18).

Case 1: Fig. 14.19.

Case 2: Fig. 14.20.

Case 3: Fig. 14.21.

Case 4: Fig. 14.22.

Case 5: Fig. 14.23.

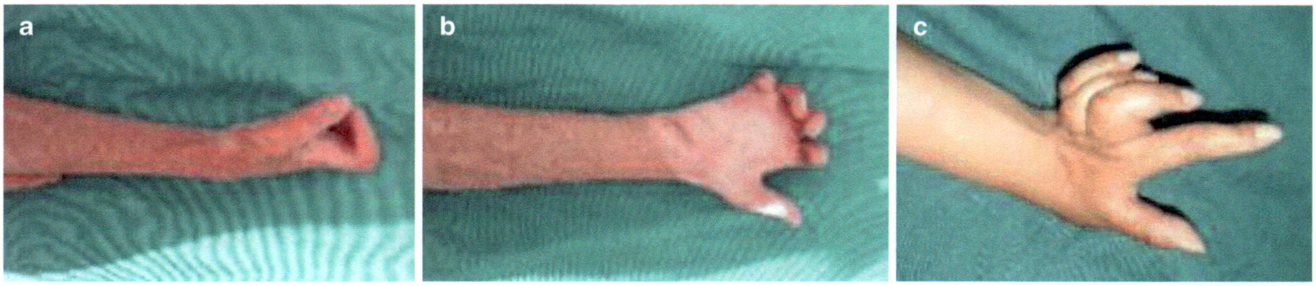

Fig. 14.18 (**a**, **b**) Burn of forearm and hand. (**c**) Posttraumatic scar contracture on the dorsal side of the left hand with extreme dorsiflexion deformity of the metacarpophalangeal joint

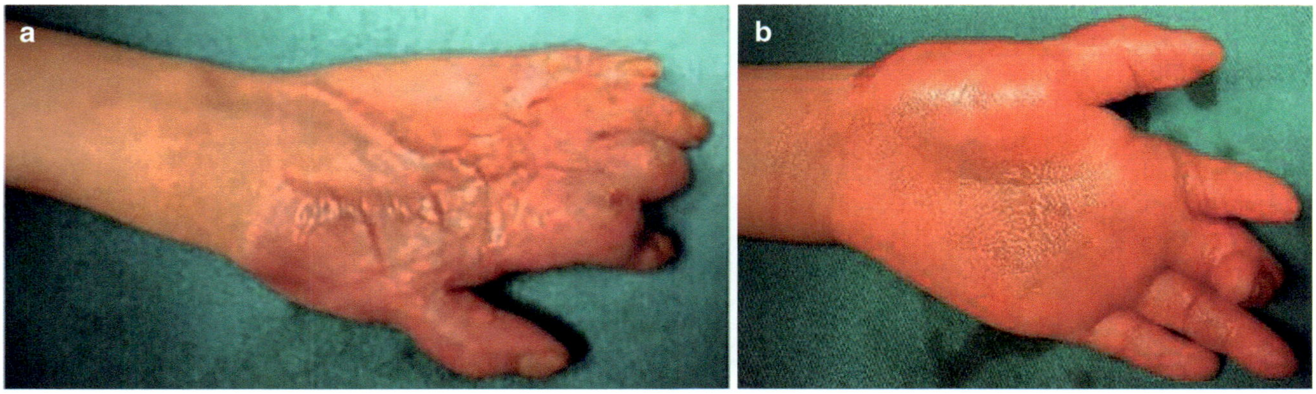

Fig. 14.19 (**a**) The patient was scalded on the left hand when he was young, and then developed scar contracture on the dorsal side of the hand, with the fingers connected together and the tiger's mouth narrowed. (**b**) Palmar contracture is mild

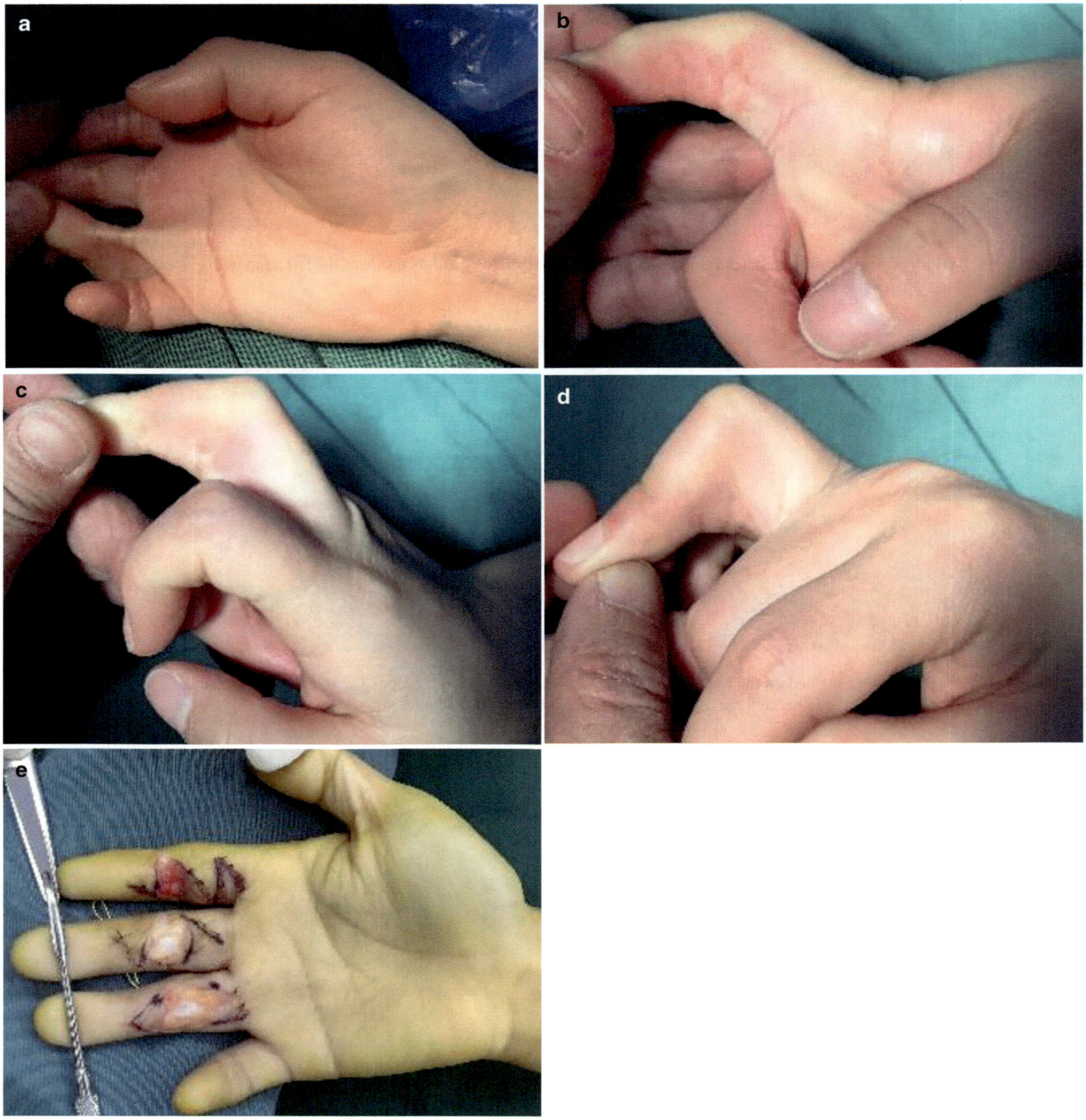

Fig. 14.20 (**a**) Scar contracture of the flexor skin of the index, middle, and ring fingers after crush injury of the right hand. (**b**) Scar contracture palmar index finger. (**c**) Scar contracture of palmar middle finger. (**d**) Palmar scar contracture of ring finger. (**e**) The finger flexion contracture was relieved after surgical release, and the residual skin defect was planned to be covered by free skin graft

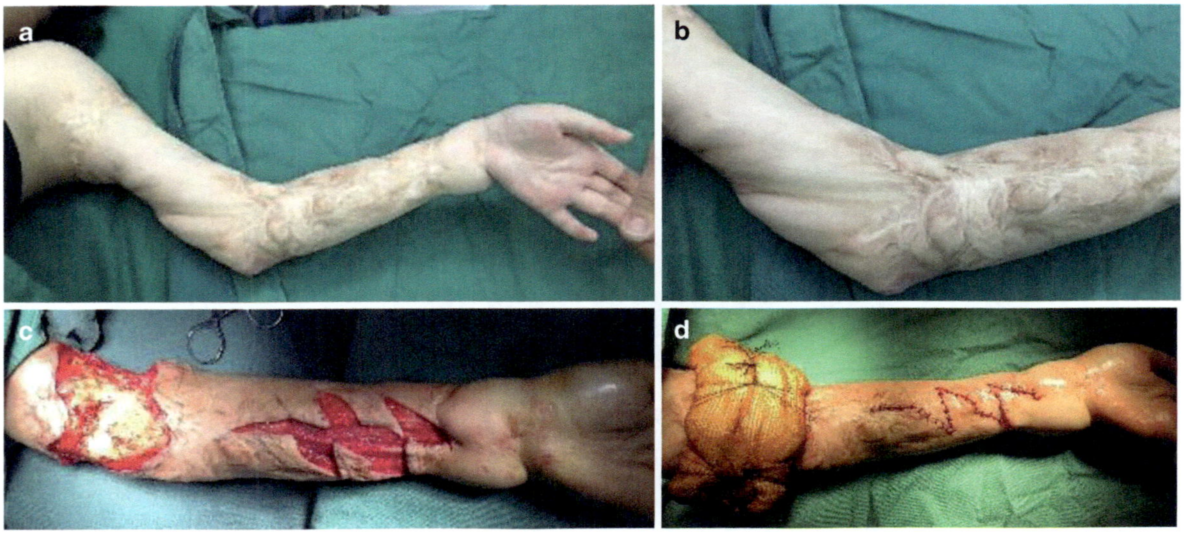

Fig. 14.21 (**a**) Extensive scar contracture of left upper limb after traffic accident. (**b**) Elbow joint contracture. (**c**) After release of scar on elbow and forearm. (**d**) After scar release (Z-shaped formation of forearm scar, scar excision, release, and free skin graft coverage on the volar side of elbow joint)

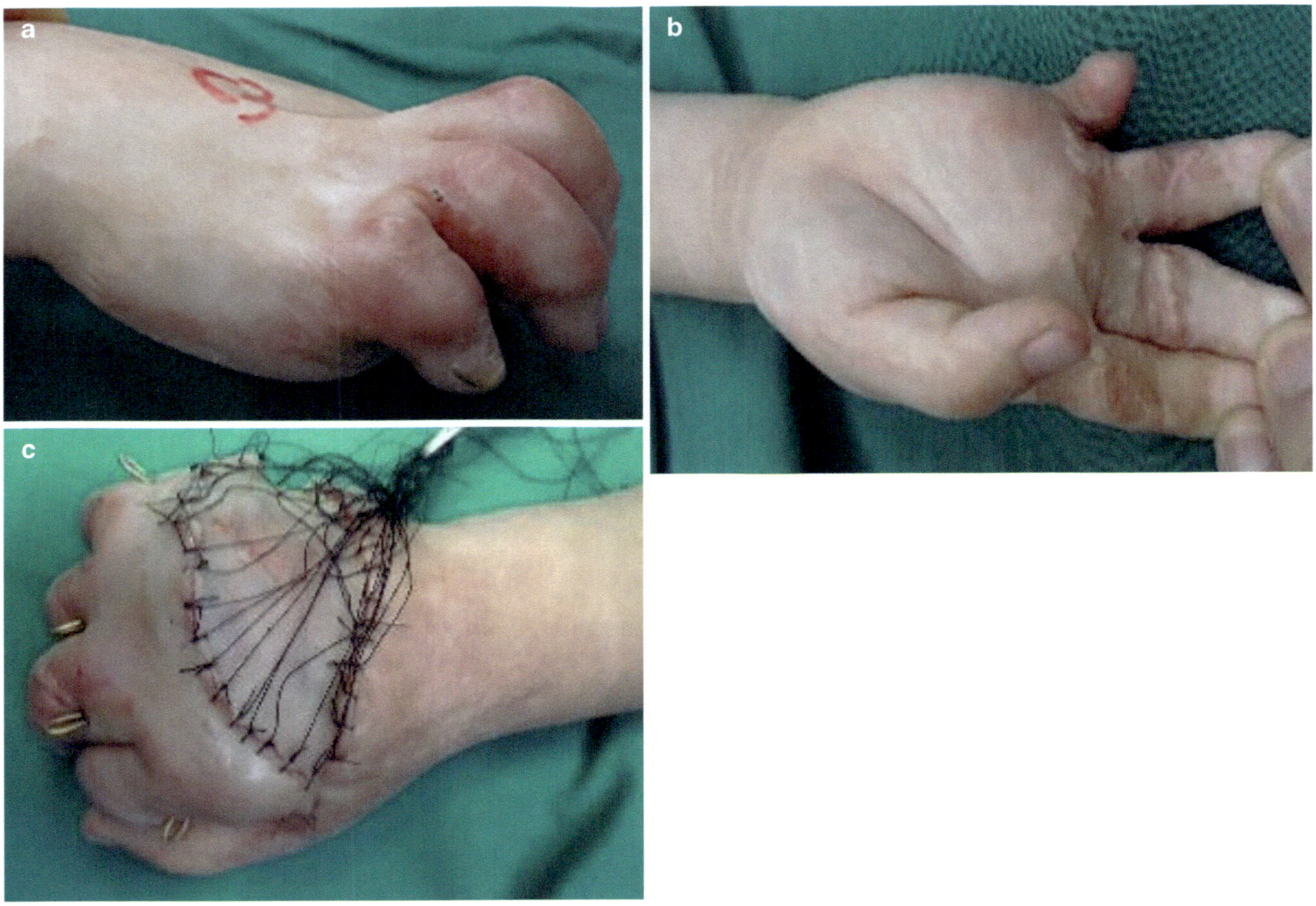

Fig. 14.22 (**a**) Scar contracture on the dorsal side of the scalded right hand, resulting in hyperextension contracture of the metacarpophalangeal joint and limitation of active and passive flexion. (**b**) Release of palmar contracture completed. (**c**) Metacarpophalangeal joints of fingers were fixed in flexion with Kirschner wire after scar release and skin grafting on the dorsum of the hand

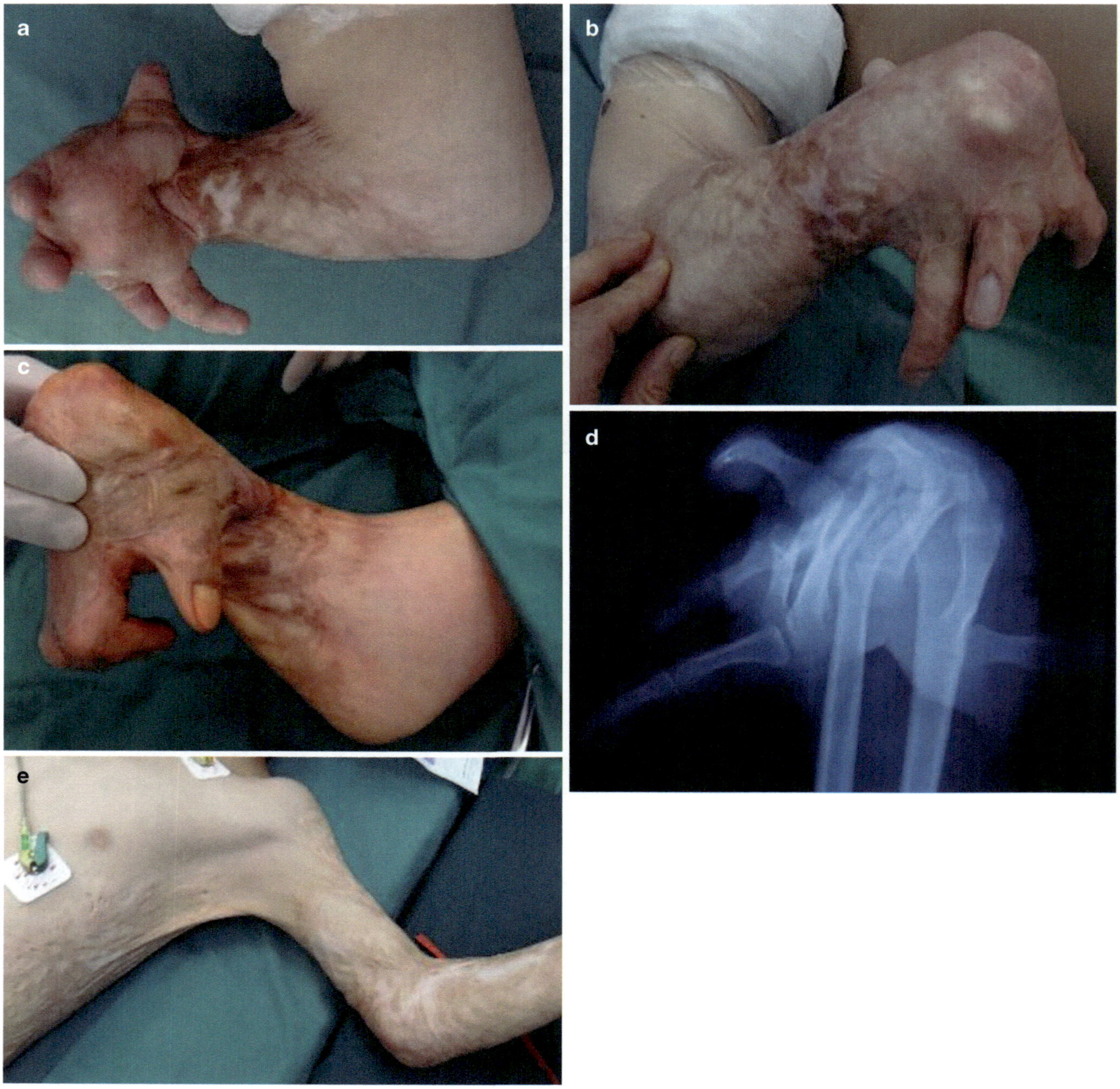

Fig. 14.23 (**a**) Scar contracture of multiple joints after trauma in both upper extremities of a child. This is a palmar view of the right upper extremity. (**b**) Ulnar view of the right upper limb, hyperextension of the metacarpophalangeal joint, and extreme flexion contracture of the wrist joint. (**c**) Radial view of right upper limb with severely flexed wrist joint. (**d**) The X-ray film of the right hand shows that the bone and joint are extremely deformed and deformed. (**e**) Scar contractures were found in the left upper limb and trunk of the child, and "axillary web" like contractures were formed in the shoulder joint

14.6 Cubitus Varus, Cubitus Valgus, and Related Deformities

14.6.1 Elbow Valgus

When the normal elbow joint is fully extended, there is a mild eversion, about 10° in men and 15° degrees in women. This eversion angle is called the carrying angle. If this angle is increased, the forearm is too abducted, which is called cubitus valgus deformity.

14.6.1.1 Etiology

Fractures of the medial and lateral condyles of the humerus in children that fail to be reset in time or have poor reset, premature closure of the lateral condylar epiphysis of the humerus or ischemic necrosis, and elbow dislocation that has not been reset or has poor reset can all lead to cubitus valgus.

14.6.1.2 Clinical Manifestation

Elbow valgus, when the elbow joint is extended, the elbow valgus angle increases, up to more than 30°. Generally, there is no obvious obstacle to the movement of the elbow joint, and the injury of the articular surface of the elbow joint in the late stage can cause pain. For patients with severe hallux valgus, because the ulnar nerve is in a high-tension traction state, or the ulnar nerve is often rubbed due to adhesion after trauma, delayed ulnar neuritis may occur, and the manifestations of ulnar nerve injury may occur, that is, unconsciously, tingling and sensory disturbance (half of the little finger and ring finger) occur in the area dominated by the ulnar nerve of the hand, and the intrinsic muscles of the hand are weak and atrophic (Fig. 14.24).

14.6.1.3 Treatment Principle

Cubitus valgus, if asymptomatic, generally does not require surgical treatment. Patients with high requirements for appearance, obvious symptoms of joint pain and weakness, affecting the function of elbow joint, arthritis or ulnar nerve symptoms should be actively corrected by surgery (Fig. 14.24).

14.6.2 Cubitus Varus

For children Supracondylar fracture of humerus, the most common complication is about 80%.

14.6.2.1 Etiology

Most of them are caused by supracondylar fracture of humerus, total epiphyseal separation of distal humerus and epiphyseal injury of medial condyle.

14.6.2.2 Clinical Manifestation

That is to say, after treatment or without treatment of elbow joint injury, the varus angle of elbow joint in extension position increases significantly, which can reach 15–35° in severe cases. At this time, the triangular relationship behind the elbow changes, and the distance between the lateral condyle and the olecranon widens. The general activities of the elbow joint were basically normal, but the muscle strength was weakened to varying degrees.

14.6.2.3 Treatment Principle

Treatment of cubitus varus aims to eliminate pain, improve function, and correct deformity. It is generally believed that surgical correction is not necessary for patients with small elbow varus angle, slight elbow pain, and good elbow function. Surgical treatment is needed for patients with severe deformity, varus angle greater than 20°, severe pain, and elbow dysfunction affecting daily work and life. The application of supracondylar osteotomy of humerus to correct cubitus varus deformity and restore the valgus angle can often achieve the purpose of eliminating pain and improving function (Fig. 14.25).

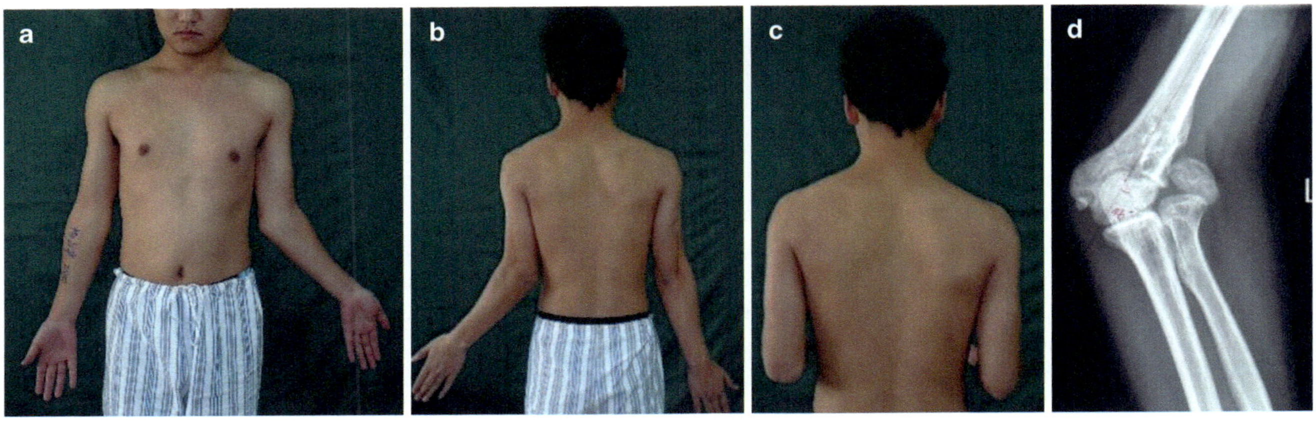

Fig. 14.24 Left cubitus valgus deformity caused by juvenile trauma. (**a**) Cubitus valgus palmar; (**b**) cubitus valgus dorsal; (**c**) combined with upper arm shortening; (**d**) preoperative radiograph showed an old fracture of the lateral condyle of the humerus

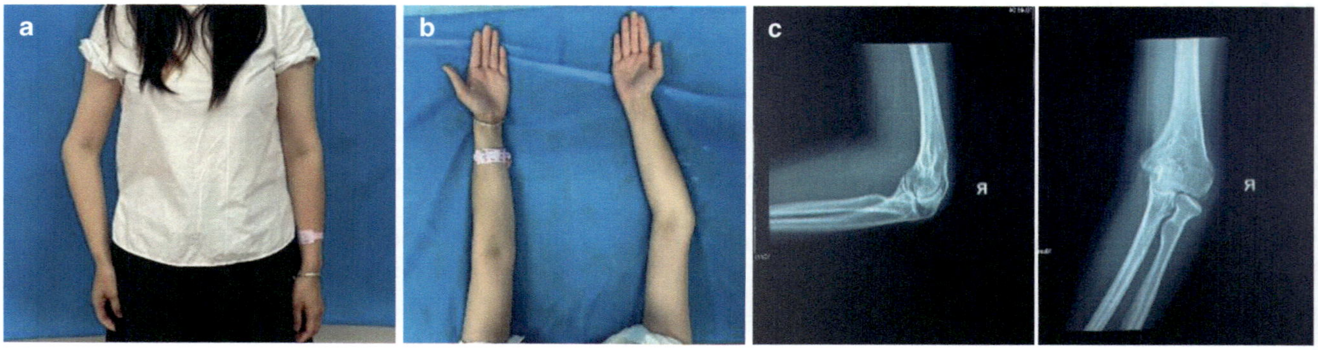

Fig. 14.25 Clinical and X-ray manifestations of right cubitus varus deformity. (**a**, **b**) Upper limb appearance of cubitus varus; (**c**) examination of varus deformity of distal humerus by UNK1 X line

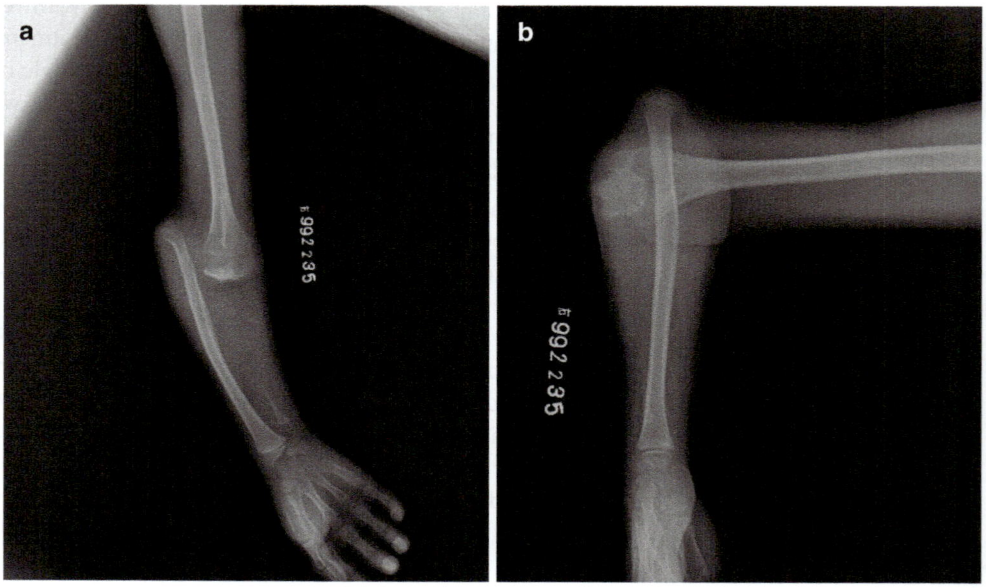

Fig. 14.26 Severe superior dislocation of radial head due to infective ulnar defect in childhood. (**a**) X-ray anteroposterior film of dislocation of radial head; (**b**) lateral radiograph showing flail joint

14.6.3 Dislocation of Radial Head

Simple dislocation of the radial head is very rare in clinic.

14.6.3.1 Etiology

Dislocation of the radial head can be caused by trauma and congenital conditions such as ulnar dysplasia or loss in children.

14.6.3.2 Clinical Manifestation

Limitation of pronation and supination of forearm and pain after injury can be diagnosed by X-ray lateral film. Congenital dislocation of the radial head has little effect on the rotation function of the forearm. Due to the short development of the ulna, especially when the elbow joint is flexed, the radial head may protrude.

14.6.3.3 Treatment

Closed reduction of acute dislocation is generally successful, and open reduction is required if closure fails. The radial head may be resected after delayed treatment in adults. Shortening due to ulnar dysplasia may be achieved by lengthening the ulna to move the radial head downward and improve function (Fig. 14.26).

14.6.4 Forearm Pronation Deformity

Congenital deformities and acquired diseases can lead to arm pronation deformity. Cerebral palsy is the most common upper limb spasm, often accompanied by wrist and hand compound deformities, and affects each other.

14.6.4.1 Etiology

It is mainly caused by contracture of pronator teres muscle or spasm and contracture of pronator quadratus muscle, resulting in dynamic imbalance of forearm. In severe cases, secondary dislocation of radial head aggravates the pathological changes of pronation deformity.

14.6.4.2 Clinical Manifestation

Forearm pronation deformity, loss of active supination function, accompanied by wrist, finger flexion, elbow flexion and other complex deformities, wrist or upper limb dysfunction.

14.6.4.3 Treatment

Simple correction of forearm pronation deformity is rare, and combined surgical correction of upper limb compound deformity is often needed to achieve satisfactory results. In most cases, tendon release and transposition were performed to improve forearm rotation and wrist extension (Fig. 14.27).

14.6.5 Elbow Stiffness

Trauma or disease of the elbow joint causes a decrease in the range of motion of the elbow joint, which cannot reach the normal range of motion.

14.6.5.1 Etiology

(1) Fracture of elbow joint, mainly intra-articular fracture with poor reduction; (2) Periarticular myositis ossificans; (3) Inappropriate treatment after elbow trauma, including long-term fixation of the joint, residual bone fragments in the joint and injuries caused by strong activities, etc. (4) Many other factors, such as elbow joint infection, muscle, tendon, ligament and joint capsule injury, can easily cause extensive and severe adhesion, followed by calcification and ossification.

14.6.5.2 Clinical Manifestation

The main manifestation is that the range of motion of elbow flexion and extension is reduced, which can be manifested as

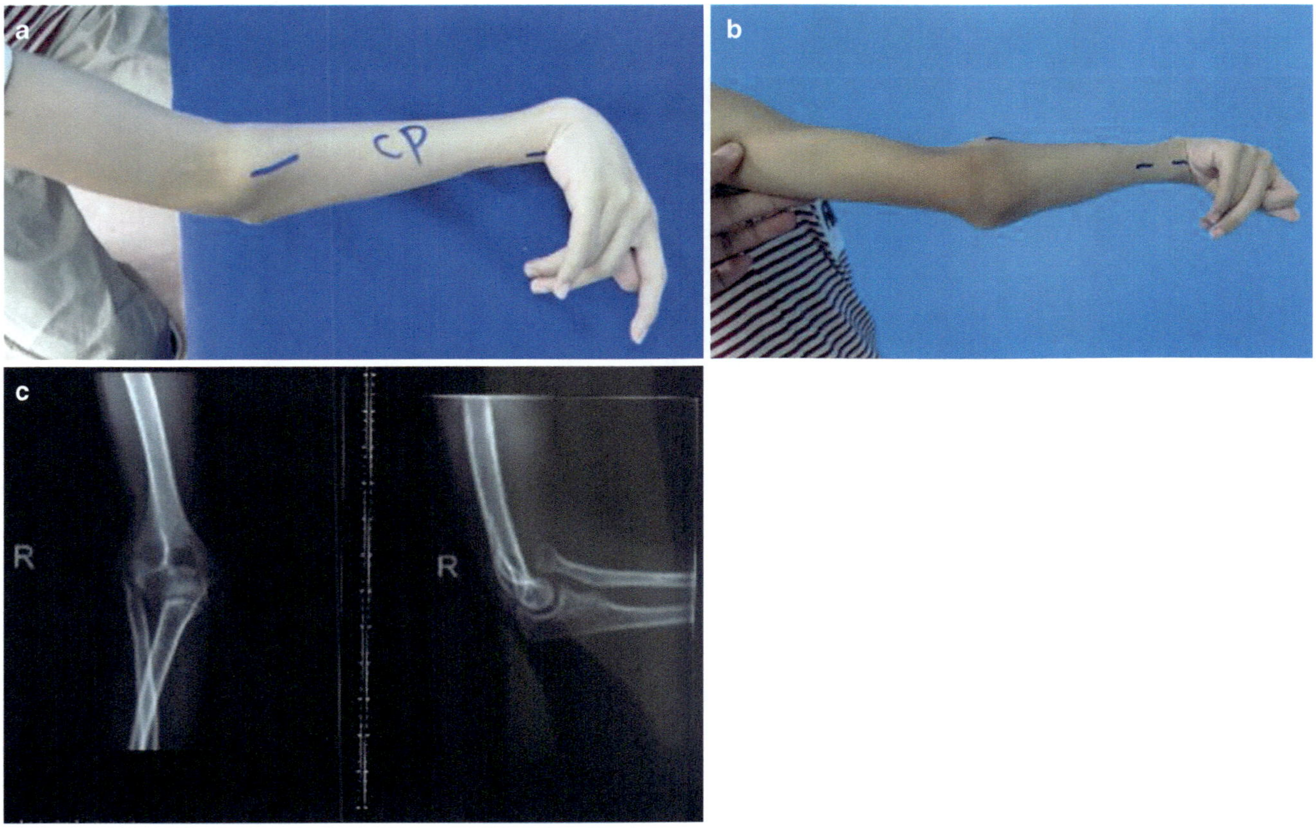

Fig. 14.27 Appearance of forearm pronation deformity. (**a**, **b**) Appearance of forearm pronation in cerebral palsy; (**c**) X-film showed dislocation of the radial head

elbow extension disorder, and elbow flexion is not affected. It can also be manifested as elbow flexion disorder, and the extension is not affected. Some patients have both extension and flexion disorders.

14.6.5.3 Treatment Principle

Elbow flexion and extension range of motion directly affects the degree of upper limb dysfunction. Patients with mild fibrous stiffness of elbow joint and unaffected elbow flexion function may not be treated. If the fibrous stiffness of the elbow joint affects the function of the upper limb, the elbow joint can be released, combined with Ilizarov technique, to increase the range of motion of the elbow joint and improve the function of the elbow joint (Fig. 14.28).

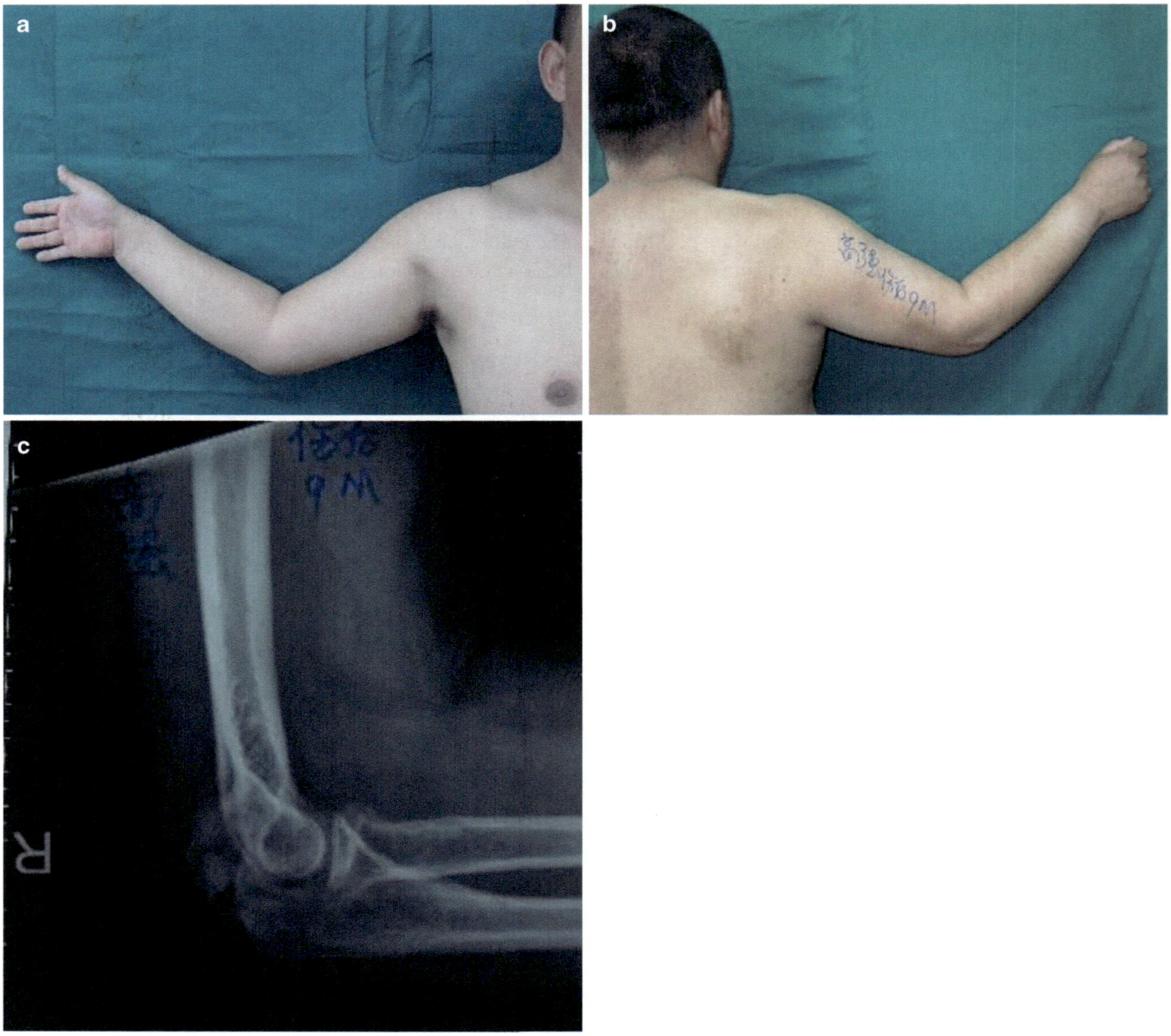

Fig. 14.28 Incomplete fibrous stiffness of elbow joint after trauma. (**a**) Incomplete stiffness of the elbow joint, frontal appearance; (**b**) back view; (**c**) preoperative X-ray

14.7 Upper Limb-Hand Deformity Caused by Comprehensive Causes

14.7.1 Scleroderma

Scleroderma is a connective tissue disease characterized by inflammation, degeneration, thickening and fibrosis of the skin leading to sclerosis and atrophy, which can cause multi-system damage. In addition to the degenerative lesions of skin, synovium and finger (toe) arteries, the internal organs such as digestive tract, lung, heart, and kidney can also be involved in systemic sclerosis.

14.7.1.1 Etiology

The etiology of scleroderma is still unclear. It may be that under the action of genetic, environmental factors (viral infection, chemicals such as silicon, etc.), female hormones, cellular and humoral immune abnormalities, fibroblasts synthesize and secrete collagen, leading to fibrosis of skin and viscera. Chemical or viral infections are environmental factors that affect susceptibility to disease. People who are frequently exposed to silica in their work have an increased relative risk of the disease.

14.7.1.2 Clinical Manifestation

The early clinical manifestation of specific scleroderma is swelling and thickening of the skin, beginning in the fingers and hands. In the early stage of the disease (edema stage), the skin shows mild redness and swelling, some patients have erythema, itching and edema. The early finger edema stage can last for a long time. The skin changes stop at the distal end of the upper limb, and can also spread to the forearm, chest, abdomen, back and face. With the progress of the disease, the skin is tight and shiny, the normal wrinkles and skin folds disappear, and the facial skin is thin and dull. The lips are thin and tight, the mouth opening is restricted, and systemic melanin appears at the same time, or even earlier in some cases. Patchy telangiectasia and subcutaneous calcification may occur in fingers, face, lips, tongue, and forearms, with fingertips being the most common, ranging from small spots to large masses of varying sizes covering knees, elbows or other most prominent parts. When scleroderma progresses to the sclerotic stage, the skin becomes thicker and the dryness of the skin causes itching. This stage is progressive and lasts for 1–3 years or longer. Finally, the inflammation and fibrosis stop and the skin atrophies and thins. The fibrotic tissue clings to the subcutaneous tissue and is not easy to pinch with the hand. Bony ulcers may occur at the site of flexion contracture, such as near the finger (toe) joint (Fig. 14.29).

14.7.1.3 Classification

According to the degree of skin invasion, scleroderma can be divided into two subtypes: (1) Patients with localized scleroderma only have skin thickening in the distal extremities, and the trunk is not invaded. CREST syndrome includes calcinosis, Raynaud's phenomenon, esophageal dysfunction, fingertip sclerosis and telangiectasia, which belongs to the category of localized scleroderma. (2) Patients with diffuse scleroderma showed thickening of the skin of the distal and proximal extremities and/or trunk.

14.7.1.4 Treatment Principle

(1) Early diagnosis and early treatment are beneficial to prevent disease progression, and the principles are vasodilation, anti-fibrosis, immunosuppression and immunomodulation. (2) For patients with secondary bone and joint deformity, on the basis of treatment of primary disease, bone and joint deformity should be corrected to improve the function of affected limbs.

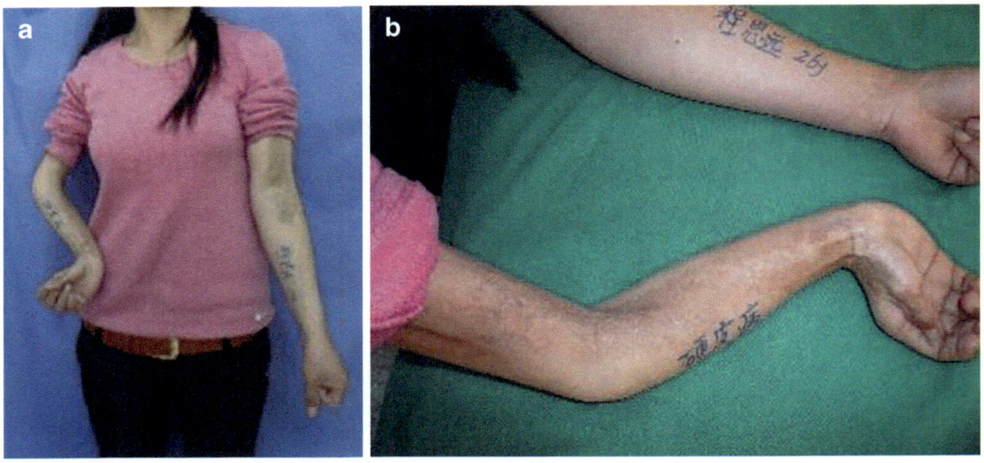

Fig. 14.29 (1) Holistic view; (2) local view. Elbow flexion, wrist dorsiflexion, and radial deviation caused by scleroderma of the right upper limb

14.7.2 Lupus Erythematosus Hand Deformity

Case 1: Fig. 14.30.

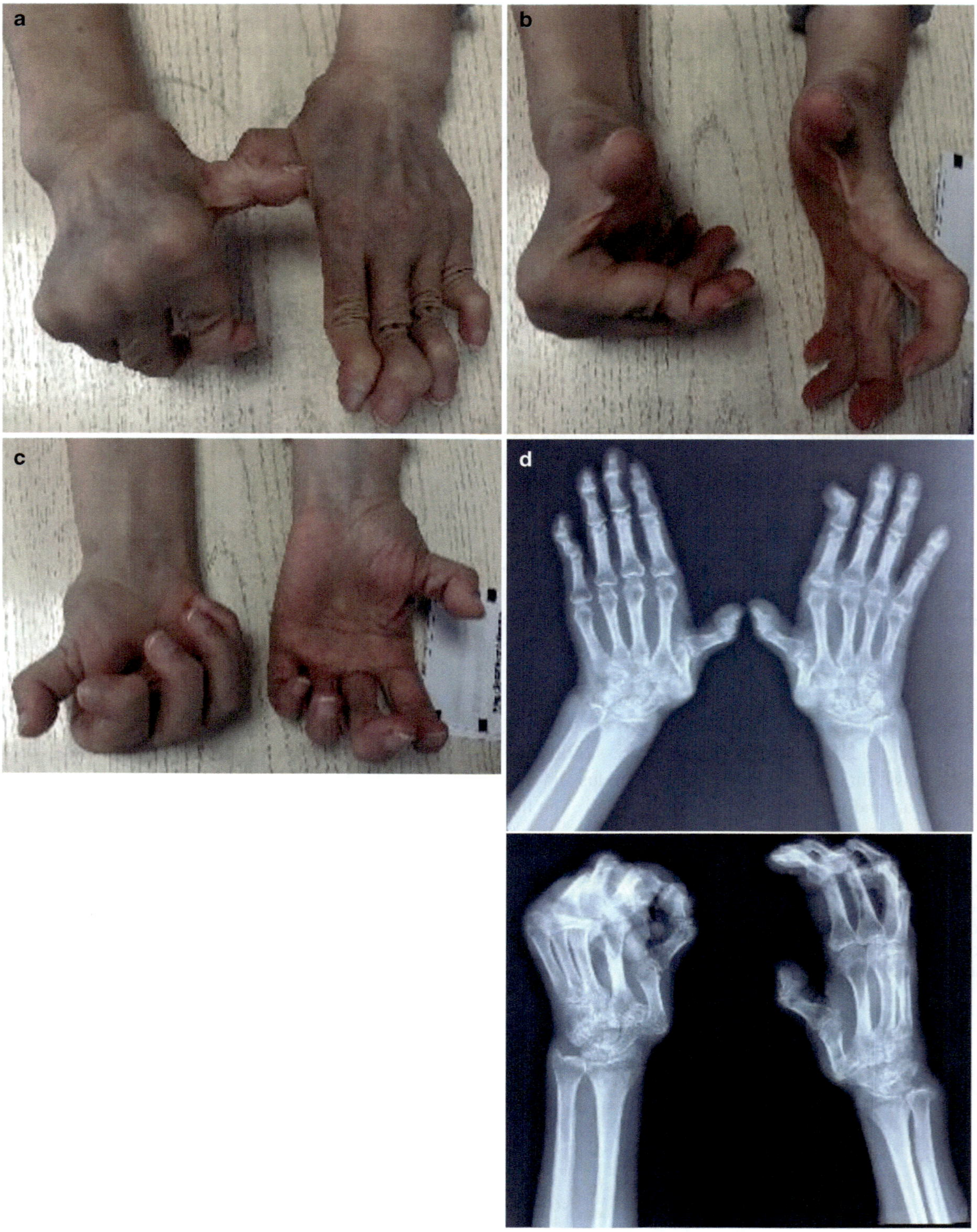

Fig. 14.30 (**a**) Patient A is an adult male who has been diagnosed with "lupus erythematosus arthritis" for 10 years. At present, the joints of both hands are deformed, the right hand has flexion contracture, and the left hand has secondary gooseneck deformity. (**b**) Side view. (**c**) Palmar view. (**d**) X-ray film of both hands shows severe deformation and dislocation of bone and joint

14.7.3 Rheumatoid Arthritis

Case 1: Fig. 14.31.

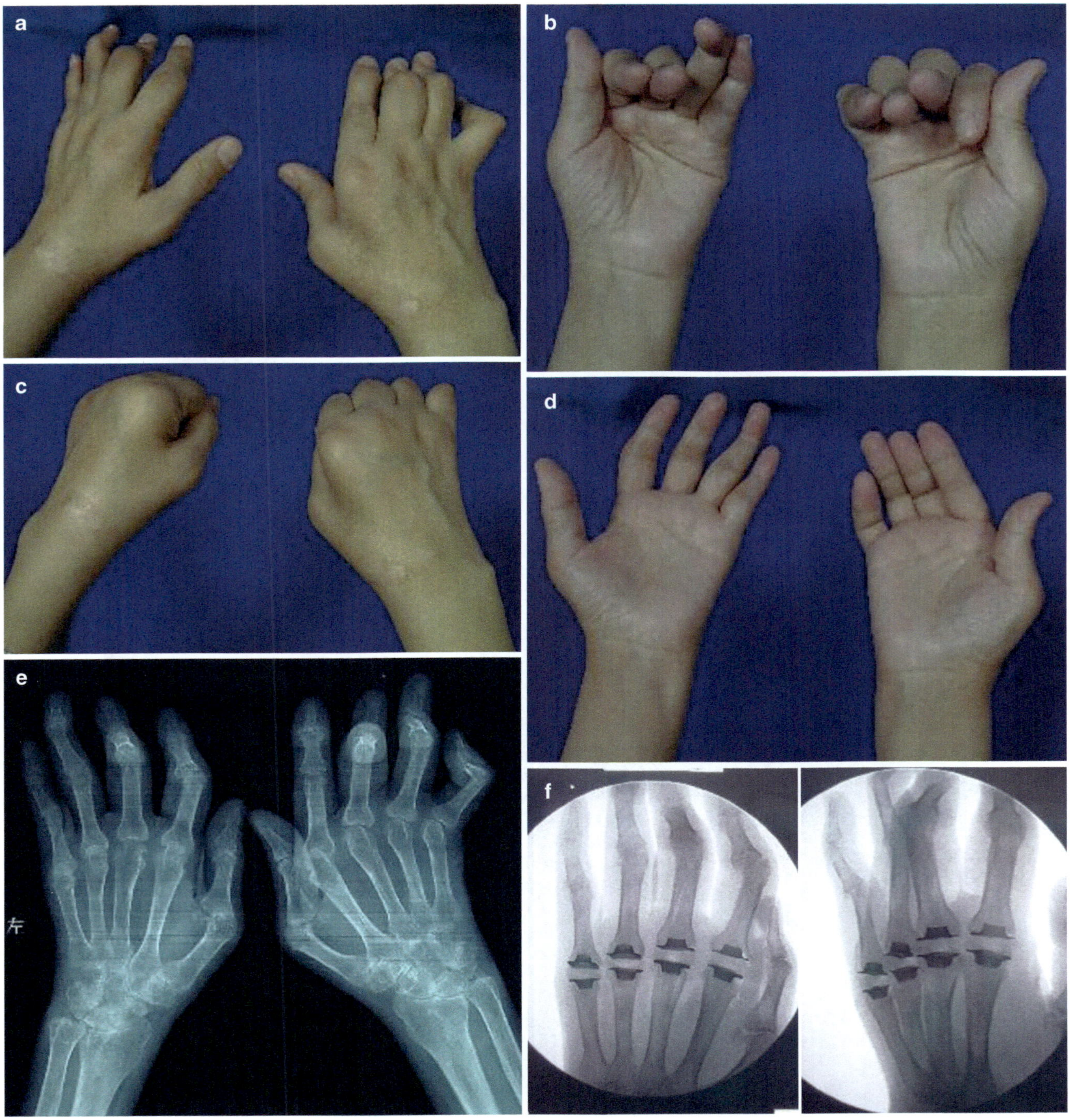

Fig. 14.31 (**a**) Patient is an adult female with rheumatoid arthritis of both hands for 20 years. The hand joints are severely deformed. The metacarpophalangeal joints of the fingers are flexed ulnaris and the interphalangeal joints are flexed. (**b**) Palmar view of finger flexion. (**c**) Dorsal view of finger in flexion. (**d**) Limited finger straightening. (**e**) X-ray film showed that the osteoporosis of both hands was severe, the space of each joint (including wrist joint) was narrowed, the bone was destroyed, and some joints were dislocated and deviated. (**f**) Deformity of the left metacarpophalangeal joint was significantly improved after prosthetic replacement

14.7.4 Gout Finger Deformity

Case 1: Fig. 14.32.

Crystals aggregate to form a "mass".

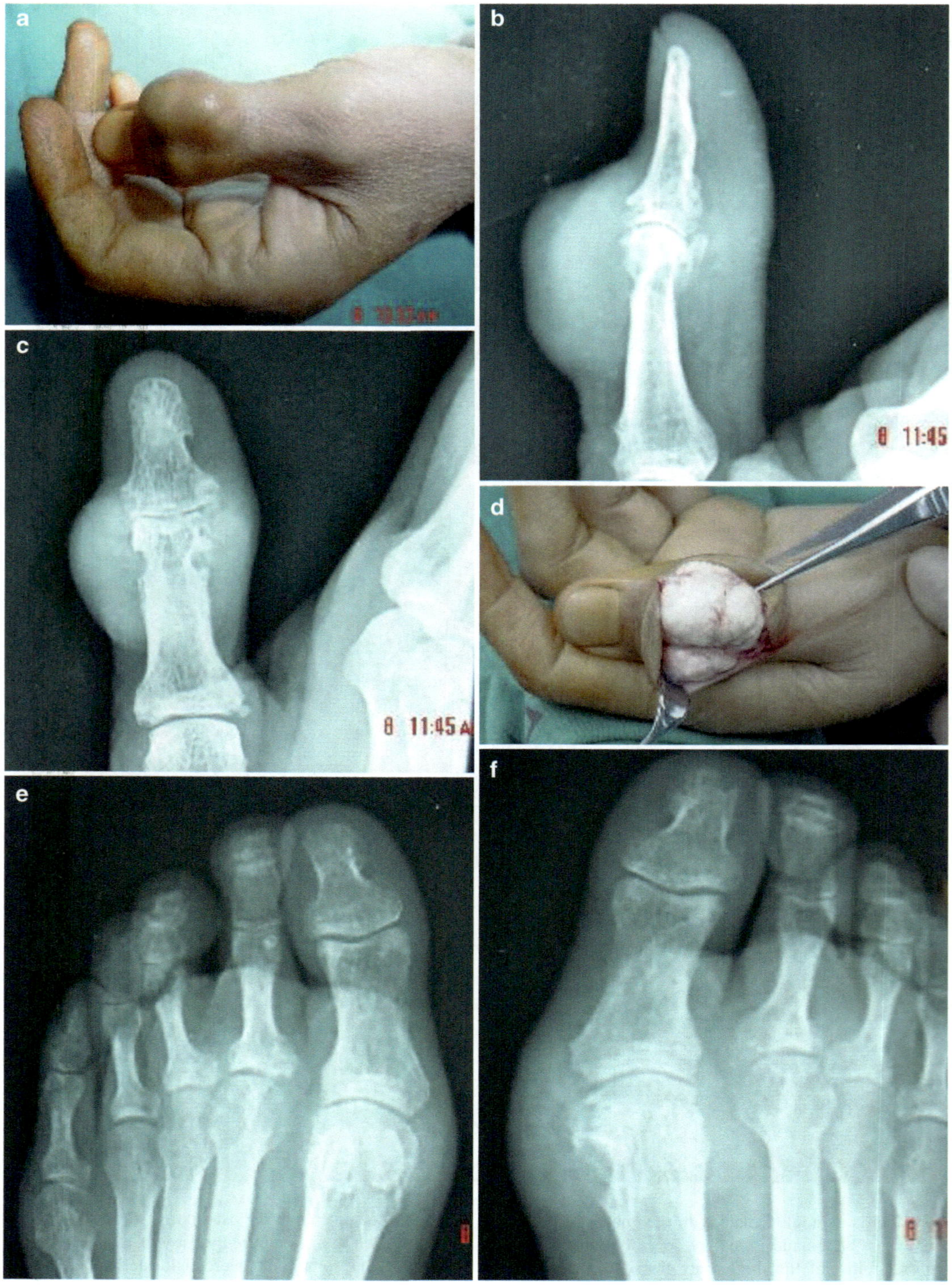

Fig. 14.32 (**a**) Patient is an adult male with gout for 10 years. The left interphalangeal joint of the thumb has a gout nodule on the dorsal side. The lateral X-ray film of (**b**) shows that the bone of the interphalangeal joint of the thumb is severely destroyed. (**c**) Anteroposterior radiograph shows bone destruction and joint space narrowing. (**d**) Surgical exploration reveals urate on the dorsal interphalangeal joint. (**e**) X-ray film of the patient's foot (left side). The destruction of bone and joint is similar to that of the affected hand. (**f**) X-ray film of F patient's foot (right side)

14.7.5 Pathological Changes of Fingers in Waxy Drop Osteopathy

Case 1: Fig. 14.33.

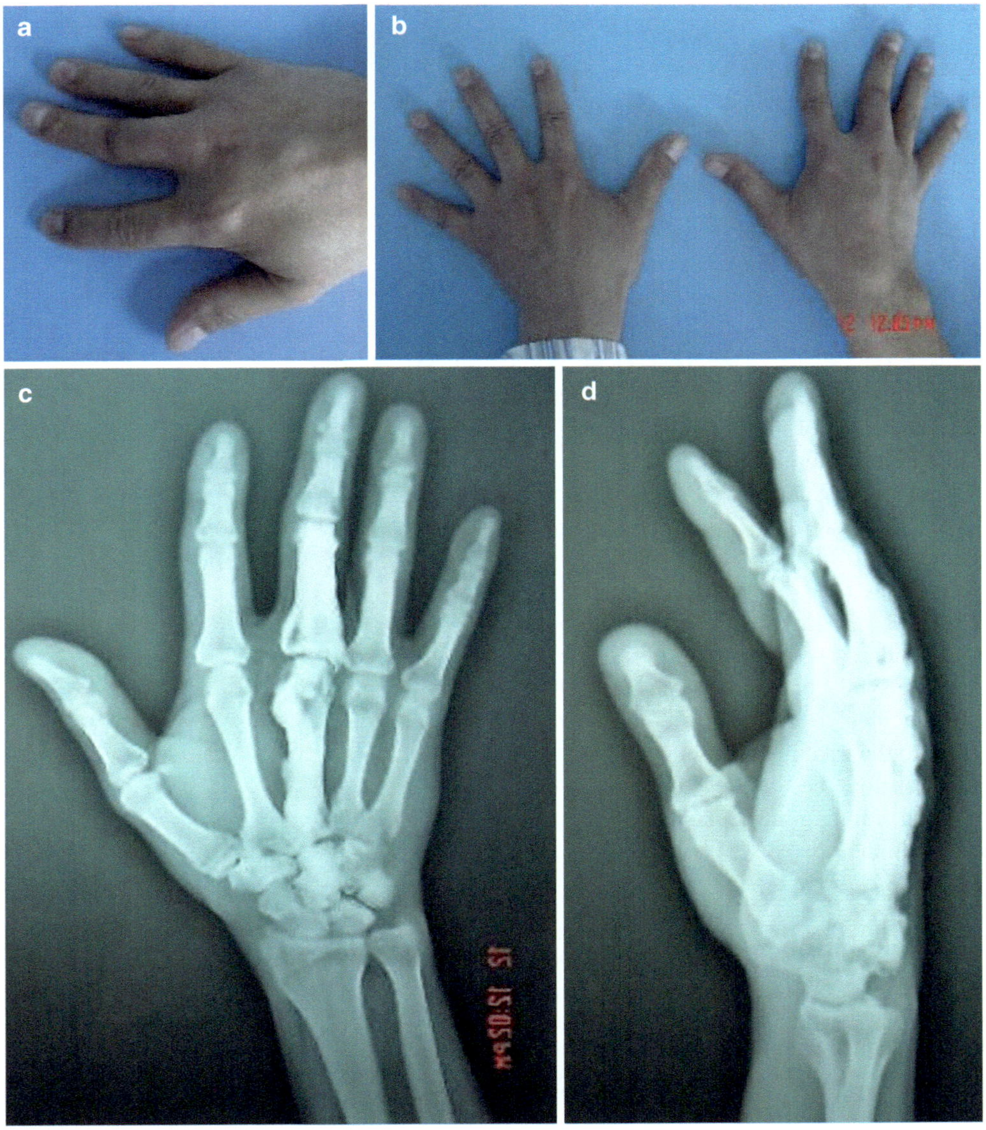

Fig. 14.33 (**a**) The patient is an adult female. The middle finger of the right hand is found to be partially deformed and thickened for 15 years. Localized bulges can be seen on the back of the hand and the back of the wrist. (**b**) Comparison of both hands. (**c**) X-ray shows that the phalanx bone of the right middle finger is irregularly sclerotic, and the proximal end of the lesion extends to the carpal bone, which is a typical wax-drop change

GPSR Compliance

The European Union's (EU) General Product Safety Regulation (GPSR) is a set of rules that requires consumer products to be safe and our obligations to ensure this.

If you have any concerns about our products, you can contact us on ProductSafety@springernature.com

In case Publisher is established outside the EU, the EU authorized representative is:

Springer Nature Customer Service Center GmbH
Europaplatz 3
69115 Heidelberg, Germany

Batch number: 10731661

Printed by Printforce, the Netherlands